GERALD E. SWANSON, M.D.
9601 UPTON ROAD
MINNEAPOLIS, MN 55431
TELE: 881-6869

CURRENT THERAPY IN INFECTIOUS DISEASE - 2

Current Therapy Series

Bayless:
Current Therapy in Gastroenterology and Liver Disease
Bayless, Brain, Cherniack:
Current Therapy in Internal Medicine
Brain, Carbone:
Current Therapy in Hematology-Oncology
Callaham:
Current Therapy in Emergency Medicine
Cameron:
Current Surgical Therapy
Cherniack:
Current Therapy of Respiratory Disease
Dubovsky, Shore:
Current Therapy in Psychiatry
Ernst, Stanley:
Current Therapy in Vascular Surgery
Foley, Payne:
Current Therapy of Pain
Fortuin:
Current Therapy in Cardiovascular Disease
Garcia:
Current Contraceptive Management
Garcia, Mastroianni, Amelar, Dubin:
Current Therapy of Infertility
Garcia, Mikuta, Rosenblum:
Current Therapy in Surgical Gynecology
Gates:
Current Therapy in Otolaryngology—Head and Neck Surgery
Glassock:
Current Therapy in Nephrology and Hypertension
Grillo, Austen, Wilkins, Mathisen, Vlahakes:
Current Therapy in Cardiothoracic Surgery
Jeejeebhoy:
Current Therapy in Nutrition
Johnson:
Current Therapy in Neurologic Disease
Kass, Platt:
Current Therapy in Infectious Disease
Krieger, Bardin:
Current Therapy in Endocrinology and Metabolism
Lichtenstein, Fauci:
Current Therapy in Allergy, Immunology and Rheumatology
Long:
Current Therapy in Neurologic Surgery
McGinty, Jackson:
Current Therapy in Orthopaedics
Nelson:
Current Therapy in Neonatal-Perinatal Medicine
Nelson:
Current Therapy in Pediatric Infectious Disease
Parrillo:
Current Therapy in Critical Care Medicine
Provost, Farmer:
Current Therapy in Dermatology
Resnick, Kursh:
Current Therapy in Genitourinary Surgery
Rogers:
Current Practice of Anesthesiology
Trunkey, Lewis:
Current Therapy of Trauma
Welsh, Shephard:
Current Therapy in Sports Medicine

CURRENT THERAPY IN INFECTIOUS DISEASE - 2

EDWARD H. KASS, PH.D., M.D., SC.D.(HON.), M.A. (HON.)

William Ellery Channing
Professor of Medicine
Director, Channing Laboratory
Harvard Medical School

Senior Physician
Brigham and Women's Hospital
Boston, Massachusetts

RICHARD PLATT, M.D.

Assistant Professor of Medicine
Harvard Medical School

Associate Hospital Epidemiologist
Brigham and Women's Hospital

Hospital Epidemiologist
New England Deaconess Hospital
Boston, Massachusetts

1986

B.C. DECKER INC • Toronto • Philadelphia
The C.V. MOSBY COMPANY • Saint Louis • Toronto • London

Publisher

B.C. Decker Inc.
3228 South Service Road
Burlington, Ontario L7N 3H8

B.C. Decker Inc.
P.O. Box 30246
Phildelphia, Pennsylvania 19103

Sales and Distribution

United States and Possessions	**The C.V. Mosby Company** 11830 Westline Industrial Drive Saint Louis, Missouri 63146
Canada	**The C.V. Mosby Company, Ltd.** 5240 Finch Avenue East, Unit No. 1 Scarborough, Ontario M1S 4P2
United Kingdom, Europe and the Middle East	**Blackwell Scientific Publications, Ltd.** Osney Mead, Oxford OX2 OEL, England
Australia	**Holt-Saunders Pty. Limited** 9 Waltham Street Artarmon, N.S.W. 2064 Australia
Japan	**Igaku-Shoin Ltd.** Tokyo International P.O. Box 5063 1-28-36 Hongo, Bunkyo-ku, Tokyo 113, Japan
Asia	**Holt-Saunders Asia Limited** 10/F, Inter-Continental Plaza Tsim Sha Tsui East Kowloon, Hong Kong

Current Therapy in Infectious Disease - 2 ISBN 0-941158-46-2

Library of Congress catalog card number: 85-062981

10 9 8 7 6 5 4 3 2 1

CONTRIBUTORS

MARK D. ARONSON, M.D.

Associate Professor, Division of General Medicine, Department of Medicine, Beth Israel Hospital, Harvard Medical School, Boston, Massachusetts
Pharyngitis

ELIA M. AYOUB, M.D.

Professor and Chief, Department of Pediatrics, University of Florida College of Medicine, J. Hillis Miller Health Center, Gainesville, Florida
Immunodeficiency Disorder in Infants and Children

ANN SULLIVAN BAKER, M.D.

Assistant Professor, Harvard Medical School; Associate Physician, Infectious Disease Unit, Massachusetts General Hospital, Consultant, Infectious Disease, Massachusets Eye and Ear Infirmary, Harvard Medical School, Boston, Massachusetts
Endophthalmitis

DAVID W. BARNES, M.D.

Associate in Medicine, Division of Infectious Diseases, University of Alabama School of Medicine, University of Alabama at Birmingham, Birmingham, Alabama
Herpes Simplex Virus Infection

DOUGLAS J. BARRETT, M.D.

Associate Professor of Pediatrics, University of Florida College of Medicine, J. Hillis Miller Health Center, Gainesville, Florida
Immunodeficiency Disorder in Infants and Children

JOHN G. BARTLETT, M.D.

Professor of Medicine, The Johns Hopkins University School of Medicine, Baltimore, Maryland
Intra-abdominal Abscess

SETH F. BERKLEY, M.D.

Respiratory and Special Pathogens Epidemiology Branch, Division of Bacterial Diseases, Centers for Disease Control, Atlanta, Georgia
Toxic Shock Syndrome

RAMÓN H. BERMÚDEZ, M.D., F.A.C.P.

Associate Professor of Medicine, University of Puerto Rico School of Medicine; Chief, Infectious Disease Section, Veterans Administration Medical Center, San Juan, Puerto Rico
Infection Caused by Intestinal Helminths

ALAN L. BISNO, M.D.

Professor of Medicine, University of Tennessee College of Medicine; Attending Physician, The University of Tennessee Medical Center, Memphis, Tennessee
Nonsuppurative Sequelae of Group A Streptococcal Infection

GERALD P. BODEY, M.D., F.A.C.P., F.A.C.C.P., F.R.S.M., F.R.S.H.

Professor of Medicine, Baylor College of Medicine; Internist, The University of Texas System, Cancer Center, M.D. Anderson Hospital and Tumor Institute, Houston, Texas
Solid Tumors - Associated Infection

DONALD L. BORNSTEIN, M.D.

Associate Professor of Medicine; Chief, Infectious Disease Section, State University of New York Health Sciences Center at Syracuse, Syracuse, New York
Tetanus

JOEL G. BREMAN, M.D., D.T.P.H.

Chief, Malaria Control Activity, Division of Parasitic Diseases, Center for Infectious Diseases, Centers for Disease Control, Atlanta, Georgia
Malaria

JAMES W. BROOKS, Jr., M.D.

Fellow, Division of Infectious Diseases, University of Alabama School of Medicine, University of Alabama at Birmingham, Birmingham, Alabama
Myocarditis and Pericarditis

WARD E. BULLOCK, M.D.

Professor of Medicine; Director, Infectious Diseases Division, University of Cincinnati College of Medicine, Cincinnati, Ohio
Leprosy

JOHN F. BURKE, M.D.

Helen Andrus Benedict Professor of Surgery, Harvard Medical School; Chief, Trauma Services, Massachusetts General Hospital, Boston, Massachusetts
Infection Following Burn Injury

DAVID CHARLES, M.D., F.R.C.O.G., F.A.C.O.G.

Professor and Chairman, Department of Obstetrics and Gynecology, Marshall University School of Medicine; Chief of Obstetrical Service, St. Mary's Hospital, Huntington, West Virginia
Infection in Pregnancy

JAMES CHIN, M.D., M.P.H.

Clinical Professor of Epidemiology, University of California, School of Public Health; Chief, Infectious Disease Branch, California Department of Health Services, Berkeley, California
Medical Requirements and Recommendations for International Travelers

GERALD W. CHODAK, M.A., M.D.

Associate Professor of Surgery/Urology, University of Chicago, Division of the Biological Sciences, Pritzker School of Medicine, Chicago, Illinois
Prostatitis, Epididymitis, and Balanoposthitis

SANFORD CHODOSH, M.D.

Associate Professor of Medicine, Boston University School of Medicine; Chief of Medicine, Veterans Administration Outpatient Clinic, Boston, Massachusetts
Bronchitis

ANTHONY W. CHOW, M.D., F.R.C.P.(C), F.A.C.P.

Professor of Medicine, University of British Columbia Faculty of Medicine; Head, Division of Infectious Diseases, Vancouver General Hospital, Vancouver, British Columbia
Vulvovaginitis, Cervicitis, and Pelvic Inflammatory Disease

CHIN HAK CHUN, M.D.

Assistant Professor of Medicine, University of Louisville School of Medicine; Chief, Infectious Diseases, Veterans Administration Medical Center, Louisville, Kentucky
Biliary Tract Infection

C. GLENN COBBS, M.D.

Professor of Medicine and Director, Division of Infectious Diseases and Allergy, University of Alabama School of Medicine, University of Alabama in Birmingham, Birmingham, Alabama
Myocarditis and Pericarditis

WILLIAM A. CRAIG, M.D.

Professor of Medicine, University of Wisconsin; Chief, Infectious Diseases, William, S. Middleton Memorial Hospital, Veterans Administration Hospital, Madison, Wisconsin
Antibacterial Chemotherapy

DONALD E. CRAVEN, M.D.

Associate Professor of Medicine, Boston University School of Medicine; Hospital Epidemiologist, Department of Medicine, Division of Infectious Diseases, Boston City Hospital, Boston, Massachusetts
Gram-Negative Bacteremia

CHARLES E. DAVIS, M.D.

Professor of Pathology, University of California, San Diego, School of Medicine; Director of Microbiology Laboratories, University of California Medical Center, San Diego, California
Trypanosomiasis: African (Sleeping Sickness) and American (Chagas' Disease)

RICHARD D. DIAMOND, M.D.

Professor of Medicine, Boston University School of Medicine; Chief of Infectious Diseases, Boston University Medical Center, Boston, Massachusetts
Antifungal Chemotherapy

R. BRUCE DONOFF, D.M.D., M.D.

Professor of Oral and Maxillofacial Surgery, Harvard School of Dental Medicine; Chief, Oral and Maxillofacial Surgery Service, Massachusetts General Hospital, Boston, Massachusetts
Infection of the Mouth, Salivary Glands, and Neck Spaces

HERBERT L. DUPONT, M.D.

Professor of Medicine, Director, Program in Infectious Diseases and Clinical Microbiology, University of Texas Medical School, Houston, Texas
Infectious Diarrhea: A Patient Outside the United States

ASIM K. DUTT, M.D., F.R.C.P.(Glas), F.A.C.P.

Professor of Medicine, University of Arkansas for Medical Sciences; Director, Respiratory Therapy, John L. McClellan Veterans Administration Medical Center; Consultant, Tuberculosis Program, Arkansas Department of Health, Little Rock, Arkansas
Tuberculosis

DENIS A. EVANS, M.D.

Assistant Professor of Medicine, Harvard Medical School; Associate in Medicine, Brigham and Women's Hospital, Boston, Massachusetts
Bacteriuria and Pyelonephritis

BARRY M. FARR, M.D., M.Sc.

Assistant Professor of Internal Medicine, University of Virginia School of Medicine; Physician, University of Virginia Hospital, Charlottesville, Virginia
Common Cold

C. STEPHEN FOSTER, M.D.

Associate Professor of Ophthalmology, Harvard Medical School; Associate Surgeon, Director, Immunology and Uveitis Unit, Director, Hilles Immunology Laboratory, Massachusetts Eye and Ear Infirmary, Boston, Massachusetts
Keratitis

LAWRENCE R. FREEDMAN, M.D.

Professor of Medicine, UCLA School of Medicine; Chief, Medical Service, Veterans Administration Wadsworth

Medical Center, Los Angeles, California
Infective Endocarditis and Mycotic Aneurysm

RUTH K. FREINKEL, M.D.

Professor of Dermatology, Northwestern University Medical School, Chicago, Illinois
Acne Vulgaris

JACOB K. FRENKEL, M.D., Ph.D.

Professor of Pathology and Oncology, University of Kansas School of Medicine; Staff, University of Kansas Medical Center, Kansas City, Kansas
Toxoplasmosis

GERALD H. FRIEDLAND, M.D.

Associate Professor of Medicine, Albert Einstein College of Medicine of Yeshiva University; Director, Medical Service, Montefiore Medical Center, Bronx, New York
Fever and Lymphadenopathy
Acquired Immunodeficiency Syndrome

NELSON M. GANTZ, M.D., F.A.C.P.

Professor of Medicine and Microbiology, University of Massachusetts Medical School; Clinical Director of Infectious Disease, Hospital Epidemiologist, University of Massachusetts Medical Center, Worcester, Massachusetts
Listeriosis

GARY E. GARBER, B.Sc., M.D., F.R.C.P.(C)

Senior Fellow, Division of Infectious Disease, Department of Medicine, University of British Columbia and Vancouver General Hospital, Vancouver, British Columbia, Canada
Vulvovaginitis, Cervicitis, and Pelvic Inflammatory Disease

RICHARD A. GARIBALDI, M.D.

Professor of Medicine, University of Connecticut School of Medicine; Vice Chairman, Department of Medicine, Hospital Epidemiologist, University of Connecticut Health Center, Farmington, Connecticut
Postoperative Wound Infection

W. LANCE GEORGE, M.D.

Associate Professor of Medicine, UCLA School of Medicine; Assistant Chief, Infectious Disease Section, Wadsworth Division, West Los Angeles Veterans Administration Medical Center, Los Angeles, California
Crepitus and Gangrene

ANNE A. GERSHON, M.D.

Professor of Pediatrics, Columbia University College of Physicians and Surgeons, New York, New York
Childhood Exanthems

ROGER I. GLASS, M.D.

Medical Officer, Laboratory of Infectious Diseases, National Institute of Allergy and Infectious Diseases, National Institutes of Health, Bethesda, Maryland
Amebiasis and Giardiasis

DAVID J. GOCKE, M.D.

Professor of Medicine and Microbiology; Chief, Division of Immunology and Infectious Diseases, University of Medicine and Dentistry of New Jersey Rutgers Medical School, Piscataway, New Jersey
Viral Hepatitis

ELLIE J.C. GOLDSTEIN, M.D.

Associate Clinical Professor of Medicine, Director, R.M. Alden Research Laboratory, UCLA School of Medicine, Los Angeles, California; Staff Physician, Santa Monica Hospital and Medical Center, Santa Monica, California
Animal Bite Infection

ELLIOT GOLDSTEIN, M.D.

Professor of Medicine and Chief, Division of Infectious and Immunologic Diseases, University of California School of Medicine, Davis, California
Infection Following Trauma

ERNESTO GONZALEZ, M.D.

Assistant Professor of Dermatology, Harvard Medical School; Associate Dermatologist, Chief, Dermatology Ambulatory Care Center, Massachusetts General Hospital, Boston, Massachusetts
Superficial Fungal Infection

BARNEY S. GRAHAM, M.D.

Fellow in Infectious Diseases, American College of Physicians Teaching and Research Scholar, Department of Medicine, Metropolitan Nashville General Hospital, Vanderbilt University School of Medicine, Nashville, Tennessee
Hospital-Acquired Pneumonia

RICHARD L. GUERRANT, M.D.

Professor of Medicine, Division of Geographic Medicine, Department of Internal Medicine, University of Virginia School of Medicine, Charlottesville, Virginia
Infectious Diarrhea: A Patient in the United States

JACK M. GWALTNEY, Jr., M.D.

Professor of Internal Medicine, University of Virginia School of Medicine; Physician, University of Virginia Hospital, Charlottesville, Virginia
Common Cold

RICHARD HARRIS, M.D.

Assistant Professor of Medicine, Baylor College of Medicine; The Methodist Hospital, Houston, Texas
Sternal Wound Infection and Mediastinitis

HARLEY A. HAYNES, M.D.

Associate Professor of Dermatology, Harvard Medical School; Director, Dermatology Division, Department of Medicine, Brigham and Women's Hospital, Boston, Massachusetts, Chief of Dermatology, Veterans Administration Hospital, West Roxbury, Massachusetts
Ectoparasitic Infection

SETH HETHERINGTON, M.D.

Assistant Professor of Pediatrics, Albany Medical College of Union University; Attending Physician, Albany Medical Center Hospital, Albany, New York
Infection in the Newborn

MARTIN S. HIRSCH, M.D.

Associate Professor of Medicine, Harvard Medical School; Associate Physician, Infectious Disease Unit, Massachusetts General Hospital, Boston, Massachusetts
Viral Encephalitis

JAN V. HIRSCHMANN, M.D.

Associate Professor of Medicine, University of Washington School of Medicine; Assistant Chief, Medical Service, Seattle Veterans Administration Center, Seattle, Washington
Systemic Prophylactic Antibiotics in Surgery

DAVID D. HO, M.D.

Instructor, Department of Medicine, Harvard Medical School; Assistant in Medicine, Infectious Disease Unit, Massachusetts General Hospital, Boston, Massachusetts
Viral Encephalitis

DONALD R. HOPKINS, M.D., M.P.H.

Visiting Lecturer, Department of Tropical Public Health, Harvard School of Public Health, Boston, Massachusetts; Adjunct Professor of Preventive Medicine and Biometrics, Uniformed Services University of the Health Sciences School of Medicine, Bethesda, Maryland; Clinical Associate Professor of Community Medicine and Family Practice, Morehouse School of Medicine, Atlanta, Georgia; Deputy Director, Centers for Disease Control, Atlanta, Georgia
Nonvenereal Treponematosis

DON WALTER KANNANGARA, M.D., Ph.D.

Assistant Professor of Medicine, Division of Infectious Diseases and Clinical Microbiology, Hahnemann Medical College and Hospital, Philadelphia, Pennsylvania
Bacterial Arthritis

EDWARD H. KASS, Ph.D., M.D., Sc.D.(Hon.), M.A.(Hon.)

William Ellery Channing Professor of Medicine; Director, Channing Laboratory, Harvard Medical School; Senior Physician, Brigham and Women's Hospital, Boston, Massachussets
Nontuberculosis (''Atypical'') Mycobacterial Infections

JEROME O. KLEIN, M.D.

Professor of Pediatrics, Boston University School of Medicine; Director, Division of Pediatric Infectious Diseases, Boston City Hospital, Boston, Massachusetts
Childhood Immunization

JOSEPH J. KLIMEK, M.D.

Associate Professor of Medicine, University of Connecticut School of Medicine, Farmington, Connecticut; Associate Director of Infectious Diseases, Hospital Epidemiologist, Hartford Hospital, Hartford, Connecticut
Postoperative Wound Infection

VERNON KNIGHT, M.D.

Professor of Medicine, Baylor College of Medicine; Senior Attending Physician, The Methodist Hospital, Houston, Texas
Ornithosis

ANTHONY L. KOMAROFF, M.D.

Associate Professor of Medicine, Harvard Medical School; Chief, Division of General Medicine, Physician, Brigham and Women's Hospital, Boston, Massachusetts
Pharyngitis

STEPHEN J. KRAUS, M.D.

Assistant Clinical Professor of Dermatology, Emory University School of Medicine; Clinical Research Investigator, Division of Sexually Transmitted Disease, Centers for Disease Control, Atlanta, Georgia
''Minor'' Sexually Transmitted Disease

BRYAN LARSEN, Ph.D.

Associate Professor of Obstetrics/Gynecology and Microbiology, Marshall University School of Medicine, Huntington, West Virginia
Infection in Pregnancy

JACK L. LEFROCK, M.D.

Scientific Director, Therapeutic Research Institute Inc., Sarasota, Florida
Bacterial Osteomyelitis
Bacterial Arthritis

MARTHA L. LEPOW, M.D.

Professor of Pediatrics, Albany Medical College of Union University; Attending Physician, Albany Medical Center Hospital, Albany, New York
Infection in the Newborn

PHILLIP I. LERNER, M.D.

Professor of Medicine, Case Western Reserve University School of Medicine; Chief, Infectious Disease, Mount Sinai Hospital, Cleveland, Ohio
Prosthetic Valve Endocarditis

MYRON M. LEVINE, M.D., D.T.P.H.

Professor of Medicine and Pediatrics, Head, Division of Geographic Medicine, Head, Division of Infectious Diseases and Tropical Pediatrics, Director, Center for Vaccine Development, University of Colorado School of Medicine, Denver, Colorado
Typhoid Fever and Enteric Fever

EDWARD B. LEWIN, M.D.

Associate Clinical Professor of Pediatrics and Communicable Diseases, University of Michigan Medical School; Head, Division of Pediatric Infectious Diseases, Henry Ford Hospital, Ann Arbor, Michigan
Epiglottitis (Supraglottitis)

CARLOS E. LOPEZ, M.D.

Clinical Assistant Professor of Medicine, Emory University School of Medicine; Infectious Disease Consultant, Piedmont Hospital, Atlanta Georgia
Leptospirosis

TOM MADHAVAN, M.D., F.A.C.P.

Chief, Infectious Diseases, Medical Director, Research and Infection Control, Providence Hospital, Southfield, Michigan
Tularemia

LAURI E. MARKOWITZ, M.D.

Respiratory and Special Pathogens, Epidemiology Branch, Bacterial Diseases Division, Centers for Disease Control, Atlanta, Georgia
Lyme Disease

KENNETH H. MAYER, M.D.

Assistant Professor of Medicine, Brown University Program in Medicine, Providence, Rhode Island; Head, Division of Infectious Diseases, Memorial Hospital, Pawtucket, Rhode Island
Infection Associated with Hematologic Malignancy

WILLIAM R. McCABE, M.D.

Professor of Medicine and Microbiology, Director, Division of Infectious Diseases, Boston University School of Medicine; Director, Maxwell Finland Laboratory, Boston City Hospital, Boston, Massachusetts
Gram-Negative Bacteremia

RICHARD H. MEADE III, M.D.

Professor of Pediatrics, Tufts University School of Medicine, Boston, Massachusetts
Kawasaki Syndrome

JACK MENDELSON, M.D., M.S., F.R.C.P.C.(C)

Professor of Medicine and Microbiology, McGill University Faculty of Medicine; Senior Physician, Sir Mortimer B. Davis–Jewish General Hospital, Montreal, Quebec, Canada
Aseptic Meningitis

RICHARD D. MEYER, M.D.

Professor of Medicine, UCLA School of Medicine; Director, Division of Infectious Diseases, Cedars-Sinai Medical Center, Los Angeles, California
Lung Abscess

ABDOLGHADER MOLAVI, M.D.

Associate Professor of Medicine, Hahnemann University School of Medicine, Philadelphia, Pennsylvania
Bacterial Osteomyelitis

MAURICE A. MUFSON, M.D.

Chairman and Professor of Medicine, Professor of Microbiology, Marshall University School of Medicine; Chief of Staff for Research and Development, Veterans Administration Medical Center, Active Staff, St. Mary's Hospital and Cabell-Huntington Hospital, Huntington, West Virginia
Pleural Effusion and Empyema

EILEEN MURPHY, M.D.

Fellow in Infectious and Immunologic Diseases, Department of Medicine, University of California, School of Medicine, Davis, California
Infection Following Trauma

GARY D. OVERTURF, M.D.

Professor of Pediatrics, University of Southern California School of Medicine; Director, Communicable Disease Service, Los Angeles County-USC Medical Center, Los Angeles, California
Meningitis in Children

MICHAEL N. OXMAN, M.D.

Professor of Medicine and Pathology, University of California, San Diego, School of Medicine; Chief, Infectious Diseases Section, San Diego Veterans Administration Medical Center, La Jolla, California
Guidelines for Antiviral Chemotherapy

JAMES E. PENNINGTON, M.D.

Associate Professor of Medicine, Harvard Medical School; Physician, Brigham and Women's Hospital, Boston, Massachusetts
Organ Transplantation-Associated Infection

RONALD L. PERKINS, M.D.

Professor of Medicine, Director, Division of Infectious Diseases, The Ohio State University College of Medicine, Columbus, Ohio
Actinomycosis

CLARENCE JAMES PETERS, M.D.

Associate, Department of Immunology and Infectious Diseases, School of Hygiene and Public Health, The Johns Hopkins University School of Medicine, Baltimore, Maryland; Chief, Disease Assessment Division, U.S. Army Institute of Infectious Diseases, Fort Detrick, Frederick, Maryland
Viral Hemorrhagic Fever

RICHARD PLATT, M.D.

Assistant Professor of Medicine, Harvard Medical School; Associate Hospital Epidemiologist, Brigham and Women's

Hospital, Hospital Epidemiologist, New England Deaconess Hospital, Boston, Massachusetts
Adult Immunization

THOMAS C. QUINN, M.D.

Associate Professor of Medicine, The Johns Hopkins University School of Medicine, Baltimore, Maryland; Senior Investigator, Laboratory of Immunoregulation, National Institute of Allergy and Infectious Diseases, National Institutes of Health, Bethesda, Maryland
Infection other than AIDS in Homosexual Men

MARTIN J. RAFF, M.D., M.S., F.A.C.P.

Professor of Medicine, Assistant Professor of Microbiology and Immunology, Chief, Section of Infectious Diseases, Department of Medicine, University of Louisville School of Medicine, Louisville, Kentucky
Biliary Tract Infection

CARLOS H. RAMIREZ-RONDA, M.D., F.A.C.P.

Professor of Medicine, University of Puerto Rico School of Medicine; Associate Chief of Staff for Research and Development, Veterans Administration Medical Center, Director, Infectious Diseases Program, San Juan Veterans Administration Hospital and University Hospital, San Juan, Puerto Rico
Diphtheria

ARTHUR L. REINGOLD, M.D.

Assistant Branch Chief, Respiratory and Special Pathogens Epidemiology Branch, Division of Bacterial Diseases, Centers for Disease Control, Atlanta, Georgia
Toxic Shock Syndrome

PETER A. RICE, M.D.

Associate Professor of Medicine and Microbiology, Boston University School of Medicine; Associate Physician, Medical Service, Boston City Hospital, Boston, Massachusetts
Disseminated Gonococcal Infection

RICHARD B. ROBERTS, M.D.

Professor of Medicine, Cornell University Medical College; Attending Physician, New York Hospital, New York, New York
Bacterial Meningitis in Adults

JOHN A. ROMANKIEWICZ, Pharm.D.

President, Scientific Therapeutics Information, Fort Lee, New Jersey
Bacterial Meningitis in Adults

MARIA C. SAVOIA, M.D.

Assistant Adjunct Professor of Medicine, University of California, San Diego, School of Medicine; Assistant Chief, Medical Services, San Diego Veterans Administration Medical Center, La Jolla, California
Guidelines for Antiviral Chemotherapy

WILLIAM SCHAFFNER, M.D.

Professor of Medicine and Chief, Division of Infectious Diseases, Vanderbilt University School of Medicine, Nashville, Tennessee
Hospital-Acquired Pneumonia

EDWARD J. SEPTIMUS, M.D.

Associate Clinical Professor of Medicine, Program in Infectious Diseases and Clinical Microbiology, University of Texas Health Science Center at Houston; Director Infectious Diseases Program, Memorial Hospital System, Houston, Texas
Nocardial Infection

ALEXIS SHELOKOV, M.D.

Senior Associate, Department of Epidemiology, School of Hygiene and Public Health, The Johns Hopkins University School of Medicine, Baltimore, Maryland; Director of Vaccine Research, The Salk Institute, Government Services Division, Swiftwater, Pennsylvania
Viral Hemorrhagic Fever

PAUL A. SHURIN, M.D.

Assistant Professor of Pediatrics, Case Western Reserve University School of Medicine; Associate Director, Pediatric Infectious Diseases, Cleveland Metropolitan General Hospital, Cleveland, Ohio
Otitis Media

BRUCE R. SMITH, Pharm.D.

Therapeutic Research Institute Inc., Sarasota, Florida
Bacterial Osteomyelitis

CHARLES B. SMITH, M.D.

Professor and Associate Chairman of Medicine, University of Utah College of Medicine; Chief, Medical Service, Salt Lake Veterans Administration Hospital, Salt Lake City, Utah
Nonbacterial Arthritis Syndrome

MARGARET H.D. SMITH, M.D.

Professor Emeritus of Pediatrics, Tulane University School of Medicine, New Orleans, Louisiana
Pertussis

DAVID R. SNYDMAN, M.D.

Associate Professor of Medicine, Tufts University School of Medicine; Hospital Epidemiologist and Physician, Department of Medicine, New England Medical Center, Boston, Massachusetts
Intravenous Catheter-Associated Infection

PHILIP J. SPAGNUOLO, M.D.

Associate Professor of Medicine, Case Western Reserve University School of Medicine; Director, Division of Infectious Diseases, Cleveland Metropolitan General Hospital, Cleveland, Ohio
Plague

PETER SPEELMAN, M.D.

Fellow in Infectious Diseases, University of Washington School of Medicine, Seattle, Washington
Amebiasis and Giardiasis

WALTER E. STAMM, M.D.

Associate Professor of Medicine, University of Washington School of Medicine; Head, Infectious Disease Division, Harborview Medical Center, Seattle, Washington
Acute Dysuria in Women and Urethritis in Men

WILLIAM W. STEAD, M.D., F.A.C.P.

Professor of Medicine, University of Arkansas College of Medicine; Director, Tuberculosis Program, Arkansas Department of Health, Little Rock, Arkansas
Tuberculosis

ALLEN C. STEERE, M.D.

Associate Professor of Medicine, Yale University School of Medicine, New Haven, Connecticut
Lyme Disease

NEAL H. STEIGBIGEL, M.D.

Professor of Medicine, Albert Einstein College of Medicine; Head, Division of Infectious Diseases, Montefiore Medical Center, Bronx, New York
Acquired Immunodeficiency Syndrome

RHOADS ELLIOTT STEVENS, M.D.

Clinical and Research Fellow, Massachusetts Eye and Ear Infirmary, Cornea Service, Harvard Medical School; Eye Research Institute of the Retina Foundation, Boston, Massachusetts
Infection of the Conjunctiva, Eyelids, and Lacrimal Apparatus

HERBERT BERNARD TANOWITZ, M.D.

Associate Professor of Pathology and Medicine, Albert Einstein College of Medicine; Associate Attending in Medicine and Pathology, Bronx Municipal Hospital Center, Hospital of Albert Einstein College of Medicine, Bronx, New York
Babesiosis

ROBERT R. TIGHT, M.D.

Associate Professor of Medicine, University of North Dakota School of Medicine; Chief, Infectious Diseases, Fargo Veterans Administration Hospital, Fargo, North Dakota
Syphilis

RONALD G. TOMPKINS, M.D., Sc.D.

Instructor in Surgery, Harvard Medical School, Boston, Massachusetts; Research Associate, Massachusetts Institute of Technology, Cambridge, Massachusetts; Assistant in Surgery, Massachusetts General Hospital, Boston, Massachusetts
Infection Following Burn Injury

KENNETH L. TYLER, M.D.

Assistant Professor of Neurology, Instructor of Microbiology and Molecular Genetics, Harvard Medical School; Clinical Assistant in Neurology, Massachusetts General Hospital, Boston, Massachusetts
Localized Infection of the Central Nervous System

GEORGE VAN HARE, M.D.

Instructor, Department of Pediatrics, Case Western Reserve University School of Medicine; Instructor, Department of Pediatrics, Cleveland Metropolitan General Hospital, Cleveland, Ohio
Otitis Media

BORIS VELIMIROVIC, M.D., D.T.P.H.

Professor of Medicine, University of Graz; Director, Institute of Social Medicine, Graz, Austria
Anthrax

BURTON A. WAISBREN, B.S., M.S., M.D., F.A.C.P., F.A.S.I.D.

Director of Waisbren Clinic and Clinical Cell Biology Laboratory, Milwaukee, Wisconsin
Sinusitis

RICHARD JAMES WALLACE, Jr., M.D.

Associate Professor of Research and Clinical Medicine and Chief, Department of Microbiology, University of Texas Health Center, Tyler, Texas
Nocardial Infection

JOHN W. WARREN, M.D.

Associate Professor of Medicine, Division of Infectious Diseases, University of Maryland School of Medicine; Attending Physician, University of Maryland Hospital and Psychiatric Institute, Baltimore, Maryland
Catheter-Associated Urinary Tract Infection

KENNETH S. WARREN, M.D.

Director, Health Sciences Division, Rockefeller Foundation, New York, New York
Schistosomiasis

CHATRCHAI WATANAKUNAKORN, M.D., F.A.C.P., F.C.C.P.

Professor of Internal Medicine, Northeastern Ohio Universities College of Medicine, Rootstown, Ohio; Chief of Infections Disease Section, Department of Internal Medicine, St. Elizabeth Hospital Medical Center, Youngstown, Ohio
Community-Acquired Pneumonia

CYNTHIA S. WEIKEL, M.D.

Assistant Professor of Medicine, Division of Geographic Medicine, Department of Internal Medicine, University of Virginia School of Medicine, Charlottesville, Virginia
Infectious Diarrhea: A Patient in the United States

RICHARD J. WHITLEY, M.D.

Professor of Pediatrics and Microbiology, University of Alabama School of Medicine, University of Alabama, Birmingham, Alabama
Herpes Simplex Virus Infection

TEMPLE W. WILLIAMS, Jr., M.D.

Professor of Medicine and Microbiology-Immunology, Baylor College of Medicine, Houston, Texas
Sternal Wound Infection and Mediastinitis

MURRAY WITTNER, M.D., Ph.D.

Professor of Pathology and Medicine, Albert Einstein College of Medicine; Director of Parasitology and Tropical Disease, Albert Einstein Affiliated Hospital, Attending Physician Bronx Municipal Hospital Center and Hospital of Albert Einstein College of Medicine, Bronx, New York
Babesiosis

THEODORE E. WOODWARD, M.D., M.A.C.P.

Professor Emeritus of Medicine, University of Maryland School of Medicine, Baltimore, Maryland
Rickettsial Infection

DAVID J. WYLER, M.D., F.A.C.P.

Professor of Medicine, Tufts University School of Medicine; Physician, New England Medical Center Hospital, Boston, Massachusetts
Leishmaniasis

THOMAS T. YOSHIKAWA, M.D.

Professor, Department of Internal Medicine, UCLA School of Medicine; Chief, Division of Geriatric Medicine and Clinical Director of Geriatric Research, Education and Clinical Center, West Los Angeles Veterans Administration Medical Center, Los Angeles, California
Cellulitis and Soft Tissue Infection

EDWARD J. YOUNG, M.D.

Associate Professor of Medicine, Microbiology and Immunology, Baylor College of Medicine; Chief of Staff, The Veterans Administration Medical Center, Houston, Texas
Human Brucellosis

DORI F. ZALEZNIK, M.D.

Instructor in Medicine, Harvard Medical School; Assistant in Medicine, Beth Israel Hospital, Associate Physician, Brigham and Women's Hospital, Boston, Massachusetts
Fever and Rash

MOHSEN ZIAI, M.D.

Chairman, Department of Pediatrics, The Fairfax Hospital, Falls Church, Virginia
Trachoma

STEPHEN H. ZINNER, M.D.

Professor of Medicine, Brown University Program in Medicine; Director, Division of Infectious Diseases, Roger Williams General Hospital, Providence, Rhode Island
Infection Associated with Hematologic Malignancy

PREFACE

The kind reception accorded the original volume, *Current Therapy in Infectious Disease* prompted the preparation of this new volume. The present work is radically changed from the preceding one. Virtually all of the authors are different, not because of inadequacies of their predecessors, but rather to bring to our readers a wider range of viewpoints on the complexities of management of infectious disease. New topics have been added, some combined, and others reorganized.

We have, however, maintained the basic thrust of the earlier volume by insisting, wherever it was appropriate, that the authors eschew the common practice of using permissive and occasionally ambiguous recommendations. Instead, we asked them to tell us *what they do* in the specific circumstances under discussion. This principle was outlined in the preface to the previous volume, from which we now quote liberally.

Many, if not most, textbooks and manuals are written by experts and try to earn the approbation of fellow experts in the field. Since some disagreement within a field is necessary and reasonable, recommendations for treatment usually contain wide ranges of dosages and broadly permissive statements, such as, "may sometimes be helpful" or "is often recommended." For the busy practitioner, who cannot take the time to thread through all the details of current controversy or uncertainty, such distressingly common statements are perplexing in the least and frustrating in the extreme. If to this problem is added the contemporary one of the new antimicrobial drugs that are appearing on the market with staggering frequency, difficult problems of choice and awareness are posed. In addition, given that each new product is usually marketed forcefully and convincingly by its respective purveyors, the plight of the practitioner is further compounded.

It seems reasonable, therefore, to assemble a volume on treatment and prevention of infectious disease that attempts to cut through the problems of choice and of consensus by adhering to two simple principles. The first is that experts in their respective fields would be asked to state what they did when faced with a patient with the disease under discussion. Second, the recommendations would be given in straightforward terms, especially when dosages, routes, difficulties, and reasons for a given choice were concerned. If there were acceptable alternatives, these were to be stated in order of preference. Where there were disagreements, these could be mentioned, but only in relation to a statement of the author's preference.

Therefore, this is a manual intended for the busy practitioner. It gives only enough diagnostic information to offer a rational framework for treatment. It is our hope that future editions will offer recommendations from different experts, thereby reflecting occasional differences of approach.

We are most appreciative of the helpful suggestions that we have received; we have tried to respond to as many of them as possible. We hope that the present effort will elicit constructive comments from our readers. We have tried to make the presentations succinct, and in so doing have sometimes edited the individual contributions. Errors and misinterpretations in the presentations are ours, but we shall be ready to amend and to add to these topics in response to our readers.

We are particularly grateful to the contributors who have provided their expert views on the various topics that are presented; they have put up with our queries and editorial comments with good humor and constructive response. Because most of them are members of the Infectious Diseases Society of America, we have, as in the past, attempted to express our appreciation by contributing to the Lectureship Fund of the IDSA, from the royalties of these volumes. However, the Society has no official involvement with this work, has neither approved nor disapproved of it, and is in no way responsible for any of the opinions and judgments expressed.

Our particular gratitude goes to Joan Daniels for her perceptive contributions to this volume, to Julie McIntyre Curran for her helpful assistance in ways too numerous to mention, and to the publisher, Brian Decker, for his many valuable suggestions.

Edward H. Kass
Richard Platt
December, 1985

PREFACE

CONTENTS

Infections Affecting More Than One System and Caused by Parasites or Fungi

Nosocomial Infections

GENERAL THERAPEUTICS

ANTIVIRAL CHEMOTHERAPY

MARIA C. SAVOIA, M.D.
MICHAEL N. OXMAN, M.D.

Until recently, chapters on antiviral chemotherapy were missing from major textbooks of medicine and even from major texts on infectious diseases. Our traditional approach to the control of viral diseases has been to prevent infection either by limiting exposure or by immunization, techniques of unquestionable merit and unparalleled cost-effectiveness. When virus infections did occur, few if any therapeutic options were available. The recent development of effective antiviral agents has altered this situation. Many compounds are being developed that take advantage of virus-specific metabolic reactions to inhibit virus replication selectively without significant toxicity for host cells. Five antiviral drugs with proven efficacy and acceptable therapeutic to toxic ratios have already been licensed for use in the United States, and many additional agents are currently being evaluated.

While vaccines that prevent infection will continue to be our most important and cost-effective weapons in the battle against viral diseases, physicians will now also have access to an ever-increasing array of therapeutic agents. This chapter is concerned primarily with antiviral agents that are currently approved for use in the United States, but investigational agents and indications for use that are likely to gain such approval are also considered. Guidelines for the use of these agents are summarized in Table 1.

Readers of this chapter should keep in mind the following general principles:

1. *Use of any antiviral agent requires a specific virologic diagnosis.* More than 500 different viruses—belonging to at least 17 distinct virus families—cause disease in humans. Since individual antiviral agents rely for their selective antiviral activity upon virus-specific metabolic reactions that are often unique to individual viruses or virus families, the choice of an appropriate antiviral agent requires a specific virologic diagnosis. Clinical diagnosis is often unreliable because many different viruses may cause the same clinical syndrome. Fortunately, rapid progress is being made in the development and application of laboratory techniques for the quick and accurate diagnosis of viral infections. Physicians should soon be able to obtain reliable diagnostic information early enough to permit the effective utilization of available antiviral agents.

2. *Most viral infections are acute and self-limited.* In many cases, peak virus multiplication and dissemination occur late in the incubation period and rapidly diminish after the onset of symptoms. Since most antiviral agents act by inhibiting virus multiplication, they can only be effective if administered at a time when progression of disease is dependent upon continuing virus replication. In general, this means that antiviral therapy must be initiated very early in the course of the disease. Moreover, the natural history of the untreated infection and the status of host-defense mechanisms are important considerations in selecting patients who might benefit from antiviral therapy. For example, in immunologically normal patients with recurrent mucocutaneous herpes simplex, host defenses rapidly terminate virus replication and lesions quickly resolve without treatment, whereas in immunocompromised patients, lesions may progress and virus multiplication may continue at high levels for many weeks. Clearly, an agent that inhibits herpes simplex virus replication will have a much greater impact on the course of the disease in immunocompromised patients.

3. *Antiviral agents should be reserved for situations in which clinical benefit has been demonstrated.* Anecdotal experience, case reports, and uncontrolled trials often lead to false impressions of clinical efficacy and can encourage both physicians and patients to use ineffective and harmful remedies. In most virus diseases, the efficacy and toxicity of an antiviral agent can be evaluated only by randomized, double-blind, placebo-controlled studies involving proven cases.

4. *The indiscriminate use of antiviral agents will hasten the emergence of resistant viruses.* Just as the use of antibiotics has led to the emergence of antibiotic-resistant bacteria, resistance to antiviral agents will develop with their widespread use. Although the clinical importance of this phenomenon may not become apparent for some time, antiviral agents should be used judiciously to minimize the selection of resistant viruses.

AGENTS USEFUL IN THE TREATMENT OF RESPIRATORY VIRUS INFECTIONS

Amantadine (1-adamantanamine hydrochloride)

In 1966, amantadine (Symmetrel), a symmetric tricyclic amine, became the first antiviral agent licensed for systemic use by the U.S. Food and Drug Administration

TABLE 1 Indications for the Use of Available Antiviral Agents

Indication	*Antiviral Agent*	*Route*	*Dose*	*Comments*
Treatment of influenza A virus infection	Amantadine	Oral	Adults: 100–200 mg/day (see text) for 5–7 days; children ≤9 years: 4.4–8.8 mg/kg/day for 5–7 days not to exceed 150 mg/day)*	Normal persons >65 years of age should receive 100 mg/day
Prophylaxis against influenza A virus infection	Amantadine	Oral	Adults: 100–200 mg/day (see text); children ≤9 years: 4.4–8.8 mg/kg/day (not to exceed 150 mg/day)*	Should be continued for the duration of the epidemic *or* for 2 weeks in conjunction with influenza vaccination (until vaccine-induced immunity develops); normal persons >65 years of age should receive 100 mg/day
Treatment of herpes simplex virus (HSV) encephalitis†	Acyclovir	IV	10 mg/kg (1 hour infusion) every 8 hours for 10 days‡	Recent comparative studies demonstrate that although IV vidarabine (15 mg/kg by continuous infusion over 12 hours each day for 10 days) is effective, morbidity and mortality are significantly lower in patients treated with acyclovir than with vidarabine
Treatment of neonatal herpes	Vidarabine	IV	30 mg/kg/day (continuous infusion over 12 hours) for 10 days§	Efficacy of vidarabine is established; vidarabine and acyclovir currently being compared in controlled clinical trials
	or			
	Acyclovir	IV	10 mg/kg (1 hour infusion) each 8 hours for 10 days‡	
Treatment of mucocutaneous herpes simplex in immunocompromised hosts	Acyclovir	IV	250 mg/M² (1 hour infusion) every 8 hours for 7 days‡	Choice of topical, oral, or intravenous preparation depends upon clinical severity and setting; topical acyclovir is appropriate only when it can be applied to all lesions; it does not affect untreated lesions or systemic symptoms
	or			
	Acyclovir	Oral	200 mg 5 times/day for 10 days	
	or			
	Acyclovir	Topical	5% ointment; 4–6 applications/day for 7 days or until healed	
Prophylaxis against mucocutaneous herpes simplex during periods of intense immunosuppression	Acyclovir	Oral	200 mg 4 times/day‖	Oral therapy most convenient; lesions recur when therapy stops
	or			
	Acyclovir	IV	250 mg/M² every 8 hours or 5 mg/kg every 12 hours (1 hour infusion)‡	Lesions recur when therapy stops
Treatment of initial genital HSV infections	Acyclovir	Oral	200 mg 5 times/day for 10 days‖	Drug of choice in most clinical settings; treatment has no effect on subsequent recurrence rates
	or			

TABLE 1 Indications for the Use of Available Antiviral Agents—Continued

Indication	*Antiviral Agent*	*Route*	*Dose*	*Comments*
	Acyclovir	IV	5 mg/kg (1 hour infusion) each 8 hours for 5–7 days‡	When severity of infection merits hospitalization, or with neurologic or other visceral complications
	or			
	Acyclovir	Topical	5% ointment, 4–6 applications/day for 7–14 days	May cause stinging on contact; does not affect constitutional symptoms, new lesion formation, or untreated sites of infection
Treatment of recurrent genital herpes#	Acyclovir	Oral	200 mg 5 times/day for 5 days‖	No effect on subsequent recurrence rates; efficacy greater if used early in attack
Prophylaxis against frequently recurring genital herpes#	Acyclovir	Oral	200 mg 3 times/day for up to 6 months‖	May promote emergence of resistance; occasional "breakthrough" attacks and/or asymptomatic virus shedding during treatment; not recommended for periods exceeding 6 months
Treatment of HSV keratitis	Trifluridine	Topical	One drop of 0.1% ophthalmic solution every 2 hours while awake (up to 9 drops/day)	3% acyclovir ointment (ophthalmic) is equal or superior to idoxuridine, vidarabine and trifluridine for treatment of HSV keratitis, but is not available in the United States
	or			
	Vidarabine	Topical	One-half-inch ribbon of 3% ophthalmic ointment 5 times/day	
	or			
	Idoxuridine	Topical	One-half-inch ribbon of 0.5% ophthalmic ointment 5 times/day	
Treatment of varicella in immunocompromised hosts	Acyclovir	IV	500 mg/M² (1 hour infusion) every 8 hours for 7 days‡	In the absence of comparative data, acyclovir is preferred because of its ease of administration and lower toxicity
	or			
	Vidarabine	IV	10 mg/kg/day (continuous infusion over 12 hours) for 5 days§	
Treatment of severe localized or disseminated herpes zoster in immunocompromised hosts	Acyclovir	IV	500 mg/M² or 5–10 mg/kg (1 hour infusion) every 8 hours for 5–7 days‡	Comparative trials in severe localized and disseminated herpes zoster are underway; pending results, acyclovir is preferred because of its ease of administration and lower toxicity
	or			
	Vidarabine	IV	10 mg/kg/day (continuous infusion over 12 hours) for 5–7 days§	

* Dosage adjustment required in patients with renal insufficiency (see Table 2).
† Brain biopsy is required to rule out other diagnoses that require different modalities of therapy.
‡ Dosage adjustment required in patients with renal insufficiency (see Table 3).
§ In patients with severe renal insufficiency (creatinine clearance ≤10 ml/minute/1.73M²), the dose should be reduced by 25%.
‖ In patients with severe renal insufficiency (creatinine clearance ≤10 ml/minute/1.73M²), the dose should be reduced to 200 mg every 12 hours.
Appropriate only for carefully selected patients.

(FDA). Amantadine specifically inhibits the multiplication of influenza A viruses and is clinically effective in the prophylaxis and treatment of influenza A virus infections. Its efficacy is strictly limited to influenza A virus strains. Although its mechanism of action is not precisely known, amantadine acts at an early stage of virus replication; it appears to prevent the uncoating of the viral genome that normally follows attachment and penetration of the virus into the host cell.

Many clinical trials have demonstrated that administration of amantadine within 24 to 48 hours after the onset of symptoms of naturally occurring or experimentally induced influenza A virus infection shortens the duration of illness; fever and systemic symptoms resolve in approximately half the time in treated patients. Subtle abnormalities in peripheral airway function also resolve more quickly in patients with uncomplicated influenza A who are treated with amantadine. However, the efficacy of amantadine in treating or preventing pneumonia due to influenza A virus has not yet been established. Therapeutic responses have also been demonstrated in patients with uncomplicated influenza A treated with aerosolized amantadine—a cumbersome method of delivery, but one that produces higher concentrations of amantadine in respiratory secretions than does oral administration.

Administered prophylactically, amantadine has about the same efficacy as vaccination in preventing influenza A virus infection (50% to 90%). Amantadine recipients who do develop influenza A have milder illnesses.

Pharmacology and Toxicology

Amantadine, which is available in capsules and syrup, is well absorbed following oral administration. The usual dosage for both treatment and prophylaxis is 200 mg per day in healthy adults and 4.4 to 8.8 mg per kilogram per day in children up to 9 years of age. These dosages produce plasma concentrations that average 0.6 to 0.8 μg per milliliter, two- to fourfold higher than the concentration required to inhibit most strains of influenza A virus in vitro. The concentration of amantadine in respiratory tissues and secretions appears to equal or exceed that in the plasma.

Amantadine is excreted unmetabolized in the urine, with a mean plasma half-life of 12 to 18 hours in healthy adults. Plasma half-life increases in elderly individuals and in patients with impaired renal function, necessitating dosage adjustment (Table 2). Orally administered amantadine at dosages of 6 mg per kilogram per day in children and 200 mg per day in healthy adults is generally well tolerated.

No serious hepatic, hematopoietic, or renal toxicity has been documented. Adverse effects appear to correlate with plasma levels of amantadine and to be limited, with few exceptions, to minor gastrointestinal and central nervous system symptoms that disappear when the drug is discontinued. Complaints such as nausea, loss of appetite, nervousness, insomnia, difficulty in concentrating, drowsiness, lightheadedness, confusion, and mildly diminished intellectual and motor function have been noted in 1 to 10 percent of previously healthy recipients of amantadine, but their incidence in many studies has not differed significantly in amantadine and placebo recipients.

Symptoms of central nervous system toxicity have been observed in up to 20 percent of elderly patients receiving amantadine, probably reflecting higher plasma levels associated with age-related decreases in glomerular filtration rate. Symptoms frequently resolve despite continued administration of the drug, and they may often be avoided by giving amantadine at bedtime rather than in the morning or by administering one-half of the daily dose each 12 hours. Since recent studies indicate that 100 mg per day of amantadine may be just as effective as 200 mg per day, the use of the lower dosage is recommended for prophylaxis in elderly patients.

High doses of amantadine are teratogenic in certain laboratory animals, and thus amantadine is not considered safe for use during pregnancy.

Recommended Usage

Because amantadine is not effective against other agents that may be responsible for flu-like symptoms, including influenza B viruses, its use should be reserved for situations in which infection with an influenza A virus is proven or probable. Thus, amantadine usage is only appropriate when epidemiologic and virologic evidence indicates that influenza A virus infection is prevalent in the community.

Prophylactic administration of amantadine is recommended for individuals at increased risk of complications from influenza A who have not been vaccinated against the prevalent virus strain(s) or who may be expected to have responded poorly to vaccination (e.g., immunocompromised patients). The target population of high-risk individuals includes elderly persons (65 or more years of age), especially those in nursing homes and other institutions; hospitalized patients; and children and adults with underlying pulmonary, cardiovascular, neuromuscular or immunodeficiency disorders. Additional recommended recipients include unvaccinated children and adults with other chronic diseases and malignancies; unvaccinated physicians, nurses, and other health care workers who

TABLE 2 Dosage Adjustment for Oral Amantadine in Patients with Impaired Renal Function

Creatinine Clearance (ml/minute/1.73M²)	*Suggested Oral Maintenance Regimen After 200 mg (100 mg BID) on the First Day*
≥ 80	100 mg BID
60–80	100 mg BID alternating with 100 mg daily
40–60	100 mg daily
30–40	200 mg (100 mg BID) twice weekly
20–30	100 mg 3 times each week
10–20	200 mg (100 mg BID) alternating with 100 mg every 7 days
< 10	100 mg every 7 days

Note: Modified from Horadan et al. Ann Intern Med 1981; 94:454–458.

have extensive contact with high-risk patients; unvaccinated household and institutional contacts of persons with influenza A; and unvaccinated persons who provide essential community services. Prophylaxis should begin as soon as influenza A is identified in the community and must be continued throughout the period of its prevalence (usually 4 to 8 weeks). Influenza vaccine should be administered simultaneously with the initiation of amantadine prophylaxis in unvaccinated individuals. This will provide protection against influenza B as well as influenza A and, in most recipients, reduce the required duration of amantadine administration to 10 to 14 days (i.e., until vaccine-induced immunity develops). Amantadine prophylaxis may also be used as a supplement to vaccination for better protection in immunodeficient and debilitated patients.

Treatment with amantadine is appropriate for patients at increased risk (see above) who develop an illness compatible with influenza during a period of known or suspected influenza A virus activity in the community. Treatment should be initiated as soon as possible (preferably within 48 hours of onset) and continued until 48 hours after the resolution of signs and symptoms. Though its efficacy in this setting remains to be established, it is also reasonable to administer amantadine to patients with life-threatening influenza A virus pneumonia.

Rimantadine (α-methyl-1-adamantanemethylamine hydrochloride)

Rimantadine, a structural analogue of amantadine, has been shown to be effective in the prophylaxis and treatment of infections caused by influenza A viruses. Though similar in their mechanism of action and spectrum of antiviral activity, amantadine and rimantadine differ in several respects. Rimantadine is not as well absorbed as amantadine when given orally, but its plasma half-life is nearly twice as long. Less than 10 percent of the administered dose of rimantidine is recovered unchanged in the urine (versus more than 90% with amantadine), and elevated plasma levels are less of a problem in elderly patients and patients with renal insufficiency. When given in equal doses, both drugs are almost equally effective, but rimantadine is associated with fewer central nervous system adverse effects, probably reflecting lower plasma concentrations. Rimantadine, like amantadine, is successful in reducing the symptoms of illness even when it is not successful in preventing infection. Rimantadine is not yet approved for general use by the FDA.

Ribavirin (1-β-D-ribofuranosyl-1,2,4-triazole-3-carboxamide)

Ribavirin (Virazole) is a synthetic guanosine analogue that inhibits the in vitro replication of a wide range of RNA and DNA viruses. Its mechanism of action is not well understood, but it appears to interfere with the synthesis of messenger RNA. The effect of orally administered ribavirin on influenza A and B virus infections has been evaluated in several clinical trials, and no consistent prophylactic or therapeutic efficacy has been documented. Aerosolized ribavirin has been shown to reduce the severity of illness and virus shedding in young adults with naturally acquired influenza A and B virus infections and in infants hospitalized with respiratory syncytial virus bronchiolitis and pneumonia. The need for prolonged periods of aerosol treatment (from 12 to 20 hours per day for 3 to 6 days) is a disadvantage. Parenteral ribavirin is currently also being evaluated in the treatment of bunyavirus and arenavirus infections (including Lassa fever) and in patients infected with the human retrovirus responsible for the acquired immune deficiency syndrome (AIDS).

Oral ribavirin may cause reversible increases in serum bilirubin, serum iron, and uric acid concentrations, as well as reticulocytosis after cessation of therapy. Aerosolized ribavirin may cause conjunctival injection, but it is generally well tolerated. It has recently been approved by the FDA for treatment of infants hospitalized with bronchiolitis and pneumonia caused by influenza and respiratory syncytial virus.

AGENTS USEFUL IN THE TREATMENT OF HERPESVIRUS INFECTIONS

Acyclovir (9-[2-hydroxyethoxymethyl]guanine)

Acyclovir (Zovirax) is an acyclic purine nucleoside analogue that is useful in the treatment of infections caused by herpes simplex virus types 1 and 2 (HSV-1 and HSV-2) and varicella-zoster virus (VZV). It is a safe and effective drug because it is phosphorylated selectively by a virus-specific thymidine kinase and thus concentrated in infected cells. Cellular enzymes convert acyclovir monophosphate to acyclovir triphosphate, which interferes with viral DNA synthesis by selectively inhibiting viral DNA polymerase. Some acyclovir is also incorporated into viral DNA, where it acts as a chain terminator.

Of the five human herpesviruses, HSV-1, HSV-2, and VZV are sensitive to acyclovir because they encode their own thymidine kinase and possess a sensitive DNA polymerase. In vitro, most strains of HSV-1 are inhibited by acyclovir at concentrations of 0.2 μg per milliliter or less, most strains of HSV-2 by concentrations of 0.4 μg per milliliter or less, and most strains of VZV by concentrations of 2 μg per milliliter or less.

Acyclovir also exhibits some activity against Epstein-Barr virus (EBV), which lacks thymidine kinase but possesses a very sensitive DNA polymerase. This indicates that acyclovir can be phosphorylated to some extent by cellular thymidine kinases and that some acyclovir triphosphate is formed in uninfected cells.

Unfortunately, acyclovir is not useful in the treatment of infections caused by cytomegalovirus (CMV), another member of the herpesvirus family that lacks thymidine kinase, presumably because CMV DNA polymerase is not inhibited by the low concentrations of acyclovir triphosphate formed in the absence of a viral thymidine kinase.

Pharmacology and Toxicology

Acyclovir is available in the United States in intravenous, oral, and topical forms. After intravenous infusion of 5 mg per kilogram every 8 hours, peak and trough plasma concentrations average 9.8 μg per milliliter and 0.7 μg per milliliter, respectively. The concentration of acyclovir in cerebrospinal fluid is approximately one-half of the plasma concentration. Only 15 to 30 percent of an oral dose of acyclovir is absorbed, with bioavailability decreasing slightly with increasing oral doses in the 200- to 600-mg range. Steady-state peak concentrations of acyclovir average 1.4 μg per milliliter in adults given 200 mg orally five times a day. Percutaneous absorption of acyclovir ointment (5% acyclovir in a polyethylene glycol base) is low. Excretion of acyclovir occurs both by glomerular filtration and tubular secretion, with an average plasma half-life of 2.9 hours in normal adults. Sixty to 90 percent of an administered dose may be recovered unmetabolized in the urine. Dosage adjustments are therefore required in patients with diminished renal function (see Table 3).

Acyclovir has been associated with relatively few adverse effects. Phlebitis may occur with extravasation of intravenous acyclovir. When given in high doses (more than 5 mg per kilogram every 8 hours) intravenously, acyclovir has been associated with reversible renal dysfunction in a small percentage of patients, probably due to deposition of acyclovir crystals in renal tubules. Preexisting renal insufficiency, dehydration, and rapid infusion appear to be risk factors. Encepalopathic changes, manifested by lethargy, obtundation, tremors, hallucinations, delirium, seizures, and coma, have been observed in approximately 1 percent of acyclovir recipients, but these have generally resolved following cessation of treatment. Oral acyclovir is generally very well tolerated. It is infrequently associated with nausea and headache. Topical acyclovir may cause transient burning when applied to active genital lesions. Acyclovir is not teratogenic in animals, but safety in human pregnancy has not been established. The safety of chronic administration of acyclovir for prolonged periods in reproductively active young adults also remains to be determined.

Herpes Simplex Virus Infections

All three forms of acyclovir have demonstrated efficacy in the treatment of at least some infections caused by HSV-1 and HSV-2. However, the magnitude of clinical benefit varies with the natural history of the untreated infection, the acyclovir preparation, and the status of the host's defenses. Because of its more reliable absorption and the higher plasma levels achieved, intravenous acyclovir is preferred whenever the severity of the disease warrants hospitalization.

TABLE 3 Dosage Adjustment for Intravenous acyclovir in Patients with Impaired Renal Function

Creatinine Clearance (ml/minute/1.73M²)	*Percentage of Standard Dose*	*Dosing Interval (Hours)*
> 50	100	8
25–50	100	12
10–25	100	24
0–10*	50	24

* Administered after hemodialysis.

Herpes Simplex Encephalitis. Two recent randomized studies comparing the efficacy of intravenous acyclovir (30 mg per kilogram per day) and vidarabine (15 mg per kilogram per day) in patients with herpes simplex encephalitis (HSE) have demonstrated the superiority of acyclovir. Mortality, expected to exceed 70 percent without treatment, was reduced to approximately 24 percent in recipients of acyclovir compared with 52 percent in vidarabine recipients. In addition, the proportion of the survivors who returned to normal life was twice as high among recipients of acyclovir as among vidarabine recipients. With either drug, the outcome was best in patients treated early, (i.e., before they had lapsed into semicoma or coma). These data indicate that intravenous acyclovir is now the treatment of choice for HSE.

The safety and ease of administration of acyclovir and the importance of early treatment have led some physicians to treat patients on the basis of a presumptive diagnosis of HSE without confirming the diagnosis by brain biopsy. This approach is dangerous because nearly two-thirds of patients begun on therapy on the basis of a presumptive diagnosis of HSE prove on brain biopsy not to have this disease, and nearly one-third of these biopsy-negative patients have an alternative diagnosis revealed by the brain biopsy that requires another form of therapy. The morbidity and mortality resulting from failure to recognize and treat other treatable diseases are far greater than the morbidity and mortality of brain biopsy. Acyclovir treatment may be initiated prior to brain biopsy, but this crucial diagnostic procedure should not be delayed.

Neonatal Herpes. Like HSE, neonatal herpes is a disease with high morbidity and mortality. Efficacy has already been demonstrated for vidarabine (see below), and a trial comparing intravenous acyclovir with vidarabine is nearing completion.

Mucocutaneous Herpes Simplex in Immunocompromised Hosts. In immunocompromised hosts, mucocutaneous HSV infections are characterized by persistent progressive lesions and prolonged virus replication. Several controlled trials have demonstrated that intravenous acyclovir (5 mg per kilogram or 250 mg per square meter each 8 hours for 7 days) markedly reduces the duration of virus shedding, decreases pain, and accelerates healing of mucocutaneous HSV infections in organ allograft recipients and other immunocompromised patients. Uncontrolled trials indicate that oral acyclovir

(200 mg five times daily) is also effective. Topical acyclovir (5% acyclovir in polyethylene glycol ointment administered six times daily) has been shown to accelerate the healing of cutaneous lesions in immunocompromised patients with mucocutaneous HSV-1 infections when the lesions are accessible to therapy.

Prophylactic administration of intravenous acyclovir (250 mg per square meter each 8 hours beginning before immunosuppressive therapy) has been shown to prevent reactivation of latent HSV infections in seropostive patients undergoing bone marrow transplantation and remission induction chemotherapy for acute leukemia. Comparable results have been obtained with oral acyclovir (200 mg every 6 hours). Unfortunately, prophylaxis with acyclovir does not eliminate latent HSV infection, and the majority of these patients develop symptomatic HSV infections after acyclovir is stopped.

Genital Herpes. Primary genital herpes is usually more severe than recurrent infection; most patients experience fever, headache, malaise and myalgia, new lesions continue to appear for a week or more, virus shedding continues well into the second week, and complete healing may take several weeks. In patients with first episodes of genital herpes severe enough to warrant hospitalization, intravenous acyclovir (5 mg per kilogram every 8 hours for 5 days) has been shown to reduce the duration of virus shedding, new vesicle formation, local and constitutional symptoms, and time of healing when compared with placebo. Oral acyclovir (200 mg five times daily for 10 days) was similarly effective in outpatients with primary genital herpes. Topical acyclovir (5% acyclovir in polyethylene glycol ointment applied four times daily for 7 days) reduces the duration of virus shedding and shortens the clinical course of local disease in patients with primary genital herpes. However, in contrast to oral and intravenous acyclovir, topical acyclovir does not decrease formation of new lesions or reduce the duration of dysuria, vaginal discharge, or constitutional symptoms. Oral acyclovir is the treatment of choice for most patients with primary genital HSV infections.

Oral and topical acyclovir have been evaluated by means of double-blind, placebo-controlled studies for the treatment of recurrent genital herpes, a self-limited disease of variable but generally mild severity in immunologically normal adults. Therapy with oral acyclovir (200 mg five times daily for 5 days) is associated with statistically significant decreases in the duration of virus shedding, new lesion formation, and time to healing, especially when treatment is begun early. Actual clinical benefits are modest in most patients because of the short duration of the illness even without treatment. Oral acyclovir is useful in some patients whose episodes of recurrent genital herpes are particularly severe or frequent, especially when prodromal symptoms permit treatment to be initiated before the development of vesicular lesions. However, the expense, potential adverse effects, and possible selection and transmission of acyclovir-resistant HSV mutants should discourage the indiscriminate use of oral acyclovir. Topical acyclovir offers no significant clinical benefit to normal hosts with recurrent genital herpes.

Daily prophylactic administration of oral acyclovir (200 mg three to five times daily) to immunocompetent patients with frequently recurring genital herpes has been shown to markedly reduce the frequency and severity of recurrences. Once the drug is stopped, however, recurrences resume, and there is some suggestion that the first recurrence following a period of acyclovir suppression may occur more quickly and be somewhat more severe than that in placebo recipients.

Neuronal HSV latency appears to be established early in the course of primary HSV infections, probably before the onset of symptoms. Once established, latent HSV infection is not abolished by prolonged treatment with intravenous or oral acyclovir. Thus, treatment of primary or recurrent episodes of genital herpes does not appear to affect the rate of subsequent recurrences. Genital herpes invariably recurs when treatment is stopped, even after prolonged and successful suppression with daily acyclovir. Chronic administration of acyclovir has also been associated with the emergence of acyclovir-resistant mutants of HSV. The clinical significance of these mutants, many of which may have reduced virulence, remains to be determined.

Herpes Labialis. Controlled trials of topical acyclovir (either 5% or 10% acyclovir in polyethylene glycol ointment) have failed to demonstrate any clinical benefit for normal hosts with recurrent herpes labialis.

Ocular HSV Infections. Topical acyclovir (3% ophthalmic ointment) is probably the most effective treatment for primary keratoconjunctivitis and recurrent epithelial keratitis caused by HSV. Deep infections, such as stromal disease or uveitis, respond poorly to topical acyclovir or any other topical antiviral agent. Acyclovir ointment is well tolerated. A small proportion of patients develop punctate keratopathy, a problem that also occurs in patients treated with other topical antiviral agents. The ophthalmic preparation of acyclovir is not available in the United States.

Other HSV Infections. Eczema herpeticum, HSV-infected burns, herpetic whitlow, and complications of primary oropharyngeal or genital HSV infections that appear to involve continued viral replication (e.g., cutaneous dissemination, HSV meningitis, sacral radiculopathy) should probably be treated with intravenous (5 mg per kilogram or 250 mg per square meter every 8 hours) or oral (200 mg five times daily) acyclovir for 5 to 10 days. This recommendation is not based upon the results of placebo-controlled clinical trials (which have yet to be carried out), but represents the authors' opinion.

Varicella-Zoster Virus Infections

Varicella. Though generally benign in normal children, varicella may be severe and life-threatening in immunocompromised children and adults. Intravenous acyclovir (500 mg per square meter each 8 hours for 7 days) has been shown to markedly reduce the frequency of visceral complications in immunocompromised children with varicella. Vidarabine is also effective in this setting (see below). Until the results of studies directly comparing the two agents are available, we prefer to use acyclovir because of its lower toxicity and ease of administration.

Herpes Zoster (Shingles). A randomized, double-blind, placebo-controlled clinical trial has demonstrated that intravenous acyclovir (500 mg per square meter each 8 hours for 7 days) shortens the period of virus shedding, decreases acute pain, and reduces the incidence of visceral and progressive cutaneous dissemination in immunocompromised patients with acute herpes zoster. These results are similar to those obtained with intravenous vidarabine (see below) and a direct comparison of the two drugs is currently underway. Until results are available, we prefer to use acyclovir because of its lower toxicity and ease of administration.

In normal hosts with herpes zoster, intravenous acyclovir (either 5 mg per kilogram or 500 mg per square meter each 8 hours for 5 days), if administered within 72 to 96 hours of onset, has been shown to shorten the period of virus shedding and new vesicle formation, accelerate healing, and decrease acute pain. However, there was no effect upon the incidence of postherpetic neuralgia, the most troublesome complication of herpes zoster in the normal host. Thus, in uncomplicated herpes zoster in normal hosts, the inconvenience and expense of intravenous acyclovir treatment appear to outweigh its clinical benefits. A placebo-controlled trial of high-dose oral acyclovir, with and without prednisone, is currently underway in elderly patients with herpes zoster.

Other Herpesviruses

Even at doses high enough to cause some bone marrow and neurologic toxicity, intravenous acyclovir has shown no clinical benefit in immunocompromised patients with cytomegalovirus (CMV) infections.

Intravenous acyclovir has been administered to patients with a variety of Epstein-Barr virus (EBV) associated diseases. Despite transient suppression of EBV shedding, intravenous acyclovir has not been observed to alter significantly the clinical course of the disease in patients with severe infectious mononucleosis. There have been anecdotal reports of transient remissions following treatment with acyclovir in immunocompromised patients with EBV-associated lymphoproliferative disorders, including EBV-associated B-cell lymphomas. However, beneficial effects have generally been transient and their relationship to acyclovir therapy unproven, and other similar patients treated with acyclovir have failed to respond. Controlled trials of acyclovir in normal hosts with infectious mononucleosis are currently underway.

Vidarabine (9-β-D-arabinofuranosyladenine, adenine arabinoside, ara-A)

Vidarabine (Vira-A), an analogue of adenine deoxyriboside, was the first drug licensed by the FDA for systemic treatment of herpesvirus infections. It is available in the United States as an intravenous preparation and as a 3 percent ophthalmic ointment. Its mechanism of action is not completely understood, but it is phosphorylated by cellular enzymes to vidarabine triphosphate, which competitively inhibits herpesvirus DNA polymerase to a greater extent than cellular DNA polymerases. It also acts as a chain terminator and is incorporated into both viral and cellular DNA. Vidarabine inhibits the in vitro replication of HSV-1, HSV-2, VZV, and EBV, but has variable activity against CMV. Vidarabine's water solubility is low (0.45 mg per milliliter at 25 °C), and thus it must be administered in dilute solutions by slow intravenous infusion. The large volumes of fluid required may complicate treatment of patients who ordinarily require fluid restriction or who have herpes simplex encephalitis.

Following intravenous administration, vidarabine is rapidly deaminated to hypoxanthine arabinoside (ara-Hx), which has only 2 to 3 percent of the antiviral activity of vidarabine. Approximately one-half of the total daily dose of vidarabine is excreted in the urine as ara-Hx and 1 to 3 percent as vidarabine. Dosage adjustment is necessary in renal failure. Dose-related gastrointestinal toxicity is common, manifested by anorexia, nausea, vomiting, and diarrhea and/or weight loss. High doses may be associated with megaloblastic changes in the bone marrow and sometimes with anemia, leukopenia, or thrombocytopenia. Thrombophlebitis at the infusion site, the syndrome of inappropriate secretion of antidiuretic hormone, and rash have also been reported. Tremor, myoclonus, ataxia, alterations in mental status, pain syndromes, and, rarely, seizures and coma have been reported during vidarabine therapy and occur more frequently in the presence of preexisting renal or hepatic insufficieny or with concomitant administration of interferon or, possibly, allopurinol. Vidarabine is oncogenic, mutagenic, and teratogenic in some experiental systems, and its systemic use should be reserved for the treatment of serious infections.

A number of randomized, double-blind, placebo-controlled studies have documented the therapeutic efficacy of vidarabine in severe HSV and VZV infections. In such a study, intravenous vidarabine (15 mg per kilogram per day for 10 days) was shown to decrease mortality in patients with biopsy-proven herpes simplex encephalitis from 70 percent in placebo recipients to 40 percent, with the most favorable outcomes observed in young patients treated early, before the onset of semicoma or coma. At the same dose, intravenous vidarabine reduced the mortality in newborns with disseminated and localized central nervous system HSV infections from 74 to 38 percent. Intravenous acyclovir has now supplanted vidarabine for the treatment of HSE and the two drugs are being compared for treatment of neonatal herpes.

Intravenous vidarabine (10 mg per kilogram per day for 5 days) significantly decreased new vesicle formation, fever, and the incidence of visceral complications in immunocompromised patients with varicella. In immunocompromised patients with herpes zoster, intravenous vidarabine administered within 72 hours of onset of rash reduced new vesicle formation, cutaneous and visceral dissemination, and central nervous system complications. Vidarabine also appeared to reduce the duration of acute pain and postherpetic neuralgia. Intravenous vidarabine and acyclovir are currently being compared in immunocompromised patients with VZV infection.

Intravenous vidarabine, especially when administered in conjunction with interferon, reduces hepatitis B virus replication in patients with chronic active hepatitis B. However, the long-term effect on clinical outcome remains to be determined.

Topical vidarabine (3% ophthalmic ointment) is effective treatment for HSV keratoconjunctivitis and is less allergenic than idoxuridine. Topical vidarabine is of no benefit in the treatment of genital or oral HSV infections.

Idoxuridine (5-iodo-2′-deoxyuridine, IDU, IUdR)

Idoxuridine (Stoxil, Dendrid, Herplex) is an iodinated thymidine analogue that inhibits viral DNA synthesis and is incorporated into both viral and cellular DNA. Idoxuridine was administered intravenously in early attempts to treat HSE, but a randomized, double-blind, placebo-controlled study revealed that the drug was ineffective and, in addition, caused life-threatening hematopoietic toxicity. In the United States, idoxuridine is approved only for the topical treatment of HSV keratitis, and a 0.5 percent ophthalmic ointment is available. Resistance to the antiviral effect of IDU may develop during treatment. Adverse reactions include pruritus, pain, inflammation, and edema of the eye or lids as well as rare allergic reactions.

Trifluridine (5-trifluoromethyl-2-′-deoxyuridine trifluorothymidine)

Trifluridine (Viroptic) is an analogue of deoxythymidine, that also inhibits viral DNA synthesis. Viral thymidine kinase is not necessary for its action, and thus it is active against thymidine kinase–negative strains of HSV that are resistant to acyclovir. Its usefulness as an antiviral agent is limited to the topical treatment of ocular HSV infections because of unacceptable toxicity with systemic administration. It is available as a 1 percent ophthalmic solution. Clinical trials suggest that its efficacy is superior to that of idoxuridine and comparable to that of vidarabine. Patients who have not responded to the other topical antivirals may respond to trifluridine. Adverse reactions include stinging upon instillation, palpebral edema, and, rarely, superficial punctate or epithelial keratopathy and hypersensitivity reactions.

NEW ANTIVIRAL AGENTS

At present, a number of promising new antiviral agents are under investigation. These include bromovinyldeoxyuridine (BVDU), which is highly active against VZV and HSV-1; acyclic nucleosides like 9-(1,3-dihydroxy-2-propoxymethyl) guanine (DHPG), which may be effective in CMV infections; 2-fluoroarabinosylnucleosides (FIAC, FIAU, FMAU), with in vitro activity similar to that of acyclovir; arildone, a phenoxyl diketone with in vitro activity against a variety of DNA and RNA viruses; phosphonoacetic acid and phosphonoformic acid, which inhibit HSV DNA polymerase; benzimidazole derivatives, which inhibit picornavirus replication; and 3′-azido-3′ deoxythymidine, which inhibits the retrovirus responsible for AIDS. Human interferons have already been shown to have therapeutic efficacy in severe human papillomavirus infections, HSV keratitis, respiratory virus infections, varicella and herpes zoster in immunocompromised patients, and chronic hepatitis B virus infections. The therapeutic efficacy of various human interferon preparations (alone or in combination with other antiviral agents) is currently under active investigation in patients with a variety of viral and neoplastic diseases.

USE OF UNPROVEN THERAPIES

Over the years, many forms of therapy have been advocated for various virus infections, especially infections for which no treatment of proven efficacy was readily available. Nowhere is this more obvious than in recurrent genital herpes. Unfortunately, the remarkable variability in the natural history of recurrent genital herpes, as well as most other viral infections, renders completely uninterpretable data from uncontrolled trials and anecdotal case reports. When unproven forms of therapy, such as 2-deoxy-D-glucose, L-lysine, photodynamic inactivation with neutral red or proflavine and light, topical idoxuridine, topical vidarabine, ether, levamisole, BCG vaccine, or multiple smallpox vaccinations have been carefully evaluated with randomized, placebo-controlled clinical trials, they have been found to be ineffective. Many have actually been harmful. Thus, it is imperative that physicians avoid exposing their patients to the hazards and expense of any form of therapy until its safety and efficacy have been demonstrated by means of randomized, placebo-controlled studies involving adequate numbers of proven cases.

ANTIBACTERIAL CHEMOTHERAPY

WILLIAM A. CRAIG, M.D.

The prime objective of antimicrobial chemotherapy is to aid in eradicating invading bacteria by delivering an optimal amount of drug to the focus of infection. The choice of antibacterial agent is dependent not only on the drug's activity against the known or suspected pathogen, but also on its ability to reach and maintain effective concentrations at sites of infection. In 1985, nearly 50 years after the introduction of sulfanilamide and the beginning of the modern era of chemotherapy, we are blessed, or possibly cursed, by the availability of an exceedingly large number of antibacterial agents. Many drugs have only small differences in antibacterial activity and pharmacology. Yet, if one listens to the pharmaceutical industry, these differences are important in drug selection. The authors of other chapters in this book give specific drug and dosage regimens for the various types of infections. The primary purpose of this chapter is to review the general pharmacodynamic and pharmacokinetic principles on which these recommendations are based. The kinetics of antibacterial action, the penetration of drugs to various sites of infection, the impact of different dosage regimens, and the cost of therapy can all be important determinants of antibacterial drug selection.

ANTIBACTERIAL PHARMACODYNAMICS

Pharmacodynamics is concerned with the pharmacologic and toxicologic effects of drugs and their mechanisms of action. The value of a drug as an antibacterial agent is due to its selective toxicity for the infecting bacteria, but not for mammalian cells.

Mechanisms of Action

Antibacterial drugs are often classified according to their mechanism of action, as outlined in Table 1. The beta-lactam antibiotics (penicillins and cephalosporins), vancomycin, bacitracin, and cycloserine inhibit bacterial cell wall synthesis. This inhibition also results in the activation of enzymes that cause lysis of the bacterial cell. Thus, these drugs demonstrate bactericidal activity. The polymyxin drugs (polymyxin B, colistin, and colistimethate) bind to phospholipids in the bacterial cell membrane, leading to increased cellular permeability. This detergent-like disruption of the cell membrane accounts for their bactericidal activity. Unfortunately, the polymyxins also bind to the cytoplasmic membranes of mammalian cells, resulting in a significant incidence of toxicity with systemic use of these drugs. On the other hand, since mammalian cells have no structure analogous to the bacterial cell wall, there is minimal direct toxicity from inhibitors of cell wall synthesis, such as the penicillins and cephalosporins.

A variety of different antibacterial agents inhibit bacterial protein synthesis. Some impair the function of ribosomes, where proteins are assembled, whereas others act earlier in the process by impairing the synthesis or function of the nucleic acids that direct or code for protein synthesis. The drugs that impair ribosomal function can be further divided into two groups. The aminoglycoside antibiotics inhibit protein synthesis irreversibly and exhibit bactericidal activity. In contrast, tetracycline, chloramphenicol, clindamycin, and erythromycin tend to produce reversible inhibition of protein synthesis. These drugs exhibit primarily a bacteriostatic effect except with very high concentrations or when the organism is exquisitely sensitive to the drug. For example, in vivo concentrations of chloramphenicol are bactericidal for most strains of *Hemophilus influenzae* and *Streptococcus pneumoniae*. Sulfonamides interfere with nucleic acid synthesis by inhibiting bacterial folic acid production. This inhibition is rarely complete and these drugs are bacteriostatic. Trimethoprim is more effective in inhibiting folic acid synthesis and tends to be bactericidal, especially when combined with a sulfonamide. Rifampin, nalidixic acid and its derivatives, and metronidazole act directly on nucleic acid synthesis or function and are bactericidal.

TABLE 1 Classification of Antibacterial Agents by Mechanism of Action

Mechanism of Action	*Antibacterial Agents*	*In Vivo Activity*
Impaired cell wall synthesis	Penicillins, cephalosporins, vancomycin, bacitracin, cycloserine	Bactericidal
Cell membrane damage	Polymyxins	Bactericidal
Impaired ribosome function	Aminoglycosides	Bactericidal
	Tetracyclines, chloramphenicol, erythromycin, clindamycin	Bacteriostatic
Impaired nucleic acid synthesis or function	Sulfonamides, trimethoprim	Bacteriostatic or bactericidal
	Rifampin, nalidixic acid, metronidazole	Bactericidal

Whether a drug is bacteriostatic or bactericidal has little importance for many infections. The antimicrobial agent needs only to slow or inhibit the growth of the organism, as the body's host defenses will kill and eliminate the infecting pathogen. However, endocarditis, meningitis, and osteomyelitis are infections that occur in areas of impaired host defense. Bactericidal drugs are required for effective therapy for these infections. Patients with neutropenia or significant defects in neutrophil function should also receive bactericidal drugs.

Knowledge of whether a drug is bactericidal or bacteriostatic can also be useful when using drugs in combination to enhance antibacterial activity. The combination of two bactericidal drugs may produce a more rapid or complete bactericidal effect. Two bacteriostatic drugs (e.g., trimethoprim plus a sulfonamide) can even result in bactericidal activity. However, the combination of a bactericidal with a bacteriostatic drug frequently results only in a bacteriostatic effect. Such combinations should generally be avoided for the treatment of infections in patients or at sites with impaired host defenses where bactericidal activity is more critical.

Quantitation of Antimicrobial Activity

The standard method for quantitating antibacterial activity in vitro is by determining the minimal inhibitory and minimal bactericidal concentrations (MIC and MBC). By definition, the MIC is the lowest concentration of drug that prevents visible bacterial growth over an 18- to 24-hour incubation period. The MBC is the lowest concentration that kills 99.9 percent of the organisms over the same period. In the past, these determinations were too complicated and time consuming to be routinely used in clinical microbiology laboratories. Instead, qualitative methods, such as the Kirby-Bauer disk diffusion test, were used to classify organisms as "susceptible" and "resistant." However, more automated techniques now allow many laboratories to report MIC values routinely. MBC determinations are also more readily performed, but are usually reserved for those infections where bactericidal activity is mandatory.

Although specific MIC and MBC values for different antibacterial agents can facilitate drug selection, they may be insufficient in predicting therapeutic success or failure. It should be appreciated that constant exposure of a relatively small number of bacteria (10^5 to 10^6) to an antibacterial agent in MIC and MBC determinations differs considerably from the in vivo situation in which larger numbers of bacteria are usually exposed to fluctuating levels of drug. Furthermore, the MBC does not express the rate at which bactericidal activity occurs. For some drugs, such as the aminoglycosides, bactericidal activity is rapid and concentration dependent. The higher the aminoglycoside level, the faster the rate of killing. On the other hand, bacterial killing with penicillins and cephalosporins is slower, with little dependence on the concentration of drug. Thus, the extent of killing with beta-lactams is dependent more on the duration of exposure. In addition, sub-MIC concentrations of many antibacterial agents can alter bacterial morphology and slow the rate of growth. These sub-MIC effects could delay the regrowth of organisms when serum and tissue levels decrease below the MIC.

Another potentially important pharmacodynamic parameter not assessed by MIC and MBC determinations is the postantibiotic effect (PAE). This term refers to a persistent suppression of bacterial growth after limited exposure to an antimicrobial. This phenomenon has been observed since the early years of penicillin. It is a feature of all antibacterial agents with gram-positive cocci and for inhibitors of protein and nucleic acid synthesis with gram-negative bacilli. In contrast, very short or no PAEs are observed with beta-lactam antibiotics with gram-negative bacilli. Like sub-MIC effects, the PAE prevents regrowth of organisms when drug levels at foci of infection decrease below the MIC.

As a general rule, for an antibacterial agent to be effective, it should produce a concentration at the site of infection that exceeds the MIC or MBC for at least several hours during each dosage interval. However, MIC and MBC testing in broth does not reflect the inhibitory effects of drug binding to serum and tissue proteins. For example, the MIC of dicloxacillin against staphylococci is about 0.1 μg per milliliter in broth, but 3 to 5 μg per milliliter in human serum, as 97 percent of the drug is bound to serum proteins. Thus, proper interpretation of an MIC requires knowledge of the expected concentration of free, unbound drug at the site of infection. For most infections it is not known to what extent drug levels need to exceed the MIC and for what period. Maximal killing by antibacterial agents in cerebrospinal fluid requires levels that are 10 to 20 times the MBC. Studies in cancer patients with gram-negative bacteremia have shown that peak serum concentrations that remain bactericidal following at least an eight-fold dilution in 50 percent serum (this takes into consideration the effect of protein binding) are associated with improved outcome. However, it is not clear from these studies if the peak level is the critical parameter or whether a high peak level simply reflects the persistence of inhibitory or bactericidal levels for a longer portion of the dosage interval. The relationship of pharmacokinetic parameters, such as peak level and the duration of time levels exceed the MIC or MBC, to therapeutic efficacy will be discussed in a later section on dosing regimens.

ANTIBACTERIAL PHARMACOKINETICS

Pharmacokinetics deals with the absorption, distribution, metabolism, and excretion of antibacterial agents and their metabolites. These factors, in combination with the dosage regimen, determine the time course of drug concentrations in serum and tissues. Of primary concern with antibacterial chemotherapy is the time course of drug concentrations at the site of infection.

Absorption

In order for a drug to have adequate oral absorption, it must initially dissolve in the gastrointestinal secretions, resist degradation by gastric acid, and be sufficiently lipid-soluble to diffuse passively across the lipid barrier of the gastrointestinal epithelium. Several antibacterial agents such as amoxicillin, oral cephalosporins, trimethoprim, sulfamethoxazole, chloramphenicol, metronidazole, clindamycin, doxycycline, minocycline, and rifampin have relatively complete absorption. The majority of these drugs are quite lipid soluble. Amoxicillin and the oral cephalosporins are better absorbed than one would expect on the basis of their lipid solubility, and some studies suggest active transport of these drugs across the gastrointestinal epithelium. To enhance the absorption of other drugs, pharmaceutical companies have made ester derivatives (e.g., bacampicillin, indonyl carbenicillin, erythromycin estolate), which are more lipid soluble and resistant to acid degradation. These drugs are then de-esterified in tissues and serum to yield the parent drug. Although food tends to decrease the absorption of most antibacterial drugs, it enhances the absorption of most ester derivatives. Thus, one can improve the absorption of these drugs by giving them with meals. The systemic bioavailability of rifampin after oral dosing can be improved by giving a large, single daily dose. Lower doses at more frequent intervals do not surpass the ability of the liver to extract rifampin from the portal circulation (i.e., first-pass effect).

The high oral bioavailability of certain antibacterial agents makes oral therapy an acceptable alternative to parenteral therapy for certain moderately severe infections. For example, oral therapy of acute staphylococcal osteomyelitis in children is highly effective, provided that therapy is appropriately monitored. When treating more significant infections with oral therapy, one should ensure that the patient has normal gastrointestinal function and choose the best-absorbed drug among different analogues. For example, dicloxacillin and cloxacillin are better absorbed than are oxacillin and nafcillin, and amoxicillin and bacampicillin are better absorbed than is ampicillin.

Distribution

The ability of an antibacterial agent to penetrate into tissues and body fluids is dependent on many physiochemical and pharmacologic properties. Serum protein binding appears to be one of the important determinants since only unbound drug molecules can readily pass through capillary pores into tissue fluids. Highly bound drugs would tend to remain within the intravascular compartment, giving rise to high serum levels but lower tissue levels. A variety of human studies, by use of implanted subcutaneous threads, skin-blister fluid, and wound exudates, documented the inhibitory effect of protein binding on tissue penetration. However, a major decrease in tissue concentrations is not observed at binding values less than 80 percent.

The actual drug concentration obtained in various tissues and body fluids is dependent on the ratio of the diffusing capillary surface area to the volume of fluid. In most tissues, the surface area of the capillaries is quite large in relationship to the small volume of interstitial fluid. Antibacterial drug concentrations at these sites show little lag and closely approximate free drug levels in serum. On the other hand, large inflammatory collections of pleural, peritoneal, or synovial fluids, as well as abscesses, have a smaller diffusing area relative to the volume of fluid. Changes in drug levels at these sites lag behind those in serum. Peak levels are generally lower and occur later than those in serum. Furthermore, drug elimination from these foci is somewhat slower, resulting in higher concentrations in the fluids than in serum towards the end of a dosing interval. However, the mean level and area under the concentration-verus-time curve of free drug in these tissue sites would be relatively similar to those in serum. Since standard doses of highly protein-bound antibacterial drugs provide serum concentrations of free drug in excess of the MIC of susceptible organisms, it is not surprising that highly bound antibacterials are just as clinically effective as lowly bound drugs.

Penetration of antimicrobials into tissues lacking a porous capillary bed, such as the central nervous system and ocular vitreous humor, is much more dependent on the lipid solubility of the drug than on its pharmacokinetics in serum. Active transport systems at these sites can further reduce the concentration of drugs, especially for beta-lactam antibiotics. The most important factor for increasing antibacterial concentrations in cerebrospinal fluid is inflammation. For drugs such as ampicillin and penicillin G, inflammation not only enhances the influx of drug into CSF, but also reduces the active transport of drug from the CSF. As the inflammation resolves, the degree of drug penetration into the CSF will decrease. Thus, intravenous administration of full doses should continue for the entire period of therapy in order to prevent relapse of the infection. Antibacterial drugs can be divided into three groups, as shown in Table 2: those that penetrate the normal meninges, those that only achieve therapeutic levels in the presence of inflammation, and those that provide marginal or inadequate levels in the CSF. Use of some marginal drugs, especially in adults, may require direct administration into the CSF.

Elimination

Antibacterial agents and their metabolites are eliminated from the body in urine or bile. A useful way of grouping drugs is according to the major site of clearance of the parent compound. Drugs with predominant hepatic clearance include antimicrobials excreted primarily in bile or extensively metabolized by the liver even though the metabolites may be excreted in urine. Drugs with predominant renal clearance are excreted primarily unchanged in the urine. Some drugs are eliminated significantly by both mechanisms. Table 3 provides a classification of antibacterial agents according to their major routes of elimination. Such a grouping is useful in determining whether a drug will need dosage modification in the presence of renal or hepatic dysfunction. Drugs with predominant hepatic elimination do not require dosage modification in renal disease unless metabolites excreted in the urine are toxic. Although the dosage of these drugs should be reduced in severe liver disease, there is no simple test for the quantitation of hepatic function as there is for renal function. Since most studies have shown a doubling of the half-life of these drugs in patients with severe hepatic dysfunction, dosage may only need to be reduced 50 percent.

TABLE 2 Antibacterial Penetration into Cerebrospinal Fluid

Category	*Antibacterial Agent*	
Adequate penetration with normal meninges	Chloramphenicol Doxycycline Metronidazole Minocycline	Rifampin Sulfonamides Trimethoprim
Therapeutic levels achieved with inflamed meninges	Ampicillin Azlocillin Carbenicillin Cefotaxime Ceftazidime Ceftizoxime Ceftriaxone Cefuroxime	Methicillin Mezlocillin Moxalactam Nafcillin Penicillin G Piperacillin Ticarcillin
Marginal or inadequate penetration with inflamed meninges	Aminoglycosides* First-generation cephalosporins Cefamandole Cefonicid Cefoperazone	Ceforanide Cefoxitin Clindamycin Erythromycin Vancomycin*

* Intrathecal administration may be necessary.

TABLE 3 Major Route of Antibacterial Drug Elimination

Hepatic	Chloramphenicol Clindamycin Erythromycin	Minocycline Rifampin
Dual (renal and hepatic)	Azlocillin Mezlocillin Piperacillin Sulfonamides Trimethoprim Cefoperazone	Ceftriaxone Cloxacillin Dicloxacillin Doxycycline Nafcillin Oxacillin
Renal	Aminoglycosides Ampicillin Carbenicillin First- and second-generation cephalosporins Cefotaxime Ceftazidime	Ceftizoxime Methicillin Moxalactam Polymyxin Tetracycline Ticarcillin Vancomycin

Drugs with predominant renal elimination require modification in renal disease, but not in the presence of hepatic dysfunction. There are numerous formulas, tables, nomograms, and computer programs that one can use to facilitate dosage adjustment in renal impairment. Cefotaxime, cephalothin, and cephapirin require less dosage modification than other renally excreted cephalosporins because approximately half of the drug is metabolized to a less active desacetyl derivative. Dosage modification with drugs with dual mechanisms of elimination is dependent on which route is predominant. In Table 3, the first column of drugs with dual elimination have greater renal elimination and do require some dosage modification in severe renal impairment. The second column of drugs have equal or greater hepatic clearance and require no dosage modification in renal disease. None of these drugs requires significant dosage modification in hepatic impairment. Virtually all antibacterial drugs require dosage adjustment in the presence of combined hepatic and renal dysfunction.

Excretion of drugs into the urine occurs by either glomerular filtration or tubular secretion. Penicillins and most of the older cephalosporins are eliminated predominantly by tubular secretion. However, several of the new third-generation cephalosporins, such as cefoperazone, ceftazidime, ceftriaxone, and moxalactam, are excreted primarily by glomerular filtration. The absence of a probenecid effect supports the relative lack of tubular secretion. It is well known that protein binding reduces the rate of drug elimination by glomerular filtration. With the exception of cefoperazone, which is eliminated primarily in bile, the half-life of these cephalosporins is directly related to the degree of protein binding. This varies from 1.5 hours for ceftazidime (low binding) to 8 hours for ceftriaxone (high binding). If ceftriaxone did not have high protein binding, its filtration clearance would increase and the half-life would start to approach that of ceftazidime. By slowing elimination of primarily filtered drugs, protein binding can have a positive effect on drug distribution by producing higher and more sustained serum concentrations.

The biliary excretion of unchanged drug is minimal for most antimicrobials. However, it does not require much drug to be eliminated in the bile to provide adequate biliary concentrations. For example, 1 percent of a 1-g dose of drug in 500 ml of bile would provide a mean biliary concentration of 20 μg per milliliter. However, the excretion of antibacterial drugs into bile is markedly reduced by biliary tract disease. The biliary excretion of several new beta-lactam antibiotics is quite high. As much as 75 percent of cefoperazone, 45 percent of ceftriaxone, and 30 percent of azlocillin, mezlocillin, and piperacillin is eliminated in the bile. The mechanism of enhanced biliary excretion of these drugs is not known, but may be related to molecular weight. Cefoperazone has the highest molecular weight among cephalosporins and is predominantly eliminated in bile. Azlocillin, mezlocillin, and piperacillin have the highest molecular weights among the penicillins. Although enhanced biliary excretion can provide high bile levels even in the presence of hepatic dysfunction, there are currently no data that demonstrate that biliary concentrations are an important determinant of clinical outcome in biliary tract infections.

DOSAGE REGIMENS

Most current dosage regimens for antibacterial agents are empiric and have not been tested in dose-response clinical trials. Dosage schedules are usually designed by matching a drug's MICs against commonly encountered bacteria with its pharmacokinetic profile in serum, obtained primarily in normal volunteers. The dose and dosing interval chosen is designed to maintain serum concentrations above the MIC of most organisms for a major portion of the dosage interval. Although this approach has been successful for most infections, it does not necessarily mean that these "best guess" regimens are optimal ones.

Penicillins and Cephalosporins

The current available information, based on in vitro and animal studies and even some human trials, suggests that the duration during which serum levels exceed the MIC or MBC is an important pharmacokinetic parameter for beta-lactam antibiotics. As stated earlier, bactericidal activity of these drugs exhibits little dependence on concentration, but is related primarily to the duration of exposure. Furthermore, these drugs do not exhibit significant postantibiotic effects with gram-negative bacilli. It would seem desirable to continually maintain inhibitory or killing concentrations at foci of infection with these drugs. As the penicillins and older cephalosporins have relatively rapid elimination half-lives, a dosing regimen providing continuous exposure would require frequent doses every 4 to 6 hours or continuous intravenous infusion. Several newer cephalosporins have significantly longer half-lives as well as much lower MICs. The longer dosage intervals recommended for these drugs, such as once daily dosing for ceftriaxone and cefonicid and twice daily dosing for cefoperazone and moxalactam, are rational since continuous exposure would still occur with these drugs at the wider dosing intervals. For treatment of many infections, continuous exposure may not be required because the postantibiotic effect prevents regrowth of the organism for several hours when inhibitory concentrations are not present. Studies have also shown that organisms in the postantibiotic phase are more susceptible to the antibacterial activity of human neutrophils.

Aminoglycosides

Aminoglycosides, on the other hand, exhibit concentration-dependent killing and produce long periods of postantibiotic suppression of bacterial growth with gram-negative bacilli. Peak level or area under the concentration-versus-time curve rather than the duration of time that serum levels exceed the MIC appears to be the important pharmacokinetic parameter for these drugs. Clinical trials have demonstrated that peak aminoglycoside levels greater than 5 μg per milliliter for gentamicin and tobramycin and greater than 20 μg per milliliter for amikacin are associated with less mortality in gram-negative bacillary bacteremia. Even higher peak levels, 6–8 μg per milliliter for gentamicin and tobramycin and 24–28 μg per milliliter for amikacin, appear to enhance clinical efficacy in gram-negative bacillary pneumonia. Intermittent exposure of pathogens at infected foci should be possible with the aminoglycosides since the long postantibiotic effect would prevent regrowth after serum and tissue levels decrease below the MIC. In animal infection models, 12 hourly or even once daily dosing of the same total amount of aminoglycoside is as effective, or possibly more so, than regimens that continuously maintain inhibitory concentrations. Human studies have also failed to show any benefit of continuous infusion of aminoglycosides over the 6 and 8 hourly regimens currently used to treat serious infections. Would 12 or 24 hourly dosing of aminoglycosides be as effective in humans as in animals? One might anticipate so since half-lives of these drugs are considerably longer in humans than in animals. Currently available human data have shown comparable efficacy for 8 and 12 hourly dosing regimens. Clinical trials of once daily dosing are just underway.

One of the advantages of more intermittent administration of large doses of an antimicrobial is that effective concentrations at sites of infection are reached more quickly than with more continuous dosing. A potential disadvantage with the aminoglycosides is that 12 or 24 hourly administration of large doses would produce very high peak levels that might induce toxicity. However, studies in animals have shown that intermittent exposure to very high aminoglycoside levels is less nephrotoxic and possibly less ototoxic than continuous exposure to therapeutic concentrations. Thus, this author currently sees no value for continuous administration of aminoglycosides and would use 8 hourly dosing regimens in serious infections and 12 hourly dosing regimens in moderately severe infections.

Monitoring Antibiotic Activity

Determinations of peak aminoglycoside levels are necessary to ensure effective concentrations as the pharmacokinetics of these drugs exhibits significant individual variation. Multiple serum-level determinations allow for more pharmacokinetic individualization of aminoglycoside dosing, and there are some data to suggest that this process will result in greater efficacy as well as lower toxicity. Peak serum bactericidal activity testing (Schlicter test) has been recommended by some investigators for monitoring therapy of endocarditis, osteomyelitis, and serious gram-negative infections. The goal has been to obtain a titer of at least 1:8. However, there are no data to suggest that this test provides more information with single-agent therapy than does a drug level. Penicillin and cephalosporin serum concentrations are not routinely available, but as stated previously, higher levels above the MBC are not associated with significantly faster rates of kill. The primary value of the peak bactericidal activity test with beta-lactam usage is that a titer of at least 1:8 signifies that concentrations above the MIC or MBC will be maintained for most of the dosing interval.

COMBINATION THERAPY

As stated previously, a primary reason for using drugs in combination is to enhance antimicrobial activity. Although there is a large literature on the in vitro synergy of antibacterials, in only a few situations have drug combinations been associated with greater efficacy in humans. The major examples are penicillin plus an aminoglycoside for enterococcal endocarditis and an antipseudomonal penicillin plus an aminoglycoside for pseudomonas infections in neutropenic patients. Both of these examples represent sites or patients with impaired host defenses.

Antibacterial combination are also used to treat mixed infections (e.g., intra-abdominal infections due to both aerobes and anaerobes), to broaden coverage of infections with unknown etiology, and to prevent the emergence of resistant organisms. Tuberculosis is the primary infection where drug combinations have been shown to prevent the emergence of resistant organisms. However, the emergence of resistant bacteria has also been documented during treatment of gram-negative bacillary infections with a variety of antibacterials. This phenomenon is commoner when beta-lactams are used alone to treat infections due to *Enterobacter* and *Serratia* species and *Pseudomonas aeruginosa*. Studies in animals and a few in humans suggest that the concomitant use of an aminoglycoside can reduce the emergence of resistant strains. It is possible that much of the clinical synergy for the combinations of a beta-lactam and an aminoglycoside in pseudomonas infections may be due to the prevention of the emergence of resistance.

fections may be due to the prevention of the emergence of resistance.

COST OF ANTIBACTERIAL CHEMOTHERAPY

With the current climate of cost containment and the financing of health care by fixed payments and prospective reimbursement schemes, the cost of antibacterial chemotherapy has become an increasingly important determinant of drug selection. With the large number of antibacterials being marketed today, frequently a number of drugs with equivalent efficacy could be used to treat the same infection. The term ''drug of choice'' has become at a minimum the ''antibacterial class of choice.'' Knowledge of the cost of different antibacterial agents would enable the physician to select the most cost-effective agent.

Hospital charges for intravenous antibacterials are inconsistently calculated and vary enormously. While some hospitals use actual drug acquisition costs to calculate patient charges, others use a wholesale price guide, which often overestimates the drug cost. Many hospitals add a markup and/or a dispensing fee for each dose. Furthermore, most hospitals add a preparation charge for each piggyback infusion setup. In a recent nationwide survey of hospital charges for intravenous antibacterial agents, the acquisition drug cost to the pharmacy accounted for only one-fourth to one-third of the charge to the patient. In this same study, the mean preparation charge for the infusion setup was approximately (U.S.) $9. Thus, a drug that can be administered only once daily would cost $27 less to the patient per day than one that had to be given four times daily. Therefore, many of the newer cephalosporins that have longer half-lives may provide significant savings over equivalent cephalosporins and penicillins because of fewer drug preparation charges. With combination drug therapy, admixing compatible drugs (e.g., clindamycin and an aminoglycoside) in the same piggyback setup should halve preparation charges.

Finally, home or outpatient intravenous therapy for patients requiring prolonged treatment has been shown to be efficacious, well tolerated and cost-effective. This form of therapy has predominantly been used in patients with osteomyelitis and soft tissue infections. Oral therapy of moderately severe infections provides another means of reducing cost, but this should only be used when clinical trials have shown it to have equal efficacy to parenteral treatment.

ANTIFUNGAL CHEMOTHERAPY

RICHARD D. DIAMOND, M.D.

Because of the nature of the organisms involved, several important differences exist between antibacterial and antifungal chemotherapy. Perhaps the major determining factor in this regard is the fact that fungi, like mammalian cells, are eukaryotic. Thus, though diverse groups of antibiotics exploit well-characterized structural and metabolic differences between prokaryotic bacterial cells and mammalian cells, far fewer agents are available that act with the necessary selectivity against fungal cells. Compared with the broad range of generally safe and effective antibacterial drugs in common use, available antifungal agents are relatively fewer in number, less dramatically effective, and more often require toleration of significant adverse effects. However, with increased recognition of the clinical significance of mycoses in recent years, the choice of potentially effective antifungal agents has begun to widen, and this trend is likely to continue.

CURRENTLY AVAILABLE ANTIFUNGAL AGENTS

Fungal cell walls differ considerably from those of bacteria, so that major antibacterial antibiotics that bind to cell-wall constituents and interfere with cell-wall synthesis lack antifungal activity. Although it seems reasonable that unique features of fungal cell walls (e.g., chitin, carbohydrates such as glucans or mannans, and glycoproteins) might be useful targets of antifungal drugs, clinically effective agents employing such mechanisms are yet to be defined. Rather, to act selectively against mycoses, effective antifungal agents thus far have exploited other differences between fungi and host cells. In particular, these targets of action include cell-membrane sterols as well as enzymes that control cellular metabolic activity and nucleic acid synthesis. The mechanisms of action of the major classes of antifungal drugs and their range of activities are summarized in Table 1. Forms of these (and some other) drugs currently available for topical antifungal therapy are listed in Table 2. Agents for the treatment of systemic mycoses are noted in Table 3.

COMBINATIONS OF AGENTS

Though combination drug therapy of systemic mycoses is a reasonable concept, efficacy has been established only for the use of amphotericin B with flucytosine for cryptococcal meningitis. The rationale for this combination is that amphotericin B prevents emergence of resistance to flucytosine (an all-too-common event when flucytosine is used alone), whereas flucytosine permits the use of a lower (and, therefore, less toxic) dose of amphotericin B (0.3 instead of 0.4 to 0.6 mg per kilogram per day). By analogy, largely based on in vitro data, combined amphotericin B-flucytosine therapy has been used

TABLE 1 Currently Marketed Antifungal Agents (1985)

Class of Drug	Forms Sold in United States	Routes of Administration	Proposed Mechanism of Action	General Spectrum of Activity: Dermatophytes	General Spectrum of Activity: Systemic Mycoses
Polyenes	Amphotericin B Nystatin Pimaricin	IV, topical Topical Topical (ophthalmic)	Membrane: preferential binding to fungal sterols (ergosterol) causing increased permeability	No	Most (not *Pseudo-allescheria boydii*)
Imidazoles (*N*-substituted imidazoles and amino-triazoles)	Miconazole Ketoconazole Clotrimazole Econazole Ticonazole	IV, topical Oral Topical Topical Topical	Membrane: interference with synthesis of ergosterol by blockade of demethylation of lanosterol to ergosterol; enzyme and oxidative metabolism inhibition	Yes	In vitro activity against most (limited or none against *Aspergillus* species and fungi causing mucomycosis)
Nucleic acid analogues	5-Fluorocytosine (flucytosine)	Oral	Interference with RNA and DNA synthesis	No	Only *Candida, Cryptococcus, Torulopsis,* and fungi causing chromomycosis
Hydroxypyridones	Cyclopirox	Topical	Interference with fungal energy metabolism	Yes	Mainly *Candida*
Iodides	Saturated (1 g/ml) potassium iodide	Oral	Unknown (organisms grow in vitro in drug solutions	No	Lymphocutaneous sporotrichosis only
Other antibiotics	Griseofulvin	Oral	Interference with cell division	Yes	No

for other mycoses including meningeal cryptococcosis, candidiasis, torulopsosis, and invasive aspergillosis (where higher than usual doses of amphotericin B are used). Thus far, insufficient clinical evidence is available to support the use of other combinations of systemic antifungal drugs. For some potential combinations (e.g., amphotericin B and imidazoles), available data from in vitro and animal experiments have been conflicting as to whether synergistic, additive, neutral, or antagonistic effects occur. Efficacy and toxicity of imidazoles combined with flucytosine are similarly uncertain.

GENERAL GUIDELINES IN THE USE OF SYSTEMIC ANTIFUNGAL DRUGS

The major adverse effects of antifungal agents are summarized in Table 4. Acute toxic effects to amphotericin B generally are manageable and need not prevent the use of the drug in situations where it may be lifesaving. Acute nephrotoxicity due to amphotericin B usually is reversible after completion of therapy. Loading of salt-depleted patients with saline may decrease amphotericin B-induced renal failure. Permanent nephrotoxicity is related to total dose of the drug used (e.g., 75% of patients receiving over 4 g total dose of amphotericin B have residual decreased creatinine clearances). Among antimicrobial agents, amphotericin B is unique in that it causes renal failure yet does not accumulate in blood at increased levels as renal function declines. Thus, to maintain therapeutic levels of amphotericin B, some acute nephrotoxicity (e.g., creatinine rises in serum to 3.0 to 3.5 mg per deciliter) must be tolerated. Other nephrotoxic agents must be used concomitantly with extreme caution, and particular care must be taken in monitoring levels of other drugs that, unlike amphotericin B, do accumulate during renal failure. This is especially true when flucytosine and amphotericin B are used in combination, as serious flucytosine adverse effects (marrow suppression and colitis) appear to be commoner with high (>100 μg/ml) peak blood levels of flucytosine. Figure 1 summarizes procedures for use of amphotericin B. Imidazoles, in general, are less toxic than amphotericin B. However, ketoconazole has been associated with severe and even fatal "side" effects (e.g., hepatitis, perhaps as often as 1:10,000 cases and hormonal effects that may lead to azoospermia and sterility, possibly persisting even after discontinuation of the drug). Like amphotericin B, neither miconazole nor ketoconazole is excreted significantly by the kidneys, and does not require dose modification in renal failure.

TABLE 2 Topical Antifungal Drugs Available for the Treatment of Cutaneous Mycoses

Type of Organism	Drug	Formulation
Dermatophytes and *Candida*	Clotrimazole	Cream, solution, oral and vaginal troches
	Miconazole	Cream, lotion
	Econazole	Cream
	Ticonazole	Cream
	Ciclopirox	Cream
Dermatophytes only	Haloprogin	Cream, solution
	Tolnaftate	Cream, solution, powder, aerosol, gel
	Undecylenic acid	Cream, lotion ointment, soap, powder aerosol
Candida only	Nystatin	Cream, ointment, powder
	Amphotericin B	Cream, lotion, ointment

PATTERNS OF INFECTION BY FUNGI

For general purposes, including projection of likely outcomes and requirements for specific therapeutic mo-

TABLE 3 Systemic Antifungal Agents

Drug	*Route of Administration*	*Daily Dose*	*General Indications/Adverse Effects*
Amphotericin B	IV	0.3–0.6 (up to 1.0–1.5) mg/kg*	Most systemic mycoses; Coccidioidal meningitis
	intrathecal	0.5 mg (thrice weekly or more)†	
Flucytosine	PO	150 mg/kg in divided doses q6h (decreased with low creatinine clearance)	Chromomycosis; combined with amphotericin B in cryptococcosis and some cases of disseminated candidiasis and torulopsosis
Miconazole	IV	0.6–3.6 g (in divided doses q8h)‡	Pseudoallescheriosis (petriellidiosis); alternative therapy for coccidioidomycosis, paracoccidioidomycosis, and some other mycoses
Ketoconazole	PO	200–1,200 mg§	Paracoccidioidomycosis; some cases of histomycosis, coccidioidomycosis, blastomycosis, localized candidiasis
Hydroxystilbamidine	IV	225 mg	Alternative treatment of mild cases of blastomycosis
Saturated solution of potassium iodide	PO	9–12 ml/day (highest dose tolerated by patient)	Lymphocutaneous sporotrichosis only
Griseofulvin	PO	500–1,000 mg# (or single dose of 3 g for some cases of tinea capitis)	Dermatophyte infections refractory to topical therapy

*Standard dose for systemic mycoses is 0.3 mg/kg/day to start, increased over 3–7 days to 0.6 mg/kg/day. In unresponsive, rapidly progressive aspergillosis or mucormycosis, doses may be increased to 1.0–1.5 mg/kg/day (in divided doses q8–12h). Some patients with localized infections unresponsive to topical therapy (e.g., Candidal esophagitis) respond to low doses for short durations (e.g., 5–15 mg/kg/day for 1–2 weeks).

†Begin with 0.1 mg and increase in increments of 0.05–0.1 mg per injection.

‡Lower end of dose range for paracoccidioidomycosis, highest for coccidioidomycosis or pseudoallescheriosis.

§ 200 mg/kg/day for paracoccidioidomycosis; 400 (or 800, if needed) mg/kg/day for histoplasmosis, blastomycosis, localized candidiasis; 800–1,200 (or even higher) for coccidioidomycosis.

#Nail involvement requires higher dose for 4–6 months or more; lower dose is often sufficient for at least some cases of tinea corporis, tinea cruris, and some cases of tinea capitis. Ultramicronized griseofulvin is given in one-half the dose (250–500 mg/day) of the standard, micronized preparation.

TABLE 4 Major Adverse Effects of Systemic Antifungal Agents

Amphotericin B	*Flucytosine*	*Miconazole*	*Ketoconazole*	*2-Hydroxystilbamidine*	*Griseofulvin*	*Iodides*
Anorexia Nausea Vomiting Chills Fever Thrombophlebitis Nephrotoxicity* (acute and chronic azotemia, renal tubular acidosis, hypokalemia, hypomagnesemia) Cardiotoxicity (rapid infusions)* Anemia Possible pulmonary toxicity in combination with leukocyte transfusions	Anorexia Nausea Vomiting Diarrhea (colitis)* Leukopenia* Anemia Thrombocytopenia* Paracytopenia* Hepatic dysfunction (slight increases in serum transaminases and/or alkaline phosphatase, usually asymptomatic)	Nausea Vomiting Pruritis Phlebitis Fever Chills Drowsiness Erythrocyte aggregation Anemia Thrombocytopenia Hyperlipidemia Hyponatremia Skin rash Cardiac arrhythmias* Anaphylaxis*	Nausea Vomiting Abdominal pain Diarrhea Skin rash Itching Depressed ACTH response Depressed testosterone synthesis Gynecomastia Mild hepatic dysfunction (asymptomatic increases in serum enzymes) Acute hepatitis* Anaphylaxis*	Hypotension (with rapid infusions) Anorexia Nausea Rash Paresthesia Headache Mild hepatic dysfunction	Increased warfarin requirements Allergic rash Paresthesia Nausea Vomiting Epigastric pain Diarrhea Headache Confusion Photosensitivity Leukopenia*	Lacrimation Parotitis Abdominal cramping Nausea Vomiting Acneiform rash

* May be irreversible or incompletely reversible and/or life threatening in some patients.

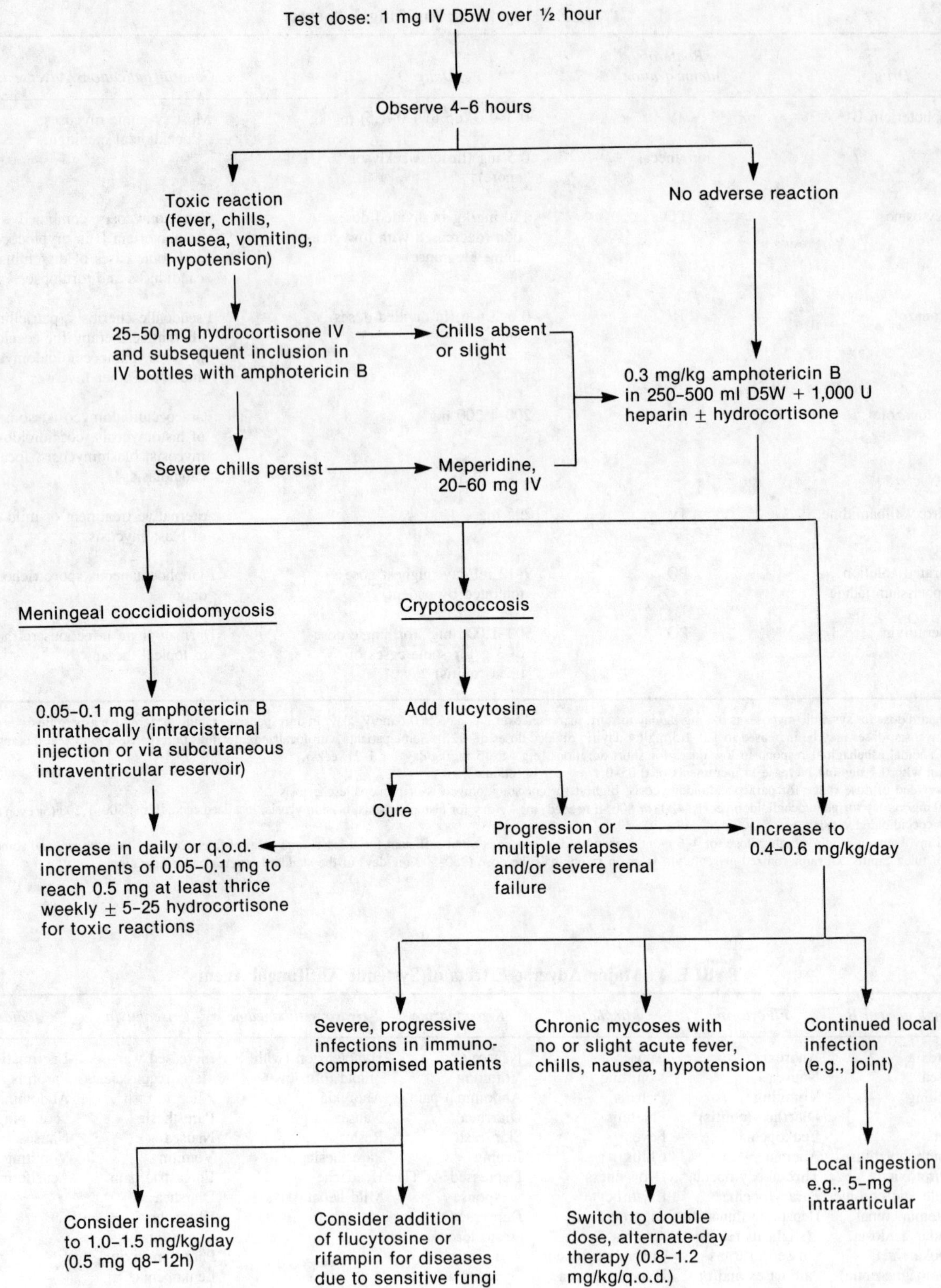

Figure 1 Recommended procedures for therapy with Amphotericin B.

dalities, it is useful to classify mycoses as either superficial (i.e., limited to skin and subcutaneous tissues) or systemic (i.e., involving deeper tissues such as bone and viscera).

Superficial Mycoses

In determinations of likely therapeutic requirements, it is useful to separate further these main categories. For example, superficial mycoses restricted to surface skin and mucous membranes may respond favorably to topical therapy, whereas mycoses extending to subcutaneous tissues and deeper structures require parenteral therapy with specific antifungal agents (Fig. 2). Even in immunocompromised patients, superficial mycoses rarely disseminate to deeper structures. Thus, though patients may be deeply troubled by local discomfort or disfiguring lesions, this general group of infections is seldom life threatening. Therefore, the general rules for therapy involve trials of less toxic therapeutic agents first. Examples of broad guidelines for the management of mycoses restricted to cutaneous structures are outlined in Figure 3.

Though significant experience indicates that ketoconazole is a highly effective agent for the treatment of dermatomycoses, routine, large-scale, primary usage of a drug with potentially fatal effects (even if relatively uncommon) cannot be justified for an infection that is not life threatening. Ultimately, the judgment as to exactly when and how potentially toxic antifungal therapies are used rests upon subjective weighing of three major factors: the assessment of the degree of morbidity caused by a mycosis in an individual patient, the lack of responsiveness to safer therapeutic agents, and the known risks of the drug to be used (e.g., the occurrence of severe, sometimes fatal, drug-induced hepatitis in addition to possible azoospermia and sterility in patients receiving ketoconazole). These issues are discussed in greater detail in the chapter *Superficial Fungal Infection*.

Systemic Mycoses

In the case of systemic mycoses, it is useful to consider separately those fungi often affecting normal hosts from fungi that are primarily opportunistic, causing infections in immunocompromised patients. Of course, some of the former group of more pathogenic fungi cause infections of greater severity in patients with specific predisposing factors. Thus, for example, severe disseminated coccidioidomycosis (especially with meningitis) is more likely to occur in association with pregnancy or immunosuppression, rapidly progressive disseminated histoplasmosis most often occurs in infants or immunosuppressed adults, and severe cryptococcosis is characteristically seen in immunocompromised patients (especially those receiving corticosteroid therapy and having underlying lymphoreticular malignancy or acquired immunodeficiency syndrome). Overall, then, the pattern of disease observed (and the therapy required) depends on underlying host factors in addition to the specific causative organism (Fig. 4).

Mycoses occurring in immunocompromised patients (e.g., those receiving corticosteroid or cytotoxic drug therapy or having hematologic malignancy or hereditary or acquired immunodeficiency states) often are caused by fungi that rarely produce systemic infections in normal hosts. Thus, local and then disseminated mycoses may ensue (Fig. 5).

THERAPY FOR SYSTEMIC MYCOSES

Antifungal Chemotherapy

The choice of therapy for mycoses involving deep tissues (i.e., subcutaneous or systemic) again depends on the severity of individual infections balanced against the

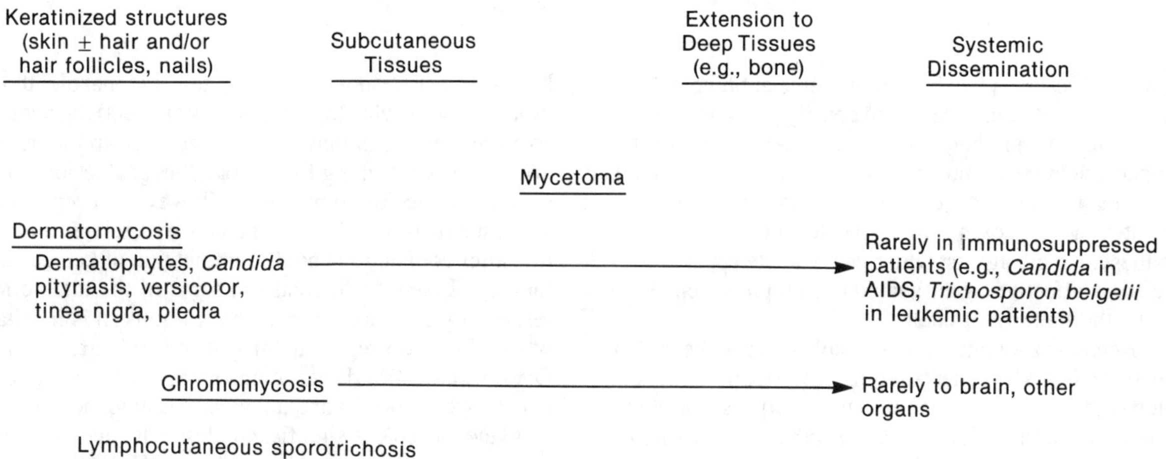

Figure 2 Patterns of infection in superficial mycoses.

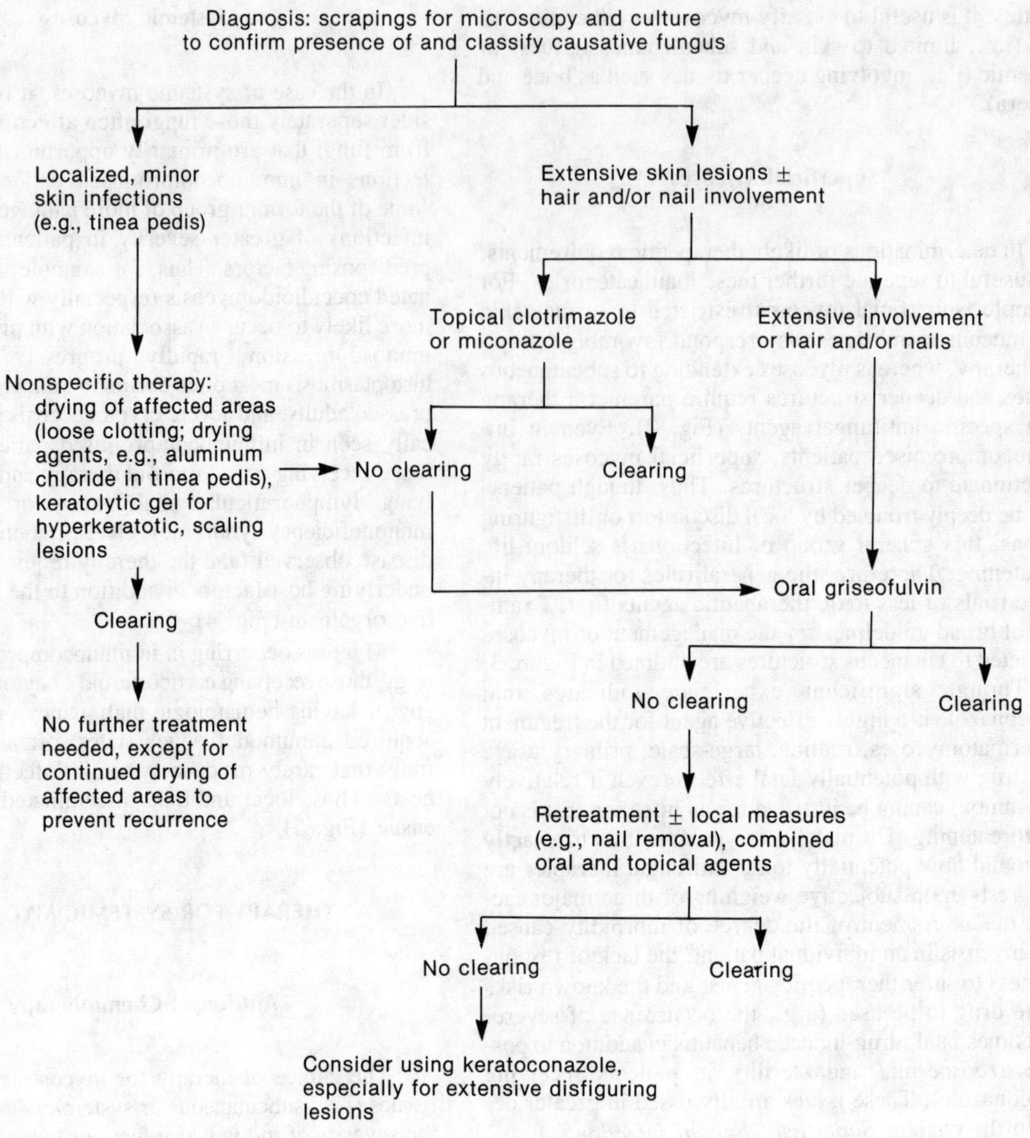
Diagnosis: scrapings for microscopy and culture to confirm presence of and classify causative fungus
Localized, minor skin infections (e.g., tinea pedis)
Extensive skin lesions ± hair and/or nail involvement
Topical clotrimazole or miconazole
Extensive involvement or hair and/or nails
Nonspecific therapy: drying of affected areas (loose clotting; drying agents, e.g., aluminum chloride in tinea pedis), keratolytic gel for hyperkeratotic, scaling lesions
No clearing
Clearing
Oral griseofulvin
Clearing
No further treatment needed, except for continued drying of affected areas to prevent recurrence
No clearing
Clearing
Retreatment ± local measures (e.g., nail removal), combined oral and topical agents
No clearing
Clearing
Consider using keratoconazole, especially for extensive disfiguring lesions

Figure 3 Treatment of cutaneous mycoses.

relative efficacy and toxicity of available antifungal drugs. In general, ketoconazole is more easily administered and less toxic than amphotericin B, but is less effective than amphotericin B for most indications and not effective at all in many situations (e.g., meningitis). Thus, for life-threatening mycoses (with the exception of pseudoallescherosis, against which miconazole appears to be the most effective agent available), amphotericin B remains the therapy of choice.

Ketoconazole thus far has established a niche in therapy of mycoses in patients requiring systemic treatment, but who have relatively chronic, milder forms of systemic fungal infections (Fig. 6). *Paracoccidioides brasiliensis* is especially sensitive to ketoconazole; the drug can be used in low doses (200 mg per day) to treat paracoccidioidomycosis. Patients with histoplasmosis and some with blastomycosis respond favorably to ketoconazole, though usually at somewhat higher doses (400 to 800 mg per day). Even higher doses may be required, but are sometimes effective in controlling focal, nonmeningeal lesions in disseminated coccidioidomycosis. However, recent reports suggest a disturbingly high incidence of relapse of infection after completion and discontinuation of ketoconazole therapy. Likewise, increase in some of the toxic effects (especially effects on hormone metabolism) is inevitable when high-dose regimens of ketoconazole are required. Overall, although direct, controlled, experimental comparisons of efficacy are unavailable, evidence suggests that ketoconazole is significantly less effective than is amphotericin B for most deep mycoses. However, even if relapses occur, a trial of ketoconazole in mycoses that are not immediately life threatening may, without major ad-

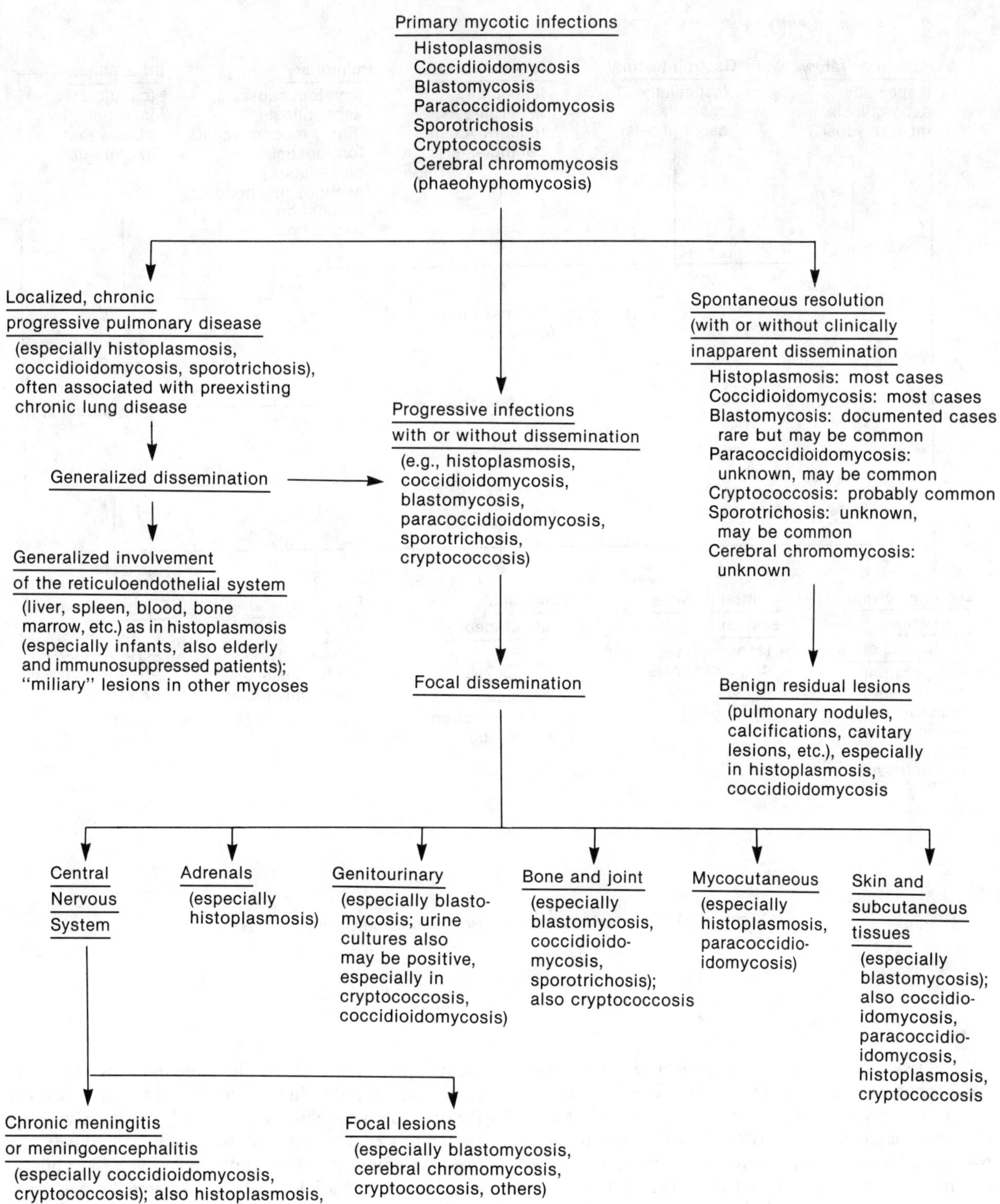

Figure 4 Patterns of systemic mycosis occurring in the absence of obvious immunocompromise.

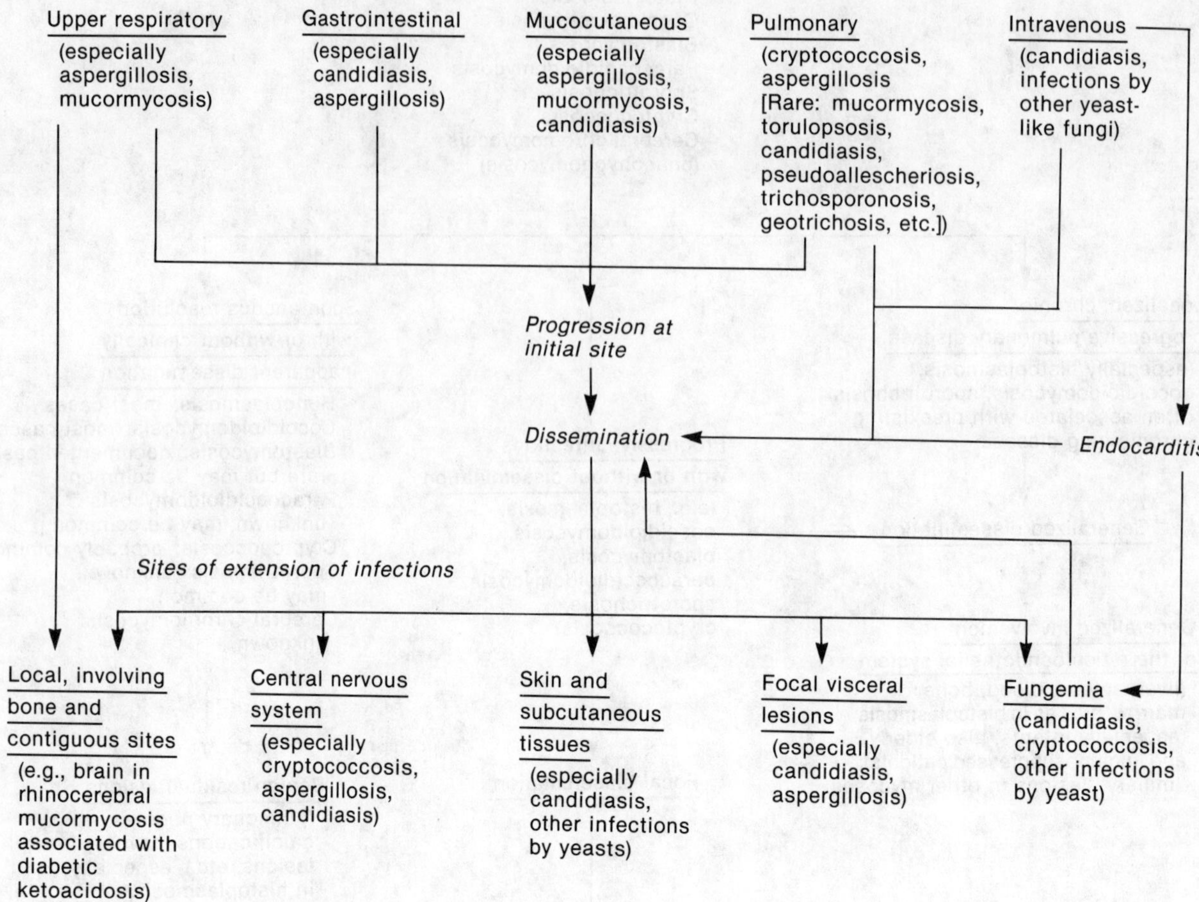

Figure 5 Patterns of systemic mycoses in immunocompromised hosts

ditional risks, spare at least some patients the risk of taking amphotericin B. Even if some chronic lesions are not completely cured (as may occur in some cases of coccidioidomycosis treated with any antifungal agent), the relative added comfort and convenience of ketoconazole therapy make it preferred over amphotericin B for most patients when there is a choice.

In the treatment of immunocompromised patients, the underlying status of the host is a major factor determining the outcome of infection. Infections in such patients often progress rapidly, and even the best available antifungal therapy falls far short of ideal. Thus, institution of appropriate antifungal therapy early in the course of opportunistic mycoses may be critical in preventing early deaths.

However, specific diagnoses of mycoses are especially difficult to achieve in these patients. In many cases, uncorrectable thrombocytopenia, hypoxia, or other factors are severe enough to preclude the invasive diagnostic procedures required to establish definitely the presence of invasive fungal infections. Even when biopsy procedures are feasible, specimens often fail to yield evidence of the presence of a specific causative organism. For example, in invasive aspergillosis, samples obtained from involved tissues may show evidence of hemorrhage, necrosis, and infarction without revealing the culprit fungus that invaded nearby blood vessels to cause the lesions. As a consequence of this, empiric therapy with amphotericin B has been used in many medical centers. In some hospitals, where the incidence of opportunistic mycoses has been particularly high, evidence has been cited justifying the addition of amphotericin B therapy in patients who fail to defervesce or have advancing pulmonary infiltrates despite the use of broad-spectrum antibacterial agents. However, in other centers, where the incidence of mycoses has been lower, more stringent criteria for commencement of amphotericin B therapy should be employed.

To a great extent, as long as neither diagnostic procedures nor therapies are ideally safe and effective, criteria for commencement of empiric use of amphotericin B inevitably will vary according to the experience in different institutions and even according to the specific histories and needs of individual patients. Likewise, because the effectiveness of amphotericin B is limited in immunocompromised patients, the therapeutic goals generally are limited to containment of opportunistic mycoses until such time as there might be reversal of the immunodepressed state (e.g., hematologic remission after chemotherapy). Only then does complete cure of the infection become truly feasible.

When mycoses progress despite the use of amphoteri-

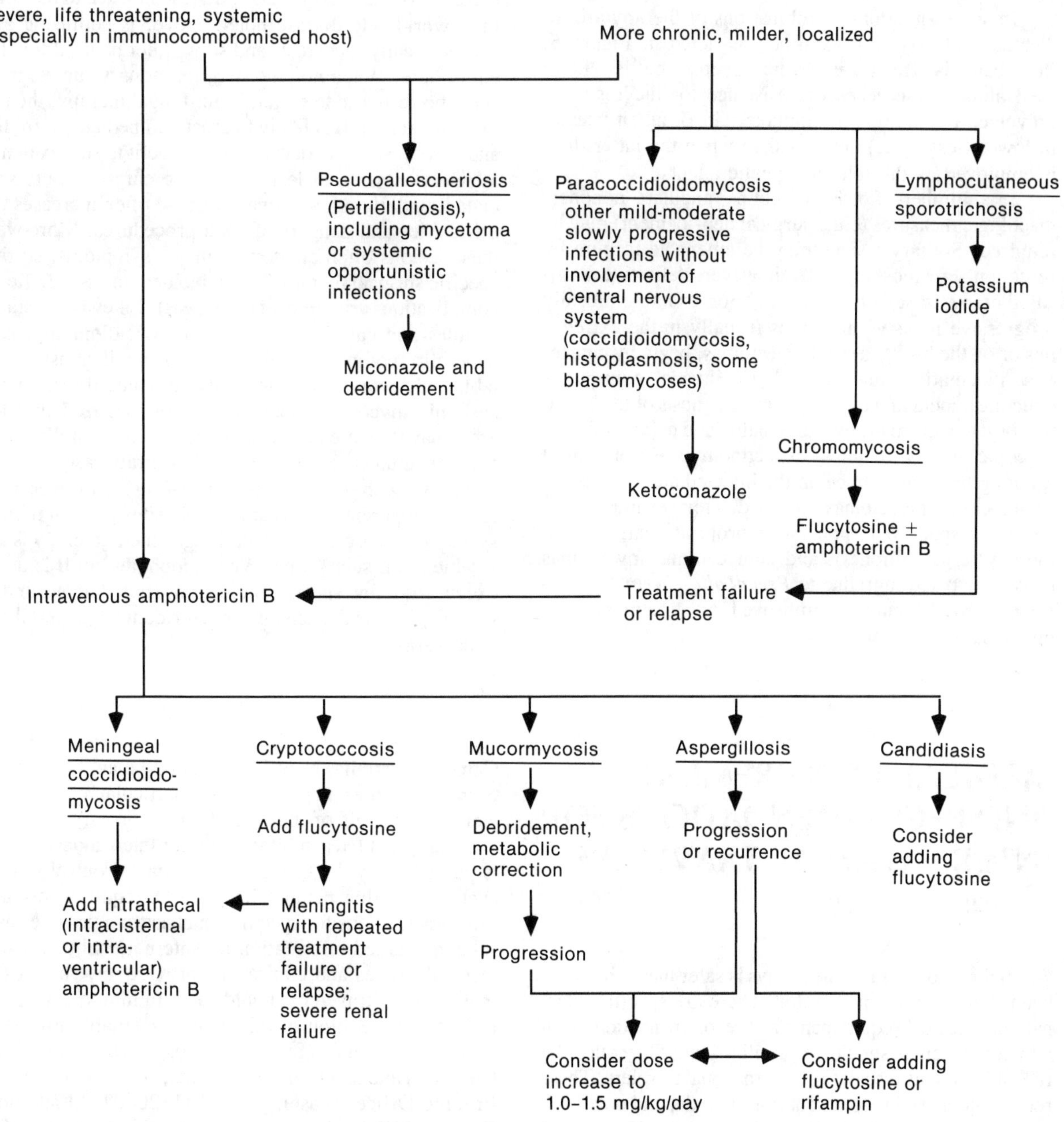

Figure 6 Choice of therapy for invasive and subcutaneous mycoses.

cin B, especially in cases of invasive aspergillosis as noted in Figure 6, higher doses of amphotericin B have been tried and other drugs (flucytosine or rifampin) have been added. Although experience in humans has not established that such measures are effective, especially with failure to respond to conventional doses of amphotericin B alone, such trials seem reasonable given the almost invariably dire outcome for these patients.

Ideally, then, the most important consideration in the management of mycoses complicating the course of an immunocompromised patient is, whenever possible, to eliminate the predisposing immunologic factor, for example, correct metabolic abnormalities in diabetics, withdraw iatrogenic immunosuppression, induce a hematologic remission in patients with malignancy.

In some situations, combinations of therapy are indicated routinely. For example, as noted in Figure 6, flucytosine is effective in several mycoses but is seldom used alone. Emergence of resistance to flucytosine is prevented by addition of amphotericin B, albeit usually in lower (less toxic) dosages than when the latter drug is employed as the sole therapeutic agent.

In a number of other infections, ancillary nonpharmacologic measures (e.g., surgical debridement) may be required. Solitary lesions may be amenable to cure by resection. For most mycoses, however, definitive surgical therapy is seldom practical. For example, locally progressive invasive infections (usually in the extremities or on the back), termed mycetomas, begin by cutaneous inoculation and spread to invade contiguous structures, including bone. Specific diagnosis of the causative organism is made by examination and culture of macroscopic grains (clumps of actinomycetes or fungi) draining from sinus tracts in the infected area. Some actinomycotic mycetomas (caused, for example, by *Nocardia* species) respond to appropriate antibacterial therapy (e.g., sulfones), and eumycetoma (mycetomas caused by true fungi) due to *Pseudoallescheria (Petriellidium) boydii* may be improved by treatment with miconazole.

Surgical Therapy

For some causative organisms, no effective antifungal agents are yet available. However, in all cases of mycetoma, ancillary surgical therapy is critically important. Since the causative organisms seldom disseminate to distant sites, amputation of involved limbs, though a last resort, often represents the only possibility for cure.

Surgical therapy also has some role in the treatment of other mycoses. *Aspergillus* and other saprophytic fungi may colonize previously damaged areas of the lung with no (or, occasionally, minimal) invasion of surrounding tissue. Such "fungus balls" in cavitary pulmonary lesions often have been referred to as mycetomas in clinical literature. This latter term bears little resemblance to the common worldwide disease noted above, is confusing and mycologically incorrect, and so will not be used for this entity here. When noninvasive, pulmonary fungus balls show no response to systemic antifungal therapy, the use of amphotericin B is likely to create immediate morbidity and leave residual toxicity without benefit to such patients. Surgical excision of lesions may be curative, but associated, underlying pulmonary disease often increases the difficulties and dangers of such procedures. Moreover, these lesions often create few major symptoms, so that specific surgical therapy is best avoided unless significant complications arise (e.g., hemoptysis). Likewise, residual nodules and cavities (e.g., due to coccidioidomycosis) generally require no interventions if the diagnosis is established securely. Occasionally, in some disseminated systemic mycoses, apparent solitary localized infected areas have been excised or debrided successfully, with apparent total cure of the patient (e.g., rare cases of cryptococcosis with solitary lysis bone lesions). However, clinically inapparent lesions at multiple sites are common in systemic mycoses, so that antifungal chemotherapy is advisable in all such cases. When amphotericin B is used, except for a few specific indications (noted above and in Fig. 6), surgical excision or debridement generally is unnecessary.

MEDICAL REQUIREMENTS AND RECOMMENDATIONS FOR INTERNATIONAL TRAVELERS

JAMES CHIN, M.D., M.P.H.

International travel these days is safer than it has ever been, but it can be made safer. There are specific international medical requirements and recommendations with which physicians should be familiar that will reduce the risk of infectious diseases for international travelers. These requirements and recommenations will depend on a traveler's itinerary and schedule. Very few apply to travel to Europe and other industrialized countries such as Canada, Australia, New Zealand, and Japan. Other areas of the world present greater risks, particularly if the traveler ventures off of the main tourist routes.

A manual (Health Information for International Travel) is published by the Centers for Disease Control (CDC) each year. This manual lists health requirements and recommendations for specific countries and provides useful and detailed information for international travel. All medical offices and clinics that provide any services to international travelers should, at a minimum, have the most current edition of this manual available for reference. This manual is for sale at a cost of U.S. $5.00 from the Superintendent of Documents, U.S. Government Printing Office, Washington, D.C. 20402. In addition, most local health departments and travel agencies receive special international health alerts that describe recent problems. The Quarantine Division, Centers for Disease Control, Atlanta, GA 30333, distributes a weekly blue sheet listing countries reporting cholera, yellow fever, and plague and issues advisory memoranda on various disease risks for travelers when new problems arise. Health care providers will need to have all of this information, updated, to provide appropriate advice, drugs, and immunobiologics (vaccines, toxoids, and immune globulins) for international travelers. Computerized services (such as IMMUNIZATION ALERT), which provide detailed and up-to-date information on disease risks and recommendations for international travel, are becoming available. Physicians and clinics that provide services to international travelers may wish to explore the availability and utility of such computerized systems.

GENERAL HEALTH ADVICE

To avoid last minute problems and frustrations, prospective travelers should determine their health needs several months in advance of a trip. If necessary, however, most of the required and recommended vaccines and medications can be given or prescribed during the last week before departure. However, it must be appreciated that some vaccines, such as those for hepatitis B and rabies, achieve effective protection only after a full primary series of doses over a period of several weeks to several months.

If the traveler has a known health problem, it would be prudent to determine before the patient leaves on a planned trip whether any changes in medications are indicated. A written summary of the patient's problem should be carried by the traveler on his or her trip. The traveler should be advised to keep all personal medications in separate, well-marked containers stating their content, indications, and the dosage schedule. Travelers should also be advised to inquire about the availability of essential medications abroad, including birth control pills, and to be safe, to take an adequate supply with them.

Aside from the discomfort of mosquito and other insect bites, such bites may also transmit parasitic and viral disease. Avoidance of mosquito bites is the only preventive measure available for dengue, which is endemic in most of the tropical countries of Asia and Africa. Dengue has also been reported in most South Pacific island groups and many countries in the Carribean, Mexico, and in some Central and South American countries. Travelers should be advised to take general measures to prevent or reduce numbers of mosquito bites; such measures include not being outdoors at dusk and in the early evening when possible, wearing long pants and long-sleeved shirts, using mosquito repellents on exposed skin, or sleeping in screened rooms or under netting when indicated.

Travelers should be advised to report immediately any unexplained fever or symptoms that may develop during or after the trip, especially if they have visited tropical and developing countries. Figure 1 presents a general guide to the requirements and recommendations for travel to various areas of the world.

VACCINES

International Certificate Requirements

International certificates of vaccination are available at many local health departments, some travel agencies, passport offices, and medical clinics and offices that provide services for international travel. They can be purchased directly from the U.S. Government Printing Office Washington, D.C. 20402. Validation of the certificate, which is required by quarantine authorities for yellow fever and cholera vaccines, can be obtained at most local health departments or from physicians who possess a Uniform Stamp, which some states issue upon application. However, yellow fever vaccine must be given at an officially designated yellow fever vaccination center, and the certificate must be validated by the center that administered the vaccine. Local health departments can provide the location of these centers within their jurisdiction.

Yellow Fever Vaccine

Yellow fever vaccine is universally recommended for travel in nonurban areas of countries designated endemic zones for yellow fever (primarily the tropical and subtropical regions of Africa and South America (see Table 1). The risk of yellow fever to travelers who limit their itineraries to the urban areas of yellow fever zones is extremely low. However, a number of countries require travelers to present an international certificate of vaccination against yellow fever if they have come from or through any country in the officially designated yellow fever endemic zone. Requirements of individual countries vary widely. Therefore, it is prudent to provide travelers with a valid international certificate to facilitate travel to and from any country where yellow fever may be present. An international certificate of vaccination against yellow fever is valid for 10 years, beginning 10 days after primary vaccination or on the date of revaccination if within 10 years of first injection.

Pregnant women who must travel to areas where the risk of yellow fever is high should be vaccinated. However, if international travel regulations constitute the only reason to immunize a pregnant woman (or patient who is hypersensitive to eggs), then the physician can consider providing a letter of waiver outlining the contraindication to yellow fever vaccine. Such a letter of waiver (written on the physician's letterhead and bearing the stamp used by health departments and officially designed centers to validate the international certificates of vaccination) has been acceptable to some countries. Under these circumstances, it is prudent to obtain specific, authoritative advice from the embassies or consulates of countries to be visited.

Cholera Vaccines

These are only marginally effective, and the requirement for cholera vaccine was dropped from the interna-

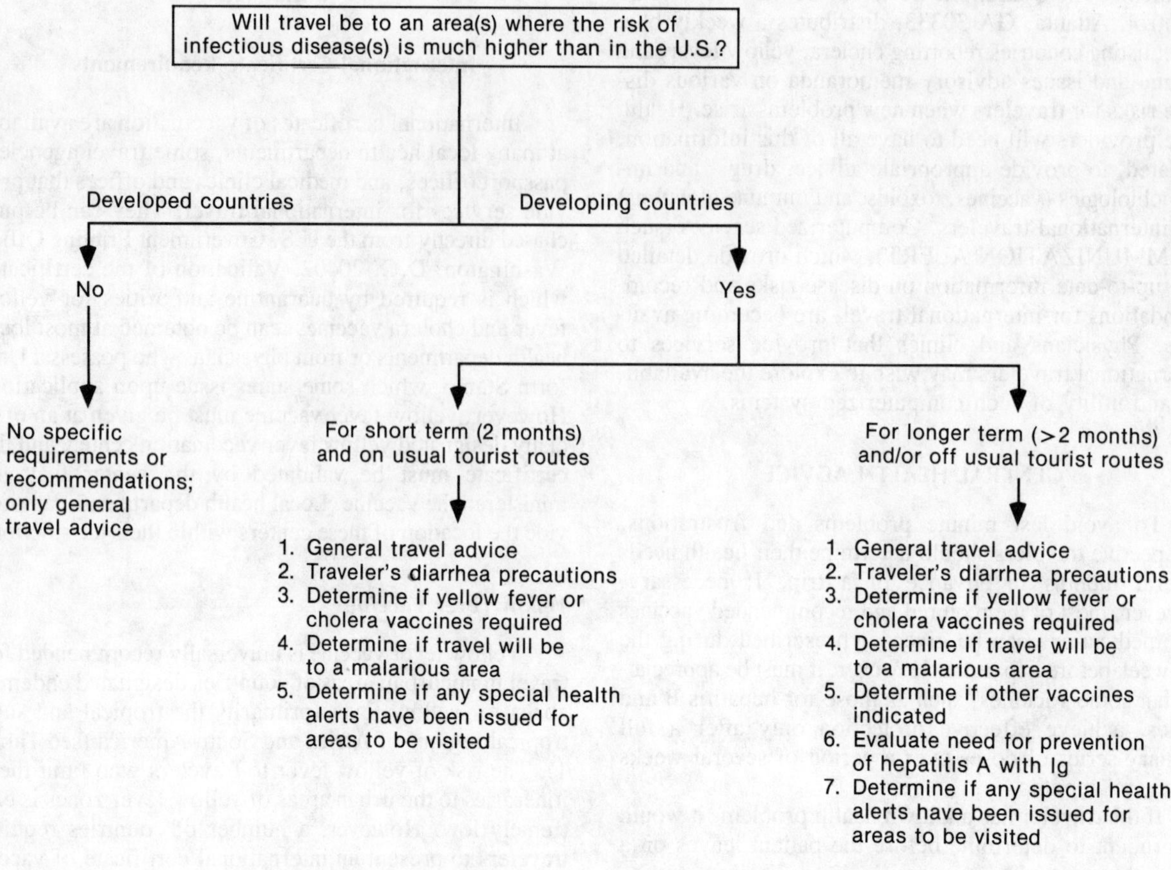

Figure 1 Medical information for international travelers.

tional health regulations in 1973. However, many countries still require travelers to present an up-to-date international certificate of vaccination against cholera

TABLE 1 Countries Reporting Yellow Fever and Cholera to the World Health Organization, April 1985

Yellow Fever	*Cholera*	
Bolivia	Benin	Mauritania
Brazil	Burkina Faso*	Mozambique
Burkina Faso*	Burundi	Nigeria
Colombia	Cameroon	Philippines
Ecuador	Djibouti	Rwanda
Gambia	Equatorial Guinea	Senegal
Ghana	Ghana	Somalia
Nigeria	India	South Africa
Peru	Indonesia	Swaziland
Sudan	Ivory Coast	Tanzania
Zaire	Kenya	Thailand
	Liberia	Vietnam
	Malaysia	Zaire
	Mali	

Note: Additions to and deletion from this listing can occur at any time but changes, especially for yellow fever, are generally not frequent. Refer to the blue sheet Summary of Health Information for International Travel, distributed every other week by the Quarantine Division, CDC, for the most up-to-date information.

* Formerly Upper Volta.

when arriving from or traveling to cholera-infected areas (see Table 1). A current international certificate is thus needed to facilitate travel to and from these countries. An international certificate of vaccination against cholera is valid for 6 months, beginning 6 days after one injection of vaccine or on the date of revaccination if within 6 months of the first injection.

Smallpox Vaccination

Vaccination against smallpox is no longer required by international health regulations because smallpox has been eradicated. Every country has officially dropped the requirement for an international certificate of vaccination against smallpox.

Other Vaccine Recommendations

No immunizations are required for travelers entering or coming back into the United States. However, international travelers should be urged to have all of their children's routine immunizations (poliomyelitis, diphtheria, tetanus, pertussis, measles, rubella, and mumps) current.

The majority of adult U.S. citizens planning international travel on the usual tourist routes will not need any additional immunization, except for a Td (tetanus/diphtheria) booster if more than 10 years have elapsed since their last dose. Travel to Europe, Canada, New Zealand, and Australia does not present any increased risks. However, travelers to developing countries who venture to smaller cities off of the usual tourist routes and those who stay in villages or rural areas for extended periods are at much higher risks of acquiring many infectious diseases, and the following vaccines may be indicated for some of them. All vaccines for international travel are summarized in Table 2.

Poliovirus Vaccine

Travel to tropical and subtropical areas with poor sanitation poses increased risk of exposure to polioviruses. Children and adults who have completed an oral (OPV) or an inactivated (IPV) poliovirus vaccine series should have one additional dose of OPV prior to departure. No additional doses are then needed for any subsequent travel. For adults who have never had any poliovirus vaccine or who have had an incomplete series, the recommendations are more involved. For previously unimmunized adults, IPV is indicated. However, if less than 4 weeks are available before protection is needed, a single dose of OPV is recommended. Travelers who have previously received less than a full primary course of OPV or IPV should be given the remaining required doses of either vaccine, regardless of the interval since the last dose and the type of vaccine previously received. Those who have previously received a primary series of IPV should receive a dose of either OPV or IPV. If IPV is used exclusively, an additional dose may be given every 5 years if exposure continues or recurs, although the need for these boosters has not been established.

TABLE 2 Vaccines for International Travel

Vaccine	*Primary Schedule and Booster(s)*	*Comments*
Yellow fever (live, attenuated virus, 17-D strain)	1 dose SC 6 days to 10 years before travel; booster every 10 years	Avoid during pregnancy unless risk of yellow fever is very high; only available at officially designated yellow fever centers; many states designate physician's offices or clinics as an official center upon application
Cholera (inactivated bacterial vaccine)	2 0.5-ml doses SC or IM or 2 0.2-ml doses ID 1 week to 1 month apart; booster doses (0.5 ml IM or 0.2 ml ID) every 6 months	1 dose generally satisfies international health regulations; however, some countries may require validation of complete primary series (2 doses) or booster dose given within 6 months of arrival
Inactivated poliovirus (IPV) or live oral poliovirus (OPV)	IPV:3 doses SC 4 weeks apart, a 4th dose 6 to 12 months after the 3rd; for those with a completed primary series booster can be given with either OPV or IPV	IPV preferred for primary immunization of adults; if immediate protection needed, OPV can be given; IVP or OPV can be given during pregnancy if risk of infection is high
Typhoid (inactivated bacterial vaccine)	2 0.5-ml doses SC 4 or more weeks apart, booster 0.5 ml SC or 0.1 ml ID every 3 years if exposure continues	Immunization should not be considered as alternative to continued careful selection of food and water
Human diploid cell rabies (HDCV) (inactivated, whole-virion and split-virion)	Preexposure: 2 doses 1 week apart; 3rd dose 3 weeks after 2nd; if exposure continues, booster 2 years later or an antibody titer determined and booster dose given if titer inadequate	Preexposure immunization does not eliminate need for postexposure treatment following rabies exposure; it only reduces postexposure regimen
Meningococcal polysaccharide (bivalent A, C and quadravalent A, C, Y, and W-135	1 dose in volume and by route specified by manufacturer; need for booster(s) unknown	Avoid during pregnancy unless there is substantial risk of infection
Plague (inactivated bacterial vaccine)	3 IM doses; first dose 1.0 ml; 2nd dose 0.2 ml 1 month later; 3rd dose 0.2 ml 5 months after 2nd; Give 2 booster doses, each 0.1–0.2 ml at 6-month intervals, thereafter booster doses (0.2 ml) at 1–2 year intervals if exposure continues	Do not give during pregnancy unless there is substantial and unavoidable risk of exposure; prophylactic antibiotics are likely still indicated for definite exposure whether vaccine received or not
Hepatitis B inactivated virus vaccine (HBV)	2 doses IM 4 weeks apart; 3rd dose 5 months after 2nd; need for booster(s) unknown	Indicated primarily for long-term travelers to areas where hepatitis B is very prevalent and where they expect to have very close (i.e., blood, household, and/or sexual) contact with local population
Japanese encephalitis (inactivated viral vaccine)	Recommended schedule will probably be 3 doses, each given 1 week apart	As of late 1985, only available in the U.S. as experimental vaccine; contact state health departments for local availability

Typhoid Vaccine

For travelers to areas where typhoid is prevalent and environmental conditions and hygiene are poor, typhoid vaccine is not required, but is generally recommended. However, it is not usually given routinely to short-term travelers (i.e., < 2 months) to such areas if they will be staying at standard tourist accommodations primarily in urban areas. Typhoid vaccine should be considered for travelers to smaller cities and villages or rural areas off of the usual tourist itinerary in areas endemic for typhoid. However, even travelers who elect to receive this vaccine should be advised to exercise caution in selecting food and water. For persons who have never received this vaccine, the primary series consists of two doses given 4 or more weeks apart. If there is insufficient time, then three doses can be given at weekly intervals, but this latter schedule may be less effective. A booster dose is needed every 3 years to maintain protection; this may be given subcutaneously (0.5 ml) or intradermally (0.1 ml). Typhoid immunization often results in 1 to 2 days of discomfort at the site of injection; this local reaction may be accompanied by fever, malaise, and headache.

Meningococcal Vaccine

This vaccine may be indicated for some travelers to countries where an epidemic of meningococcal disease is occurring. Most large epidemics of meningococcal disease are usually due to serogroup A, although epidemics attributable to groups B and C have been observed in recent years. Two meningococcal polysaccharide vaccines—a bivalent A, C and a quadrivalent A, C, Y, and W-135 vaccine—are licensed for use in the United States. No vaccine is yet available against serogroup B. Only one dose of vaccine is needed to confer adequate protection.

Plague Vaccine

Immunization against plague is not indicated for most travelers to countries of Africa, Asia, and South America reporting cases, particularly if travel is limited to urban areas and usual tourist accommodations are used, and this vaccine is not required by any country as a condition of entry. Plague vaccine, which is only partially effective, might be considered for persons who will have direct contact with wild rodents or rabbits in plague-enzootic areas and for persons who will reside in plague-enzootic rural areas where avoidance of rodents and fleas is impossible. The full primary series (three doses) of vaccine should be given over a minimal period of 8 weeks and, optimally, over 3 to 4 months.

Rabies Vaccine (Human Diploid Cell Vaccine, HDCV)

Rabies vaccine is indicated only for travelers who will be in areas for at least a month where rabies is a constant threat. Although information on the incidence of rabies in such areas is not reliable, the World Health Organization estimates that thousands of human deaths attributable to rabies occur in large areas of Africa, Central and South America, the Philippines, Sri Lanka, and Indonesia. In India alone, several-hundred thousand persons are treated annually because of possible exposure to rabies. For preexposure immunization, three 1.0-ml injections of HDCV need to be given intramuscularly on days 0, 7, and 21 or 28. Because HDCV is expensive (about $50 per 1-ml dose), the intradermal route of administration, utilizing 0.1 ml per dose, has been explored for preexposure immunization. Results in the United States have generally been good, but the mean antibody response is somewhat lower and may be of shorter duration than with the 1.0-ml intramuscular dose. Antibody response in some groups given preexposure immunization by the intradermal route outside of the United States has been found inadequate. Preliminary data suggest that concurrent administration of malaria chemoprophylaxis may be a factor in the poor antibody response of persons overseas given this vaccine by the intradermal route. It should be emphasized that preexposure immunization does not eliminate the need for prompt postexposure prophylaxis following an actual exposure to rabies; preexposure immunization only reduces the postexposure regimen.

Japanese Encephalitis Vaccine (JEV)

This was, as of November 1985, not available as a licensed vaccine in the United States. Immunization against this mosquito-borne viral infection is only indicated for those travelers who will be in epidemic or endemic rural areas for more than 2 to 3 months. Epidemics of this disease occur principally in the rural areas of India, Bangladesh, the eastern USSR, Korea, China, and northern Thailand. In other more tropical areas of Southeast Asia, the virus is endemic, causes sporadic cases in the indigenous populations, and is transmitted at higher rates during the rainy season. A JEV produced and routinely used in Japan has been made available as an investigational new drug to selected medical centers and offices in the United States. It is anticipated that after completion of this investigational phase, this vaccine will be made more accessible to those few travelers for whom it might be indicated. The recommended schedule will probably consist of three doses, each given a week apart. State health departments can be contacted for information regarding availability of JEV.

HEPATITIS

Prevention of Viral Hepatitis

Viral hepatitis includes type A (infectious), type B (serum), and non-A, non-B hepatitis. Recommendations and immunobiologics for the prevention and/or modification of types A and B are available, but are not available for non-A, non-B hepatitis.

Type A Hepatitis

Viral hepatitis, type A is an infection that may be spread through contaminated food and water. It is much commoner in tropical areas and developing countries than it is in the United States. A vaccine for the prevention of type A hepatitis is not yet available, but immune globulin (Ig or gamma globulin) can provide temporary protection. However, even travelers who receive Ig should be advised to exercise caution in selecting food and water.

Travelers to areas where environmental sanitation is low and where the incidence of traveler's diarrhea is high are at increased risk for hepatitis A. If travel to such an area is of short duration (less than 2 months) and usual tourist accommodations and restaurants are used, Ig for the prevention of hepatitis A is not routinely indicated. However, Ig should be offered to travelers to these areas who travel either outside major cities or within major cities, but using nontourist facilities. For short-term travel (less than 2 months) such travelers should be given Ig (less than 50 pounds, 0.5 ml; 50 to 100 pounds, 1.0 ml; and over 100 pounds, 2.0 ml) shortly before their departure. The dosage of Ig for persons planning travel for more than 2 months is approximately double that for short-term travel and needs to be repeated at 4- to 5-month intervals while abroad. Frequent international travelers to such areas should be tested for antibody to hepatitis A (anti-HAV IgG), and if antibody is present, then Ig is not needed for the prevention of hepatitis A.

Type B Hepatitis

Viral hepatitis, type B is an infection transmitted by percutaneous exposure to infectious blood (e.g., by needlestick) or by very close and intimate contact with the blood or secretions of an infected person. Most international travelers are not considered to be at an increased risk of hepatitis B infection. However, hepatitis B vaccine should be considered for persons who plan to reside in areas with high levels of endemic hepatitis B (particularly areas of Asia and sub-Saharan Africa) for more than 6 months and who will have close contact with blood from or sexual contact with local residents. Travelers intending only a short stay but who are likely to have similar contact are also at risk of acquiring a hepatitis B viral infection. It should be emphasized to all travelers who may be at increased risk of hepatitis B that they must allow 6 months before travel in order to complete the primary immunization series.

ADMINISTRATION OF REQUIRED OR RECOMMENDED IMMUNOBIOLOGIES

Many immunobiologics, such as some vaccines, require more than one dose for full protection. In addition, periodic booster doses of some preparations are needed to maintain adequate protection. The average international traveler will usually not require many different immunobiologics for his or her travel. If several are indicated, their administration should be spaced appropriately. Some data have indicated that persons given yellow fever and cholera vaccines simultaneously or 1 to 3 weeks apart have lower-than-normal antibody responses to both vaccines. Unless there are time constraints, cholera and yellow fever vaccines should be administered with a minimal interval of 3 weeks. If the vaccines cannot be administered at least 3 weeks apart, then they should preferably be given simultaneously. Yellow fever vaccine and Ig (commercially available in the United States) may be given simultaneously. Ig and other antibody-containing blood products do not appear to interfere with the immune response to OPV.

Although not optimal, most of the usually required and/or recommended immunobiologics can be given or started concurrently. For example, a traveler can be given yellow fever vaccine, cholera vaccine, Ig (all at separate sites), and OPV during one office visit.

MALARIA

Prevention of Malaria

Malaria is the most serious health threat to the international traveler. From 1973 through 1983, more than 2,500 U.S. citizens contracted malaria during travel abroad, and more than 30 of these died (primarily from falciparum malaria). Malaria can be prevented by using repellents and insecticides to avoid mosquito bites, in conjunction with antimalarial drugs for chemosuppression of disease.

Risk of Malaria

There is no risk of malaria in Canada, Europe, Australia, New Zealand, Japan, and most Pacific Islands. Areas of risk include parts of Mexico, Haiti, Central America, South America, Africa, the Middle East, Turkey, the Indian subcontinent, Southeast Asia, People's Republic of China, the Indonesian archipelago, and Oceania. *Plasmodium falciparum* and *Plasmodium vivax* are found in many endemic areas; *Plasmodium ovale* is seen mainly in West Africa. Malaria due to *P. falciparum* strains, refractory to cure with the 4-aminoquinolines (such as chloroquine), occurs in the tropical portions of both hemispheres. In countries with malaria, the risk is usually not uniform, but varies with local conditions such as the density of mosquitoes, the presence of human cases of malaria, weather, and altitude. Malaria risks can change suddenly, however, resulting in contradictory information from different official sources.

Recommendations for Chemoprophylaxis

Recommendations for the prevention of malaria in American travelers were significantly changed by the Centers for Disease Control in April 1985. Prior to this, it was recommended that routine chloroquine chemoprophylaxis be given for any travel to any malarious area, even if travel was for only one night. In addition, if chloroquine-resistant *P. falciparum* was known to be present in the area, then routine weekly doses of Fansidar were also recommended. However, as a result of detailed analysis of the documented risk of malaria, especially chloroquine-resistant *P. falciparum*, to American travelers during the past few years and the increasing reports of severe (including a few fatal) reactions to Fansidar, routine chemoprophylaxis for malaria is now recommended only for those areas and/or situations where the risk of malaria transmission is considered moderate to high. These revised recommendations place increased responsibility on individual travelers and their physicians to estimate the extent of exposure to malaria, especially chloroquine-resistant malaria, that the traveler may experience. The revised recommendations are presented in an outline form in Figure 2, and alternative drug regimens for the prevention of chloroquine-resistant *P. falciparum* malaria are present in Table 3.

Chemoprophylaxis With Chloroquine Phosphate

For suppression of malaria in travelers to areas where the risk of transmission is moderate to high, chloroquine phosphate (Aralen) should be started 1 to 2 weeks prior to travel. Chloroquine is still recommended as the primary prophylactic drug of choice even in areas where there is documented chloroquine resistance. This is because there are usually other species of *Plasmodium (P. vivax, P. ovale, P. malariae)*, as well as some chloroquine-sensitive strains of *P. falciparum* for which chloroquine remains effective.

Aralen comes in two tablet sizes–150 mg base (250 mg salt) or 300 mg base (500 mg salt). The adult dose is one of the larger tablets once a week or two of the smaller tablets once a week. Patients should be advised to take these tablets on the same day(s) each week. This medication should be continued for at least 6 weeks after exposure in a malarious area. Alternatively, amodiaquine (Camoquin, which is licensed but not available in the United States) at approximately the same dosage can be used once weekly. Pregnancy is not a contraindication to these two drugs. For infants and children, the dosage is 5 mg base per kilogram of body weight once weekly, never to exceed the adult dose regardless of weight; the duration of administration is the same as that for adults. Because of the bitter taste of chloroquine, the tablets must be crushed or broken and then dissolved, preferably in syrup, for administration to young children. Liquid formulations of chloroquine sulfate (Nivaquine), or amodiaquine (Basoquin) can be purchased outside of the United States and should be considered for use in children staying for prolonged periods in malarious areas.

Adverse effects of chloroquine in prophylactic doses are rare and usually restricted to mild gastric discomfort. This reaction can be minimized by advising travelers to take tablet(s) after meals. Long-term administration of chloroquine carries the risk of retinopathy once the total cumulative dose exceeds 100 g of base. However, it would take more than 6 years of weekly chloroquine chemoprophylaxis to reach such a dose.

Prevention of Relapsing Malaria

Routine prophylactic use of chloroquine does not prevent delayed attacks of the nonfatal relapsing species (*P. vivax* and *P. ovale*) after chloroquine is discontinued. Whether there is a need to prevent such delayed attacks should be made on an individual basis, taking into account both the duration of the traveler's exposure to *P. vivax* or *P. ovale* and the potential risk of toxic reactions to the drug primaquine, which is used for such treatment.

To eliminate the hepatic stages and later relapses of vivax or ovale malaria, primaquine, 0.25 mg base per kilogram per day (15 mg base or 26.3 mg of primaquine phosphate for the average adult) for 14 days may be given concurrently with or following the suppressive drug. Larger daily doses (22.5 mg base) may be required for some Southeast Asian and Southwest pacific strains. Alternatively, primaquine, 0.75 mg base per kilogram (45 mg base or 79 mg primaquine phosphate for the average adult) once weekly for 8 weeks may be given.

Prior to primaquine administration, the patient should be tested for possible glucose-6-phosphate dehydrogenase (G6PD) deficiency. Primaquine should not be given during pregnancy. Instead, continue chloroquine weekly for the duration of the pregnancy and administer primaquine, if indicated, after pregnancy. All patients should be observed for drug-induced hemolysis; this is most likely to occur in individuals with G6PD deficiency, commoner among persons from eastern Mediterranean, African, and Southeast Asian areas.

The routine use of primaquine for prophylaxis (or presumptive terminal treatment) is controversial, but this issue should not be confused with its use in treatment of a diagnosed infection with one of these species. Routine primaquine prophylaxis might be indicated for individuals such as missionaries or Peace Corps volunteers returning home from extended periods of heavy exposure in areas where *P. vivax* and *P. ovale* are prevalent. For the average traveler, however, primaquine prophylaxis is generally not indicated unless transmission of relapsing species is at a high level, e.g., rural India or Bangladesh.

Prevention of chloroquine-resistant P. falciparum infection

Travelers to certain areas of South America, Panama, the Indian subcontinent, Southeast Asia, the Indonesian archipelago—including the Philippines and Papua New Guinea—and East Africa are at some risk for exposure to strains of *P. falciparum* that have varying degrees of resistance to chloroquine. In areas where resistance oc-

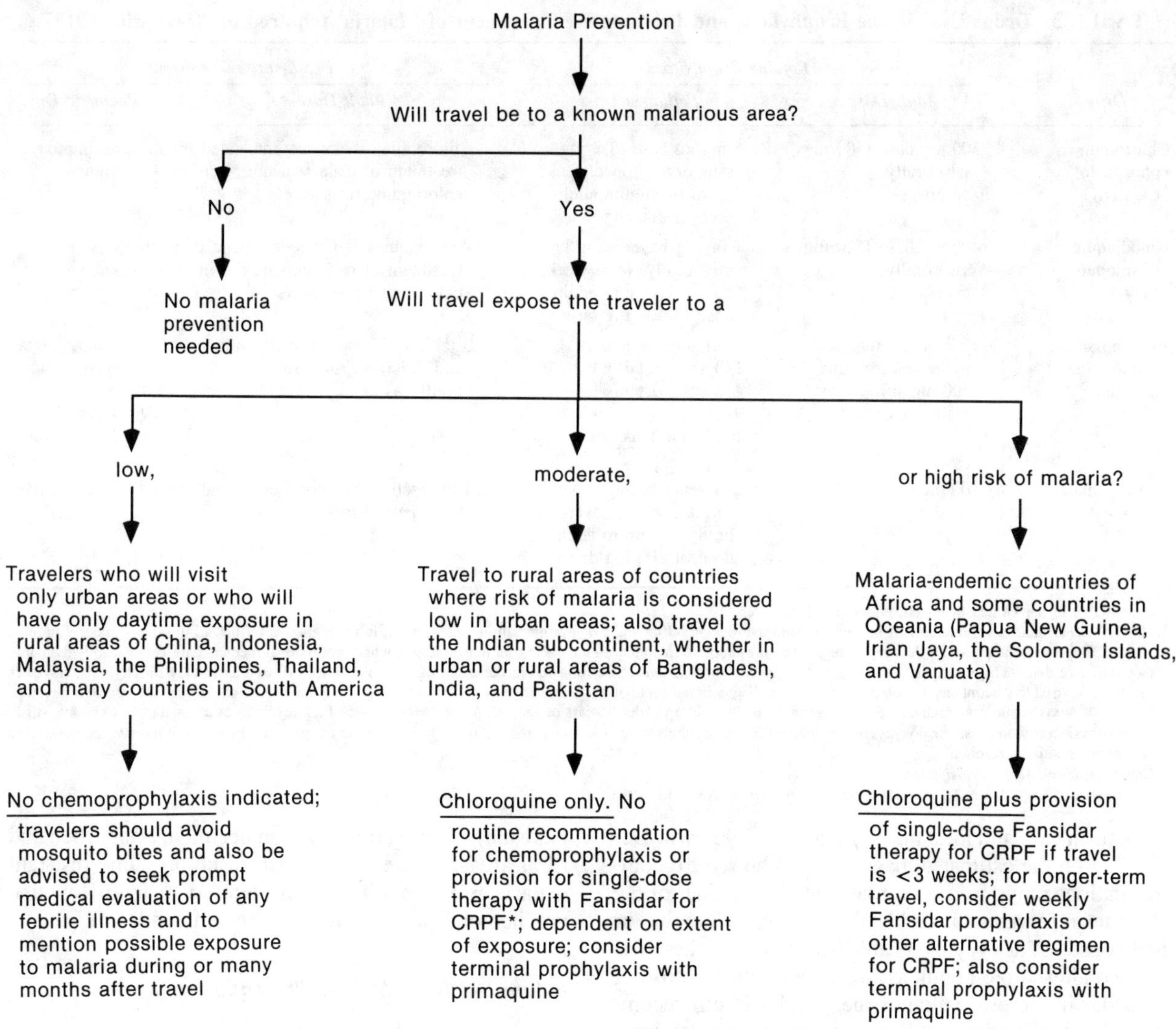

Figure 2 A general guideline for advising travelers of recommendations for malaria prevention. Specific recommendations for each traveler need to be individualized according to factors such as specific areas to be visited as well as the living conditions and duration of travel.

curs, prior recommendations were to give travelers a fixed combination of pyrimethamine (25 mg) and sulfadoxine 500 mg [Fansidar] in addition to each weekly chloroquine dose. However, strains resistant to this combination are being increasingly reported and infection with chloroquine-resistant *P. falciparum* may develop even if chloroquine and Fansidar are used. Because of the increasing documentation in American travelers of severe reactions to weekly doses of Fansidar—reactions such as drug fever and photodermatitis, jaundice, toxic epidermic necrolysis, agranulocytosis and Stevens-Johnson syndrome—with at least six deaths since 1982, the continued prophylactic use of this drug combination is now considered for use only in areas where the transmission of chloroquine-resistant malaria is very high.

The transmission of chloroquine-resistant *P. falciparum* infection is particularly intense in malarial endemic areas of Africa. Even in such areas, only chloroquine prophylaxis is recommended if travel will be less than 3 weeks. However, physicians should consider giving these travelers (except for those with a known intolerance to sulfonamides or pyrimethamine) a single treatment dose of Fansidar to take with them on their trip (Table 3). They should be cautioned not to take this treatment dose unless they experience a febrile illness during or shortly after their travel to these areas and for which they cannot promptly obtain professional medical care.

For longer-term travel in chloroquine-resistant malarial areas of Africa, there is a much higher risk of acquiring a resistant infection. Recommendations for such travelers have to be individualized, taking into account such factors as living conditions, availability and access

TABLE 3 Drugs Used in the Prophylaxis and Presumptive Treatment of Malaria Acquired in Areas with CRPF‡

	Routine Prophylaxis		*Presumptive Treatment*	
Drug	*Adult Dose*	*Pediatric Dose*	*Adult Dose*	*Pediatric Dose*
Chloroquine phosphate (Aralen)	300 mg base (500 mg salt) orally, once/week	5 mg/kg base (8.3 mg/kg salt) orally, once/week, up to maximum adult dose of 300 mg base	Chloroquine is not recommended for the presumptive treatment of malaria acquired in areas of known chloroquine resistance.	
Amodiaquine (Camoquin Flavoquine)*	400 mg base (520 mg salt) orally, once/week	7 mg/kg base (9 mg/kg salt) orally, once/week, up to maximum adult dose of 400 mg base	Amodiaquine is not recommended for the presumptive treatment of malaria acquired in areas of known chloroquine resistance.	
Pyrimethamine-sulfadoxine (Fansidar) †	1 tablet (25 mg pyrimethamine and 500 mg sulfadoxine) orally, once/week	2–11 mos: 1/8 tab/wk 1–3 yrs: ¼ tab/wk 4–8 yrs: ½ tab/wk 9–14 yrs: ¾ tab/wk >14 yrs: 1 tab/wk	3 tablets (75 mg pyrimethamine and 1,500 mg sulfadoxine), orally, as a single dose	2–11 mos: ¼ tab 1–3 yrs: ½ tab 4–8 yrs: 1 tab 9–14 yrs: 2 tabs >14 yrs: 3 tabs as a single dose
Doxycycline§	100 mg orally, once/day	>8 years of age: 2 mg/kg of body weight, orally/day up to adult dose of 100 mg/day	Tetracyclines are not recommended for the presumptive treatment of malaria.	

* Unavailable in the United States but widely available overseas

† The use of Fansidar is contraindicated in persons with histories of sulfonamide or pyrimethamine intolerance, in pregnancy at term, and in infants under 2 months of age. Physicians who prescribe the drug to be used as presumptive treatment in the event of a febrile illness when professional medical care is not readily available should ensure that such prescriptions are clearly labeled with instructions to be followed in the event of a febrile illness. If used as weekly prophylaxis, travelers should be advised to discontinue the use of the drug immediately in the event of a possible adverse effect, especially if any mucocutaneous signs or symptoms develop.

§ The use of doxycycline is contraindicated in pregnancy and in children under 8 years of age. FDA considers the use of tetracyclines as antimalarials to be investigational. Physicians who prescribe doxycycline as malaria chemoprophylaxis should advise their patients to limit direct exposure to the sun to minimize the possibility of a photosensitivity reaction.

‡ Chloroquine-resistant *P. falciparum*

Note: Reprinted from *Morbidity and Mortality Weekly Report*, April 12, 1985.

to medical care and local malaria patterns, if known. Dependent on the estimated magnitude of the risk, recommendations range from a regimen identical to that for the short-term traveler to weekly doses of Amodiaquine or daily doses of doxycyline (Table 3). Even with these latter two alternative regimens, a single treatment dose of Fansidar in the possession of the traveler is still recommended. Weekly doses of Fansidar, which were routinely recommended prior to April 1985, may be considered if the magnitude of risk of resistant malaria is sufficiently high. However, travelers given prophylactic doses of Fansidar need to be alerted to immediately discontinue use if any mucocutaneous signs or symptoms develop: pruritis, erythema, rash, orogenital lesions, or pharyngitis. The above recommendations are also applicable for travel to many areas of Papua New Guinea, Irian Jaya, the Solomon Islands, and Vanuata where the transmission of chloroquine-resistant *P. falciparum* is also very intense.

Travelers to all other areas where resistant strains may be present, such as areas in the People's Republic of China, Indonesia, Malaysia, the Philippines, Thailand, and many countries in South America, are considered at minimal risk of exposure to malaria, including resistant malaria, especially if their travel is largely confined to urban areas and they avoid rural areas from dusk till dawn. For these travelers, no malarial chemoprophylaxis (not even chloroquine) is recommended. However, travelers to these countries who will have outdoor exposure in rural areas during evenings and nightime hours should be placed on regimens similar to those detailed in Africa. In some areas of the Indian subcontinent (Bangladesh, India, and Pakistan), malaria transmission occurs in both urban and rural areas. However, the risk of chloroquine-resistant malaria as of late-1985 is considered sufficiently low that no chemoprophylaxis for it is recommended (Fig. 2).

Future Drugs for Malaria Prevention

Members of the phenanthrene methanol and quinazoline families, which may be effective against chloroquine-resistant strains of *P. falciparum* are under active development. Mefloquine, a quinoline methanol effective against all types of human malarias, including chloroquine-resistant, is not yet licensed in the United States. It may become available within the next several years, but recommendations for its use in the chemoprophylaxis of malaria will have to be carefully developed to try to avoid the rapid emergence of resistance to this drug.

OTHER DISEASES

Travelers who venture off the usual tourist routes are at much higher risk for many other infectious diseases in addition to those already described. Preventive measures for most of these infections are either not available, not practical, or not specific.

Infections such as amebiasis and giardiasis can be avoided by following the same general precautions as those recommended for prevention of traveler's diarrhea. Exposure to arthropod-borne infections such as dengue, trypanosomiasis, Rift valley fever, typhus, and filariasis can be minimized by preventing insect and tick bites.

Schistosomiasis has been reported in travelers returning from East Africa. Schistosomiasis has occurred in river-rafters and persons bathing in streams and lakes. Risk of schistosomiasis can be diminished by iodinating or chlorinating (1 ppm for 30 minutes) or heating (to at least 50 °C [122 °F] for 5 minutes) drinking and bathing water from untreated sources. These procedures kill the infective cercariae. If body contact with presumably contaminated water occurs, brisk, thorough towel drying within 10 minutes of exposure may remove and kill schistosomal cercariae before they can penetrate the skin.

CHILDHOOD IMMUNIZATION

JEROME O. KLEIN, M.D.

Immunization for children can be divided according to products recommended for all children and products recommended for special children or special situations. Seven products are considered routine immunization; these include diphtheria and tetanus toxoids and pertussis whole cell vaccine; measles, mumps, and rubella live vaccines; and oral poliovirus vaccine. Special products include influenza virus vaccine, pneumococcal, meningococcal and *Hemophilus influenzae* type B polysaccharide vaccines, bacille Calmette-Guerin (BCG), hepatitis B vaccine, and live rabies vaccine. Immune globulins are available for prevention and treatment of measles, hepatitis A and B, varicella-zoster, rabies, and tetanus.

Recommendations for immunization in the United States are provided by the Committee on Infectious Diseases of the American Academy of Pediatrics (AAP) and published in the Report of the Committee (revised every 3 to 4 years) and the Advisory Committee on Immunization Practices of the United States Public Health Service, published in the *Morbidity and Mortality Weekly Report* (MMWR). In most circumstances the recommendations of the two groups coincide. Current recommendations for immunization of adults (18 years of age and older) are provided in a recent MMWR supplement (September 28, 1984; vol. 33, no. 1S).

RECOMMENDATIONS FOR IMMUNIZATION OF NORMAL INFANTS AND CHILDREN

The schedule recommended by the AAP and ACIP for active immunization of normal infants and children is provided in Table 1.

Diphtheria and Tetanus Toxoids and Pertussis Vaccine (DTP)

The primary series of DTP is given at 2, 4, 6, and 18 months, with a booster administered between 4 and 6 years. The primary series of DTP is carried out up to the seventh birthday. After the seventh birthday primary immunization should consist of adult-type tetanus toxoid and reduced dose of diphtheria toxoid (Td). A lapse in the schedule does not require restarting the schedule; subsequent doses are given at the recommended time intervals. Although the optimal age for beginning immunization in infants who are born prematurely is unknown, available data suggest that DTP can be administered at the same chronologic age to premature as to term infants.

The preferred site of administration for DTP and other products administered by the intramuscular route is the anterolateral aspect of the upper thigh (preferred in infants because it is the largest muscle mass) and the deltoid muscle of the upper arm (appropriate for most older children). For routine usage, the buttocks should be avoided as a site for injection. Large volumes may require use of the buttocks; the site should be the upper outer mass of the gluteus maximus to avoid injury to the sciatic nerve.

Approximately one-half of children who receive DTP vaccine have local (tenderness, pain) and systemic (fever, irritability) adverse effects; seizures occur, with or without fever, in approximately one in 2,000 children who receive DTP, and brain damage has been identified 1 year later at a frequency of one in 310,000 doses. These effects are associated with the whole-cell pertussis component of the vaccine. Most public health experts agree that, on balance, the benefits of pertussis vaccine far outweigh the risks and it should be administered as part of the routine schedule. However, concern about toxicity of whole-cell pertussis vaccine has led to reconsideration of contraindications of its use in children. Deferral of DTP is recommended for children who have previously had convulsions (febrile or nonfebrile) until it can be determined whether an evolving neurologic disorder is present. If an evolving disorder is identified, infants or children should be given DT rather than DTP. Pertussis vaccine is also contraindicated if the child has a history of severe reaction following a prior dose (usually within 48 hours). Severe reactions include shock, collapse, persistent screaming episodes, temperature of 40.5 °C (105 °F) or greater, alterations of consciousness, generalized or local neurologic signs, or systemic allergic reactions.

Measles, Mumps, and Rubella Live Vaccines (MMR)

Live attenuated vaccines for measles, mumps, and rubella are administered in a combined vaccine. Single

TABLE 1 Recommended Schedule for Active Immunization of Normal Infants and Children

Recommended Age	Vaccine	Comments
2 months	DTP; OPV	Can be initiated earlier in areas of high endemicity
4 months	DTP; OPV	
6 months	DTP; (OPV)	OPV optional for areas where polio may be imported
15 months	MMR	
18 months	DTP; OPV	
4–6 years	DTP; OPV	Up to the 7th birthday
14–16 years	Td	Adult tetanus toxoid (full dose); diphtheria toxoid (reduced dose); repeat every 10 years

Abbreviations: DTP = diphtheria, tetanus, pertussis; OPV = oral poliovirus vaccine; MMR = measles, mumps, rubella; Td = tetanus, diphtheria.

vaccines are also available for special use. A single dose of MMR provides durable protection with minimal side effects when administered at 15 months of age. Reimmunization is not recommended except for children who received immunization at earlier age (under 12 months for measles vaccine), with other products (killed measles vaccine), or in modified dosage or form (administered with gamma globulin).

Rubella vaccine results in viremia and infection of the placenta and fetus, but available data indicate vaccine virus is not a teratogen. Use of rubella vaccine is encouraged for susceptible nonpregnant women in the childbearing age group.

Immunization after exposure to disease may be of value for measles, but not for mumps or rubella. Measles virus vaccine administered as late as 5 days after exposure is protective in a majority of individuals. Administration of immune globulin is preferred for infants 12 months of age and younger who are exposed to measles because of the chance of vaccine failure in this age group.

Oral Poliovirus Vaccine (OPV) and Inactivated Poliovirus Vaccine (IPV)

OPV is administered at ages 2, 4, 18 months, and 4 and 6 years of age. In areas where exposure to wild virus is possible (some of the states in the Southwest), an additional dose at 6 months is recommended.

Paralytic poliomyelitis has resulted from administration of live vaccine to children with immune defects. Live virus vaccines, including OPV, should not be administered to children with known or suspected immunodeficiency. Because the vaccine virus is excreted by the vaccinee and may infect contacts, the live vaccine should not be used in families with a member who is immunodeficient. Inactivated poliovirus vaccine (IPV) should be used in children with immune defects and members of their households.

Routine immunization against poliovirus is not recommended for susceptible adults. For parents or travelers who may be exposed to wild or vaccine virus, IPV should be administered. The primary series of IPV consists of four doses; the first three may be given at the same time as DTP (in a separate syringe); the fourth dose is given 6 to 12 months after the third or on entry to school for children.

VACCINES FOR SPECIAL CHILDREN OR SPECIAL CIRCUMSTANCES

Hepatitis B Vaccine for Prevention of Perinatal Infection

Mothers who are hepatitis B antigen (HBsAg)–positive may infect their newborn infant. The initial infection is usually asymptomatic, but about 25 percent of infant carriers may ultimately develop chronic active hepatitis, cirrhosis, and, possibly, primary hepatocellular carcinoma. The severity and chronicity of the disease warrant protection of any infant born to a mother who is hepatitis B antigen–positive. The recommended schedule combines hepatitis B immune globulin (HBIg) and hepatitis B vaccine. HBIg, 0.5 ml intramuscularly, is administered as soon after birth as possible. The vaccine, 0.5 ml intramuscularly, is given before the infant leaves the hospital or within 1 week after birth and at 1 and 6 months of age. The first dose of vaccine may be given at the same time as HBIg at a separate site.

Pneumococcal Vaccine

A 23-valent polysaccharide vaccine against disease due to *Streptococcus pneumoniae* was licensed in the United States in 1983, replacing the 14-valent vaccine introduced in 1977. Although the vaccine contains serotypes responsible for most pneumococcal disease in children, the immune response to most types for children under 2 years of age is limited. Because of the lack of immunogenicity, the vaccine is not recommended for infants. The vaccine should be used for children 2 years of age and older who are at increased risk for pneumococcal disease; these include children with anatomic or functional asplenia, those with sickle cell disease, nephrotic syndrome, cerebrospinal fluid leaks, and conditions associated with immunosuppression. The vaccine may have some value in prevention of recurrent episodes of otitis media in the older children. Duration of immunity is uncertain; until data are available, reimmunization is not recommended.

Meningococcal Vaccine

A polysaccharide vaccine for groups A, C, Y and W-135 is now available as a quadrivalent product. Group A vaccine produces satisfactory immune response in infants as young as 5 months, but the other group polysaccharides are poor immunogens for infants younger than 18 months of age. Immunity is group-specific, and protective levels of antibody are achieved in 1 week. The duration of immunity is uncertain, but is estimated to be 1 to 3 years. Group B meningococcus is the most prevalent group in the United States today; the polysaccharide is a poor immunogen and does not elicit protective antibody. Current indications in children older than 18 months of age (or younger if disease due to group A is to be prevented) include control of epidemic disease, use for travelers to endemic or epidemic areas, and prolonged prophylaxis for household contacts (because one-half the secondary family cases occur more than 5 days after the primary case).

Hemophilus Influenzae Type B Vaccine

A polysaccharide vaccine against invasive disease caused by *H. influenzae* type B was introduced in the spring of 1985 in the United States. Infants under 18 months of age respond infrequently and with less antibody than do older children. The efficacy of the vaccine was documented in a clinical trial in Finland: the protective efficacy of the vaccine was 90 percent in children 18 to 71 months of age; the vaccine was not effective in children under 18 months of age. Current recommendations for vaccine use include immunization of all children at 24 months of age; optional immunization of children 18 to 23 months of age who are known to be at high risk, including those with sickle cell disease, asplenia, malignancies associated with immunosuppression, and children who attend day-care facilities; and usage in children not previously immunized between 24 months and 59 months of age. New vaccines with improved immunogenicity for children under 18 months of age, including *H. influenzae* type B polysaccharide–protein conjugate vaccines, are now in clinical trial.

Influenza Vaccine

Influenza is a mild illness in most children, and, therefore, there is no basis for routine immunization. Annual immunization with current influenza vaccines is recommended for children with chronic disorders of the cardiovascular or pulmonary systems that are severe enough to have required regular follow-ups or hospitalization during previous years. If the physician believes the child would be harmed if infected, influenza vaccine should be used. Current influenza vaccines are prepared in eggs and contain trace amounts of egg antigens. Children known to be allergic to eggs should not receive influenza vaccine.

Bacille Calmette-Guerin (BCG)

Selective usage of BCG vaccine may be of value in infants and children: those in a household with repeated exposure to patients with infectious tuberculosis; and those in groups with excessive rates of new infection and for whom usual medical care is not feasible. BCG should not be given during INH administration since multiplication of the bacillus is inhibited by the drug. Skin test with purified protein derivative is done 2 months after vaccination; if skin test is negative, BCG is repeated.

Rabies Vaccine

Human diploid cell vaccine (HDCV) and human rabies immune globulin (HRIg) are recommended following bite by a wild animal of a species known to carry the virus (skunk, fox, coyote, raccoon, bat, and other carnivores) unless the animal is proved to be virus-negative by laboratory test. HDCV and HRIg are also recommended if a domestic animal—dog or cat is known or suspected to be rabid. If the animal's health is unknown or the animal has escaped, consultation with a local public health official is important to provide information on the risk of rabies in the area (see chapter *Animal Bite Infection).*

Human Immune Globulin

Immune globulin (Ig) is prepared from pooled serum of adults. Ig is of value for prophylaxis against hepatitis A and measles. Special preparations of high-titer immune globulin are available for prevention or treatment of disease due to varicella, hepatitis B, rabies, and tetanus. Dosage schedules for immune and hyperimmune globulins are given in Table 2. Immune globulins are administered intramuscularly; 1 to 5 ml are administered at one site, depending on the size of the muscle mass.

Ig can be administered to susceptible children who are exposed to measles and is effective for prevention or modification of disease. Ig should be administered to children during the first year of life, to older children who have been exposed for more than 5 days (too late for use

TABLE 2 Dosage Schedules for Immune Globulins for Prevention and Treatment of Disease

Agent	*Condition*	*Preparation*	*Dose*
Measles	Normal children	Ig	0.25 ml/kg
	Immunodeficient children	Ig	0.5 ml/kg
Hepatitis A	Household contacts	Ig	0.02 ml/kg
	Day care contacts	Ig	0.02 ml/kg
Hepatitis B	Newborn infants	HBIg	0.5 ml
	Exposure to infected blood	HBIg	0.06 ml/kg
Varicella	Immunodeficient children	VZIg	125 units/10 kg
	Newborn infants	VZIg	125 units
Rabies	Postexposure	HRIg	20 IU/kg; ½ dose IM ½ dose at wound
Tetanus	Postexposure	HTIg	250–500 units IM

Abbreviations: Ig = immune globulin; HBIg = hepatitis B immune globulin; VZIg = varicella-zoster immune globulin; HRIg = human rabies hyperimmune globulin; HTIg = human tetanus immune globulin.

of vaccine), and to immunocompromised children. Vaccine should be given 3 or more months after administration of Ig to immunocompetent children.

Ig is recommended for prevention of hepatitis A in households and day care centers. Ig should be administered to all household contacts of a clinical case. If a case of hepatitis A occurs in a child or member of the staff of a day care center or in the households of two or more attendees, Ig should be given to children and staff of the center. Exposure in schools is not a reason for administration of Ig.

Hepatitis B immune globulin is administered to infants of mothers who are HBsAG-positive and to children or adults who are exposed to infected blood.

Varicella-zoster immune globulin should be used for immunocompromised children, for newborns of mothers with peripartum varicella (within 5 days before and 48 hours after delivery) and for premature infants with significant postnatal exposure.

Human rabies hyperimmune globulin should be administered with rabies vaccine (except for those who have been previously immunized). It provides antibody until the initial doses of vaccine have stimulated an immune response. Vaccine and human rabies hyperimmune globulin are administered via the intramuscular route in different sites. If feasible, one-half the dose of human rabies hyperimmune globulin is infiltrated in the area of the wound and one-half, intramuscularly.

Human tetanus immune globulin is indicated for patients whose tetanus toxoid immunization is unknown, those who have received an incomplete series of toxoid immunizations, and those whose wound is older than 24 hours.

ADULT IMMUNIZATION

RICHARD PLATT, M.D.

The indications for immunization of adults include a number of factors—principally, the individual's age, prior immunization history, exposures to specific pathogens, underlying health problems and availability of newly developed vaccines. The table lists vaccines and immune globulins that are currently available and recommended for use under appropriate circumstances in adults. Most of these preparations are discussed in the separate chapters in this book that address these diseases.

The Advisory Committee on Immunization Practice (ACIP) provides periodic recommendations for use of these agents. These are published as they are developed in *Morbidity and Mortality Weekly Reports*, available from the National Technical Information Service and also from several private publishers. In addition, the American College of Physicians has recently published a *Guide for Adult Immunization*. This guide provides recommendations for adults of different ages, special groups such as pregnant women, health care personnel, day care workers, and homosexually active men, immunologically compromised hosts, and travelers. It also provides discussions of specific vaccines. Single copies may be obtained for $10.00 from the American College of Physicians, Adult Immunization, P.O. Box 7777–R0325, Philadelphia, PA 19175.

Four vaccines merit broad use in various age groups of the general population.

TETANUS/DIPHTHERIA

Tetanus/diphtheria toxoids, provided as a single preparation, should be used for all individuals. For adults the Td (tetanus toxoid) preparation should be used. This contains less diphtheria toxoid than DT, which, along with DPT (diphtheria, pertussis, and tetanus) is routinely used for children. Most young adults have been immunized against tetanus, but a substantial proportion of those over 60 years of age do not have antibody. Individuals who are not known to have completed a three-dose primary immunization series should receive three 0.5-ml doses of Td. The second dose should be given 4 weeks after the first; the third should be given 6 to 12 months after the second. Additional doses should be given approximately every 10 years. The mid-decade birthdays (25, 35, 45 years, etc.) have been suggested as reminders for giving these booster doses.

For postexposure prophylaxis, for instance after wounds, no antitetanus therapy is indicated if the individual has completed a primary immunization course or had received a booster within the preceding 5 years (10 years for a minor wound). If longer intervals have occurred, Td should be given. Therapy should be given as soon as possible after injury occurs. Those who have not completed a primary series should begin one. In addition, individuals who have not completed a primary series should ordinarily receive tetanus immune globulin. The dose of immune globulin depends on the severity of the wound. Tetanus toxoid and tetanus immune globulin should be given at separate sites using different syringes. Adsorbed rather than fluid toxoid should be used if immune globulin is used.

MEASLES/MUMPS/RUBELLA

These are attenuated live virus preparations. They are available singly and in combination. A single dose of each or of the combination is sufficient. Administration of these vaccines to individuals who are immune is not associated with significant adverse effects. Measles and mumps vaccines should not be given to individuals who are allergic to eggs. None of these vaccines should be given to immunocompromised individuals.

Rubella

The principal reason for rubella vaccination is prevention of congenital rubella. Nonpregnant women of childbearing age who do not have documentation of prior vaccination or serologic evidence of immunity should be immunized. Although the risks of vaccination during pregnancy are not known to be great, women should be counseled not to become pregnant within 3 months after immunization. In general, the trivalent preparation should be used for rubella immunization unless the individual is known to be immune to measles and mumps or is allergic to eggs. Rubella immunization should not be given less than 14 days before immune globulin, or within 6 weeks after.

Transient arthralgias or arthritis occur after immunization in a substantial minority of susceptible individuals. This is believed to be a manifestation of mild infection. Other adverse effects, including frank arthritis, have been reported extremely rarely.

Measles

Measles vaccine is indicated for individuals born after 1956 who are not known to be immune. Immunity is likely if live virus vaccine was given after the first birthday or if clinical measles was diagnosed by a physician. In part because the U.S. national measles eradication program has reduced the occurrence of natural measles, the existing cohort of unimmunized young adults has provided a new focus for outbreaks, a number of which have occurred on college campuses in recent years.

Postexposure immunization is most likely to be effective if given within 72 hours. Immune globulin may also be used within 6 days to attentuate or possibly prevent infection, especially for individuals who cannot receive the vaccine.

Individuals who are allergic to eggs should not receive measles vaccine. The principal adverse reactions, occurring in 5 to 15 percent of recipients, are fever, usually lasting 1 to 2 days, and rash. Adverse reactions, including local reactions, are commoner among individuals who have received killed measles vaccine (no longer available).

Mumps

Most adults are immune to mumps virus; however, adults who are suspected to be susceptible should be immunized. The vaccine should not be used for individuals with allergy to eggs. The same time frame before and after immune globulin should be observed as the rubella vaccine.

TABLE 1 Diseases in Adults for Which Immunoprophylaxis Is Available

Cholera
Hepatitis A (immune serum [gamma] globulin)
Hepatitis B (vaccine and immune globulin)
Influenza
Measles (vaccine and immune serum [gamma] globulin)
Meningococcal disease
Mumps
Plague
Pneumococcal pneumonia
Poliomyelitis
Rabies (vaccine and immune globulin)
Rubella
Tetanus (toxoid and immune globulin)
Tuberculosis (BCG)
Typhoid fever
Varicella-Zoster (immune globulin)
Yellow fever

Notes: 1. Except for the preparations discussed in the text, the use of specific agents should be reserved for individuals who are at special risk.
2. The efficacy of some of these, e.g., BCG, and cholera and typhoid vaccines, is either not proved or known to be modest.

INFLUENZA

Influenza vaccine is recommended for all individuals over 65 years of age and for younger individuals with serious underlying diseases or for those who have a substantial occupational exposure, such as health care workers. The vaccine is a killed virus preparation that is not contraindicated in immunosuppressed individuals. The vaccine is reformulated each year to include virus strains that are believed likely to be prevalent during the ensuing season. Vaccination should be repeated each year, during the autumn or early winter.

The vaccine should not be given to individuals with allergy to eggs. Adverse effects include usually mild local reactions and rare constitutional symptoms.

PNEUMOCOCCAL PNEUMONIA

Pneumococcal vaccine contains antigens for the 23 commonest types of pneumococcus. It is indicated for essentially the same individuals who should receive influenza vaccine, except for health care workers. If possible, it should be administered before splenectomy.

Mild local and systemic side effects occur infrequently. Neither allergy to egg nor immunosuppression are contraindications to immunization. The vaccine should be given only once. Unlike the other vaccines discussed here, revaccination is contraindicated at present. A summary of the contents of this chapter is provided in Table 1.

SYSTEMIC INFECTIONS

FEVER AND RASH

DORI F. ZALEZNIK, M.D.

The presentation of the patient in the emergency room with complaints of fever and rash is common. The dilemma for the clinician is to distinguish among the vast array of diseases with these two presenting signs and to initiate therapy in cases in which immediate action is required. Despite the teaching that the morphology of the lesions provides the best basis for making these distinctions, the appearance of the rash may well be confusing and, in the absence of a constellation of historical and physical findings, may be misleading. A more reliable approach to this clinical problem combines careful history that includes information about others in the community who may have a similar illness, physical examination—with thorough assessment of appearance and extent of the rash—and, often, a diagnostic evaluation. Despite these efforts, the clinician is frequently faced with a diagnosis of exclusion.

For an accurate assessment of fever and rash it is desirable to view as many rashes as possible and to formulate patterns of recognition that suggest the diagnosis. To attempt to provide a framework, this chapter discusses emergency problems that present with fever and rash, essential diagnostic maneuvers, entities with similar presentations that may cause confusion, and diagnostic and therapeutic options that may prove helpful.

SKIN RASHES ASSOCIATED WITH SYSTEMIC ILLNESSES

Five major diagnoses require urgent evaluation and treatment: meningococcemia, Rocky Mountain spotted fever, septic embolic lesion with a major bacteremic episode, toxic shock syndrome, and rapidly spreading cellulitis. Morphology alone does not distinguish any of these rashes from other entities. A series of questions and observation of the lesions provide assistance in making a diagnosis. Table 1 lists some of the most helpful features.

Conventional teaching dictates that petechial and purpuric rashes are of major concern. However, the presentation of the patient with a petechial rash, for example, does not make a diagnosis of meningococcemia. Among the various dangerous illnesses with rashes, meningococcemia is the entity most likely to lead to rapid death of the patient if left unrecognized. Other features, in addition to the appearance of the rash, help in diagnosis. It is not uncommon for a patient with meningococcemia to present with vague symptoms of pharyngitis, low-grade fever, a maculopapular rash, and muscle tenderness. Headache may or may not be prominent. Unlike a rash due to a viral syndrome, however, the rash in meningococcemia progresses rapidly and within hours becomes petechial; these petechiae may coalesce to form large purpuric lesions. Fever then becomes prominent. The change in the character of the lesions and the rapidity of spread are major characteristics of meningococcemia.

In contrast, Rocky Mountain spotted fever, which may result in a rash similar in appearance to the rash of meningococcemia, has several different characteristics. One determining feature of the diagnosis of Rocky Mountain spotted fever is that the rash does not appear at the time of onset of symptoms. Unlike most bacterial and many viral processes, rickettsial diseases, such as Rocky Mountain spotted fever, begin with fever and severe headache, and only days into the illness (mean, 4 days) does a rash appear. The rash of Rocky Mountain spotted fever, which may be petechial at the onset, characteristically begins around the ankles and wrists and progresses centrally. Involvement of the trunk is usually late. Unlike the situation in another tick-borne disease to be discussed below, Lyme disease, patients with Rocky Mountain spotted fever usually are aware of a prior tick bite.

TABLE 1 How to Distinguish Emergency Situations From Other Syndromes

Time course of the rash
- Onset with or after fever
- Change in character of rash (papular changing to petechial lesions are of concern)
- Rapidity of spread or change (faster progression is more worrisome)

Whether the patient has traveled (exposure to ticks, for example)

Epidemiologic setting (other similar disease in the community or isolated case)

Morphology of rash (petechial/purpuric lesions of particular concern)

Extent of lesions (particularly, involvement of palms and soles)

One can see from the examples of meningococcemia and Rocky Mountain spotted fever how distinctions can be drawn in illnesses in which the rashes appear much the same. Individual lesions of disseminated gonorrhea can resemble lesions of meningococcemia. However, prodromal pharyngitis and fever are unusual. The rash of gonorrhea is generally not widespread, but occurs as individual lesions or small clusters, and the patient generally appears less toxic. In addition, the skin manifestations of disseminated gonorrhea generally occur as small petechiae or apparent septic lesions, rather than developing as a maculopapular rash. A pustular or necrotic center may be seen in the lesions of gonococcal bacteremia.

Involvement of the palms and soles in a patient with a rash often signals a worrisome entity such as meningococcemia or Rocky Mountain spotted fever, but several other entities need to be considered. In particular, secondary syphilis characteristically presents with involvement of palms and soles. Syphilitic lesions are maculopapular and usually not petechial. In contrast, a number of viral processes, especially coxsackie A, may present with petechial lesions involving the palms and soles as well as a widespread rash. Patients with viral syndromes may look quite toxic, and the differential diagnosis may well include meningococcemia. In these patients, however, mucous membrane involvement is often prominent, with lesions in the mouth and on the genitalia that may appear to be vesicular. Hand-foot-and-mouth disease, another viral process, can present with similar lesions, but unlike those of coxsackie A, these lesions are not usually petechial.

The rashes in meningococcemia and Rocky Mountain spotted fever are generally widespread. Solitary or widely scattered purplish lesions that do not blanch and often have a slightly necrotic center prompt the clinician to consider the diagnosis of septic embolus associated with bacterial bloodstream infection. The presence of these lesions on the digits is particularly characteristic. Ecthyma gangrenosum is a lesion of this type associated especially with *Pseudomonas aeruginosa* bacteremia, but may be found with other organisms as well. Septic emboli to the skin are particularly common in *Staphylococcus aureus* bacteremia and also in disseminated fungemia caused by *Candida albicans*. Septic peripheral manifestations of subacute bacterial endocarditis, which are not observed as frequently as in the past, may be found in some individuals upon careful examination of the soles of the feet.

Though the likely pathogenesis of many skin lesions associated with bacteremia is a septic embolus, bacteria may not be found in aspirates of the lesion. Nevertheless, this maneuver is useful for diagnosis when results are positive. Insertion of a tuberculin syringe with a 25-gauge needle into the center of the lesion, aspiration, and mixture of any contents with a small volume of sterile saline that is subsequently Gram stained can lead to a rapid diagnosis if bacteria are observed. Another rapid diagnostic approach that can be highly useful in early detection of bacteremia is Gram stain of the buffy coat of the blood. Identification of an organism on a Gram stain of the buffy coat can help to direct early therapy and confirm a clinical suspicion of the bacteremia. In *S. aureus* bacteremia, the urine may also contain the organism. The appearance of large gram-positive cocci, whether or not in clusters, in the urine of a patient thought to have bacteremia should raise the possibility of *S. aureus* as an etiologic agent, since this organism is an unusual find in a urinary tract infection, except in patients who have a urinary catheter in place. Not all solitary lesions with slightly necrotic centers result from a septic embolus, however. Some animal bites, particularly the bite of the brown recluse spider, can appear in this fashion, again making the patient's history and associated physical findings essential.

The relatively newly described entity, toxic shock syndrome (discussed in a separate chapter), is another example of an illness with fever and rash that requires urgent attention. The scarlatiniform rash may be difficult to appreciate, since it will often look like a sunburn, especially on the chest and abdomen. The "strawberry tongue" (also seen in Kawasaki's disease and scarlet fever) is frequently found in toxic shock syndrome, and conjunctival hyperemia is an additional diagnostically helpful finding. The presence of these findings in a patient with hypotension, especially with evidence of multisystem derangement, should raise the diagnostic possibility of toxic shock syndrome. The organism is usually penicillin-resistant and should be eradicated using a beta-lactamase-resistant penicillin.

CELLULITIS

Unlike the other entities discussed thus far in which the appearance of the rash raises a number of diagnostic possibilities, cellulitis is not difficult to identify. In general, cellulitis caused by group A streptococci or *S. aureus* is not difficult to treat with penicillin, for the former, and a semisynthetic penicillin, for the latter; therapy may be administered orally if the disease is not far advanced. An issue of diagnostic concern in cellulitis is whether infection is confined to the surface or whether extension to deeper structures, including fascia and underlying muscle, is present. Mixed synergistic gangrene or a rapidly spreading fasciitis can be life threatening. *Clostridium perfringens* is the single organism most frequently considered to cause this type of infection, particularly when there is gas formation in the tissues. However, a mixture of organisms, particularly anaerobic and aerobic gram-positive cocci and facultative aerobic gram-negative rods, is the more likely etiology. Radiologic examination of the soft tissues will often show gas formation. If present or if a deeper infection is suspected, surgical exploration is necessary to define the deepest structure infected. Wide surgical debridement is necessary if muscle or fascia is involved. As with aspiration of a septic embolic lesion, aspiration of the margin of advancing cellulitis with a tuberculin syringe, or even an injection of a small amount of nonbacteriostatic saline into the margin of involved skin and subsequent aspiration, may yield fluid for Gram stain. If an organism is observed on Gram stain, therapy may be tailored to cover this bacterium. Failure to appreciate an organism is not helpful, but the procedure requires little time and may limit use of toxic antibiotics if results are positive.

Diabetics are a subset of patients in whom the treatment of cellulitis and ulcers merits special attention. In these hosts, unusual organisms, such as aerobic gram-negative rods, and anaerobes, such as *Bacteroides fragilis* are encountered in addition to aerobic gram-positive organisms. Surface swabs yielding organisms from the base of an ulcer, for example, may not reflect the underlying pathogen. If a diabetic with cellulitis or a foot ulcer fails to respond to apparently adequate therapy, further diagnostic evaluation with biopsy and culture of tissue for aerobes and anaerobes is warranted. In the case of an ulcer, it may also be necessary to evaluate the patient for underlying osteomyelitis.

DIAGNOSTIC DILEMMAS

The entities most often confused with fever and rash due to a bacterial cause are noninfectious diseases, such as drug eruptions or vasculitis, and viral exanthems. These diagnoses, particularly drug eruptions, must always enter into the differential diagnosis, since the morphology of lesions varies widely. There is virtually no rash with which a patient presents that could not be attributed to a drug. Rashes range from the classic maculopapular, widespread eruption that is characteristic of a drug rash to pustular and even vesicular or bullous eruptions. Patients may present with high fever and may even look quite toxic. Since therapy of a drug rash is quite different from therapy of bacteremia, for instance, it is always important to elicit a history of recent medications. Even if the patient has been taking a medication for a substantial period, it is possible that a rash could be due to this drug.

Viral exanthems also can be wide ranging in appearance, although the commonest presentation is a maculopapular eruption. In general, these patients appear less toxic, and rash is almost always apparent at the time of presentation. Infectious mononucleosis caused by Epstein-Barr virus is a notable exception in which rash often appears following ampicillin therapy. These patients may mistakenly be diagnosed as allergic to ampicillin. The mechanism of the development of this common rash is unclear. Though patients with viral illness may be febrile at the time of presentation, it is distinctly uncommon for rash and fever to linger for more than 3 or 4 days. Viral cultures may help to confirm a diagnosis, but these cultures are costly and results not rapidly available. Therefore, clinical diagnosis is not substantially enhanced by such cultures.

Vasculitis of the skin is recognizable morphologically, but determination of the cause of the rash—whether systemic collagen vascular disease or other systemic process—requires further assessment. In particular, for suspected vasculitis or drug eruptions, skin biopsy often can be diagnostic and should be performed.

Despite all of the previous caveats, there are certain instances in which the morphology of the rash helps to focus differential diagnosis. Petechial lesions, though not exclusive to a single entity, as discussed above, do help to narrow diagnostic possibilities. In addition, nodular lesions strongly favor other diagnostic categories, including mycobacterial disease, fungal disease, tumors such as Kaposi's sarcoma (now seen more commonly in patients with AIDS), and parasitic disease. These lesions generally arise over time, and travel history, exposure history, or some other helpful historical information may be elicited from the patient. Nodules virtually always need to be biopsied for firm diagnosis, and since onset is generally subacute, treatment may be delayed until a diagnosis is made.

Several other rashes are morphologically characteristic, but the entities are associated with a number of infectious and noninfectious causes. Erythema nodosum, which appears as painful, tender, red nodules mainly confined to the shins, is associated with a wide variety of other disease. A partial differential diagnostic list includes tuberculosis, fungal processes such as histoplasmosis or coccidioidomycosis, yersiniosis, beta-hemolytic streptococcal infection, lymphogranuloma venereum, or noninfectious causes such as sarcoidosis, inflammatory bowel disease, or drug therapy with antibiotics (notably, sulfonamides and penicillin) and with oral contraceptives. An entity known as nodular liquefying panniculitis, which is associated with pancreatitis, may be confused with erythema nodosum. These lesions are generally tender but movable, commoner on the legs (but not necessarily the shins), and may be more widespread. Associated laboratory abnormalities such as abnormal amylase or lipase may be helpful, and biopsy is quite distinct, with fat necrosis present in new nodules.

Erythema multiforme, characteristically presenting as target lesions that are often found on the palms, is also associated with a wide range of other diseases. Usually, no etiology or associated disease is clear in a patient presenting with erythema multiforme. However, it is common to see this skin disease with herpes viral or other viral infections, mycoplasmal infection, or in patients taking certain drugs, such as penicillin, sulfonamides, dilantin, and barbiturates.

Another characteristic rash that may or may not be associated with fever is erythema chronicum migrans, which is found in patients with Lyme disease. This rash has large erythematous lesions, often having serpiginous borders and marked central clearing, and may start surrounding a small nodular lesion at the site of a tick bite. It occurs after the bite of a tick, which is small and brown in color. Patients, therefore, may not be able to provide a history of a bite. This disease, caused by a newly described spirochete, is important to recognize. Treatment with tetracycline or penicillin during the stage of the skin rash has been shown to limit extracutaneous later manifestations, such as arthritis or cardiac or neurologic manifestations.

DIAGNOSTIC OPTIONS

A number of diagnostic options are available for evaluation of patients with rash and fever. The easiest initial approach is aspirating the lesion. This procedure is simple and cannot be harmful to the patient. Negative results, however, are not diagnostic. Since the object of aspirating a lesion is to see bacteria on Gram stain, the settings of a possible septic lesion or cellulitis are the most helpful circumstances in which to perform this procedure. Skin biopsies, which can be performed rapidly but will not have results available to assist with immediate management, are most helpful in differentiating noninfectious from infectious causes of rash and fever. Drug reactions and vasculitis are most easily distinguished with this procedure. In addition, tumors of the skin and other subacute infectious causes of rash may be appreciated on skin biopsy. If the differential diagnosis is between bacteremia and vasculitis, antibiotic therapy may need to be initiated while the results of a skin biopsy are awaited.

Several adjunctive tests are essential in evaluating patients with fever and rash. Blood cultures are crucial for diseases with septic emboli to the skin; these include subacute bacterial endocarditis, meningococcemia, and gonococcemia. Blood cultures obviously are very helpful even if negative. Gram stain of the buffy coat has been mentioned as a helpful tool for rapid diagnosis of bacteremia, but only if positive. A cervical swab with Gram stain can be helpful in making a diagnosis of gonorrhea or of toxic shock syndrome. Viral cultures, though confirmatory of a diagnosis of a viral process, are not helpful in acute diagnosis and management and tend to be costly.

Though diagnostic tools are available and helpful, there is no substitute for careful history and physical examination in the evaluation and management of patients with the common presenting findings of fever and rash.

FEVER AND LYMPHADENOPATHY

GERALD H. FRIEDLAND, M.D.

The logical evaluation of a patient with fever and lymphadenopathy requires that four questions be answered:

1. Is the adenopathy local or generalized?
2. Is the process acute or chronic?
3. Is the etiology infectious or noninfectious?
4. Is there a primary peripheral lesion?

To answer the first question a thorough physical examination of all accessible major lymph-node-bearing areas should be performed. These include the nodes of the head and neck, the axillary, epitrochlear, and inguinal nodes. Radiologic studies are necessary to define the two other clinically important major node-bearing areas: the mediastinum and hilum of the lung and the retroperitoneum. The somewhat arbitrary period of one month separates acute and chronic lymphadenopathy in adults. In children, a period of two or three months is more reasonable. Although they are less common, noninfectious etiologies should be considered in puzzling cases, and in localized lymphadenopathy, a primary lesion should always be sought. See Figure 1 for an overview of guidelines to the differential diagnosis of fever and lymphadenopathy.

GENERALIZED LYMPHADENOPATHY

Generalized lymphadenopathy is present if nodes in two or more noncontiguous major lymph-node-bearing areas are enlarged.

Acute generalized infectious lymphadenopathy is most commonly viral and rarely bacterial in origin. Generalized lymph node enlargement is a constant feature of many of the common viral infections of childhood, including rubella, measles, and varicella. It may be present during the prodromal period in hepatitis A and B and is a common feature of infectious mononucleosis, cytomegalovirus mononucleosis, toxoplasmosis, and enteroviral infections as well. In all of these infections the nodes are typically tender, discrete, firm to touch, and without fluctuance. The tenderness and enlargement as well as the fever gradually subside over a period of days to a few weeks without specific therapy.

Acute generalized noninfectious lymphadenopathy is frequently due to hypersensitivity reactions, most commonly drug-induced. Among those agents known to cause fever and lymphadenopathy are the sulfonamides, hydralazine, and phenytoin. The syndrome rapidly disappears with the withdrawal of the drug. Collagen-vascular diseases, including rheumatoid arthritis and systemic lupus erythematosus, may be causes of acute generalized lymphadenopathy and fever. The mucocutaneous lymph node syndrome (Kawasaki's disease) a disease of uncertain origin, must be considered in children with lymphadenopathy, fever, mucosal inflammation, and peripheral rash with desquamation.

Chronic generalized infectious lymphadenopathy is much less commonly encountered but raises more serious diagnostic possibilities. If the fever and lymphadenopathy have been present for a month or longer in adults and three months in children, viral etiologic agents become unlikely. Disseminated bacterial and fungal diseases must be considered including tuberculosis, syphilis, histoplasmosis, cryptococcosis, and coccidiomycosis. The lymph nodes are firmer than those in cases of acute infection and there may be fusion and matting of adjacent nodes. Infection with HTLV III/LAV virus is associated with chronic generalized lymphadenopathy. When present in association with characteristic immuno-

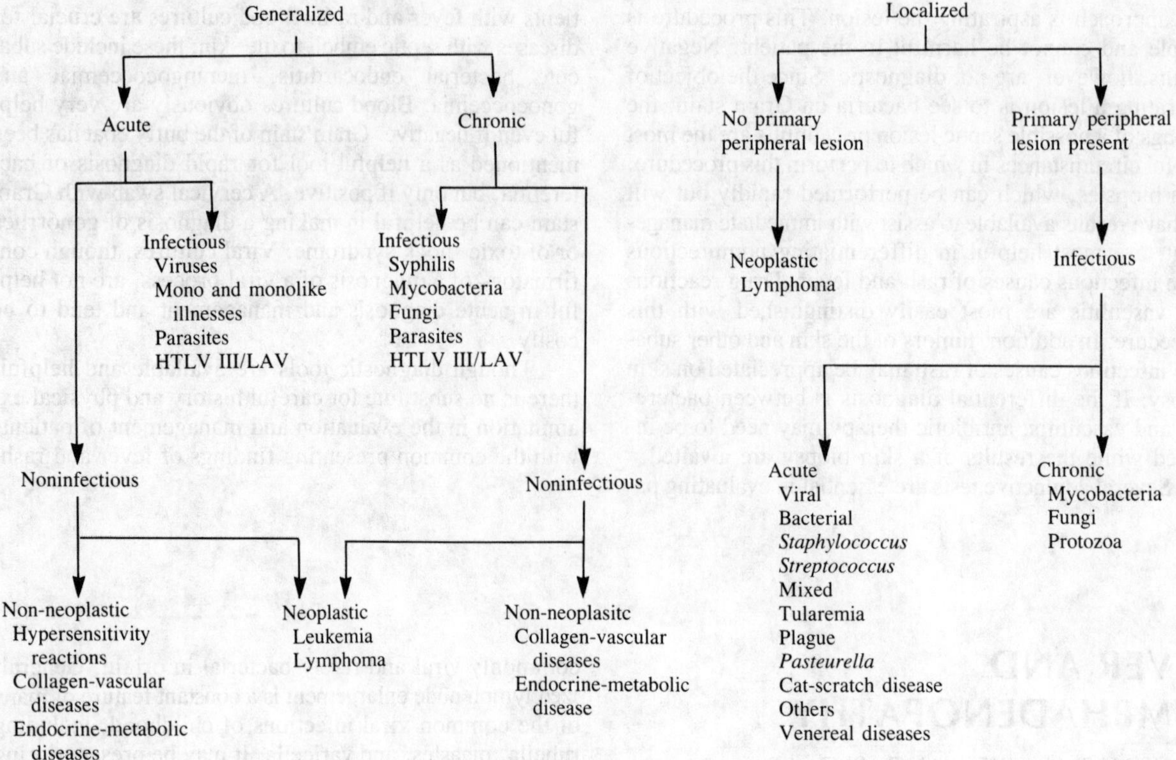

Figure 1 Differential diagnostic scheme for fever and lymphadenopathy

logic abnormalities, the term AIDS-*related complex* or ARC is used.

Chronic generalized noninfectious lymphadenopathy is most often neoplastic in origin. Lymphoreticular neoplasms (Hodgkin's disease, lymphosarcoma, chronic lymphatic leukemia) predominate. In patients with neoplastic generalized lymphadenopathy, fever may be due either to the underlying malignant process or to secondary infection. This is always a difficult clinical situation, made increasingly so by the frequency with which such patients' host defenses are altered by chemotherapy, radiotherapy, or immunosuppressive agents. Infrequently, hyperthyroidism may present with generalized lymphadenopathy and signs and symptoms suggesting infection.

AIDS

The recently described acquired immunodeficiency syndrome must be considered in patients with chronic weight loss, malaise, fever, generalized lymphadenopathy, and lymphopenia. Such patients typically are homosexual men, intravenous drug abusers, recipients of multiple transfusions or clotting factors, or heterosexual partners of individuals in the above groups. Oral candidiasis is often encountered. An immunopathy consisting of depressed T helper/inducer cells, cutaneous anergy, and hypergammaglobulinemia is found. By definition, these patients have life-threatening opportunistic infections and/or Kaposi's sarcoma (see AIDS chapter).

Lastly, hyperthyroidism may present with generalized lymphadenopathy and signs and symptoms suggesting infection.

LOCALIZED LYMPHADENOPATHY

Localized lymphadenopathy is present if not more than two contiguous lymph-node-bearing areas are involved. Anatomically and clinically the local node-bearing areas are divided into five major groups: the nodes of the head and neck, the axilla, the inguinal area, the mediastinal-hilar areas, and the retroperitoneal para-aortic nodes. The physician again must consider both infectious and noninfectious etiologic agents. A further question will help distinguish between these categories: Is there a primary peripheral lesion?

Noninfectious local adenopathy is not associated with a primary peripheral lesion. The most likely cause is lymphoproliferative neoplasm, particularly if the lymphadenopathy is chronic.

Infectious local adenopathy is usually associated with a primary peripheral lesion and requires an appreciation of the anatomic areas which each nodal area drains. The evaluation of localized lymphadenopathy should always include a thorough examination of these areas. In the following sections each nodal area will be discussed separately, with particular reference to those infections that are most characteristic in each area. This is a convenient separation but is somewhat artificial, since many of the infections discussed may present in any of the anatomic sites. Any regional group of nodes may be involved in a disease producing generalized lymphadenopathy, and it is worth stressing again that careful examination of other areas is always indicated.

The lymph nodes of the head and neck can be further divided into several more local anatomic and clinical areas.

The *occipital* and *posterior auricular* nodes drain large areas of the scalp and face, and drain in turn into the posterior and inferior cervical nodes. Careful examination of the scalp is essential when these nodes are enlarged. A small primary lesion may be overlooked when the hair is thick. In children, secondarily infected insect, tick or spider bites and ringworm are common causes. Posterior auricular and occipital adenopathy is a feature of many acute viral illnesses.

The *anterior auricular* nodes drain the eyelids, the palpebral conjunctivae, the external auditory meatus, and the pinna. Primary infections in these sites must be sought in patients with involvement of these nodes. A large number of organisms have been reported to produce the "oculoglandular syndrome" (conjunctivitis and anterior auricular adenopathy) by direct inoculation of the conjunctiva, including the gonococcus *Francisella tularensis*, the presumed agent of cat-scratch fever and epidemic keratoconjunctivitis.

The *"tonsillar," submaxillary, and submental* nodes drain the tonsils and other structures of the pharynx and mouth and as such are of great clinical significance. Involvement of these nodes requires careful inspection and often palpation of the mouth, teeth, and pharynx. The "tonsillar" nodes belong to the superior deep cervical node group and lie below the angle of the mandible. They drain the posterior and lateral pharynx, including the tonsils. The submaxillary nodes lie within the submaxillary fascial compartment, surrounded by the deep cervical fascia. Some of the nodes are imbedded within the submaxillary gland and are often indistinct on palpation even in acute infections. This important group of nodes drains the lateral margins of the tongue, the gums, the angle of the mouth and cheek, the lateral part of the lower lip and the entire upper lip, and the medial aspect of the conjunctiva. They are commonly involved in dental infections, and they, in turn, drain into the deep cervical nodes. The submental nodes drain the floor of the mouth, the tip of the tongue, the central part of the lower lip, and the skin of the chin. They drain into the submaxillary nodes and are also commonly involved in dental infections.

The *posterior cervical* nodes are located in the occipital triangle of the neck above the inferior belly of the omohyoid muscle and posterior to the sternomastoid. They are commonly involved in scalp infections and are often prominently involved in the generalized lymphadenopathy of infectious mononucleosis and monolike syndromes. Involvement of these nodes is highly unlikely in localized infections of the mouth and pharynx.

The *inferior deep cervical nodes* lie below the level of the inferior belly of the omohyoid muscle and both posterior (the supraclavicular nodes) and anterior (the scalene nodes) to the sternomastoid muscle. Those nodes receive drainage from the scalp, the superior deep cervical nodes, the axillary nodes, and also from the nodes of the hilum of the lung, mediastinum, and abdominal viscera. Their enlargement may signify primary disease at any of these distant sites. Adenopathy in this area not readily palpable may be detected by performance of the Valsalva maneuver.

Acute cervical adenopathy is most likely to be of pyogenic bacterial or viral origin. Staphylococci and streptococci predominate among bacterial etiologic agents, the former from primary skin sites and the latter from oral and dental infections. Infections of the tonsils, pharynx and skin are the most frequent primary sites in children, whereas dental infections more commonly result in cervical adenopathy in adults. Appreciation of the primary site of infection, as well as aspiration, Gram stain, and culture of fluctuant or grossly enlarged and tender nodes are of therapeutic as well as diagnostic importance. Penicillin is prescribed in those infections of oral and dental origin. A semisynthetic penicillinase-resistant penicillin is used when the primary site of infection is in the skin. Rupture of cervical nodes into their fascial spaces may additionally require surgical drainage if there is fluctuance, impingement on vital structures, or both.

Chronic cervical adenopathy raises the possibility of granulomatous infections, particularly *Mycobacterium tuberculosis* and atypical mycobacterial infection. Toxoplasmosis may cause chronic cervical lymphadenopathy, particularly involving the posterior cervical nodes.

The importance of histologic as well as microbiologic diagnosis in all chronic infections, as well as the need to exclude lymphoproliferative neoplasm, require that surgical excision of an entire intact node be carried out in cases of chronic cervical lymphadenopathy. More specific indications for surgical excision will be discussed later in this chapter.

The *mediastinal and hilar nodes* are rarely involved in acute suppurative disease. The structures drained include the lungs, pleura, and mediastinal contents. Of particular importance diagnostically is the continuity of these nodes with the inferior deep cervical nodes (supraclavicular and scalene groups) and axillary nodes, since these represent an accessible area for both examination and biopsy. Biopsy at this site in the presence of intrathoracic disease may yield a diagnosis in from 30 percent to 80 percent of selected cases. Anatomically, the drainage remains on the homolateral side except for the left lower lobe, where drainage is to both lateral nodal areas via the interbronchial nodes. Since the nodes within the thorax and their drainage areas are not readily accessible to direct examination, more indirect methods must be used to elicit a diagnosis. In addition to the history and general physical examination, the radiologic characteristics or absence of coexistent pulmonary lesions and examination of sputum are of obvious importance. The differential diagnosis of hilar and mediastinal adenopathy most frequently includes granulomatous disease of both infectious and uncertain origin (sarcoidosis) and lymphoproliferative disorders. In the former, *M. tuberculosis* and fungal disease predominate. In these infections, adenopathy is almost always unilateral—a useful differential diagnostic point. Bilateral hilar adenopathy is present in approximately three-fourths of patients with sarcoidosis and in 10 percent of cases of lymphoma. Looked at from another perspective, 90 percent of patients presenting with bilateral hilar adenopathy have sarcoidosis and only 10 percent have neoplastic disease. Additionally, in the absence of constitutional symptoms or peripheral adenopathy, bilateral hilar adenopathy is almost always caused by sarcoid. Transbronchial lung biopsy, inferior cervical node biopsy, or both are indicated in most patients with hilar adenopathy. Mycobacterial skin tests, sputum examination, cultures, and sputum cytology are also indicated.

Finally, it is worth noting that systemic lupus erythematosus and other collagen-vascular diseases may present with hilar adenopathy.

The *axillary nodes* drain the entire upper extremity as well as the lateral parts of the chest wall, back, and the breast. This cluster of nodes is most frequently involved in acute pyogenic infections of these drainage areas. Careful examination of the readily accessible and often obvious primary site is essential. By far the most common organisms involved are the staphylococcus and streptococcus, often associated with primary areas of cellulitis, lymphangitis, or furunculosis. The upper extremity and axillary nodes may be involved by many additional infecting organisms.

Several zoonoses (discussed in detail in other chapters) should be considered in the appropriate epidemiologic setting. Tularemia, transmitted by bite or skin contact with wild rodents, is seen most frequently in hunters and butchers. Aspiration of nodes and serologic testing will confirm the diagnosis. Agents of choice include tetracycline, chloramphenicol, and streptomycin. Plague must be considered in the southwestern United States where transmission still occurs. Aspiration of nodes should be carried out. Giemsa stain of aspirated material demonstrates the characteristic safety pin appearance of plump rodlike organisms. The organism can be cultured from buboes and blood on routine culture media. Treatment with streptomycin, tetracycline or chloramphenicol should be instituted upon suspicion of the disease.

Pasteurella multocida infections are common following cat and dog bites and scratches. The infection presents with a lesion at the primary site, lymphatitis and/or cellulitis, and tender regional adenopathy. Gram stain of the primary lesion of draining aspirated nodes reveals characteristic gram-negative coccobacillary organisms that are easily cultured. Penicillin is the drug of choice.

Cat-scratch disease may present as lymphadenopathy and fever. The diagnosis is made on the basis of history of cat contact; a papule at the inoculation site; tender regional lymphadenopathy that is often fluctuant, draining, and shows granulomatous inflammation on biopsy; and the exclusion of other definable etiologic agents. There is no specific treatment.

Inguinal lymphadenopathy is commonly encountered clinically. The inguinal nodes drain not only the lower extremities, but the lower abdominal wall, the genitalia, perineum, and perianal area as well. Careful examination of all the drainage areas is essential to a thorough evaluation of inguinal adenopathy, including a careful pelvic and rectal examination if other areas of primary infection are not apparent. Acute pyogenic bacterial infection is most common, usually caused by the same organisms enumerated in the discussion of axillary adenopathy. The drainage of the perineum and perianal area suggests the possibility that enteric aerobic gram-negative organisms and gram-positive and gram-negative anaerobic organisms may be present. Because of the drainage of the genitalia, venereal infections often involve the inguinal nodes. Those likely to present with prominent inguinal adenopathy are syphilis, lymphogranuloma venereum, chancroid, and herpes progenitalis. The appearance of the primary lesion is useful in distinguishing among these entities.

The *abdominal and retroperitoneal nodes* drain the abdominal viscera and retroperitoneal and pelvic organs and may receive drainage from the inguinal nodes as well. Neither the nodes nor the primary site of infection are directly clinically accessible, making assessment difficult. Radiologic procedures must be employed for evaluation, including the intravenous pyelogram, lymphangiogram, and CT scan. Although the nodes are involved in acute intra-abdominal systemic infections, the possibility of chronic infections, particularly tuberculosis, and of lymphoproliferative disorders involving them is the usual reason for using these diagnostic tools.

GENERAL DIAGNOSTIC APPROACHES

Indirect

In most cases of infectious and non-neoplastic lymphadenopathy with fever, the diagnosis is apparent on the bases of the history and the extranodal features of the illness on examination. This is particularly true of lymphadenopathy of less than 1 month's duration. Other clinical and laboratory findings short of biopsy often suggest the etiologic agent in the enlarged nodes. Some of these findings are:

1. Primary site of infection—clinically apparent and characteristic; streptococcal cellulitis, staphylococcal furuncle, syphilitic chancre, and so on.
2. Characteristic rash—rubella, rubeola, varicella-zoster, secondary syphilis, drug eruption, oral candidiasis.
3. Typical hematologic findings—atypical lymphocytes in mononucleosis and monolike illnesses, eosinophilia in drug hypersensitivity reactions.
4. Skin tests—tuberculosis and atypical mycobacterial disease, lymphogranuloma venereum, tularemia.
5. Serologic tests—infectious mononucleosis and mono-

like illnesses (cytomegalovirus and toxoplasmosis), hepatitis, syphilis, tularemia, fungal infections.
6. Stains and culture of material from peripheral primary lesions and pulmonary lesions—acute pyogenic infections, including staphylococci, streptococci, tularemia, plague, *P. multocida*, herpes simplex, chancroid, mycobacteria, fungi.
7. Radiologic appearance of primary sites, particularly the character of pulmonary infiltrate.

Direct

Although the diagnosis is often apparent by the methods noted above, careful evaluation of enlarged nodes is always indicated.

1. The physical characteristics of nodes often reveal important information: discrete, tender, firm nodes that are acutely enlarged suggest acute bacterial or viral infections. Chronic firm and rubbery nodes are characteristic of lymphoproliferative diseases and granulomatous infections. Matted, fluctuant nodes suggest the presence of pyogenic organisms. Hard, fixed nodes are characteristic of carcinoma.
2. Aspiration of fluctuant but nondraining nodes in palpable areas is a simple and valuable diagnostic technique that is not carried out as frequently as it is indicated. Aspirated material should be stained (Gram, Giemsa, acid-fast) and cultured for all suspected pathogens.
3. Excision of a lymph node or lymph node biopsy is usually carried out to distinguish between chronic infection and neoplasm. The indications for lymph node biopsy are often vague. The following general guidelines are intended to suggest to the clinician circumstances in which biopsy is appropriate:

Indications for Lymph Node Biopsy

1. Undiagnosed chronic lymphadenopathy (of more than 1 month's duration in adults, 3 month's in children).
2. Localized lymphadenopathy without an accessible or apparent peripheral lesion.
3. Enlarging, undiagnosed lymphadenopathy, after two weeks of observation.
4. Nontender, matted to hard lymphadenopathy.
5. Systemic signs and symptoms suggesting granulomatous or lymphoproliferative disease (prolonged fever, sweats, weight loss, fatigue).
6. Radiologic findings suggesting granulomatous disease.
7. Positive tuberculin test.
8. New adenopathy in immunocompromised patients.
9. Clinical or epidemiologic suspicion of acquired immunodeficiency syndrome.
10. Lymphadenopathy in the setting of fever of undetermined etiology.

Technique of Lymph Node Biopsy

Approximately half of lymph node biopsies lead to a specific diagnosis. All too frequently, excision of abnormal lymph nodes does not reveal the diagnosis because of technical errors. Careful attention to several rules maximizes the usefulness of this invasive diagnostic procedure.

1. Consider all of the diagnostic possibilities before performing surgey and make appropriate arrangements for the handling of the excised tissue.
2. Select the best site. Lymph nodes that are frequently involved in common minor inflammatory processes should be avoided, as they may show only nonspecific chronic inflammatory changes or fibrosis. In the presence of generalized lymphadenopathy the inferior or posterior cervical nodes are preferred. The submandibular nodes should be avoided. The axillary nodes are the next best and the inguinal nodes, except in the presence of localized adenopathy in this area, are least likely to provide a diagnosis.
3. Select the best node—the most superficial and accessible node is not necessarily the most desirable or diagnostic node. The biopsy area should be carefully explored and the largest node in a cluster of enlarged nodes should be removed.
4. Remove the node or several nodes in their entirety with their capsules intact. Bisect the nodes, sending half of the specimen to the pathology laboratory and the other half to the bacteriology laboratory for stains and culturing of common pathogens, *M. tuberculosis*, fungi, and other suspected organisms.
5. Request that the pathologist make additional sections of the tissue excised if the node is abnormal but not diagnostic.
6. Consider a repeat biopsy and the excision of more tissue if the node is abnormal but not diagnostic and the clinical picture is unclear.

Interpretation of Lymph Node Biopsy

The interested reader will find detailed histological descriptions elsewhere. Entities discussed in this chapter for which a characteristic histologic pattern exists and for which a specific or strongly suggestive diagnosis can be made histologically are lymphoma and other neoplasms, tuberculosis, fungal diseases, sarcoidosis, toxoplasmosis, acquired immunodeficiency syndrome, and cat-scratch disease. Most noninfectious, nonneoplastic disorders will show nonspecific lymphadenitis or hyperplasia only, as will most acute viral infections. However, it is important to note that a signficant number of patients with initially nondiagnostic lymph node biopsies and persistent lymphadenopathy will ultimately prove to have a serious underlying disease. If the biopsy is not initially diagnostic it is essential to follow the patient carefully and to consider repeat biopsy if adenopathy persists.

INFECTION IN PREGNANCY

DAVID CHARLES, M.D.
BRYAN LARSEN, PH.D.

In this survey of the infectious diseases that affect the gravid host, emphasis will be placed on systemic infections that present unique problems because of the pregnancy. It is probable that the gravid patient is susceptible to any infectious disease, but some of these complicate the pregnancy by threatening the baby in utero (often without the mother becoming seriously ill). Moreover, some infectious processes, although not posing a direct threat to the baby, are associated with premature delivery. Table 1 contains a summary of these infections.

A further topic addressed in this chapter is antimicrobial therapy inasmuch as the pregnant patient is characterized by pharmacodynamic and pharmacokinetic differences from the nonpregnant individual. The potential toxicity of chemotherapeutic agents to the fetus is of concern to the physician who must prescribe them during pregnancy.

VIRAL INFECTIONS DURING PREGNANCY

The deleterious potential of viral infections for the conceptus has been a major stimulus to research and has resulted in the incorporation of a series of immunologic tests into the routine assessment of the mother prior to pregnancy. Assessment of the pregnant patient for susceptibility to rubella is now standard. Other viral infections may be similarly evaluated in the gravid patient in the future. The possibility that specific viral infections may be more severe in pregnant women than among those who are not pregnant, coupled with the fact that the unborn child may be especially liable to damage by infectious agents that cross the placenta, emphasizes the importance of detecting viral infections encountered during the gravid state.

Infections responsible for perinatal mortality and morbidity may be acquired by the embryo without eliciting symptoms in the mother, but the conceptus may experience significant damage. Many viral diseases have been associated with spontaneous abortion. It should be noted that spontaneous abortion may result from the fever associated with such infections.

Approximately 20 percent of perinatal deaths are ascribed to congenital malformations; however, the identification of viral teratogens is not simple since retrospective studies may be unable to establish that infection definitely did occur, especially if the infection was subclinical. Prospective studies demand a great number of cases to provide consequential data. Congenital anomalies can, however, be correlated with the stage of gestation at which the infection was acquired.

Many prenatally acquired maternal viral infections appear to have no deleterious effect on the mother or fetus. Viral agents for which a teratogenic role is established include rubella virus, herpesvirus group, mumps virus, influenza viruses, coxsackievirus, cytomegalovirus, and Venezuelan equine encephalitis virus. Not every encounter with one of these viral agents during pregnancy results in fetal infection. Other viruses are of interest, but, as yet, they have not been assigned any embryopathic role.

Possible long-term effects of intrauterine viral infection not apparent at birth are now beginning to be documented. The congenital rubella syndrome may not manifest itself until late childhood when the child develops diabetes and has abnormal dermatoglyphics. Congenital cytomegaloviral infection may be responsible for hearing defects—originally ascribed to hypoxia—as well as some cases of mental retardation discernible only when the children enter school.

Rubella is one of the few congenital infections for which an estimate of the relative risk for congenital damage has been assigned following exposure to the virus at a given gestational age. Generally, the earlier in pregnancy the infection occurs, the greater the risk of detrimental effects to the fetus. In contrast, infection with herpesvirus hominis is likely to cause greater damage, particularly to the central nervous system, when it is acquired late in pregnancy or during parturition. Since no antiviral agent is approved for use during pregnancy, the preven-

TABLE 1 Infectious Complications of Pregnancy That Have Fetal Sequelae

Infection	*Maternal Consequence*	*Fetal Consequence*
Viral		
Influenza	Moderate to severe respiratory infection	Prematurity (?)
Hepatitis	Possibly more severe than in nonpregnant patient	Prematurity (?)
Cytomegalovirus	Mild febrile illness or no symptoms	Congenital infection
Rubella	Mild illness with rash	Congenital rubella syndrome with multisystem damage
Genital herpes	Genital lesions	Neonatal infection may be severe or fatal
Bacterial		
Syphilis	Primary or secondary lesions or no symptoms	Possibly abortion if acquired early or stigmata of congenital disease if acquired late
Listeriosis	Mild febrile illness associated with bacteremia	Abortion or stillbirth
Group B *Streptococcus*	Intrapartum vaginal colonization, postpartum endometritis	Congenital infection, lung, CSF infection
Gonorrhea	Endocervical infection, possibly disseminated gonococcal infection	Possibly premature delivery; neonatal opthalmia
Normal vaginal flora	No untoward maternal intrapartum effect, postpartum	Chorioamnionitis; neonatal septicemia, pneumonia
Pneumonia	More severe in gravid than nongravid patient	May prevent carriage to term

tion of rubella by testing for susceptibility and protecting the susceptible host by vaccination, where feasible, should be undertaken before pregnancy.

Attenuated viral vaccines are potentially harmful for the fetus despite the lack of any adverse effects upon the mother. For this reason, pregnancy is a contraindication for rubella vaccination. Rubella vaccine is unusual among immunogenic agents in that the major purpose for its introduction was for the protection of a future conceptus. The live-attenuated virus can be transferred across the placenta, but its effects on the fetus have not been determined. The duration of protection from rubella vaccination has not been established and consequently all patients who have not been recently vaccinated should be tested for susceptibility at their initial prenatal visit.

Additional live viral vaccines that are contraindicated in pregnancy are: trivalent oral poliomyelitis, mumps, rubella, yellow fever, and vaccinia. There is no indication at present for smallpox immunization.

Adverse effects ascribed to other live viral vaccines may be unpredictable and idiosyncratic. Such a reaction is illustrated by the recipients of swine influenza vaccine who developed the Guillain-Barré syndrome. This complication may be associated with vaccines other than the swine influenza preparation. Currently, vaccines are not available for varicella-zoster, herpesvirus hominis, or cytomegalovirus. The overriding concern centers on the neurotropic nature of these agents and their possible association with carcinogenesis.

Influenza vaccination should be offered to the gravid patient if the pregnancy includes a period of high influenza activity. The gravid patient may experience more severe symptoms of influenza than the nonpregnant individual. Moreoever, the influenza virus may exert adverse effects on the fetus as a result of transplacental infection. Vaccination of pregnant women is desirable, but only an inactivated vaccine should be used.

PROTOZOAL INFECTIONS

The incidence of protozoal infections during pregnancy and the relative importance of these infections as causes of fetal loss and perinatal disease remain to be determined. The risk of such pregnancy complications is dependent on geographic location and the population group being considered. Maternal infection with any species causing human malaria may result in congenital malaria.

Another common protozoal infection capable of causing congenital infection is toxoplasmosis. The reader is referred to the chapter *Toxoplasmosis* for additional information. Congenital infection has also been reported from Chagas' disease because of the transplacental transmission of *Trypanosoma cruzi*. This organism may produce hepatosplenomegaly, fetal hydrops, jaundice, seizure disorders, and cataracts. The frequency of such complications is unknown. Other protozoal infections in pregnancy may also have a deleterious effect on the fetus.

BACTERIAL INFECTIONS

It is difficult to define the incidence of bacterial infections in pregnancy, but they are a major cause of morbidity and severe illness in the gravid patient. Although the fetal risk of transplacental bacterial infection is not known, serious perinatal bacterial illnesses can result from ascending infections. Comprehensive studies of stillbirths and early neonatal deaths have shown that about one-third are associated with chorioamnionitis, and it is recognized that many bacteria encountered by the fetus during the second stage of labour—during its passage through the birth canal—can cause serious disease. Maternal genitourinary bacterial infections are recognized as a major danger to the preterm infant and contribute in large measure to neonatal morbidity and mortality.

Among the most significant systemic infections that threaten the well-being of mother and fetus during pregnancy are syphilis and listeriosis. Although these are encountered relatively infrequently in the United States, they pose a serious threat to the fetus, and prenatal care should include consideration of these diseases. Serologic testing for syphilis is a mandatory part of prenatal care, and satisfactory outcome is possible only if adequate treatment of the disease is prescribed.

Listeriosis represents a challenging problem during pregnancy primarily because the disease is usually a mild, albeit bacteremic, illness in the mother that usually does not generate concern. The physician must therefore be responsible for suspecting listeriosis, especially if the patient has an influenza-like syndrome and provides a history of contact with animals or animal products. In addition it should be noted that *Borrelia* and *Leptospira* may cause febrile illness and fetal infection, although these infections are rarely encountered in gravid patients.

An emerging problem is that of campylobacteriosis. Awareness of this disease process is beginning to develop, and, as a result, complications of pregnancy are now being recognized. A recent case, which consisted of maternal fever and chills accompanied by diarrhea, resulted in the delivery of a 900-g infant 2 weeks after the initial maternal symptoms. The mother had not consumed unpasteurized milk products, but did have a positive vaginal culture for the organism. Obstetricians and pediatricians will need to be aware that more cases of campylobacteriosis in pregnancy are likely to emerge.

URINARY TRACT INFECTION AND PYELONEPHRITIS

Urinary tract infections are among the commonest complications of pregnancy, and in former years, fulminant upper urinary tract infections were frequently associated with endotoxic shock. Since the introduction of antimicrobial agents, however, this complication is infrequently encountered. Much interest has been generated in the relationship of bacteriuria to obstetric complications. The realization that significant bacteriuria can occur in the absence of symptoms or signs of urinary tract infection and is encountered in at least 5 percent of all gravid patients has resulted in a better understanding of urinary tract infections associated with the gravid state.

The occurrence of asymptomatic bacteriuria in pregnancy is now recognized as a condition requiring therapy because in the absence of appropriate therapy, one-third of such patients will develop overt pyelonephritis. In many instances the bacteriuria antedates the gestation and, in fact, is probably no more frequent in the gravid than in the nongravid state. Furthermore, the vast majority of gravid women with asymptomatic bacteriuria can be identified by routine use of urine culture at the initial prenatal visit. Screening of prenatal patients has been facilitated by the availability of relatively inexpensive methods for the detectin of significant bacterial growth. The finding of more than 100,000 organisms per milliliter in a clean voided specimen of urine represents significant bacteriuria and, thereby, identifies individuals who require treatment.

Asymptomatic bacteriuria is observed in at least 2 percent of women. This fact justifies the routine prenatal screening of all patients and treatment of bacteriurics if clinically overt pyelonephritis is to be effectively prevented. This strategy may be important in the prevention of preterm birth. Most urinary tract infections during pregnancy are caused by *Escherichia coli*. The majority of strains of this organism are cured by a short-acting sulfonamide. Such a drug is ideal for the initial therapy of asymptomatic bacteriuria. An alternative therapeutic agent is ampicillin, although treatment should always be based on the antimicrobial susceptibility of the isolated organism.

Single-dose therapy has been studied, but one-third or more patients fail treatment on such a regimen. The majority of patients appear to be cured by a 14-day course of the agents mentioned. Urine culture should be repeated during, and again 1 week after, completion of therapy. If asymptomatic bacteriuria persists after treatment, further therapy is indicated, and the agent prescribed will depend on the in vitro susceptibility of the organism. A combination of trimethoprim-sulfamethoxazole should be avoided in the first trimester because of potential teratogenicity and, likewise, in the last trimester of pregnancy because of the small risk of kernicterus in the neonate.

The presence of underlying renal disease should always be suspected when such organisms as *Proteus, Pseudomonas,* or *Klebsiella* are isolated. Women with urinary tract infection due to these organisms should be thoroughly evaluated after the pregnancy. Approximately one-third of women with recurrent or refractory asymptomatic bacteriuria during pregnancy have some urinary tract abnormality demonstrable by excretion urography.

Acute pyelonephritis in pregnancy remains a serious complication and can result in growth retardation of the fetus, preterm birth, or intrauterine fetal death. Such infections frequently occur at the end of the first half of pregnancy. The major clinical features are high fever, chills, and flank pain. The patient may be acutely ill and may complain of headache, malaise, anorexia, vomiting, and colicky abdominal pain. Acute pyelitis almost invariably involves the right kidney and marked tenderness is elicited in the right costovertebral angle and along the course of the right ureter. The clinical manifestations may simulate acute appendicitis, but the diagnosis is readily established by urine culture.

In severe infections, aggressive treatment with parenteral antibiotics and intravenous fluids are of prime importance. The initial antibiotic therapy should consist of ampicillin, 2 g every 6 hours, until the result of the antimicrobial susceptibility testing of the organism is available. Ampicillin is usually ineffective for therapy of resistant organisms. Bacteria, such as strains of *Klebsiella* and indole-negative *Proteus* species, are susceptible to high concentrations of cephalosporins, which are readily attainable in the urine. The newer cephalosporins are highly effective and are preferred to the aminocyclitols in these individuals because of the latter's potential for nephrotoxicity and VIIIth cranial nerve involvement. Compared with the penicillins and cephalosporins, the margin between toxic and therapeutic doses of the aminocyclitols is narrow. It is especially narrow for gentamicin and tobramycin because of vestibular nerve damage and nephrotoxicity.

Although most patients with urinary tract infections respond rapidly to appropriate therapy, they are, however, liable to have further exacerbations of infection—if they have had a previous upper tract infection—unless therapy is prolonged for at least 3 weeks. Intravenous antimicrobial therapy should be continued for 5 days in patients with pyelonephritis or pyelonephritis associated with bacteremia, but before any form of oral antimicrobial therapy is substituted, urine cultures and susceptibility patterns should be repeated. In less severe cases of acute pyelitis of pregnancy, oral medication can be instituted as soon as the patient has been afebrile for 48 hours. The patient's recovery is expedited by instructing her to maintain a liberal fluid intake and to lie in the lateral recumbent position. After completion of appropriate therapy, the patient's urine should be screened at each subsequent prenatal visit for the remainder of the pregnancy.

CHORIOAMNIONITIS

Inflammation of the fetal membranes results from an ascending infection from the cervical-vaginal ecosystem. Once the bacterial colonization is established in the lower female genital tract, the periodic fluctuations in physiologic conditions—including hormonal changes, mucus secretion, menstruation, and pregnancy—influence the quantitative composition of the flora. The composition of the cervical-vaginal flora is of importance in the decisions involving therapy for neonatal sepsis following chorioamniotic infection or maternal therapy for endomyometritis, which is a sequel of chorioamnionitis. The presence of mixed aerobic and anaerobic organisms helps to guide therapy before specific microorganisms are identified. Routinely, cultures are not performed in cases of chorioamnionitis; amniotic fluid may be cultured, if available, but the results are not at hand soon enough to influence therapy. The fetus cannot be adequately treated in utero by administering parenteral antibiotics to the mother, and if chorioamnionitis threatens the fetus, expiditious delivery should be performed. Therapy of mother and fetus is instituted independently. Culture of the corporeal endometrium can be performed, but is problematic because of contamination with cervical flora even with the most exacting sampling techniques. Therefore, therapy is usually empiric and based on the normal composition of cervical-vaginal flora. There is even some interest in obtaining prenatal cultures for organisms, such as the group B *Streptococcus*, associated with particularly serious consequences for the baby. Culture for group B *Streptococcus* should be obtained in women who have previously lost an infant to group B *Streptococcus*, but is not generally advocated in routine clinical practice.

Currently, it is not possible to predict which patients will develop chorioamnionitis, although premature rupture of the fetal membranes and lower socioeconomic circumstances are obvious risk factors. Moreover, early and accurate diagnosis of impending chorioamnionitis is not presently available. Thus, diagnosis is usually made relatively late in the course of ascending intrauterine bacterial infections, and the nature of the infectious agents and subsequent therapy is based on the predicted composition of the genital microflora.

When intrauterine infection of the fetus occurs, parenteral antibiotics administered to the mother are generally ineffective for the fetus. The fetus is usually infected by aspiration of the contaminated amniotic fluid, but perfusion of the fetal lung is poor until after birth. For this reason, successful therapy cannot be assured for the intrauterine patient. In the face of serious intra-amniotic infection, it is usually preferable to deliver the fetus provided that it can be cared for in a neonatal intensive care unit. Figure 1 contains a summary of the best approaches to identifying systemic infections during pregnancy.

PREMATURITY

The problem of prematurity and preterm labor remains the single largest cause of perinatal morbidity and mortality. Among the contributing factors are economic deprivation, poor maternal nutrition, medical illness and obstetric complications, but none of these emerges as the dominant etiologic factor. The recent recognition that bacteria may produce mediators that initiate the production of prostaglandins and, hence, labor, provides an explanation for an apparent association between infections and prematurity. There is a growing consensus that subclinical chorioamnionitis is responsible for many cases of premature birth. The microorganisms usually involved are members of the microbial flora of the lower female genital tract and may include aerobic and anaerobic species that do not possess potent virulence factors causing fulminant disease. Among the organisms implicated in initiating premature labor are mycoplasmas. Finally, an association has been recorded between untreated asymptomatic urinary tract infection and low birth weight. The mediators involved in untimely delivery of infants from mothers with urinary tract infection have not been identified, but it is clear that this represents an additional area in which therapeutic intervention may improve the outcome of pregnancy.

ANTIMICROBIAL THERAPY DURING PREGNANCY

A dual danger exists in inappropriate antibiotic use in pregnancy: the fetus may be damaged by uncontrolled infection, or injury to the fetus may occur as a result of drug toxicity.

Almost all available pharmacokinetic information has been derived from nongravid patients. These data are inadequate for pregnant women because several physiologic changes take place during pregnancy that substantially alter the way in which drugs are handled. The fetal-placental unit comprises a separate compartment into which antibiotics may be transported or diffused or from which they may be excluded. The tissues of the fetus are, in some cases, more sensitive to the toxic effects of certain drugs. As noted before, perfusion of the fetal lung is poor. Other factors affecting pharmacokinetics during pregnancy are expansion of maternal plasma volume, increased glomerular filtration rate, and altered gastrointestinal motility and absorption. Blood flow to the skin, skeletal muscles, kidneys, and uterus is increased, and serum proteins are decreased. The alteration of plasma protein levels—particularly albumin, which provides most of the drug binding sites—may have a significant effect on drugs that are highly bound to plasma protein. Bound drugs are generally considered to be incapable of passage through the capillary walls into tissues. Thus, the effectiveness of a standard dose of a drug may be modified in the pregnant patient.

The absolute amount of a therapeutic agent transferred to the fetus is proportional to the amplitude and duration of the maternal plasma concentration and the rate constant for placental transfer. Low-molecular-weight drugs, such as antibiotics, are considered to be transported through the placenta by diffusion. Pathologic changes in the placenta associated with maternal hypertension and diabetes can alter placental permeability. Placental transmission of a drug may be modified by such abnormalities of the umbilical cord as velamentous insertion of the vessels or absence of one umbilical artery.

Fetal hemodynamics also affect drug distribution in the fetal compartment and characteristics of the fetal circulation whereby much of the umbilical venous blood bypasses the liver via the ductus venosus and the lungs by the ductus arteriosus and results in elevated drug concentrations in the fetal heart and central nervous system.

We are relatively ignorant of the effect and toxicity of these drugs on the intrauterine patient. The majority of antibiotics cross the placenta and attain therapeutic levels in the fetus. Some agents, however, should never be administered to the pregnant patient because of toxicity;

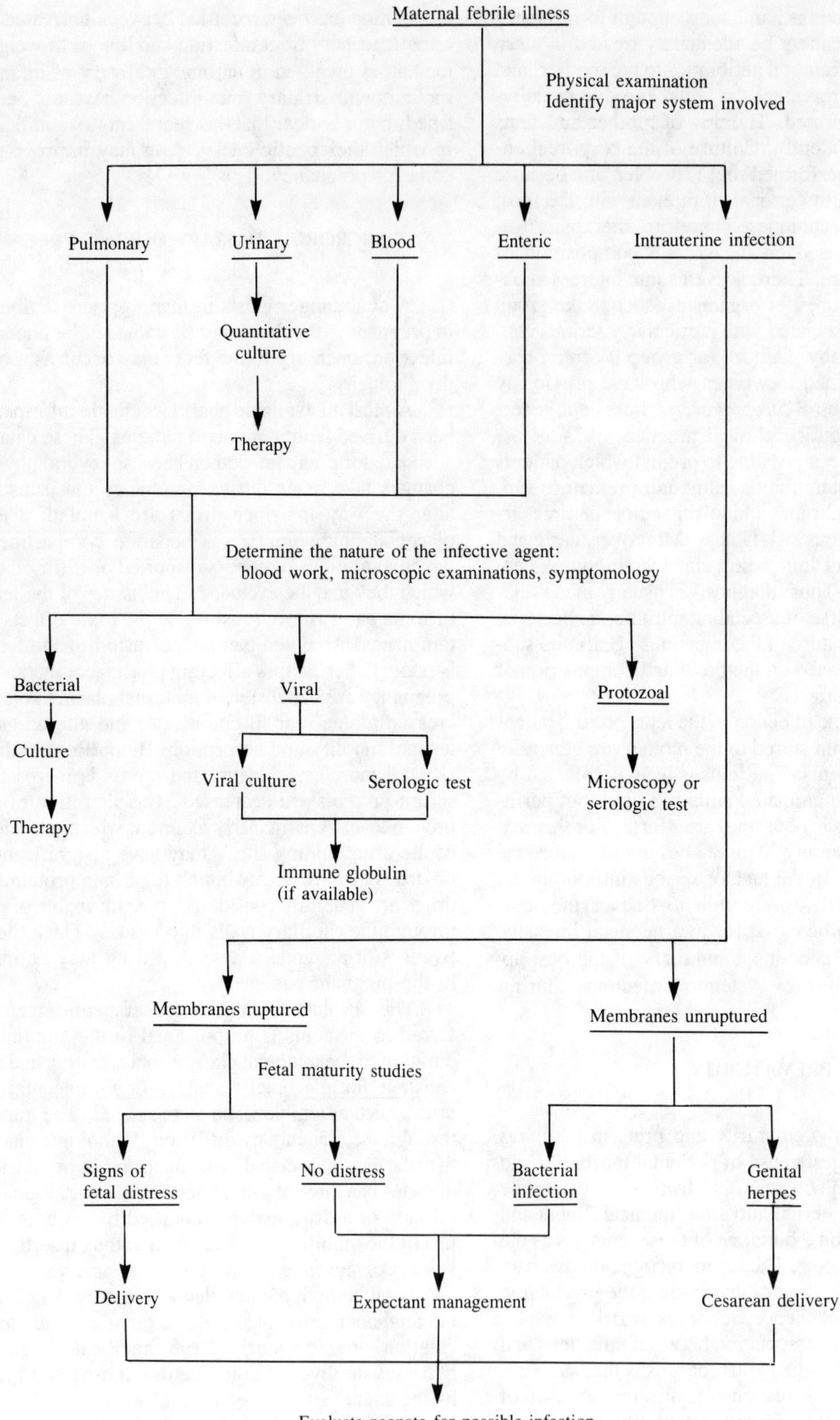

Figure 1 Identifying systemic infections during pregnancy

TABLE 2 Therapeutic Recommendations for Infections in the Pregnant or Parturient Patient

Infection	*Causative Organism*	*First Choice for Therapy*	*Alternate Therapy*
Asymptomatic bacteriuria	*E. coli*	Sulfonamides 0.5 g PO q6h	Ampicillin 500 mg q6h
Acute cystitis	*E. coli,* Group B *Streptococcus, Klebsiella*	Ampicillin 500 mg PO q6h	Trimethoprim 160 mg + sulfamethoxazole 800 mg q12h × 12–14 days
	P. aeruginosa	Amikacin 15 mg/kg/day in 2-3 divided doses IV *plus* Ticarcillin 1 g IV q6h	---
Acute pyelonephritis	*E. coli*	Ampicillin 500 mg IV q6h	Cefotaxime 1.0 g IV q6h
Mastitis	*S. aureus*	Penicillinase-resistant synthetic penicillin, e.g., methicillin 1.0 g IM q4h	Vancomycin 0.5 g IV q6h Cloxacillin 0.5 g PO q6h
Pneumonia	*S. pneumoniae*	Penicillin G 600,000 units IM q6h	Erythromycin stearate 500 mg PO q6h
	H. influenzae	Ampicillin 2.0 g PO q6h	Cefuroxime 500 mg IV q6h Cefotaxime 500 mg IV q6h
	M. pneumoniae	Erythromycin stearate 500 mg PO q6h	---
Tuberculosis	*M. tuberculosis*	Isoniazid 5 mg/kg/day PO *plus* Ethambutol 25 mg/kg/day × 2 months, then 15 mg/kg/day PO	If triple therapy add rifampin 9 mg/kg/day
Gonorrhea	*N. gonorrhoeae*	Procaine penicillin 4.8 million units IM *plus* Probenecid 1.0 g orally; for patients with penicillin allergy, erythromycin stearate 1.5 g PO followed by 0.75 g PO q6h for 5 days	Spectinomycin 2.0 g IM *or* Cefotaxime 2.0 g IM and probenecid 1.0 g PO
Syphilis	*T. pallidum*	Benzathine penicillin G 1.4 million units IM weekly × 3 weeks	For patients with penicillin allergy, erythromycin stearate 0.75 g PO q6h × 15 days; repeat course after an interval of 6 weeks
Listeriosis	*L. monocytogenes*	Ampicillin 1.0 g PO q6h	Erythromycin 750 mg PO q6h
Campylobacteriosis	*Campylobacter fetus* ssp. *jejuni*	Erythromycin 500 mg PO q6h	Clindamycin 600 mg followed by 300 mg PO q6h
Postpartum endomyometritis or septic abortion	Enterobacteriaceae *Bacteroides bivius* *Bacteroides disiens*	Cefoxitin 1.0 g IV q6h	Clindamycin 600 mg IV q6h *plus* Cefotaxime 1.0 g IV q6h
	Bacteroides fragilis	Clindamycin 600 mg IV q6h	Metronidazole* 0.5 g IV q6h

TABLE 2 Therapeutic Recommendations for Infections in the Pregnant or Parturient Patient—Continued

Infection	*Causative Organism*	*First Choice for Therapy*	*Alternate Therapy*
			plus Cefotaxime 1.0 g IV q6h
	Peptostreptococci	Piperacillin 1.0 g IV q6h	Cefotaxime 1.0 g IV q6h
Puerperal septicemia	Enterobacteriaceae *Bacteroides* species *Peptostreptococcus* *Streptococcus*	Cefotaxime 1.0 g IV q6h *plus* Clindamycin 600 mg IV q6h	Cefotaxime 1.0 g IV q6h *plus* Metronidazole* 500 mg IV q6h

* In the absence of lactation.

these are exemplified by tetracycline, which may cause hypoplasia of fetal bone and discoloration of the primary and secondary dentition. The primary reason for concern about antimicrobial agents administered to the pregnant host is not the known deleterious effects, but the lack of information about the safety of these agents.

Ampicillin achieves plasma levels in pregnant women that are approximately 50 percent of levels attained in nongravid patients. This effect persists until the third post partum day. Despite this, the levels in urine are similar in the two groups. An increased dose of ampicillin is not particularly hazardous and if the identical ratio between the plasma levels of ampicillin and the mean inhibitory concentration for the infective organism is to be attained in pregnant women, the dose should be twice that used in nongravid patients. The same applies to other antibiotics, although the actual adjustment required must be based on the measurement of serum levels and these data are as yet not available for all compounds. Although drug dosage in pregnancy probably needs to be increased for a variety of antimicrobial compounds, such adjustments need to be guided by determinations of plasma levels and consideration of potential toxic reactions associated with increased drug dosage. In some situations, such as impaired hepatic or renal function, one must be especially careful about the precise drug concentrations.

It is important for the physician managing individuals with postpartum endometritis to recognize that the hemodynamic changes and altered pharmacokinetics of pregnancy do not immediately return to normal at parturition. In the majority of instances, therefore, patients who become infected after cesarean section require 50 percent more antibiotic for the first 3 days of therapy than is recommended for the nongravid patient. Failure to observe this fact may result in prolonged morbidity.

Table 2 has been provided as a guideline for antibiotic therapy and an overall concept of the agents available that can be prescribed to the pregnant patient. The physicians who have an adequate understanding of the mechanisms of action of currently available therapeutic agents and the rationale for their use will be able to use current and future agents to the maximum advantage of their gravid patients. Finally, the effectiveness of these agents must not be viewed as license to neglect the general management of obstetric patients with infections.

INFECTION IN THE NEWBORN

MARTHA L. LEPOW, M.D.
SETH HETHERINGTON, M.D.

BACTERIAL INFECTIONS

Epidemiology

Systemic bacterial infections during the first month of life affect 0.1 to 0.5 percent of all live-born infants, with mortality rates of 20 to 60 percent. About 30 percent have associated meningitis, with mortality as high as 75 percent. As many as one-half of the survivors of neonatal meningitis develop neurologic sequelae such as hydrocephalus, motor or developmental disabilities, seizure disorder, or mental retardation. Early suspicion, diagnosis, and institution of treatment are essential for improving outcome. Each of the following sections will be divided into considerations of primary and secondary infections since etiology and management may require different diagnostic and therapeutic approaches.

Pathogenesis

Host factors

Prematurity is one of the largest risk factors because the primary host-defense systems are less adequately developed than in the term infant. Boys have a higher infection rate than girls. Significant IgG synthesis does not occur in the fetus, and there is passive and active transfer of maternal IgG in proportion to gestational age, but little occurring prior to 32 weeks. Complement levels in the neonate are 50 to 75 percent of adult levels. The bone marrow reserve of the neonate is only two to three times the circulating number of neutrophils, compared with 17 times as much for an adult. Thus, the pool is easily depleted.

Environment

Primary Infection. Here obstetrical factors are most important: (1) Premature ruptures of membranes of more than 24 hours is associated with a higher infection rate in neonates, especially in those of low birth weight and gestational age. (2) Etiologic agents are those bacteria and viruses that colonize the maternal genital tract; scalp electrodes for fetal monitoring provide a portal of entry for potential pathogens. (3) Maternal perinatal bacterial infections such as bacteremia, chorioamnionitis, or pyelonephritis may result in transplacental bacteremia. (4) Protective potential of maternal antibody for the fetus is variable. Group B streptococcal (GBS) infection is less likely in infants born of mothers colonized with GBS who are serum antibody–positive; however, maternal antibody to cytomegalovirus may not be protective. Table 1 compares early—and late—onset group B streptococcal (GBS) disease.

Secondary Infection. Invasive but necessary procedures for the premature infant, such as ventilatory support, indwelling catheters for hyperalimentation, or surgical intervention for processes such as necrotizing enterocolitis, increase the risk for nosocomial infection. Term infants requiring surgical intervention or ventilatory support have similar risks.

Organisms

Primary Infection. Over the past four decades there has been a constant incidence of neonatal infections, although the major responsible organisms have changed. The principal pathogenic organisms are those of the vaginal flora such as *Escherichia coli*, especially strains containing K-1 antigen that is associated with virulence, and group B *Streptococcus*, which has emerged in the past decade as the principal cause of intrapartum infection. Less frequently, *Listeria monocytogenes, Hemophilus influenzae*, and, rarely, *Streptococcus pneumoniae, Neisseria meningiditis*,, and anaerobes are found.

Secondary Infection. Secondary infections that are hospital acquired are most commonly due to *Staphylococcus aureus, Klebsiella* species, *Enterobacter* species, *Pseudomonas* species, *Serratia marscesans* with portals of entry in the skin and respiratory or genitourinary tract. Sepsis associated with necrotising enterocolitis probably is the result of bacterial invasion across the intestinal mucosa. *Staphylococcus epidermidis* is associated principally with indwelling catheters. *H. influenzae* may emerge as a respiratory pathogen.

TABLE 1 Comparison of Early- and Late-Onset Group B Streptococcal (GBS) Disease

Parameter	*Early*	*Late*
Age	<7 days	>7 days-3 months
Maternal complications, including premature labor	Yes	Infrequent
Clinical presentation	Pneumonia: frequent and severe (usually present at delivery)	Pneumonia: rare varied syndromes
Meningitis present	30%	Frequent
Source of GBS	Maternal	? Mother or "community"
Type	Ia, Ib, Ic, II, III	95% III

Note: *Listeria monocytogens* and *Escherichia coli* also manifest early- and late-onset disease.

Clinical Manifestations of Neonatal Sepsis

The signs of infections in the neonate are not specific and may be similar to clinical signs of respiratory, cardiac, neurologic, or metabolic diseases. These include hyper- or hypothermia, respiratory distress such as apnea or cyanosis, icterus, lethargy, poor suck, bleeding, irritability, shrill cry, vomiting, abdominal distention, and hepatosplenomegaly. Infants with meningitis may manifest seizures and a full fontanelle. Asymptomatic bacteremic states may exist, especially with anaerobic infections. The septic neonate, in comparison with the infant with respiratory distress syndrome, is more likely to be acidotic, hypotensive, more difficult to ventilate, and have a higher probability of mortality.

Laboratory Data

Rapid, detailed, complete diagnostic laboratory investigation (sepsis work-up) is essential. This includes blood culture of specimens from peripheral veins (since umbilical vessels and catheters may give false results), lumbar puncture unless contraindicated because of the infant's condition, and urine culture. If a baby requires intubation, the Gram stain and culture of the initial tracheal aspirate are helpful if there are neutrophils and a predominant bacterial species. Initial complete blood count and platelet count should be obtained and, if indicated, clotting factors should be evaluated. If the mother has received antibiotics, blood cultures from the infant may be negative, since almost all antibiotics cross the placenta. Cultures positive for pathogens from ear, throat, rectum, gastric aspirates, and placenta indicate colonization, but only a minority of such infants have septicemia.

Rapid diagnostic tests such as latex particle agglutination and countercurrent immunoelectrophoresis are most sensitive for antigens in urine and cerebrospinal fluid and less so for blood, but there may be false-positive and negative results. Such tests are available for group B *Strep-*

tococcus, H. influenzae B, N. meningitidis, and *S. pneumoniae*

Various parameters of the complete blood count have been evaluated as indicators of sepsis. All have problems of sensitivity or specificity. Several features of the white blood count may have predictive value. These include absolute neutrophil count, which may not rise because of limited bone marrow reserve, but a total white blood cell count of less than 2,500 is more significant; and band-to-segmented-neutrophil ratio greater than 0.3 or a band-to-total-neutrophil count greater than 0.2. A platelet count of less than 100,000 may be associated with sepsis.

In suspected nosocomial infections, cultures of wound sites, urine, respiratory secretions, and tips of removed vascular indwelling catheters, as well as peripheral blood, should be obtained.

Antibiotic Therapy

Prompt initiation of antibiotic therapy as soon as diagnostic studies have been performed is of critical importance. The basic principle is that for an antibiotic to be successful, an effective concentration must be present in the part of the body where the infection exists. A table of antibiotics, doses, and principal indications is included. Initial antimicrobial therapy for suspected sepsis usually consists of ampicillin and an aminoglycoside for early-onset or primary disease.

Ampicillin has a broader spectrum than penicillin against common newborn bacterial pathogens including enterococcus. Although penicillin may be more effective against anaerobic bacteria, their role in neonatal sepsis is less important. Gentamicin is less expensive than tobramycin and has equal effectiveness except for infections with some strains of *Pseudomonas*.

There are no published data in children that tobramycin is less nephrotoxic than gentamicin. Amikacin should be considered in hospitals when gram-negative organisms are frequently resistant to the other aminoglycosides. Moxalactam and ampicillin have been shown to be equal to the combination of ampicillin and amikacin for the treatment of gram-negative meningitis in newborns—a rather surprising result given the theoretically superior pharmacokinetics of the former combination. Hypoprothrombinemia and prolonged bleeding times have been associated with moxalactam and could increase the risk of intraventricular hemorrhage in the premature infant. Although cefotaxime is not implicated in coagulation disorders and is probably equivalent to moxalactam in gram-negative coverage, it has not been extensively studied in neonates.

Based on these considerations, we suggest for initial empiric therapy of the potentially septic neonate, ampicillin and gentamicin (see Table 2 for doses). Gentamicin levels must be measured after the third dose and subsequent doses adjusted accordingly. The alternative regimen of ampicillin and cefotaxime could be used if (1) an aminoglycoside-resistant organism is recovered from blood or spinal fluid and the organism is sensitive to cefotaxime; (2) the suspected organisms is *H. influenzae* by Gram stain or latex particle agglutination performed on a body fluid; or (3) there is evidence of renal dysfunction in association with aminoglycoside administration. We believe that moxalactam has been supplanted by cefotaxime and do not use the former in neonates.

In a sick infant whose circulation may be impaired, both ampicillin and aminoglycoside should be given intravenously. The relatively well infant could receive these drugs intramuscularly. If chloramphenicol is used, frequent serum level determinations are important since there is a wide individual variation in clearance.

If the initial blood culture is positive, it is best to adjust drugs based on expected sensitivity of the organism, with a final adjustment pending actual sensitivity.

If *S. aureus* is suspected as a causative organism, especially in nosocomial infections, a beta-lactamase-resistant penicillin should be given. We use oxacillin, a choice based on cost considerations alone.

Staphylococcus epidermidis is the most frequent cause of nosocomial sepsis in infants with central venous catheters, but also occurs as a major cause of late-onset sepsis in chronically ill neonates without central catheters. Since this organism is a frequent contaminant of blood cultures, more than one blood culture should be performed to confirm the diagnosis when this organism is suspected. In our hospital, one-third of *S. epidermidis* isolates are resistant to the beta-lactamase-resistant penicillins and cephalosporins. Therefore, for late-onset sepsis in the neonate with a central venous catheter or chronic illness, we initiate therapy with vancomycin and gentamicin. Vancomycin must be infused slowly over one-half hour to avoid injury to vessels, cost, and hypotension. Although both vancomycin and aminoglycosides are potentially nephrotoxic, we have not observed a rise in creatinine levels in any infant given this combination. We monitor urine output, urinalysis, and serum creatinine on days 1, 3, and 7 of therapy and weekly thereafter. Vancomycin levels must be monitored to adjust the dose and can be obtained after any dose since the drug is not cumulative.

Infections due to *Pseudomonas* have not been frequent in our nursery. Preferred therapy for this occasional pathogen is tobramycin and mezlocillin. The latter antibiotic is chosen for its synergistic effect with tobramycin for *Pseudomonas* and has replaced ticarcillin in our hospital to avoid potential platelet dysfunction and on the basis of lower cost.

Antimicrobial agents are usually discontinued after 72 hours if cultures are negative unless there are confounding factors such as maternal antibiotics, abnormal spinal fluid, or a clinical course compatible with sepsis. When cultures are positive, a 10-day treatment course is recommended.

Supportive Measures

Fluid and electrolyte balance, ventilatory and circulatory support, and provision of calories are highly important. In secondary sepsis, especially with central venous catheters, the catheter need not be immediately removed, but should be removed if cultures remain positive after 72 hours of appropriate therapy.

Careful studies have shown that neutrophil transfusions increase survival in infants with sepsis and depletion of bone marrow reserves. The optimal procedure would be to obtain a marrow aspirate from an infant with an absolute neutrophil count of less than 1,500 per cubic millimeter. If the marrow shows exhaustion, an irradiated buffy coat could be given (15 ml per kilogram). However, obtaining the marrow aspirate is often not practical, and we have given the leukocyte transfusion to infants with peripheral neutropenia, realizing that this may not truly reflect the marrow stores.

Exchange transfusions have been advocated by some on the theoretical grounds that bacterial factors could be removed (endotoxin) and host factors provided (complement and immunoglobulin). However, a significant number of leukocytes are provided and could account for the initial successes achieved with this therapy. In addition, the mortality of the procedure is not inconsequential in an ill neonate. We, therefore, do not use exchange transfusions for treatment of sepsis in our nursery. Intravenous immunoglobulins have also been advocated for the treatment of sepsis, but data are lacking, and we do not recommend this mode of therapy.

Special Measures for Meningitis

Inappropriate secretion of antidiuretic hormone may occur. Ventriculitis and obstructive hydrocephalus are frequent complications. Seizure control is important. The use of steroids and mannitol for control of cerebral edema are not ordinarily recommended.

Repeat lumbar puncture should be done in infants with gram-negative bacillary meningitis after 72 hours of treatment to assess sterility. Treatment should continue for at least 3 weeks after CSF is sterile. For all infants with meningitis, a spinal fluid examination should be done before antibiotics are discontinued to assess cell count and sugar and protein content. Computed tomographic examination should be considered at the end of therapy to assess ventricular size as well as for evidence of vascular accidents. Infants should have hearing and developmental follow-up evaluations.

Infants with ventriculoperitoneal shunts in place because of hydrocephalus are at risk for *S. epidermidis*, enterococcal, and, occasionally, gram-negative bacterial infection. Initial treatment should include vancomycin for *S. epidermidis*, both intravenously and intraventricularly (5 mg daily) or ampicillin and gentamicin, depending upon the organism. Removal of the infected shunt is imperative.

Pneumonia

Perinatal pneumonia is most commonly acquired by aspiration of infected amniotic fluid prior to or at birth. Nosocomial pneumonia may occur in infants on assisted ventilation or postoperatively. The etiologic agents are the same as those responsible for sepsis, and initial management is the same.

Chlamydia trachomatis pneumonia due to *C. trachomatis* is a result of perinatal infection and the initial infection is in the eye, with subsequent aspiration.

Skin and Soft Tissue Infections

Bacterial skin infections may present as early as the first few days of life but usually appear after a week and include pustules, furuncles, mastitis, abscesses, conjunctivitis, impetigo, and wound infections after circumcision. Occasionally, scalded skin syndrome will occur, in which there is generalized erythema followed by desquamation of large sheets of skin. The causative organism is usually *S. aureus*, although gram-negative organisms are occasionally present. Diagnosis is made by Gram stain and culture of lesions. If pustules are localized, superficial local treatment with hexachlorophene soaks and bacitracin may suffice. Systemic treatment can be initiated with oxacillin followed by oral dicloxacillin when the condition of the baby warrants it. Therapy is continued until there is clinical resolution of the infection.

Osteomyelitis

This is not frequently observed, but osteomyelitis occasionally follows superficial skin infections, heel sticks, or femoral punctures. *S. aureus*, penicillin-resistant, is the most frequent cause. Group B *Streptococcus* (late-onset), *Neisseria gonorrheae*, and other gram-negative bacteria may occasionally occur. Oxacillin and an aminoglycoside should be started and more specific treatment continued when the organism is known. The antibiotic should be given intravenously for at least three weeks, followed by an equal period of oral therapy. Local incision and drainage may be indicated.

Urinary Tract Infection

Primary urinary tract infection in the neonate may be due to septicemia. It may also be associated with congenital anomalies of the genitourinary system, especially in boys. Secondary infection occurs in babies with indwelling catheters. The commonest etiologic agent is *E. coli*, but other gram-negative organisms may be responsible for nosocomial urinary tract infections. Multiply resistant organisms may be encountered. Initial therapy is with ampicillin and gentamicin, pending results of cultures. Treatment should be for 10 days. Abdominal ultrasound and voiding cystourethrogram (VCUG) are diagnostic studies to be performed at the end of therapy. The abdominal ultrasound may be done earlier if antibiotics fail to eradicate the infection.

TABLE 2 Antimicrobial Agents Used in Neonatal Infections

Drug	Route	Daily Dose (mg/kg/24 hr) (Doses per 24 hr): Infant 0–7 Days of Age	Daily Dose (mg/kg/24 hr) (Doses per 24 hr): Infant 7–30 Days of Age	Organisms	Therapeutic Levels	Special Adverse Effects
Cephalosporins						
First-generation (cephalothin, cefazolin, cefapirin		100 (2)	150 (3)	*Staphylococcus aureus*	--	--
moxolactam	IV	100 (2)	150 (3)	Gram-negative rods resistant to aminoglycosides or in renal failure; some gram-negative bacterial meningitis	--	--
Cefotaxime	IV	100 (2)	150 (3)	Same as for moxalactam	--	--
Others						
Chloramphenicol	IV	25 (2)	50 (2)	*Hemophilus influenzae*, anaerobes, *Salmonella*, gram-negative organisms where no other drugs available, especially meningitis	Peak: 10–25 μg/ml Trough: <5 before next dose	Bone marrow depres sion; Grey-baby syndrome
Vancomycin	IV	20 (2)	30 (3)	*Staphylococcus epidermidis*	Peak <30 Trough <12	Phlebitis, renal toxicity, rash
Erythromycin	PO	--	40 (3–4)	*Chlamydia trachomatis*	--	--
Clindamycin	IV	25 mg/kg/d q8h (3)	40 mg/kg q8h	*Bacteroides fragilis* (bowel)	--	--
Antiviral agents						
Ara-A	IV	15 mg/kg/d over 12 hours for 5–10 days		Neonatal herpes simplex		May affect platelets and clotting factors
Antifungal agents						
Amphotericin B	IV	0.5 mg/kg/d (over 6 hours)		*Candida* and other fungi		Nephrotoxic
Flucytocine	PO	150 mg/kg (4)		Fungal meningitis		
Antiparasitic drugs						
Pyrimethamine and trisulfapyrimadine	PO	2 mg/kg/d × 3 d, then 1 mg/kg/d × 4 wks 100–200 mg/kg/d × 4 wks		Toxoplasmosis		Bone marrow depression rash

Penicillins						
Penicillin G	IV or IM	50,000 U (2)*	150,000 U (3)*	GBS, pneumococcus, gonococcus, meningococcus, *T. pallidum*	--	--
Ampicillin	IV or IM	50 (2)*	100 (3)*	B-Hemolytic streptococci, enterococcus, *Listeria monocytogenes, E. coli, Proteus mirabilis,* some *Salmonella, H. influenzae* (β-lactamase-negative)	--	--
Oxacillin	IV or IM	50 (2)	100 (4)	Penicillin-resistant *Staphylococcus aureus*	--	Rash, interstitial nephritis, neutropenia
Ticarcillin	IV	150 (2)	225 (3)	In conjunction with tobramycin in pseudomonas infection	--	Occasional platelet dysfunction
Mezlocillin	IV	150 (2)	225 mg/kg (3)	To cover mixed gram-negative and enterococcal infection, peritonitis, bowel surgery	--	U/A daily for interstitial nephritis
Pipercillin	IV	Newborn dosage not available		Similar to mezlocillin; consider as a second drug in pseudomonas infection resistant to ticarcillin since it is more expensive than mezlocillin	--	--
Aminoglycosides						
Gentamicin	IV or IM	5 (2)	7.5 (3)	Most gram-negative organisms except *Pseudomonas, H. influenzae, Salmonella, Shigella*	Peak 15 min p dose: 4-8 μg/ml Trough (before a dose): <2 μg/ml	Renal and ototoxicity; check creatinine twice weekly
Tobramycin	IV or IM	5 (2)	6 (3)	Same as gentamicin except more activity vs. *Pseudomonas*	Same as gentamicin	--
Amikacin	IV or IM	15 (2)	22.5 (3)	Only if organism resistant to gentamicin	Peak <40 Trough <10	--

* For treatment of meningitis, the dose should be doubled.

VIRAL INFECTIONS

Herpes Simplex, Type 2

Infants born vaginally of mothers who have active primary infection are at risk for disseminated infection. The portal of entry is frequently ocular, oral, or pulmonary. Recurrent disease in the mother is a lesser risk. The mothers of 40 percent of infected newborns have a negative history.

The infant may show similar signs to those seen in the baby with sepsis, commencing on day 3 or 4. Frequently, vesicles are noted about the face. Diagnosis is by culture of the organisms from lesion or biopsy in tissue culture, or by fluorescent antibody staining of biopsied material. CSF should be examined and cultured for virus regardless of signs.

Current recommended treatment is with adenine arabinoside (Ara-A) 5 mg per kilogram per day (over 12 hours) intravenously for 10 days. Follow-up for neurologic and visual disorders is important. Platelets and clotting factors should be followed.

Cytomegalovirus (CMV)

One to three percent of all newborns will have congenital CMV infection. Infection may occur during intrauterine infection secondary to maternal primary infection or be acquired perinatally from an asymptomatic carrier mother. Affected infants usually have one or more of the following signs: icterus, hepatosplenomegaly, microcephaly, chorioretinitis, and hematologic findings of hemolytic anemia and thrombocytopenia. The virus may be cultured from urine. There is no antiviral treatment available.

CMV occurring after the immediate perinatal period may be nosocomial via transfusion or from other affected babies or personnel. Frequently, the presentation is respiratory, and attempts should be made to isolate the organism from the respiratory secretions.

FUNGAL INFECTIONS

Candida species may be significant nosocomial invaders in neonatal intensive care units, principally in infants who have indwelling central venous catheters and require hyperalimentation. Amphotericin B is the drug of choice. All such patients should have a lumbar puncture and echocardiography to rule out a cardiac fungal mass if an indwelling catheter is present. If meningitis is present and the organism is sensitive, flucytosine should be added and therapy continued for 6 weeks. Bone marrow suppression is rare when levels are maintained below 100 μg per milliliter. Serum creatinine levels should be monitored weekly when using amphotericin B.

OTHER CONGENITAL INFECTIONS

Toxoplasmosis usually presents at birth with hydrocephalus, hepatosplenomegaly, and jaundice. Diagnosis is by fluorescent antibody (specific IgM). Treatment should be initiated with pyrimethamine-sulfamethoxazole.

PREVENTION OF NEONATAL BACTERIAL INFECTIONS

Although beyond the scope of this paper, there are several strategies, especially for prevention of primary group B streptococcal infection: (1) Immunization of the mother. This is experimental, and optimal vaccine and technique of administration are yet to be worked out. (2) Treat the mother before delivery to eliminate colonization. This holds promise if infected women can be identified, but efficacy is not proved and recurrence, not prevented. (3) Early treatment with penicillin. In controlled trials it was not effective and one study showed emergence of resistant organisms.

For secondary infections, prevention of prematurity is the most important prophylactic measure.

IMMUNODEFICIENCY DISORDER IN INFANTS AND CHILDREN

DOUGLAS J. BARRETT, M.D.
ELIA M. AYOUB, M.D.

The normal immune system consists of four major components that aid the host in defense against infection. The four components consist of antibody-mediated immunity (B-cell), cell-mediated immunity (T-cell), the phagocytic cell system, and the serum complement system. In the normal host, these components act in concert to effect the immune response.

Cells involved in the immune system are derived from a primitive pluripotential stem cell capable of differentiating along several pathways (Fig. 1). Lymphoid stem cell progeny may migrate to the thymus gland, where they differentiate into immunologically competent thymus-derived T-cells capable of cell-mediated immune reactions. These include delayed-type hypersensitivity, lymphokine secretion, lymphocytoxicity, helper T-cell function, and suppressor T-cell function. Alternatively, some of the stem cell lymphoid progeny populate the fetal liver and later the bone marrow, where they differentiate along a separate lineage to become immunocompetent

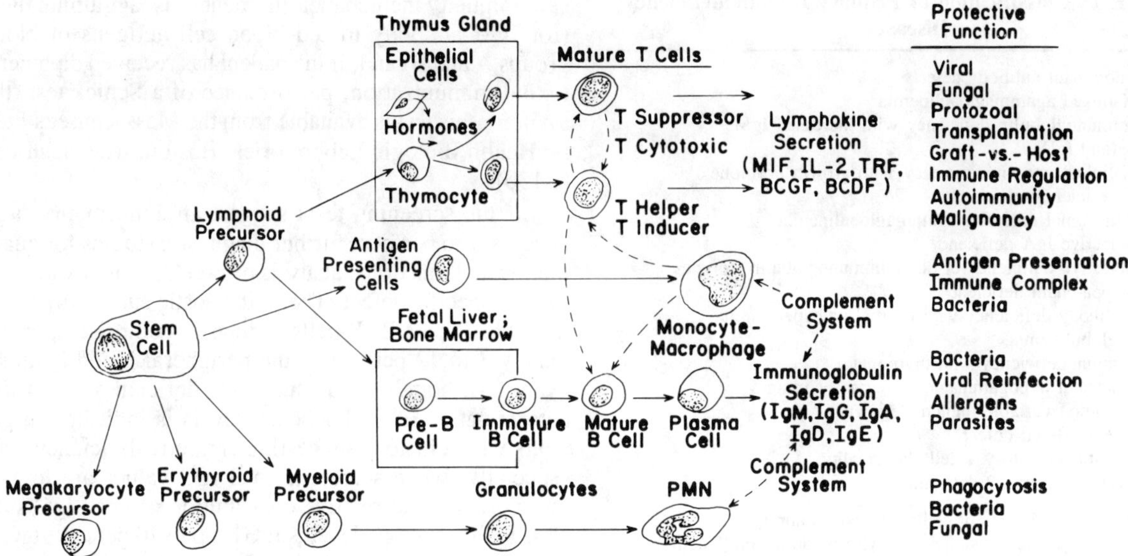

Figure 1 Schematic representation of the ontogeny and functional interaction of components of the immune system.

B-cells capable of secreting antibodies. Separate stem cell differentiation pathways lead to development of phagocytic cells, including granulocytes and monocytes/macrophages. The complement system is a series of serum proteins that interact in cascade fashion to produce active complement fragments necessary for bacterial lysis, viral neutralization, opsonization of particles, neutrophil chemotaxis, and mediation of the inflammatory response.

Congenital or acquired defects in any of the four major components of immunity will lead to one of the specific immunodeficiency states listed in Table 1.

DIAGNOSIS OF IMMUNODEFICIENCY DISEASES

General Approach

A carefully taken medical history and a detailed physical examination often lead to the suspicion of a defect in immunity. Most patients present with increased susceptibility to infection. Generally, the clinical manifestations will be related to the degree of deficiency and to the particular component of the immune system that is deficient. For example, patients with defective antibody-mediated immunity will have frequent sinopulmonary infections with pyogenic bacteria, whereas patients with defective cell-mediated immunity often present with persistent or recurrent fungal, viral, or protozoal diseases. Patients with phagocytic cell defects may have recurrent soft tissue abscesses or systemic infection with uncommon bacteria or fungi of low virulence. Patients with complement defects often present with severe recurrent pyogenic infections, recurrent neisserial infections, or conditions resembling systemic lupus erythematosus.

Physical examination should include careful attention to those features listed in Table 2. Many findings on physical examination are nonspecific and only indicate evidence of recurrent infection (e.g., lymphadenopathy, hepatosplenomegaly, or chronic pulmonary changes). However, a few findings are peculiar to a specific immunodeficiency.

Since most of the clinical findings in immunodeficiency are not sufficiently distinctive, a definitive diagnosis must include appropriate laboratory testing. Initially, the laboratory investigation should include certain nonspecific laboratory tests, including complete blood count with differential, an evaluation of cellular morphology on peripheral smear, erythrocyte sedimentation rate, platelet count, and chest roentgenogram. Before proceeding with a detailed immunologic evaluation, one should exclude nonimmunologic causes of recurrent infection, including cystic fibrosis, allergy, and ciliary dyskinesia syndromes.

Having eliminated nonimmunologic causes of recurrent infection, a detailed immunologic evaluation should assess each of the four components of immunity that are implicated by findings in the history and physical examination. Each of these components can be tested using simple and generally available screening studies. If the screening tests are all normal, immunodeficiency is usually excluded, and the patient can be assured that gamma globulin therapy or other immunotherapy is not indicated. If the screening tests are abnormal or if the history is unusually suspicious, it is then appropriate to proceed to more definitive and sophisticated diagnostic tests, some of which are available only in referral medical centers or specialized laboratories. For both screening and diagnostic studies, it is imperative to test both quantitative and qualitative (or functional) aspects of each component of immunity.

TABLE 1 Classification of Primary Immunodeficiency Diseases

Predominant antibody defects
- X-linked agammaglobulinemia
- Immunoglobulin deficiency with increased IgM (and IgD)
- X-linked immunodeficiency with growth hormone deficiency
- Autosomal recessive agammaglobulinemia
- Selective IgA deficiency
- Selective deficiency of other immunoglobulin isotypes
- Kappa-chain deficiency
- Antibody deficiency with normal or hypergammaglobulinemia
- Immunodeficiency with thymoma
- Transient hypogammaglobulinemia of infancy
- Common variable immunodeficiency
  - With B-cell defect
  - With regulatory T-cell abnormality
- Transcobalamin-2 deficiency

Predominant defects of cell-mediated immunity
- Combined immunodeficiency with predominant T-cell defect
- DiGeorge syndrome
- Purine nucleoside phosphorylase deficiency

Combined antibody and cellular immunodeficiencies
- Severe combined immunodeficiency
  - Reticular dysgenesis
  - Low T- and B-cell numbers
  - Low T-cells and normal B-cells (Swiss-type lymphopenic agammaglobulinemia)
  - "Bare-lymphocyte" syndrome
- Immunodeficiency with adenosine deaminase deficiency
- Cellular immunodeficiency with abnormal immunoglobulin synthesis (Nezelof's syndrome)
- Wiskott-Aldrich syndrome
- Ataxia-telangiectasia
- Acquired immunodeficiency syndrome (AIDS)

Phagocytic dysfunction
- Chronic granulomatous disease
- Glucose-6-phosphate dehydrogenase deficiency
- Myeloperoxidase deficiency
- Chediak-Higashi syndrome
- Job's syndrome
- Hyper-IgE with abnormal chemotaxis
- GP110, GP150 deficiency

Complement deficiency
- C1 inactivator deficiency (hereditary angioedema)
- Inherited deficiency of complement pathway component: C1q, C1r, C4, C2, C3, C4, C5, C6, C7, C8, C9
- Factor I (C3b inactivator) deficiency

Note: After WHO Scientific Group, *Clin Immunol Immunopathol* 1983; 28:450–475.

Evaluation of Antibody-Mediated Immunity

Screening tests for defects in antibody-mediated (B-cell) immunity are listed in Table 3, part A. Quantitative immunoglobulin determination is preferable to plasma electrophoresis, since exact quantitative information can be obtained about each immunoglobulin isotype. Results of immunoglobulin quantitation must be interpreted with caution because of the very marked changes that occur with age. Studies to screen for functional defects in B-cell immunity include measurement of isoagglutinin titers (for IgM antibody to red blood cell antigens of blood groups A and B) and, if the patient has received diphtheria toxoid immunization, performance of a Schick test (the toxin for this test is available from the Massachusetts Public Health Biologic Laboratories, Boston, Massachusetts 02130).

If the screening tests suggest an abnormality, it is necessary to perform further diagnostic studies for quantitation and functional analysis of B-cell immunity to identify the specific defect. These diagnostic studies are listed in Table 3, part B. B-cells ordinarily comprise approximately 8 to 12 percent of the peripheral blood lymphocytes. Although IgG subclass deficiency is rare, determination of IgG subclass levels is indicated in patients with a history suggesting antibody deficiency and, especially, when screening total IgG values are low or low-normal. The relative contribution of each IgG subclass to the total IgG level is IgG1, 60 to 70 percent; IgG2, 14 to 20 percent; IgG3, 4 to 8 percent; and IgG4, 2 to 6 percent. At present, IgG subclass level determinations are not widely available, and care must be taken to compare results with those of age-matched controls run in the same laboratory. Secretory IgA can be measured in tears or saliva.

Diagnostic studies of B-cell function include measurement of specific antibody response in serum before and after immunization with inert antigens (or before and after known infection). Ideally, antibody responses should be tested to both protein antigens (e.g., tetanus toxoid, diphtheria toxoid, streptolysin O), and polysaccharide antigens (e.g., pneumococcal polysaccharide, streptococcal group A carbohydrate, *Hemophilus influenzae* polyribose phosphate). It should be emphasized that immunization with live viral vaccines should be avoided in patients with potential or suspected T-cell immunodeficiency. The functional capacity of patient's B-cells to secrete immunoglobulin and the T-cell regulation of immunoglobulin synthesis should be tested in patients with hypogammaglobulinemia.

Evaluation of Cell-Mediated Immunity

Initial screening studies for defects in cell-mediated (T-cell) immunity are listed in Table 4, part A. Since T-cells constitute the majority of peripheral blood lymphocytes, a total lymphocyte count derived from the white blood cell count multiplied by the percentage of lymphocytes may disclose lymphopenia (fewer than 1,000 cells per cubic millimeter) in states of severe T-cell deficiency. T-cell function is best screened by use of delayed-hypersensitivity skin tests to evaluate preexisting cell-mediated immunity to antimicrobial agents or immunization. Antigens that are most useful are listed in Table 5. Delayed hypersensitivity skin tests are not generally reliable during the first year of life. False-negative results may also be due to expired lots of antigen or failure to achieve intradermal injection.

Diagnostic tests for definitive characterization of T-

TABLE 2 Features on Physical Examination Suggestive of Immunodeficiency

Site	*Abnormality*	*Associated Immunodeficiency*
General	Growth failure, short stature, dwarfism	Agammaglobulinemia, T-cell deficiencies
Skin	Eczema	Wiskott-Aldrich syndrome; T-cell deficiencies
	Candidiasis	T-cell deficiency
	Telangiectasia	Ataxia-telangiectasia
	Petechiae	Wiskott-Aldrich syndrome
Ears/mouth	Otitis media	Antibody deficiencies
	Oral ulcerations	T-cell deficiency granulocyte defects
Lymph node	Lymphadenopathy	Some antibody, T-cell, or granulocyte defects
	Absent tonsils/nodes	Agammaglobulinemia; severe combined immuno-deficiency
Integument	Sparse hair	Cartilage-hair hypoplasia syndrome
	Albinism	Chediak-Higashi syndrome
Chest	Chronic lung disease/ bronchiectasis	Antibody, T-cell, or granu-locyte defects
Heart	Congenital heart defects	DiGeorge syndrome
Abdomen	Hepatosplenomegaly	Antibody, T-cell, granulo-cyte defects
CNS	Ataxia	Ataxia-telangiectasia
Extremities	Short limbs	T-cell deficiency

cell defects should be performed in individuals who have abnormalities in the screening tests or in whom the diagnosis is highly suspected at an early age (Table 4, part B). The percentage and absolute numbers of T-cells can be quantified by their formation of rosettes with sheep red blood cells (E-rosettes) or by immunofluorescent staining using monoclonal antibodies to T-cell surface antigens. The ability to form E-rosettes is a property of both immature as well as mature T-cells. The T-cell-specific monoclonal antibodies listed in Table 6 can be used to differentiate functionally distinct T-cell subsets. Some patients may be severely deficient in T-cells as assayed by all techniques, suggesting a prethymic defect. Others may have a deficiency of mature T-cells (T3+, T4+, T8+), with increased numbers of immature cells bearing pre-T or thymocyte markers (T6+, T10+), whereas others may manifest alterations in the T-helper to T-suppressor ratio (normal T4+:T8+ = 1.8–2.2).

Diagnostic testing for T-cell function involves in vitro lymphocyte activation or transformation (blastogenesis) in response to nonspecific mitogens (e.g., phytohemagglutinin, conconavalin A, pokeweed mitogen), to soluble antigens (e.g., *Candida*, tetanus toxoid), and to cell surface alloantigens (i.e., mixed lymphocyte culture). Lymphocyte transformation assays measure the functional capability of T-cells (or T- and B-cells) to become acti-

TABLE 3 Tests for Defects in Antibody Mediated Immunity

A. Screening evaluation
- Quantitative tests
  - Quantitative immunoglobulins: IgM, IgG, IgA, and IgE
- Functional tests
  - Isoagglutinin titers
  - Schick test

B. Diagnostic evaluation
- Quantitative tests
  - B-cell enumeration
  - IgG subclass quantitation
  - Secretory IgA quantitation
- Functional tests
  - Pre- and postimmunization serum antibody levels: tetanus and diphtheria toxoids, KLH, pneumococcal and *Hemophilus* polysaccharides
  - Postinfection antibody levels: streptococcal ASO and group A carbohydrate
  - In vitro immunoglobulin secretion

TABLE 4 Tests for Defects in Cell-Mediated Immunity

A. Screening evaluation
- Quantitative tests
  - Total lymphocyte count
- Functional tests
  - Delayed hypersensitivity skin tests (see Table 5)

B. Diagnostic evaluation
- Quantitative Tests
  - T-cell enumeration: E-rosettes; monoclonal antibodies to T-cell subsets (see Table 6)
- Functional tests
  - Lymphocyte blastogenesis to mitogens and soluble antigens
  - Mixed lymphocyte culture
  - Lymphokine secretion

TABLE 5 Delayed Hypersensitivity Skin Tests

Antigen	*Dose/Dilution*
Candida (Dermatophyton)	1:100; if negative use 1:10
Mumps	1 mg/ml undiluted
Trichophyton	1:30
PPD	10 IU; if negative use 50 IU
Streptokinase/streptodornase	Under 10 years: 40 units → 100 units Over 10 years: 4 units → 40 units
Tetanus toxoid	1:100, if negative use 1:10
Diphtheria toxoid	1:100, if negative use 1:10

vated and to proliferate. Since the ability to respond to a specific antigen is detectable only with prior host sensitization to that antigen, a complete evaluation with mitogens, antigens, and allogeneic cells should be performed. Further functional studies for T-cell lymphokine generation (e.g., interleukin 2, migration inhibition factor [MIF], interferon, B-cell growth and differentiation factors) can be assessed in specialized reference laboratories.

Evaluation of the Phagocytic System

As listed in Table 7, part A, granulocytes and monocytes can be quantitated and assessed morphologically by use of the white blood cell count and differential smear. Granulocytopenia, defined as fewer than 1,500 cells per cubic millimeter, is associated with an increased risk of infection; patients with counts below 500 cells per cubic millimeter are unusually susceptible to infection with gram-positive and gram-negative bacteria as well as a variety of fungi. The finding of giant granules in neutrophils may suggest a diagnosis of the Chediak-Higashi syndrome. The simplest screening test for metabolic defects of phagocytes resulting in recurrent infection is the qualitative histochemical slide test for nitroblue tetrazolium (NBT) dye reduction. Patients with chronic granulomatous disease have less than 1 percent NBT-positive cells, whereas normal individuals generally have more than 10 percent.

Diagnostic studies for granulocyte dysfunction are listed in Table 7, part B. The qualitative presence of granulocyte and monocyte enzymes, such as alkaline phosphatase, peroxidase, and esterase, can be assessed by histochemical staining. Absence of these enzymes on the qualitative stain should be confirmed by specific quantitative assay. Monoclonal antibodies to monocyte differentiation antigens (*Leu M3, OKM1*) are also available. Fc and C3b receptors can be quantitated by rosetting with IgG-coated (EA) or complement-coated (EAC) erythrocytes, respectively. Functional defects in granulocytes include abnormalities of movement, particle ingestion, and intracellular microbicidal systems. Defects in movement, including random migration of neutrophils as well as chemotaxis toward a specific soluble attractant (e.g., C5a, *f-met-leu-phe*), can be detected by use of the modified Boyden chamber. Defects in particle ingestion and microbicidal activity are assayed by chemiluminescence and neutrophil bacterial-killing assays.

Recognition, attachment, and ingestion of opsonized particles (such as zymosan) by neutrophils leads to a respiratory burst with generation of hydrogen peroxide, superoxide ion, and singlet excited oxygen. As these high energy oxygen radicals relax to ground state, a small amount of electromagnetic energy in the form of light is emitted, a process termed chemiluminescence. This chemiluminescence correlates closely with microbicidal activity. Generation of superoxide can also be directly quantitated by cytochrome reduction assay. Granulocyte bacterial killing can be detected in a kinetic assay in which the test strain is incubated with neutrophils and opsonins from fresh serum. The number of viable intracellular organisms remaining after various times of incubation is then quantitated by culture of neutrophil lysates.

Evaluation of the Complement System

The complement system is a major effector mechanism involved in clearance of immune complexes, cytolysis, opsonization, chemotaxis, and nonspecific inflammation. Deficiencies of complement should be suspected in patients with recurrent pyogenic infections (especially *Streptococcus pneumoniae* and neisserial species) or conditions resembling systemic lupus erythematosus.

TABLE 6 Surface Markers Identifying T-Cell Subsets

T-Cell Subset	*Surface Antigen*	*Percentage Positive*		*Comments*
		Thymus	*Peripheral T-Cells*	
Total	T11	95	100	Associated with the sheep red blood cell receptor
Mature	T3	30	97	Associated with T-cell antigen receptor
Helper/inducer	T4	80	65	Present on helper and suppressor-inducer T-cells
Suppressor/cytotoxic	T8	80	35	Present on suppressor-cytotoxic T-cells
Thymocyte	T10	95	5	Present on early stem cells, activated T-cells
Pre-T/thymocyte	T6	70	0	Cortical thymocytes
Pan-T	T1	95	95	Equivalent to murine *Thy-1* antigen

TABLE 7 Tests for Defects in Phagocytic System

A. Screening evaluation
  Quantitative tests
    Total granulocyte count and morphology
    Total monocyte count
  Functional tests
    Nitroblue tetrazolium (NBT) dye reduction

B. Diagnostic evaluation
  Quantitative tests
    Histochemical staining for alkaline phosphatase, peroxidase, and esterase
    Monocyte differentiation by surface antigenic markers (*OKM1; Leu 3M*)
    C3b receptor enumeration
    Fc receptor enumeration
  Functional tests
    Random migration and chemotaxis
    Chemilumenescence of stimulated neutrophils
    Superoxide generation by stimulated neutrophils
    Granulocyte microbicidal assay

Screening assays for the complement system are listed in Table 8, part A. Serum levels of three basic components can be measured by immunoassay (radial immunodiffusion) to implicate activation or utilization of either the classical or alternative pathway. The serum C4 level is depressed with classical pathway activation, serum factor B is depressed with alternative pathway activation, and the serum C3 level is depressed when either pathway is activated, resulting in initiation of the effector phase of the complement cascade (C5 through C9). An excellent screening test for functional integrity of the entire complement system is the measurement of total hemolytic complement in the serum, expressed as 50%-hemolytic units, or CH_{50}. Although mild decreases in individual components may not be detected as a depression in CH_{50}, a low or absent CH_{50} implies a significant defect in one or more components of the classical cascade and requires further diagnostic evaluation. When there is evidence that a complement level or function is abnormal in screening assays, a definitive diagnosis of a depression or deficiency in one or more complement components or regulatory proteins can be made by quantitating the concentration of individual components by immunoassay and by measuring functional activity of individual components independently by hemolytic assays (Table 8,

TABLE 8 Tests for Defects in the Complement System

A. Screening evaluation
  Quantitative tests
    C3, C4, Factor B serum levels
  Functional tests
    Total hemolytic complement (CH_{50})

B. Diagnostic evaluation
  Quantitative tests
    Measurement of specific component levels by immunoassay: C1q, C1r, C4, C2, C3, C5, C6, C7, C8, C9, Factor P, Factor D
  Functional tests
    Assay of specific component function by factor-limited hemolytic assay

part B). These more sophisticated diagnostic assays are generally available in specialized reference or research laboratories.

Prenatal Diagnosis of Immunodeficiency

With the expansion in knowledge of specific cellular and enzymatic defects which produce immunodeficiency diseases, prenatal diagnosis of some immunodeficiency diseases has been possible. Enzymatic analysis on cultured fibroblasts obtained at amniocentesis or fetal blood sampling prior to 20 weeks' gestation has been used successfully for the diagnosis of congenital immune deficiencies. Although currently in use at only a few medical centers, these techniques should become more widely available in the near future.

THERAPY OF IMMUNODEFICIENCY

General Approach

Early diagnosis and rapid institution of specific therapy in patients with immunodeficiency disorders is imperative to prevent mortality and the morbidity of complications from recurrent opportunistic infections. Early diagnosis is possible with an aggressive and organized approach using both screening and diagnostic procedures, as outlined above. Individual specific infections should be treated with specific antibiotics, the choice being made on the basis of microbial sensitivity patterns. When the infecting agent is unknown, broad-spectrum antibiotic coverage against the most likely pathogens is indicated. Prophylactic antibiotics are generally not recommended because of the development of resistant bacterial or fungal superinfection. There are three exceptions to this general rule: penicillin prophylaxis for postsplenectomy *S. pneumoniae* infections, trimethoprim-sulfamethoxazole prophylaxis for *Pneumocystis carinii* pneumonia in patients with deficient cell-mediated immunity, and trimethoprim-sulfamethoxazole or dicloxacillin prophylaxis for patients with chronic granulomatous disease. These specific indications are discussed in more detail below.

Immunization of patients with suspected immunodeficiency should be performed with great caution. In many instances, immunization will be fruitless because the underlying immunodeficiency results in a poor antibody response. In this situation, other forms of protection must be utilized, such as passive immunization with immunoglobulin therapy. In individuals with deficiencies in cell-mediated immunity, live viral immunization (e.g., oral poliovirus, measles, mumps, rubella, smallpox, and influenza) are specifically contraindicated, since they may lead to severe or life-threatening disease in the deficient host.

Blood transfusions should be administered only for clear indications. Whole blood, packed red blood cells, unprocessed plasma, and platelets each contain viable lymphocytes and are capable of producing graft-versus-host disease in susceptible hosts with defects in cell-mediated immunity. Blood products for patients with cell-mediated immune defects should be irradiated with 3,000 rad to eliminate viable lymphocytes, which may engraft the deficient host and lead to a potentially fatal graft-versus-host disease (GVHD). The potential of GVHD can also be eliminated when blood products are processed by freezing and subsequent centrifugation.

Restoration and maintenance of adequate nutritional status is fundamental to the care of patients with immunodeficiency. At the time of diagnosis, many patients are significantly malnourished and have secondary intercurrent gastrointestinal disease, which may include *Giardia lamblia* infestation and bacterial and fungal overgrowth of the intestinal tract. Malnutrition may contribute to and complicate the immunodeficiency state, further compromising the patient. When enteral feeding is not successful, then parenteral feeding is indicated, as long as appropriate precautions to guard against infection are taken.

Therapy of Antibody-Deficiency Syndromes

Since Colonel Bruton's description in 1952 of agammaglobulinemia and its subsequent treatment with immunoglobulin, replacement therapy has been the mainstay of treatment for antibody-deficiency syndromes. Currently, there are two forms of immunoglobulin for passive administration: standard immune serum globulin for intramuscular injection and the newer intravenous immunoglobulin preparations. The latter have certain advantages over the former, including less pain on administration (particularly important in adults who require large doses for replacement), ease of achieving physiologic levels of IgG, lower risk of infection and bleeding, rapid acquisition of peak serum levels, and no impediment to frequent administration, if required. These advantages are balanced by the increased cost of the intravenous IgG replacement therapy when compared with intramuscular standard immune serum globulin.

In patients with clearly defined antibody-deficiency syndromes, intramuscular standard immune serum globulin should be administered in a dose of 0.4 ml per kilogram per dose given every four weeks. It is frequently beneficial to divide the dose into three or four separate injections to minimize the pain associated with administration of large volumes. The subsequent doses of standard immune serum globulin should be adjusted on the basis of the clinical response of the patient, since changes in total serum IgG levels are rarely observed, even with rather large intramuscular doses.

In patients who do not tolerate even maximal doses given every 3 to 4 weeks, a more frequent injection schedule using a smaller volume may be better tolerated. For patients who fail to respond, who cannot tolerate intramuscular standard immune serum globulin, or in patients who require large doses to achieve a rapid increase in serum IgG levels, intravenous gamma globulin preparations can be utilized. Doses for intravenous therapy should begin at 200 mg per kilogram per dose, given every four weeks. After a period of three to four months to allow for tissue equilibration, this dose may be increased to 400 mg per kilogram per dose depending on clinical response and serum IgG levels.

For patients receiving intravenous immunoglobulin therapy, serum total IgG levels can be monitored to achieve optimal therapy. We attempt to maintain a preinfusion IgG level that is in the range of 400 to 600 mg per deciliter, or near the lower limit of normal for age. Adverse effects of both intramuscular and intravenous immunoglobulin replacement therapy include systemic anaphylactoid reactions. These appear to be due to aggregates of IgG injected intravenously and are characterized by rise in body temperature, flushing of the face, tightness in the chest, chills, dizziness, nausea, diaphoresis, and hyper- or hypotension. These reactions are not true anaphylactic reactions (i.e., not IgE-mediated), since most patients receiving this form of therapy are deficient in their ability to make IgE antibody.

In contrast to most patients with IgG antibody-deficiency syndromes, patients with selective IgA deficiency should not be treated with gamma globulin preparations or plasma, since these patients are fully capable of forming normal antibodies of other immunoglobulin classes. Consequently, they may recognize traces of IgA contained in gamma globulin or serum as a foreign protein. The use of gamma globulin or plasma may sensitize these patients to make antibodies to IgA, which may lead to subsequent anaphylactic transfusion reactions. An exception to this rule is patients with combined IgA/IgG2 subclass deficiency. These patients may benefit from standard immunoglobulin replacement given very cautiously in a controlled setting.

Therapy of Defects in Cell-Mediated Immunity

The correction or therapy of cell-mediated immune deficiency is much more difficult and complex than is the therapy of antibody-deficiency syndromes. Patients with defects in cell-mediated immunity who also showed defective antibody synthesis will benefit from immunoglobulin replacement therapy, as outlined above. Most patients with significant impairment of cell-mediated immunity will be susceptible to *P. carinii* pneumonia. When diagnosed, this infection can be treated with trimethoprim-sulfamethoxazole in a dose of 20 mg of trimethoprim per kilogram per day plus 100 mg of sulfamethoxazole per kilogram per day, in four divided daily doses for 14 days. If not successful or not tolerated, pentamidine isethionate, 4 mg per kilogram per day intramuscularly in a single daily dose for 14 days, can be utilized. Prophylaxis against *P. carinii* should be instituted in all patients with significant cell-mediated immune deficiency using trimethoprim-sulfamethoxazole, in a dose of 5 mg per kilogram per day of trimethoprim and 25 mg per kilogram per day of sulfamethoxazole.

Precautions to prevent graft-versus-host disease (GVHD) by irradiation of blood products is indicated in patients with T-cell deficiency (see *General Approach*, outlined previously).

Severe defects in cell-mediated immunity are most effectively treated by transplantation of HLA–genotypically identical bone marrow. Complete immunologic reconstitution with this form of therapy has been documented in more than 100 patients with severe combined immunodeficiency (SCID). When an HLA-matched donor is not available, an alternative for T-cell reconstitution is transplantation of T-cell-depleted, haplotype-mismatched, parental bone marrow. In this procedure, potential GVHD-producing T-lymphocytes are eliminated from the parental marrow before transplantation by differential agglutination with the lectin soybean agglutinin or with monoclonal antibodies to T-cells. Using this approach, a small number of patients have achieved engraftment of parental marrow with subsequent immunologic reconsitution and a state of stable split chimerism.

Other alternatives utilized in the past include transplant of fetal hepatic tissue to replace putative defective stem cells, transplant of fetal thymic tissue to replace deficient stem cells and/or to provide a normal thymic microenvironment for stem cell maturation, and implantation of cultured thymic epithelium. Each of these latter therapies has been successful in a small number of patients.

In patients with severe defects in cell-mediated immunity associated with deficiency of enzymes in the purine salvage pathway, biochemical therapy is sometimes successful. In patients with adenosine deaminase deficiency, transfusion of frozen, irradiated, packed red blood cells to replace the deficient enzyme has occasionally been successful in reversing the biochemical abnormalities and partially reversing T-cell immunodeficiency.

Some patients with congenital deficiency of cell-mediated immunity appear to have defects in development or function of thymic microenvironment (DiGeorge syndrome; combined immunodeficiency with B-cells). Natural and synthetic thymic humoral factors have been prepared and tested for therapy in these patients. Encouraging preliminary results have been obtained in patients with DiGeorge syndrome and in some patients with combined immunodeficiency with B-cells, using thymosin fraction V, thymosin alpha-1, or thymic pentapeptide (TP-5). Replacement of lymphokines such as interleukin-2 or interferon (produced by recombinant DNA technology) has been utilized only in experimental situations.

Therapy of Phagocytic Disorders

At present, there is no specific therapy to increase the microbicidal-defective activity of granulocytes in chronic granulomatous disease. Management is based primarily on aggressive diagnosis of and specific antimicrobial treatment of infective episodes.

Recently, several investigators have suggested that continuous prophylactic antibiotic therapy with trimethoprim-sulfamethoxazole or dicloxacillin may be effective in decreasing the incidence or severity of infections in patients with chronic granulomatous disease. White blood cell transfusions have also been utilized as adjunctive therapies during acute life-threatening infections in patients with chronic granulomatous disease, although experience with this form of therapy is extremely limited.

Therapy of Complement Defects

Defects have been described for almost all of the complement pathway components, including C1q, C1r, C4, C2, C3, C5, C6, C7, C8, and C9 and for the complement regulatory proteins C1 inhibitor and factor I (C3b inactivator). There is no satisfactory replacement therapy for most of these deficiencies, since the catabolic rates of the proteins are very high. Impeded androgens (e.g., danazol) may decrease the frequency of attacks in patients with hereditary angioedema, presumably by increasing concentrations of C1 inactivator and C4. Therapy with fresh-frozen plasma, 10 ml per kilogram per day, may be used to restore temporarily normal complement function in patients with C3 deficiency (either primary or secondary factor I deficiency) during episodes of severe acute pyogenic infection.

Some patients with deficiencies of terminal complement components, such as C5, C6, C7, and C8 and recurrent neisserial infections, require antibiotic prophylaxis with oral penicillin.

SPECIFIC IMMUNODEFICIENCIES

Immunodeficiencies Due to Antibody Defects

This class of immunodeficiency was the first to be recognized and described. It represents the most common form of immunodeficiency. Deficiencies of all classes and subclasses of immunoglobulins have now been described. The disorders reflect marked decrease or total absence of one or more of the immunoglobulins as a result of a defect in B-cell maturation or T-cell regulation of B-cell function. The defect may be congenital or acquired, permanent or transient. In the congenital hypogammaglobulinemias, symptoms appear during first year of life, following loss of the maternal immunoglobulins acquired through transplacental transmission. The severity of symptoms varies with the degree of immunoglobulin deficiency. The hallmark of the symptoms of hypogammaglobulinemia is recurrent severe infection by pyogenic organisms. Diagnosis is established readily by quantitation of immunoglobulin isotypes in the serum. Examination of the function of the B-cells and T-cells helps in identifying the specific nature of the underlying disorder (Table 9).

X-Linked Agammaglobulinemia

(Bruton's agammaglobulinemia, congenital or infantile agammaglobulinemia, panhypogammaglobulinemia).

TABLE 9 Differential Diagnosis of Panhypogammaglobulinemia

Type of Hypogammaglobulinemia	*Predominance*	*Age of Onset*	*B-cell Plasma Cell Abnormality*	*T-Cell Abnormality*	*Response to Immunization*	*Lymph Node Histology*
X-Linked (Bruton's)	Male	>9 months	Pre-B-cells: normal B-cells: no Ig Plasma cells: absent	None	Absent	Germinal center: poorly developed
Autosomal-recessive	Female	>9 months	Pre-B-cells: normal B-cells: no Ig Plasma cells: absent	None	Absent	Germinal center: poorly developed
Common variable	Both sexes	Any age	B-cells: low-high Plasma cells: absent	Reversed T4/T8 ratio	Absent	Cortical follicles: present
Transient	Both sexes	9–30 months	B-cells: normal Plasma cells: low	Decreased T4	Normal	Normal

This is an X-linked inherited deficiency involving all classes of immunoglobulin. Total absence of immunoglobulins is rare; small amounts of immunoglobulins can usually be detected.

Pathophysiology. The deficiency in maturation of B-cells may be due to a block in the differentiation of pre-B-cells. Pre-B-cells in bone marrow are usually normal in number, but circulating B-cells or plasma cells are greatly diminished or absent. T-cells and T-cell subsets are normal in number and function.

Pre-B-cells do not have surface immunoglobulins and possess small amounts of cytoplasmic μ (heavy) chains only. In X-linked agammaglobulinemia, these μ chains appear to be smaller in size than normal μ chains and lack the protein coded by the variable heavy-chain region. An associated reduction in size of μ-chain RNA has also been described, which suggests that the defect reflects a failure to translocate the V_H region zone during cell differentiation. These B-cell defects are expressed as the inability of the patient to produce functional antibody and also as a failure to clear antigen. Thus, viral and parasitic infections in patients with X-linked agammaglobulinemia tend to persist.

Clinical Manifestations. The defect occurs only in males. Children rarely manifest clinical evidence of the disease before the age of 6 to 9 months, presumably because of acquired maternal immunoglobulins. The four characteristic manifestations of X-linked agammaglobulinemia are recurrent pyogenic infections, virtual absence of all classes of serum immunoglobulins, inability to synthesize antibody in response to immunization or infection, and absence of plasma cells from lymphoid tissue. Repeated bacterial infections are localized to the upper and lower respiratory tract and are due to pyogenic organisms, including pneumococcus, *Hemophilus influenzae*, and streptococcus. Chronic sinopulmonary infections are the major cause of morbidity in patients with agammaglobulinemia.

Although patients with X-linked agammaglobulinemia handle most viral and fungal infections relatively well, vaccine-associated poliomyelitis, persistant enteroviral encephalitis, and gastroenteritis due to rotavirus or *G. lamblia* occur with unusual frequency in these patients. *P. carinii* infections may also be the presenting infection. Some of the patients with X-linked agammaglobulinemia manifest rheumatoid arthritis and lymphoreticular malignancies.

Diagnosis. There is almost total absence of all immunoglobulin isotypes and of mature Ig-bearing B-cells in peripheral blood. The serum lacks specific antibodies, and the patients fail to respond to antigenic challenge. T-cells are normal in numbers and function. Normal numbers of pre-B-cells are present in the bone marrow. Lymph nodes show absence of plasma cells and absence or poor development of germinal centers. Thymic tissue is normal.

Treatment. Replacement therapy with human gamma globulin has proved effective in reducing morbidity and mortality in patients with agammaglobulinemia. Intramuscular or intravenous gamma globulin and supportive care should be provided, as outlined above.

X-Linked Hypogammaglobulinemia with Growth Hormone Deficiency

This immunodeficiency has been described in two children and two maternal uncles of one family. It was associated with panhypogammaglobulinemia in three of the four members affected. All had isolated growth hormone deficiency. The patients had short stature, small phallus, delayed onset of puberty, and retarded bone age. Treatment is the same as for X-linked congenital agammaglobulinemia.

Autosomal Recessive Agammaglobulinemia

A rare form of congenital agammaglobulinemia has been reported in female patients. The manifestations of the deficiency are similar to those of X-linked agammaglobulinemia. A defect in B-cell differentiation is postulated as being responsible for this disease. This condition should be suspected in females who have male and female relatives with agammaglobulinemia. The diagnostic criteria used for X-linked agammaglobulinemia apply to the autosomal recessive form. Treatment is also the same.

Common Variable Agammaglobulinemia

(Agammaglobulinemia with immunoglobulin-bearing B-lymphocytes; idiopathic late-onset immunoglobulin deficiency; acquired agammaglobulinemia)

This deficiency is also characterized by abnormally low levels or absence of all immunoglobulin isotopes. Although the term *acquired* has been used for this form of agammaglobulinemia, there is no evidence for acquisition of this deficiency. The presence of abnormal immunoglobulin levels in family members of patients with this disease, as well as a high incidence of systemic lupus erythematosus, idiopathic thrombocytopenia and hemolytic anemia in first-degree relatives suggests a hereditary influence for this condition.

Pathophysiology. Enumeration and evaluation of function of T- and B-cells in patients with common variable agammaglobulinemia suggest that this condition represents a heterogeneous disease resulting from intrinsic B-cell defects occurring at various stages of maturation of the B-cells into antibody-secreting (plasma) cells. Lymphocytes fail to differentiate into plasma cells in vitro in the presence of polyclonal B-cell activators. Immunoregulatory T-cell imbalance with reversal of helper to suppressor T-cell ratios has been described, but this may be secondary to chronic infection. In a few patients, autoantibodies to T- or B-lymphocytes have been found.

Clinical Manifestations. The agammaglobulinemia may occur at any age. Both sexes are equally affected. Patients give a history of recurrent pyogenic infections beginning several years after birth. Chronic, progressive bronchiectasis is a common presentation. A high incidence of gastrointestinal symptoms, often due to *Giardia lamblia*, and of lymphoreticular malignancy is seen in patients with this form of agammaglobulinemia. Pernicious anemia occurs in 30 percent of patients. Noncaseating granuloma of various organs is encountered and is associated with hepatospenomegaly.

Diagnosis. Patients have low or high numbers of circulating immunoglobulin-bearing B-lymphocytes. However, these cells do not differentiate into plasma cells or produce immunoglobulins in vitro, even after polyclonal stimulation. The total number of T-lymphocytes in the blood is normal, but there may be reversal of the T4/T8 subset ratio. Functional studies may demonstrate diminished helper or increased suppressor T-cell activity. Lymphocyte response to phytohemagglutinin, concavalin A, and pokeweed mitogen is significantly diminished in some. Cortical follicles in lymph nodes are present.

Treatment. Immunoglobulin administration and supportive care as for patients with X-linked gammaglobulinemia are appropriate.

Transient Hypogammaglobulinemia of Infancy

This uncommon immunodeficiency is characterized by persistent low immunoglobulin levels, below the lower normal limits for age. This abnormality persists through the first 2 years of life. Resolution is accompanied by a rise of immunoglobulin levels to normal.

Pathophysiology. This deficiency may represent a delayed maturation of the normal ontogeny of the humoral immune response. Physiologic hypogammaglobulinemia occurs at 3 to 6 months of age in normal newborns when loss of maternal immunoglobulins exceeds synthesis of antibodies to environmental antigens. This period may persist longer in premature infants. In patients with transient hypogammaglobulinemia, this period is extended to as long as 20 to 30 months. Circulating B-cells are normal in number and function; patients respond to immunization by forming specific antibodies. A numerical and functional deficiency in helper (T4-positive) lymphocytes has been described in these patients. This deficiency resolves with resolution of the hypogammaglobulinemia.

Clinical Manifestations. Two clinical patterns are recognized. The first occurs in a group of patients with no significant symptoms. All have relatives with immunodeficiencies. Immunoglobulin levels return to normal by 1 to 2 years of age. The second pattern occurs in a group with recurrent infections in early infancy that resolve in early childhood. These patients have no immunodeficient relatives. Infections are associated with unexplained febrile episodes and bronchitis. One or more of the immunoglobulin isotypes may remain below normal levels.

Diagnosis. This deficiency should be considered in a male or female infant with persistent hypogammaglobulinemia, but with normal response to antigenic challenge. Hypogammaglobulinemia involves primarily IgG. The numbers of circulating B- and T-lymphocytes is normal. T-cell subset enumeration reveals a decreased number of T4-positive lymphocytes.

Treatment. The condition is self-limited; hypogammaglobulinemia resolves by 1 to 2 years of age. No immunoglobulin administration is required except in those cases with marked hypogammaglobulinemia and severe recurrent infections.

Selective IgA Deficiency

This is the most common of the immunodeficiencies, with an incidence estimated at 1:700 of the general population. This defect is characterized by absent serum or secretory IgA or serum levels below 10 mg per deciliter.

Pathophysiology. Selective IgA deficiency may result from a maturation arrest of IgA-bearing B-cells and, in rare cases, from lack of production of secretory component. Acquired IgA deficiency may follow intake of certain drugs, such as phenytoin and penicillamine. This may be due to induction of supressor T-cells, which interfere with B-cell maturation. Serum IgA concentration may spontaneously rise to normal levels in primary IgA deficiency and return to normal following cessation of the drugs in the acquired state.

Clinical Manifestations. A majority of individuals with IgA deficiency may be totally healthy. However, some estimate that selective IgA deficiency accounts for 10 to 15 percent of symptomatic cases of immunodeficiencies. In some patients, IgA deficiency is associated with recurrent and severe infections of the respiratory, gastrointestinal, and urogenital tracts. The same pyogenic bacterial agents are involved in these infections as in other forms of agammaglobulinemia. Other patients may present only with recurrent or chronic respiratory infections or with atopic disease, while still others may have collagen-vascular or autoimmune diseases.

The propensity of patients to form antibodies to exogenous IgA is a point of serious clinical concern. Near-fatal anaphylactic reactions have followed systemic administration of human blood products to these patients. About one-half of the patients with selective IgA deficiency have antibodies to IgA in their serum.

Diagnosis. The findings of serum IgA levels lower than 10 mg per deciliter on two successive determinations after the age of 6 months establishes the diagnosis of IgA deficiency. Primary IgA deficiency may also be associated with deficiency of other classes of immunoglobulins, such as IgE or IgG2 and IgG4 subclasses. A rare deficiency in production of secretory component has been described and is associated with low levels of IgA in saliva and intestinal fluids. Familial IgA2 deficiency has been reported.

Treatment. At present there is no replacement therapy for IgA deficiency except in patients with IgG subclass deficiency. Systemic administration of human immunoglobulin to patients with IgA deficiency is contraindicated. Blood products (red cells) should be washed at least five times before administration to avoid anaphylactic reactions.

Selective IgM Deficiency

This is an extremely rare condition characterized by decreased level of serum IgM.

Pathophysiology. Normal or slightly decreased numbers of circulating IgM-bearing B-cells are seen. The underlying defect may lie in the differentiation of B-cells to immunoglobulin-secreting plasma cells. An acquired IgM deficiency has been described in patients with gluten enteropathy, which is reversed following treatment with gluten-free diet.

Clinical Manifestations. The most common infection associated with IgM deficiency is meningococcemia. Recurrent infection with other bacteria is also seen.

Diagnosis. Levels of serum IgM are subnormal. Total absence of IgM is rare.

Treatment. There is no specific therapy. Antibiotics and plasma infusions may help in serious infections.

Immunoglobulin Deficiency Associated with Elevated IgM (and IgD)

Initially thought to be X-linked, this syndrome has been observed in females and also as an acquired disease.

Pathophysiology. T-cell number and function are normal. Increased numbers of IgM-synthesizing plasmacytoid cells are present in the blood, and secrete large amounts of IgM on stimulation in vitro. Other B-cells do not synthesize or produce IgG or IgA.

Clinical Manifestations. These include recurrent pyogenic respiratory infections and autoimmune diseases, such as hemolytic anemia, thrombocytopenia, cyclic neutropenia, and lymphoproliferative disease.

Treatment. This consists of IgG replacement, which may be accompanied by regression of IgM levels and lymphoid hyperplasia in some patients.

Deficiency of Isotype Subclasses

Patients with absence or selective deficiency of one or more IgG (1–4) subclasses have been reported. There is often an associated IgA deficiency. In these patients, the total serum IgG level may be normal or below the lower normal range. Patients with subclass deficiency tend to have recurrent respiratory infections. Measurement of IgG subclasses is still not universally available. IgG replacement should be provided for those patients with isolated IgG deficiency.

Antibody Deficiency with Normal Immunoglobulin Levels

Occasional patients have been described with recurrent infections and normal immunoglobulins, but with inability to form specific antibodies following immunization or in response to antigens of infecting organisms. Some of these patients may have IgG subclass deficiency. An imbalance of the helper to suppressor T-cell ratio has been considered as the underlying defect. Because of the former association, IgG subclass determinations should be performed and replacement therapy provided if IgG subclass defect is proved.

Immunodeficiency with Hyperimmunoglobulinemia E

Several children with recurrent infections, primarily staphylococcal, and high serum IgE levels (5,000 to 30,000 IU per deciliter) have been described. In addition to recurrent skin, lung, and musculoskeletal infections, the clinical features include growth retardation and coarse facies. The patients manifest depressed antibody formation, but exquisite immediate hypersensitivity. Serum levels of other immunoglobulin isotypes are normal. T-cell number and function are also normal. Abnormal neutrophil chemotaxis has been described. A characteristic finding is the ability to absorb out serum IgE in vitro with *S. aureus* strains lacking Fc receptors on their surface. No immunoglobulin replacement therapy is indicated. Treatment of infection should include antistaphylococcal antibiotics.

DEFECTS THAT PREDOMINANTLY AFFECT CELL-MEDIATED IMMUNITY

DiGeorge Syndrome (third and fourth pharyngeal pouch syndrome)

Pathophysiology. In the embryo, the thymus gland and parathyroid glands arise from the endodermal epithelium of the third and fourth pharyngeal pouches. Dysembryogenesis involving this area during the 10th to 12th weeks of gestation may lead to aplasia, hypoplasia, or ectopia of the thymus and parathyroid glands.

Clinical Manifestations. When complete, this syndrome consists of the following features:

1. Abnormal facies with small, low-set, posteriorly rotated, dysmorphic ears, "fish-mouth" with a small mandible and a short philtrum; hypertelorism and antimongoloid slant of the eyes.
2. Congenital heart defects, especially interrupted aortic arch or truncus arteriosus, but also a variety of septal defects, patent ductus arteriosus, right-sided aortic arch, and tetralogy of Fallot.
3. Hypoparathyroidism presenting as neonatal tetany.
4. Cellular immunodeficiency, which is variable in severity from a profound deficiency of T-cells to only mild decreases in T-cell number with relatively normal T-cell function. B-cell numbers are generally normal.

The immunologic defect in DiGeorge syndrome can be corrected by fetal thymus gland transplantation, cultured thymic epithelium implantation, and, in some cases, treatment with thymosin fraction V or TP-5. These results suggest that patients with DiGeorge syndrome lack a thymic factor(s) capable of expanding their own T-cell compartment.

Combined Immunodeficiency with Predominant T-Cell Defect (Nezelof's Syndrome)

This is a variable immunodeficiency consisting of profound defects in T-cell immunity, but normal numbers of B-cells and normal to elevated immunoglobulin levels. The heterogeneity of immunologic abnormalities, the sporadic distribution or occurrence of this disorder, the fact that many cases were described before recent advances in the diagnosis of T-cell deficiencies were available, and the association of similar immunologic abnormalities with congenital cytomegalovirus all contribute to the difficulty in clearly defining this disorder. It is believed that many cases described in the past may have had purine nucleoside phosphorylase deficiency (this is discussed later).

Pathophysiology. The pathogenesis of this disorder is unknown, although the occurrence of isolated deficiency in T-cells with normal B-cell number and some immunoglobulin synthesis implicates a deficiency in the thymus gland.

Clinical Manifestations. Patients with this disorder are susceptible to recurrent viral, fungal, protozoal, and bacterial illnesses as are patients with severe combined immune deficiency (discussed later). Marked lymphadenopathy and hepatosplenomegaly clinically distinguish patients with this disease from patients with severe combined immune deficiency.

Diagnosis. A variable defect in cell-mediated immunity is present. Normal to decreased absolute lymphocyte counts are noted and moderate to severely deficient T-cell numbers are found. Lymphocyte responses to mitogens are depressed, as are the responses to allogeneic cells or soluble antigens. Immunoglobulin concentrations may be normal to increased. Total number of circulating B-cells is normal. Despite the presence of B-cells and relatively normal immunoglobulin levels—and occasionally the presence of preformed specific antibody (i.e., isoagglutinins)—there is no specific antibody formed following antigenic challenge.

Treatment. Aggressive therapy of defined infections with specific antimicrobial drugs is indicated. Gamma globulin replacement is indicated in patients who fail to mount a normal antibody response following immunization, even if serum immunoglobulins are normal. Reconstitution of T-cell immunity can be accomplished by histocompatible bone marrow transplantation or, in some cases, with thymic factors. Live viral immunization should be avoided, and blood products should be irradiated with 3,000 rad to prevent GVHD.

Purine Nucleoside Phosphorylase Deficiency

Purine nucleoside phosphorylase (PNP) and adenosine deaminase (ADA) are enzymes of the purine salvage pathway that are necessary for the metabolism of purines to uric acid. Deficiency of either of these enzymes leads to immunodeficiency (see *adenosine-deaminase deficiency*). PNP deficiency is inherited in an autosomal recessive fashion and leads to an accumulation of ionosine, guanosine, deoxyguanosine, and deoxy-GTP. This, in turn, probably results in inhibition of ribonucleotide-reductase activity, subsequent depletion of deoxyribonucleotide triphosphates, and inhibition of cellular division. Patients generally have absent T-cell immunity, normal B-cell immunity, frequent autoantibody formation, and recurrent infections, resulting in death from overwhelming viral infection in most cases. Prenatal diagnosis is now available by enzyme analysis of cultured fetal fibroblasts. Therapy with irradiated red blood cell infusions or with normal plasma has sometimes altered the metabolic accumulation of purines, but has not altered the clinical outcome. Histocompatible bone marrow transplantation is the therapy of choice for immunologic constitution and biochemical cure.

Combined Deficiencies of Cell-Mediated Immunity and Antibody-Mediated Immunity

Severe Combined Immunodeficiency

Patients with severe combined immunodeficiency (SCID) generally have recurrent fungal, viral, protozoal, and bacterial infections beginning before 6 months of age and resulting in severe disability, failure to thrive, chronic lung disease, and death, often during the first year of life. Numerous forms of SCID are recognized (see Table 2), including reticular dysgenesis, low T- and B-cell numbers (classic SCID), low T-cell number with normal B-cell number (Swiss-type lyphopenic agammaglobulinemia), "bare lymphocyte" syndrome, and SCID with adenosine deaminase deficiency. Sporadic X-linked and autosomal recessive patterns of inheritance are recognized.

Pathogenesis. The exact pathogenesis of severe combined immunodeficiency is unknown and is likely different for each of the variants described. A failure of stem cell differentiation into normal B- and T-cells may be responsible in some cases (e.g., reticular dysgenesis, classic SCID, and the "bare lymphocyte" syndrome), whereas other patients may have an intrathymic maturational defect (Swiss-type agammaglobulinemia).

Adenosine deaminase is an enzyme of the purine salvage pathway (see *PNP deficiency*), which catalyzes the conversion of adenosine and deoxyadenosine to inosine and deoxyinosine. Deficiency of ADA leads to accumulation of purine nucleosides and deoxynucleosides and deoxy-ATP, which results in inhibition of ribonucleotide reductase and inhibition of cell division.

Clinical Manifestation. Patients with SCID often present with persistent oral and gastrointestinal candidiasis, intractable diarrhea and failure to thrive, interstitial pneumonitis due to *P. carinii*, or cytomegalovirus and recurrent bacterial sepsis. With the complete lack of T-cell immunity, patients are susceptible to GVHD, which often results from (*1*) maternal T-cell engraftment in utero or during birth, (*2*) unirradiated blood products, or (*3*) attempted immunologic reconstitution.

Diagnosis. The diagnosis is confirmed by laboratory studies showing lymphopenia, eosinophilia, a marked decrease in T-cell number and function, and deficient B-cell function. Some patients with SCID appear to lack all T-cell markers (classic SCID), whereas others (e.g., with Swiss-type agammaglobulinemia) may have lymphocytes that express early thymocyte markers (T6, T10), but fail to express mature T-cell markers (T3, T4, T8). Diminished T-cell function is shown by abnormal lymphocyte blastogenesis with mitogens, soluble antigens, and allogeneic cells. Antibody-dependent cellular cytotoxicity (ADCC) and cell-mediated lympholysis are also abnormal in patients with SCID. B-cells are usually absent, but may be present in some forms (Swiss-type agammaglobulinemia). Associated immunoglobulin deficiencies may be difficult to diagnose in the first few months of life due to the presence of transplacentally derived maternal IgG. IgG values below 200 mg per deciliter are helpful in the diagnosis, and most patients with SCID will be totally lacking in serum IgM and IgA. Immunization with inert antigens produces no antibody response. Immunization with live viruses is contraindicated. Natural killer cell number and activity can be normal or decreased.

Treatment. Optimal therapy for reconstitution of the immunodeficiency is bone marrow transplantation from HLA-matched doors. With this procedure the overall survival rate is approximately 65 percent. For patients lacking histocompatible donors for bone marrow transplantation, a variety of other approaches have been attempted with limited success. Fetal liver transplantation has been partially successful in five of 43 cases; fetal thymus transplantation is also successful in 10 to 15 percent of a smaller number of cases, and the combination of fetal liver plus fetal thymus transplantation has also been successful in a few cases. More recently, the use of T-cell-depleted, haplotype-mismatched, parental bone marrow transplantation has been successful in patients with SCID. Therapy with thymic factors has not generally been successful. Since erythrocytes contain high levels of ADA, red blood cell transfusions have been useful in some patients with SCID due to ADA deficiency. This has led to reduction in the high levels of accumulated purines and a partial reversal of the T-cell defects. Some other patients, however, have not responded to red blood cell transfusions.

Wiskott-Aldrich Syndrome

Wiskott-Aldrich syndrome is characterized by severe eczema, thrombocytopenia, and susceptibility to opportunistic infections. This disorder is inherited in an X-linked-recessive fashion. Thrombocytopenia leads to severe bleeding episodes. The median survival of patients with Wiskott-Aldrich syndrome is 6 years, with death usually due to central nervous system hemorrhage, recurrent severe infections, autoimmune hemolytic anemia or vasculitis, or lymphoreticular malignancy.

Pathophysiology. The pathogenesis of this disorder is unknown, although recent studies suggest that there may be the absence of a 115,000-dalton glycoprotein from T-cell membranes and a glycoprotein 1B from platelets. This suggests that the Wiskott-Aldrich syndrome may be due to a deficiency of glycosylation.

Diagnosis. Sera from affected males show normal levels of IgG, increased levels of IgA and IgE, and deficient levels of IgM. Antibody responses to antigenic challenge are a peculiar aspect of this immunodeficiency, with affected patients showing a normal response to protein antigens, but a poor response to carbohydrate or polysaccharide antigens. Thus, the serum of these patients lacks isohemoglutinins. Autoantibodies are frequently found in patients with Wiskott-Aldrich syndrome. With age, there is a progressive attrition of T-cell number and T-cell function, with the mixed lymphocyte reaction more affected than response to nonspecific mitogens. Platelet size of affected males is approximately one-half normal.

Treatment. Although originally thought to be contraindicated in patients with Wiskott-Aldrich syndrome, splenectomy has proved useful in managing severe and life-threatening thrombocytopenia, provided that appropriate precautions are taken to avoid postsplenectomy sepsis. Steroids are generally contraindicated unless required to control autoimmune hemolytic anemia.

The T-cell, B-cell, and platelet defects in Wiskott-Aldrich syndrome can be corrected by HLA-matched sibling bone marrow transplantation. Transfer factor, thymic hormones, fetal liver or fetal thymus transplantations have not generally been useful.

For patients with severe recurrent bacterial infections

unresponsive to continuous antibiotics, therapy with intravenous gamma globulin may be instituted. Intramuscular gamma globulin therapy is contraindicated because of the risk of bleeding.

Ataxia-Telangiectasia

Ataxia-telangiectasia is a complex syndrome inherited as an autosomal-recessive trait and consisting of progressive cerebellar ataxia, retardation, cutaneous and bulbar conjunctival telangiectasias, recurrent sinopulmonary infections with bronchiectasis, and a combined immunodeficiency usually manifested by selective IgA deficiency and partial T-cell immunodeficiency. Lymphoreticular malignancies occur with an increased frequency in patients with ataxia-telangiectasia.

Pathophysiology. The pathogenesis of this condition is unknown, but may involve a basic defect in the ability to repair cellular DNA. Patients demonstrate undue susceptibility to radiation-induced cytotoxicity with an increased incidence of chromosomal breaks and translocations.

Diagnosis. Laboratory investigation reveals selective IgA deficiency in about 70 percent of patients with ataxia-telangiectasia. Other immunoglobulins may be normal to decreased. A subset of patients has combined IgA/IgG2 deficiency with an increased risk of pulmonary infections. Antibody responses to bacterial and viral antigens may be deficient. T-cell numbers are frequently, but not always, depressed, as is lymphocytic response to mitogens and antigens. T-helper-cells appear to be more affected than T-suppressor-cells.

Treatment. Aggressive supportive therapy prolongs survival; however, at present there is no cure. Gamma globulin is beneficial in patients with IgA/IgG2 deficiency and severe sinopulmonary infections. Attempts to reconstitute deficient cell-mediated immunity with thymic factors or fetal thymus gland transplants have been too limited to draw conclusions. No therapy is effective in halting central nervous system degeneration. Irradiation, including standard x-rays, should be minimized as much as possible to avoid chromosomal damage and the potential for induction of malignancy.

Immunodeficiency Due To Phagocytic Cell Defects

Phagocytosis of bacteria is a primary function of peripheral blood polymorphonuclear leukocytes. Phagocytic defects may be related to abnormalities in the number of circulating (or tissue-associated) phagocytes or due to inability of the phagocytic cells to ingest and kill bacteria. Defects in ingestion of bacteria are usually due to lack of opsonins and complement. Killing of bacteria following phagocytosis depends on an intact intracellular oxidation mechanism leading to utilization of reduced nicotinamide adenine nucleotide phosphate (NADPH) oxidase and oxygen to produce a superoxide ($O_2^{\cdot-}$ ion. This ion, together with hydrogen peroxide (H_2O_2) and intracellular myeloperoxidase and halide, catalizes the intracellular killing of bacterial organisms (Fig. 2). A defect in this pathway results in lack of microbicidal activity of the cell, with intracellular survival, persistance of bacteria and infection of tissue.

The majority of phagocytic cell defects are congenital in nature. Acquired defects are primarily due to decreased bone marrow cell production by immunosuppressive agents, destruction of the cells by antineutrophil antibodies, or increased sequestration of these cells in the spleen.

Quantitative Granulocyte Defects

Congenital granulocytopenia, cyclic, and acquired neutropenia account for the majority of defects in numbers of circulating granulocytes. Clinical manifestations may vary from total lack of symptoms to recurrent fever and mild infections or to overwhelming infections. In cyclic neutropenia, these symptoms correspond to the nadir of the peripheral granulocyte count. Diagnosis is established by performing serial white blood cell counts and differential smears twice weekly for 4 to 6 weeks. Bone marrow cytology may help differentiate various forms of granulocytopenia. Acute bacterial infection should be treated, preferably with bactericidal antibiotics.

Qualitative Granulocyte Defects

Chronic Granulomatous Disease

This is an inherited disease affecting males (X-linked). A variant has been described in females (possibly autosomal-recessive form). Clinical manifestations appear in infancy and include recurrent infections, otitis media, draining lymphadenitis, hepatospenomegaly, pneumonias, abscess formation, and osteomyelitis. Infections are usually due to organisms of low virulence.

Pathophysiology. Granulocytes of these patients possess a normal capacity to phagocytose bacteria. An enzyme deficiency involving NADPH oxidase or reductase has been found in patients with this disease. Deficiency in glutathione peroxidase and cytochrome B has been described in these patients, particularly in females. As described above, an intraphagocytic deficiency in these enzymes results in decreased formation of $O_2^{\cdot-}$, decreased H_2O_2 production, and decreased formation of the bactericidal complex of H_2O_2-myeloperoxidase-halide. Thus, bacteria that are ingested by the phagocytic cells of these patients are not killed intracellularly because of the lack of H_2O_2 needed for the formation of the bactericidal complex. This may explain why infections in the majority of patients with this defect are due to catalase-producing bacteria such as *S. aureus* and *Staphylococcus epidermidis*, *Serratia marcescens*, *Escherichia coli*, *Pseudomonas*, *Candida*, and *Aspergillus*. These organisms are not usually pathogenic in normal individuals. In contrast,

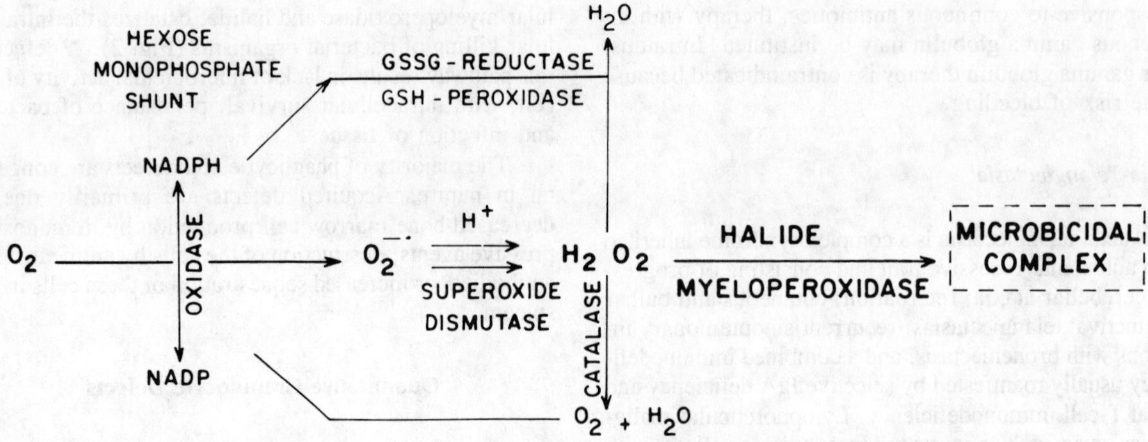

Figure 2 Oxidative pathway leading to granulocyte microbicidal activity in phagocytic cells.

bacteria that are catalase-negative and generate H_2O_2 (such as pneumococcus and streptococcus) account only rarely for infections in patients with chronic granulomatous disease because they are killed normally by the phagocytic cells of these patients.

Patients with chronic granulomatous disease are not unduly susceptible to viral infection; they have normal T- and B-cell function.

Clinical Manifestations. Onset of recurrent, prolonged infections in affected boys starts before the age of 2 years. Persistent, draining cervical adenitis is common. Generalized lymph node enlargement is seen with hepatosplenomegaly and hepatic abscesses. Infections of the lung and bone are chronic and of low-grade intensity. These infections are often not associated with severe systemic symptoms. Skin infections and subcutaneous abscesses are seen, with minimal erythema. Chronic otitis media and externa, stomatitis, and perianal abscesses are also encountered.

Diagnosis. This is usually established by examining granulocyte function. A simple screening test is the determination of nitroblue tetrazolium (NBT) dye reduction by polymorphonuclear leukocytes. If this reaction is decreased or absent, additional confirmatory studies should be performed; these include quantitative NBT, myeloperoxidase, and chemiluminescence tests. Bactericidal tests should provide definitive confirmatory evidence of this defect.

Treatment. Infections should be treated promptly with broad-spectrum bactericidal antibiotics given systemically. A semisynthetic penicillin and aminoglycoside are started empirically. Appropriate antibiotics are administered when an organism is isolated and its sensitivity determined. Chloramphenicol and rifampin have been favored by some because of their capacity to achieve high intracellular concentrations. Amphotericin B should be administered when fungal infections are encountered; if *Aspergillus* is isolated in patients with chronic lung disease, a combination of amphotericin B and rifampin is recommended. Prolonged therapy (4 to 6 weeks) is advisable for bacterial and fungal infections in these patients.

Antibiotic therapy has contributed greatly to the prolonged survival of patients with chronic granulomatous disease. Prior to the antibiotic era, most of these patients did not live beyond childhood. Prophylactic antibiotics are recommended for these patients; the most effective prophylactic agent is trimethoprim-sulfamethoxazole.

Granulocyte Deficiency Of Other Metabolic Enzymes

Patients with granulocyte dysfunction due to deficiency of other metabolic enzymes have been described. These include deficiency of glucose-6-phosphate dehydrogenase (G6PD), myeloperoxidase, and alkaline phosphatase. The bactericidal activity of the leukocytes of these patients may be only slightly decreased or totally absent—as is the case with G6PD. This defect, which is inherited as an X-linked deficiency, produces clinical manifestations similar to those of chronic granulomatous disease.

Chediak-Higashi Syndrome

This rare syndrome is characterized by the presence of giant cytoplasmic granules in white blood cells and platelets. It is inherited in an autosomal-recessive manner. The clinical manifestations consist of partial albinism, photophobia, hepatosplenomegaly, neurologic changes, anemia, and leukopenia, along with recurrent bacterial infections and a high incidence of lymphoreticular malignancies. There is delayed, but not absent, intracellular killing of all bacteria by phagocytes. Hexose monophosphate-shunt activity and H_2O_2 production are normal. Granulocyte lysosomal enzyme levels are abnormal. No treatment is available. Most patients die during childhood.

TABLE 10 Complement Deficiencies

Deficiency	*Clinical Findings*
C1q	Associated with X-linked agammaglobulinemia and severe combined immunodeficiency; urticaria; vasculitis
C1r	Systemic lupus erythematosus (SLE) syndrome; glomerulonephritis
C4	SLE syndrome
C2	SLE syndrome; glomerulonephritis; vasculitis, dermatomyositis, Schönlein-Henoch purpura; recurrent pneumococcal infection
C3	Pyogenic infections
C5	SLE syndrome; pyogenic infections; neisserial infections
C6	SLE syndrome; neisserial infections, Raynaud's phenomenon, sclerodactyly; ankylosing spondylitis; vasculitis
C8	SLE syndrome; neisserial infections
C9	Normal
C1 inhibitor	Hereditary angioedema
Factor I (C3b inactivator)	Pyogenic infections

Disorders in Leukocyte Mobility

These disorders are characterized by abnormal leukocyte chemotaxis and migration. They include the "lazy leukocyte" syndrome. Individuals present with severe bacterial infections. Abnormality of leukocyte chemotoxis has also been described in the "hyper-IgE" syndrome and in patients with glycogen- and mannose-storage diseases.

Another abnormality characterized by defective adherence and chemotaxis of neutrophils has been described recently. The leukocytes of these patients lack a surface membrane glycoprotein with a molecular weight of 150,000 to 180,000 (GP150 or GP180). The clinical manifestations include delayed separation of the umbilical cord, recurrent bacterial infections, and marked periodontitis with inability to form pus.

COMPLEMENT DEFICIENCIES

A summary of inherited complement deficiencies is presented in Table 10.

C1-inhibitor deficiency is inherited in an autosomal-dominant fashion, although all other complement-factor deficiencies are inherited in autosomal-codominant manner (heterozygotes have approximately one-half of the normal serum level). Deficiency of C1 inhibitor—the regulatory protein for C1 activation—leads to hereditary angioedema. Patients present with localized swelling and angioedema involving the subcutaneous tissue, the repiratory tract, and the gastrointestinal tract. These episodes may be severe enough to disfigure and may result in laryngeal edema and asphyxia. Two variants of hereditary angioedema are recognized: 85 percent of patients have absent C1 inactivator protein, and the other 15 percent have a functionally inactive protein that is present in normal quantities. Diagnosis is confirmed by finding low levels and/or function of C1 inhibitor. The patient may also have low C4 levels. During attacks of angioedema both C2 and C4 are further decreased. Treatment with impeded androgens (e.g., danazol) can prevent attacks of angioedema and may increase both the level and functional activity of C1 inactivator and C4. Purified human C1 inactivator is available for intravenous administration during severe acute attacks.

Deficiency of C2 is reported with increasing frequency. A lupus-like disease occurs in about 40 percent of patients. Other patients present with other collagen-vascular diseases such as Schönlein-Henoch purpura, dermatomyositis, cutaneous vasculitis, or membranoproliferative glomerulonephritis. In addition, some patients have had recurrent infections due to *Streptococcus pneumoniae*.

Treatment of C2 deficiency as well as of other complement-component deficiencies is directed toward the associated autoimmune or collagen-vascular disorder. Antibiotics are given as indicated for specific infectious illnesses.

CHILDHOOD EXANTHEMS

ANNE A. GERSHON, M.D.

MEASLES AND RUBELLA

Measles and rubella have become uncommon diseases in many developed countries today owing to widespread use of live attenuated measles and rubella vaccines introduced in 1963 and 1969, respectively. Perhaps because of the emphasis on prevention, specific antiviral therapy has never been developed for these diseases. Treatment for both thus remains symptomatic only and would include an antipyretic if indicated. Aspirin may be used to treat arthritis that often accompanies rubella in the adult. The cough of measles can be troublesome, but cough suppressants should be avoided. Prophylactic antibiotics are not indicated for either disease. Bacterial superinfections following measles, such as pneumonia and otitis media, are common, and if a superinfection has developed, it should be promptly treated with antimicrobials.

Because measles and rubella are so uncommon, it is useful to discuss diagnosis. Measles resembles a severe upper respiratory infection, such as influenza, during the first few days, with fever, cough, and coryza with no skin manifestations. Just prior to the development of rash, Koplik's spots, the pathognomonic enanthem of measles, may be seen on the buccal mucosa, usually opposite the molar teeth. The rash, which is morbilliform and then becomes confluent, begins on the face and moves down the body. Not all cases of measles fit the classic description, and since many younger physicians are unfamiliar with the disease, it is best to confirm the diagnosis serologically. To do this, 5 to 10 ml of clotted blood should be obtained as early as possible in the illness and again after 10 to 14 days. A fourfold or greater rise in serum antibody titer is, as with other viral infections, considered diagnostic. Both sera must be run simultaneously for accurate interpretation of the results.

Rubella is a milder illness than measles; as many as half the cases are subclinical. The major symptoms are a maculopapular rash, low grade fever, and cervical lymphadenopathy. Other illnesses may mimic rubella, so that the diagnosis should also be made serologically. It is particularly important to make the correct diagnosis if a women in the first trimester of pregnancy either is the patient or has been exposed to the patient.

Congenital rubella has become a rare disease in the United States, but at one time it was a major cause of fetal malformations. The decrease in incidence of congenital rubella has been attributed to improvements in diagnostic procedures, abortion policies, and live attenuated rubella vaccine. No cases of the congenital rubella syndrome as a result of inadvertent vaccination of a pregnant woman have been reported, although the vaccine virus may reach and cross the placenta. Women who have been immunized inadvertently while pregnant require careful counseling. While at one time abortion was considered mandatory, the fetal risk appears to be so small (3% or less) that each situation should be judged independently.

The best indication of immunity to rubella today is a history of receipt of live attenuated vaccine in the past. Standard serologic tests are often not sensitive enough to identify all immunes. To be safe, women of childbearing years who require immunization should refrain from becoming pregnant for at least 3 months after vaccination.

Measles, unlike rubella, poses a risk for susceptible immunocompromised patients, particularly those deficient in cellular immunity. Since measles vaccine is usually administered at 15 months of age, a situation of risk rarely arises. When there is a potential problem, however, immune serum globulin (ISG), 0.5 ml per kilogram IM, should be administered to the patient as soon as possible after the exposure. Neither measles nor rubella vaccine should be administered to immunocompromised patients. Passive immunization with ISG modifies measles; it does not prevent the congenital rubella syndrome, however, and therefore ISG is not recommended for rubella susceptible pregnant women who have been exposed to rubella.

Individuals who have received killed measles vaccine in the past are at some risk to develop the atypical measles syndrome if they are exposed to wild measles. This hypersensitivity reaction may on occasion be more severe than measles itself. Killed measles vaccine has not been available since 1968, so that persons born after that time cannot be at risk. At one time it was recommended that persons who had received killed measles vaccine be routinely revaccinated with live attenuated vaccine. Since there were many side effects, such as fever and sore arm, and since the opportunity for exposure to natural measles in the United States is now remote, revaccination is no longer routinely recommended. While measles is unusual in the United States, it still occurs frequently in other parts of the world. Thus in some instances, revaccination with live attenuated vaccine may be indicated, although live vaccine may not necessarily protect against future development of atypical measles.

Most index cases of measles in the United States are "imported" and may be the source of mini-outbreaks in unvaccinated persons. When normal, previously unvaccinated individuals have been exposed, ISG, 0.25 mg per kilogram IM, should be administered promptly.

VARICELLA

Varicella (chickenpox) and zoster are both caused by varicella-zoster (VZ) virus. Varicella is the primary infection; zoster results when latent VZ virus acquired as a result of varicella is reactivated. A vesicular skin rash is characteristic of each illness, that of varicella being generalized and zoster localized. Low-grade to moderate fever may also occur. The rash of varicella is characteristically itchy and that of zoster painful. Both diseases are usually self-limited and rarely require more than symptomatic therapy.

Immunosuppressed patients are at risk to develop severe or fatal varicella with dissemination of the virus to lungs, brain, and liver. Adults who contract varicella and newborn infants whose mothers have developed chickenpox in the 5 days before or 2 days after delivery are also at some increased risk. Passive immunization with varicella-zoster immune globulin (VZIG) can clearly modify the course of varicella. Following an intimate exposure to the virus, VZIG should be administered to varicella-susceptible, immunocompromised individuals as soon as possible (within 3 days) or, in the case of infants, at birth. An intramuscular dose of 1.25 ml per 10 kilograms is used. Adults, including pregnant women, should be passively immunized only if they are serologically proven to be susceptible to varicella, because most adults with no history of varicella are actually immune. VZIG, which contains about 20 times the amount of VZ antibody as ISG, may be obtained through local branches of the American Red Cross. VZIG is not effective for prevention of zoster in patients at high risk to develop the disease.

Pregnant women who contract varicella or zoster are at some increased risk to deliver a malformed fetus. The so-called congenital varicella syndrome, with eye, central nervous system, and limb defects is so rare, however, that most experts do not advise mandatory interruption of pregnancy after maternal VZ infection. It is a situation that requires careful weighing of the potential risks and benefits to the family involved.

Once varicella or zoster has developed, VZIG is of no therapeutic value. The antiviral drug, adenine arabinoside (Ara-A), an inhibitor of both viral and host DNA synthesis, may be used for treatment of severe VZ infections. It is administered intravenously over a 12-hour period at a dose of 10 mg per kilogram per day for 5 days. Reported toxic effects include nausea, vomiting, rash, bone marrow depression, tremors, and confusion. Toxic manifestations are more likely to occur in the setting of renal or hepatic compromise. Ara-A is licensed for treatment of herpes simplex encephalitis and not for VZ infections, but it is often employed for this purpose. Acyclovir (ACV) has also been employed successfully to treat VZ infections. ACV must be phosphorylated by a thymidine kinase present only in virus-infected cells in order to interfere with DNA synthesis. Therefore, ACV has little effect on host DNA synthesis, and it is less toxic for the host than is Ara-A. ACV is available in topical, oral, and intravenous formulations. Topical ACV is of no use for treatment of VZ infections. Until more data are available concerning the efficacy of oral ACV for VZ infections, only intravenous ACV can be recommended. The dose is 1,500 mg per square meter of body weight per day, divided into three doses. This is higher than the dose usually employed for herpes simplex viral infections. The duration of therapy is dependent upon the condition of the patient; usually a week is adequate. Toxicity is limited to phlebitis and transient increases in serum creatinine levels.

Treatment with an antiviral should begin within 3 days of onset of VZ infection for best results. Whether or not to institute antiviral chemotherapy is often a difficult decision. In many instances the illness does not become severe until a week after onset, and at that time it may be too late to institute successful therapy. The question frequently asked is whether one ought to treat all immunosuppressed patients who develop varicella or zoster. Treatment is usually recommended for varicella in immunocompromised patients who have not been passively immunized. It is wise to treat before the illness becomes severe. For zoster, no general recommendations can be given, and the decision must be made on an individual basis. It would seem prudent to be liberal in the use of antivirals in patients thought to be highly immunocompromised. It is rarely necessaary to treat otherwise normal patients with VZ with antivirals, nor is it necessary to study individuals with zoster for occult malignancy. An antiviral should be used to treat primary VZ pneumonia, which may be seen in the immunocompromised patient and occasionally in an otherwise normal adult who contracts varicella. An antiviral is of questionable use for varicella encephalitis, and it is not clear whether it is of benefit in treating encephalitis that may accompany zoster. The diagnosis of VZ encephalitis may be made by demonstrating antibody to VZ virus in cerebrospinal fluid.

Bacterial superinfections may follow varicella and should be suspected if there is a resurgence of fever or suspicious skin lesions, especially during convalescence from the illness. Prophylactic antibiotics, however, are not indicated. Superinfections are likely to be due to staphylococci or group A beta-hemolytic streptococci. Reye's syndrome rarely may follow varicella in children. Since there is increasing evidence that aspirin may also be somehow related to development of Reye's syndrome, it is recommended to refrain from treating the fever of varicella with aspirin in children under 18 years of age.

A live attenuated varicella vaccine is currently being studied for prevention of varicella. It has been highly effective in normal children, adults, and immunocompromised children. It is currently under consideration for licensure in the United States.

KAWASAKI SYNDROME

RICHARD H. MEADE III, M.D.

Increasing numbers of cases of Kawasaki syndrome (mucocutaneous lymph node syndrome) have been seen in the continental United States since 1972. Although recognized only recently as a distinct new entity, reports dating back over 100 years suggest that it is, in fact, not a new disease. Most cases have been seen in infants and children, but an increasing number have been seen in adults. Numerous causes have been suggested but none is accepted, and no specific laboratory tests for diagnosis are yet available.

EPIDEMIOLOGY

Cases of the syndrome have been seen in every month of the year, but most occur during the spring. Originally, cases were confined to the Japanese in Japan and later to those of Japanese heritage in Hawaii. In recent years cases have been seen in patients of every national origin—African, Caucasian, and Oriental. The average age of patients seen in a recent outbreak in Boston was 3.5 years, with a range from several months to 22 years. In Japan the average age was 1.5 years. Most patients are younger than 4 years (80%). Patients have ranged in age from only a few months to the late twenties.

Rug cleaners, mites, *Leptospira*, and *Rickettsia* have all been named as possible causes, but none has been confirmed. Recently, *Propionibacterium acnes* has been reported to be the cause because of its isolation from the lymph nodes of patients with Kawasaki syndrome. The occurrence of arteritis in experimental animals was cited as further evidence that this was the cause. Other studies to confirm this observation are awaited. The occurrence of most cases in the spring of the year and the restriction of cases to financially comfortable families make it hard to attribute the disease to an organism present in everyone.

The mortality rate is between 1 and 2 percent and is a consequence of coronary artery involvement. In most cases, aneurysmal rupture is the cause of death. In a few, coronary arterial occlusion with myocardial infarction has been the reason.

PATHOPHYSIOLOGY

The principal lesion is vasculitis involving much of the body, with evidence of it visible in the conjunctivae, oral mucosa, and skin. Vasculitis of all organs occurs, with clinical evidence detectable in the heart, lungs, liver, intestines, brain, and kidneys; the gall bladder and the joints are also involved. Aneurysms occur most often in the coronary arteries, but have also been found in the femoral, hepatic, iliac, axillary, and subscapular arteries. The vascular lesions are present in arteries, veins, and capillaries. There is both an acute perivasculitis with inflammation of the adventitia and an endarteritis. Infiltrating cells include both polymorphonuclear leukocytes and lymphocytes. Myocarditis accompanies coronary vasculitis.

CLINICAL ASPECTS

There are three phases in the disorder. The first is the acute stage; during this stage all of the signs of the disease occur, and fever is at its highest. The sequence in which the different manifestations appear varies. Some individuals present only with fever, some have fever and red soles and palms, and others have fever and enlarged cervical lymph nodes. Because of this diversity of initial presentation the diagnosis of some other disease is commonly made before Kawasaki syndrome is thought of. The second phase is the period in which the temperature is declining and the various signs, such as the skin rash and large nodes, are subsiding. The patient is improving during this period, but is not well. Children will not have regained their appetites, others will have persistent joint pains, and still others will have remittent fever. The third phase or convalescence begins when the temperature finally decreases to normal levels and remains there and all other signs have cleared.

The diagnosis of Kawasaki syndrome is based on the presence of certain clinical criteria:

1. All patients have fever that remains elevated for at least 5 days and is unresponsive to antipyretic drugs and antibiotic treatment. Fever is often high, but there is no specific temperature requirement as there is in toxic shock syndrome.
2. At least four of the next five criteria are required to make the diagnosis.
   a. Conjunctivitis. This consists entirely of injection of conjunctival vessels of both the bulbar and palpebral surfaces. There is no blepharitis or discharge. Uveitis occurs in up to 80 percent of patients, but can be seen only with a slit lamp. Retinal exudation is rare, but has been seen and is persistent.
   b. Abnormalities of the oral mucosa. The commonest sign is reddening of the lips. The lips can be swollen and red in some; in others, they are fissured and crusted. Inside the mouth, inflammation is usually patchy, involving the cheek, palate, or pharynx separately. The tongue may be swollen and red with hypertrophied papillae. A white coating on the surface gives the appearance of the strawberry tongue of scarlet fever. As in scarlet fever, the white coat recedes one-quarter the length of the tongue daily. By the fifth day the tongue resembles a raspberry.
   c. Polymorphous skin eruption. A variety of skin lesions are seen. (1) Scarlatiniform eruption: this rash exactly resembles that of scarlet fever. The skin of the trunk, but not the face, is red and has a diffuse follicular eruption, resulting in a "sandpaper" surface. (2) Polymorphous eruption: this is an irregularly outlined eruption on the extremities. The irregular outline is provided by the contrast between the erythema and the patches of normally colored skin. When the temperature is elevated the rash is bright red; otherwise the rash is almost invisible. (3) Erythema multiforme-like eruption: this consists of a collection of rounded, reddish brown lesions 1 to 2 cm in diameter, often with central clearing and target spot formation. These lesions are also primarily seen on the extremities, but may also be on the trunk or the face. (4) Diffuse maculopapular eruption: this is an eruption that resembles that of a viral infection. The lesions blanch on pressure, are bright red, and could be mistaken for the rash of measles. When seen alone with fever, there is no way the doctor could tell the cause of the eruption. Only when other signs of Kawasaki syndrome appear can the diagnosis be made. (5) Diaper rash: this is a bright red eczematoid eruption clustered over the groin and buttocks, seen mainly in children younger than 2 years of age. Boys have a very painful urethritis.

      Many children have severe itching with the skin eruption. This is an important symptom. Only the diaper rash looks as if it should itch. After two weeks peeling of the skin begins in most. It is often confined to the tips of the fingers and toes. Peeling occurs over the groin in those with diaper rashes and on other parts of the skin in those with scarlatiniform eruptions. In some, the peeling can be quite deep, and skin from the entire sole of the foot may be shed. After 2 months, a number of patients develop grooves in the toe or finger nails. These appear at the base, are 1 mm wide and deep and traverse the entire nail. Only one groove appears and disappears as the nail grows out.
   d. Involvement of the extremities. The commonest involvement is reddening of the soles of the feet and the palms. In addition to this, there may also be swelling of the hands and feet. This can be hard

for the doctor to see when examining a baby. The mother is able to tell that swelling is present because shoes that fit the day before have become too tight. Pain in the joints is also common and is usually seen early. Children under the age of two refuse to walk because of pain. Other joints than the ankles are involved, and swelling can be seen in the knees, wrists, and elbows. In some cases, swelling is pronounced, and when the joint is tapped, the fluid has a purulent character.

e. Lymph nodes: lymph node swelling occurs in 75 percent of patients. Node enlargement is typically cervical, although other nodes are occasionally involved. Swelling may be palpable only, but in at least 30 percent the nodes are so large that there is visible swelling on the side of the neck. The nodes are firm and moderately tender. They can be unilateral and suggest a diagnosis of suppurative adenitis.

There are a number of other clinical manifestations of Kawasaki syndrome that are not part of the diagnostic group, but are important features of the illness:

1. Central nervous system: all children under the age of 4 years are extremely irritable during the acute phase of the disease. They sleep little and fuss almost continuously. When examined, about 25 percent have signs of meningeal irritation, and when a lumbar puncture is done, most of these have an abnormal spinal fluid. From 8 to 50 cells were seen during one outbreak. In the spinal fluid, with only 8 cells, 4 were polymorphonuclear leukocytes. The sugar content is normal and the protein is also normal or slightly elevated. Uncommonly, there is a meningoencephalitis. One confused and combative child had a diffusely abnormal electroencephalogram. Cranial nerve palsy is confined to eighth nerve paralysis on one side, an abnormality seen in 4 to 5 percent of children.
2. Pulmonary system: in about 25 percent of children, the tympanic membrane is injected, making the drum look red and often leading the doctor into the diagnosis of otitis media. The drum is not immobile, however, and in this way can be distinguished from an infected one. An equal number of children have an intense, nonproductive cough often seen early in the disease where there is fever but no other sign. Roentgenography of the chest shows increased bronchovascular markings. Rarely, the roentgenogram will show a localized infiltration resembling pneumonia or pleural effusion. Both of these lesions are attributable to Kawasaki syndrome when other manifestations are present.
3. Gastrointestinal tract: occasional patients (4% to 5%) have one or more of these manifestations. Hydrops of the gallbladder occurs and is associated both with right upper-quadrant pain and moderate jaundice. Hepatitis has been seen with enough associated jaundice to lead to a mistaken diagnosis of type A hepatitis. Paralytic ileus of the small bowel occurs and is associated with marked abdominal distension and considerable pain. In contrast to the symptoms of gallbladder or liver involvement, symptoms caused by ileus can persist for as long as a week.
4. Renal system: the urinary sediment is abnormal in 50 percent of children. Both red and white cells are present in increased numbers, and albumin content is elevated. This has been attributed by one author to urethral inflammation because catheterization of the bladder in children that she studied resulted in production of normal urine. In my experience, patients have been encountered with red cell casts, and two children were seen with elevated levels of creatinine and BUN. This evidence supports the diagnosis of a mild nephritis.
5. Cardiovascular system: involvement of the heart and coronary vessels occurs in 66 percent of children studied with both electrocardiogram and two-dimensional echocardiography. Abnormalities consist of myocarditis, pericardial effusion, and impaired ventricular contraction. Twelve per cent have coronary arterial involvement, with changes ranging from occlusion to aneurysm formation. Children have died with myocardial infarction, coronary thrombosis, and aneurysm formation. More often, death is due to rupture of coronary aneurysms. Death occurs in 1 to 2 percent. Most children do not die and the coronary aneurysms heal. Healing consists of endothelial proliferation, which fills in the cavity of the aneurysm and restores a normal channel. The muscularis remains injured, although it is supported by the new growth of endothelial cells. Not all children with coronary thrombosis die. Children aged two years have been seen with classic anginal pains (hands clutched to the chest) with both ECG changes of infarction and elevation of the CPK enzyme.
6. Joints: joint involvement occurs in at least one-half of the patients. For some there is only arthralgia with pain in ankles and knees, sufficient in the 2-year-old to prevent walking.

DIFFERENTIAL DIAGNOSIS

The disease with which Kawasaki syndrome is most often confused is scarlet fever. Both the skin rash and the appearance of the tongue as well as the large cervical nodes account for this. The conjunctival changes of Kawasaki syndrome should be sufficient evidence that what the doctor is seeing is not scarlet fever. Furthermore, there is no eosinophilia as there is in scarlet fever. Viral exanthems (measles, echovirus, coxsackievirus) can produce rashes that resemble that of Kawasaki syndrome, and a mistaken diagnosis of viral disease can be made until other signs, such as conjunctivitis and oral mucosal changes, appear. Erythema multiforme is suggested by some of the skin lesions seen in some patients with Kawasaki syndrome, but the other manifestations of the syndrome exclude erythema multiforme.

The disorder that is closest to Kawasaki syndrome in appearance is the toxic shock syndrome. It produces similar changes in the eye, mouth, and nodes, and, to a certain extent, of the skin. The conjunctivitis of toxic shock syndrome, however, is associated with blepharitis and ocular discharge, and the skin eruption is usually erythematous. In toxic shock syndrome, mental confusion, diarrhea, and muscle tenderness are common. Hypotension is the rule, and cardiac involvement is rare. Shock rarely occurs in Kawasaki syndrome, and cardiac involvement is common. When used for toxic shock syndrome, steroids are rapidly effective in restoring normal temperature, clearing mental confusion, and making the patient look entirely well within hours. In Kawasaki syndrome, steroids have been associated with a marked increase in the frequency of coronary artery involvement.

LABORATORY FINDINGS

Occasional patients with Kawasaki syndrome have none of the usual laboratory abnormalities at all. They are the ones with normal white blood cell counts, normal sedimentation rates, and normal hepatic enzyme levels. The diagnosis in these patients is dependent entirely on clinical findings. In most, however, a number of abnormalities are present, some of which are of great value in establishing the diagnosis. The sedimentation rate is usually elevated. In a recent outbreak in Boston, the average level was 83 mm per hour (Westergren) with levels up to 140 mm per hour being achieved by a few. The white blood cell count is elevated to an average level of 25,000 per cubic millimeter. The differential shows an increased number of granulocytes and of band forms. The average number of bands is from 10 to 15 percent. This is in contrast with toxic shock syndrome, in which the average number of bands is 60 percent. The platelet count on hospitalization is the range of 400,000 per cubic millimeter; it rises over the next two weeks. The average platelet count then is 800,000 but counts of 2,000,000 have been seen. This is a valuable laboratory test because there are very few disorders causing such a thrombocytosis and none with the associated clinical findings.

Of great interest are laboratory abnormalities involving the lymphocytes. There are three specific abnormalities. The first is an increase in the number of helper T-cells over the normal quantity. Suppressor T-cells are decreased in number. The second is that, on culture, B-cells are found to secrete immunoglobulins of all types without stimulation. The last abnormality is that T-cells are cytotoxic toward human fibroblasts. This combination of events is not known to occur in any other disorder.

In the evaluation of patients, it is important to obtain blood cultures, to obtain blood for the measurement of antibodies to streptococcal infection or to Epstein-Barr viral infection, and to obtain cultures from both the throat and the urine. Patients thought to have Kawasaki syndrome have been found to have other diseases such as streptococcal pharyngitis, infectious mononucleosis, and even staphylococcal bacteremia.

THERAPY

Patients in the acute febrile stage should be hospitalized to permit frequent testing, especially for echocardiography to define cardiac involvement. Two features predict the likelihood of cardiac disorders: the first is an age younger than 2 years, and the second is fever lasting as long as 10 days. Cardiac involvement occurs uncommonly in older children.

Specific therapy does not exist. All that can be done is to reduce platelet aggregation. This is accomplished with aspirin in doses of 30 mg per kilogram during the acute state and in a dose of 100 mg daily thereafter. In published reports on treatment, aspirin treatment was associated with coronary arterial involvement in 12 percent, whereas prednisone treatment increased the frequency to 80 percent. During the acute state, echocardiography should be repeated no less than weekly to find out if there is cardiac involvement. If there is none when the temperature declines, then no further testing is needed. If cardiac involvement is present, tests should be done at intervals of twice a week while changes are taking place. When there is no further progression of aneurysm, pericardial fluid, or ventricular malfunction, the interval is lengthened to once a week until signs of improvement develop; this can take up to 2 months. Until improvement begins, the patient should be observed and monitored by the cardiologist. Once improvement has begun, the interval can be lengthened and the patient, sent home.

TOXIC SHOCK SYNDROME

SETH F. BERKLEY, M.D.
ARTHUR L. REINGOLD, M.D.

Although sporadic case reports of an illness resembling toxic shock syndrome (TSS) have appeared in the medical literature for years, only recently has a distinct clinical syndrome been defined. TSS is a multisystem illness associated with infection by or carriage of *Staphylococcus aureus*. Most reported cases have occurred in young menstruating women and have been associated with the use of tampons; however, it is clear that TSS can occur in a wide variety of clinical settings in individuals of both sexes and all age groups.

EPIDEMIOLOGY AND PATHOGENESIS

Cases of TSS have been found throughout the United States as well as in Europe, Asia, and Africa. As of June, 1985 more than 2,800 cases of TSS had been reported in the United States, including 122 (4%) with a fatal outcome. Although most of these cases (80%) have been in menstruating women, cases not associated with menstruation have assumed a more prominent position recently. Menstrual cases have been reported overwhelmingly in young (15 to 25 years of age) white women who use tampons. In rare instances, menstrual TSS may occur in the absence of tampon use; however, the risk of developing menstrual TSS is significantly increased in tampon users and may depend on the brand, absorbency, and chemical composition of the tampon used. Although the over all incidence of TSS is not known, the estimated incidence of menstrual TSS in the United States is five to ten cases per 100,000 menstruating women per year.

Nonmenstrual TSS can be seen in association with any of the myriad infections caused by *S. aureus*. It has been reported in both males and females in the pediatric to geriatric age groups. TSS has been associated with *S. aureus* surgical wound infections and has occurred in postpartum women with staphylococcal infections of the vagina, the breast, and cesarean section wounds. In addition, TSS has been observed in patients with primary and secondary *S. aureus* infections of skin, bone, joints, and blood. TSS has also occurred in women in association with the use of barrier-contraceptive methods such as diaphragms and contraceptive sponges.

The pathogenesis of TSS has been a subject of extensive study and is believed to be toxin-mediated. Most *S. aureus* strains recovered from patients with TSS produce a previously undescribed exoprotein, now designated toxic shock syndrome toxin-1 (TSST-1). In addition, it has been demonstrated that most patients with TSS lack antibody against TSST-1 at the onset of illness. However, the *S. aureus* strains from TSS patients also exhibit a wide range of other reasonably distinctive characteristics, and a substantial minority of such strains, particularly those from nonmenstrual cases, do not seem to make TSST-1. Thus, the exact role of TSST-1 in the pathogenesis of TSS and the possible importance of other bacterial products remain to be determined.

CLINICAL MANIFESTATIONS AND DIAGNOSIS

Because there is no currently accepted diagnostic test for TSS that is both sensitive and specific, the diagnosis remains a clinical one, based on the presence of a constellation of clinical findings. The current case definition (Table 1), although quite specific, detects only the severe form of the disease and potentially excludes milder or atypical clinical presentations. The Centers for Disease Control (CDC) defines a case as one with all four of the major criteria (fever, hypotension, rash, and subsequent desquamation), involvement of three or more organ systems, and absence of evidence of a more likely etiology. Fatal cases in which death occurs before desquamation would have been expected are also considered to have met the case definition. It is important to note that recovery of *S. aureus* from a body site is not a criterion required for diagnosis, although if searched for, the presence of *S. aureus* infection can usually be documented with proper culturing techniques.

TABLE 1 Case Definition of Toxic Shock Syndrome

Fever: temperature ≥38.9°C (102°F)

Rash: diffuse macular erythroderma

Desquamation: 1–2 weeks after onset, particularly of palms and soles

Hypotension: systolic blood pressure ≤90 mm Hg for adults or below fifth percentile by age for children younger than 16 years of age; orthostatic drop in diastolic blood pressure ≥15 mm Hg from lying to sitting; orthostatic syncope; or orthostatic dizziness

Multisystem involvement, defined as three or more of the following:
- Gastrointestinal: vomiting or diarrhea at onset
- Muscular: severe myalgia or CPK level at least twice the upper limit of normal for laboratory
- Mucous membranous: vaginal, oropharyngeal, or conjunctival hyperemia
- Renal: BUN or creatinine at least twice the upper limit of normal for laboratory or urinary sediment with pyuria (≥5 leukocytes per high-power field) in the absence of urinary tract infection
- Hepatic: total bilirubin, SGOT, SGPT at least twice the upper limit of normal for laboratory
- Hematologic: platelets ≤100,000/mm^3
- Central nervous system: disorientation or alterations in consciousness without focal neurologic signs when fever and hypotension are absent

Negative results on the following tests, if obtained:
- Blood, throat, or cerebrospinal fluid cultures (cultures may be positive for *Staphylococcus aureus*)
- Rise in titer to *Rickettsia rickettsii* (Rocky Mountain spotted fever), *Leptospira*, or rubeola virus

SGOT denotes serum aspartate transaminase; SGPT denotes serum alanine transaminase.

TSS typically presents in an acute fashion with fever, chills, malaise, and myalgias. These symptoms progress over the course of 24 to 48 hours along with headache, sore throat, nausea, vomiting, diarrhea, and abdominal pain. The rash usually appears 2 to 3 days after the onset of symptoms and is classically described as a diffuse, macular erythroderma (sunburn-like) involving the face, trunk, and extremities. However, the rash, which blanches with pressure, can be focal (limited to the face, extremities, or perineal region), subtle, or transient, and has been mistaken for the flush that sometimes accompanies fever.

Untreated, the illness usually progresses. Vomiting, diarrhea, increased insensible losses due to fever, and poor fluid intake all lead to dehydration, which contributes to the development of hypotension. Although initially manifested as orthostatic dizziness or lightheadedness, increasing hypotension may result in syncope and, in later stages, progress to shock. During this period the patient is extremely ill, and alteration in consciousness, such as confusion, delirium, or combativeness, can be seen. Other signs and symptoms seen during the acute illness include abdominal pain and muscle tenderness; hyperemia of the conjunctivae, throat, and vagina; a strawberry tongue; vaginal discharge; arthralgias; and edema of the hands and feet.

Patients who survive undergo generalized or focal desquamation 1 to 2 weeks after the beginning of their illness. The desquamation is usually most prominent over the hands and feet, where it is often full thickness, and less prominent over the face and trunk, where it usually more superficial. One to 3 months after recovery, reversible loss of fingernails and toenails and thinning of the hair are commonly seen.

COMPLICATIONS

Complications seen in TSS relate to the severity of the illness, and patients who do not receive prompt medical attention and appropriate treatment develop life-threatening, occasionally irreversible complications. Acute respiratory distress syndrome (ARDS) and refractory hypotension, the most commonly reported severe complications, are usually present and are major contributors to the outcome in fatal cases. Renal failure, which is usually due to acute tubular necrosis resulting from hypoperfusion or, occasionally, from myoglobinuria, is almost always reversible. Disseminated intravascular coagulation, profound hypocalcemia with resultant tetany, and myocardial dysfunction are among the other reported complications of TSS and should be watched for in the severely ill patient.

LABORATORY FINDINGS

Laboratory test abnormalities reflect the multiorgan involvement characteristic of the disease, and the magnitude of these abnormalities corresponds with the clinical severity of disease. Abnormalities in renal function are manifested by sterile pyuria and elevated creatinine and blood urea nitrogen (BUN). Hematologic abnormalities commonly seen include normochromic normocytic anemia, leukocytosis, lymphopenia, and thrombocytopenia with recovery thrombocytosis. Involvement of the skeletal muscles can produce an elevated creatine phosphokinase (CPK) level, and, when muscle involvement is severe, myoglobinemia, myoglobinuria, and resulting renal failure can occur. Additional laboratory abnormalities include hypocalcemia which can be profound, hypokalemia, hypophosphatemia, hyperamylasemia, and coagulation abnormalities consistent with disseminated intravascular coagulation. In severely ill patients, metabolic acidosis and hypoxemia may also be present.

Although the case definition of TSS does not require that *S. aureus* infection or colonization be demonstrated, most patients for whom appropriate cultures are performed before antibiotic therapy is initiated will be found to be culture-positive. The most common sites of *S. aureus* infection in TSS patients include the vagina, cutaneous and subcutaneous lesions, and surgical wounds. *S. aureus* bacteremia can be present but is uncommon.

DIFFERENTIAL DIAGNOSIS

The differential diagnosis depends in part on the patient's age and sex, the clinical setting, the predominant signs and symptoms, and even the geographic region in which the illness occurs (Table 2). For example, cases in children in which sore throat, fever, and rash are the predominant findings may be misdiagnosed as scarlet fever, whereas cases in young women in which vomiting, diarrhea, abdominal pain and tenderness, and fever predominate may be misdiagnosed as appendicitis or pelvic inflammatory disease. Postoperative TSS, on the other hand, can be difficult to distinguish from gram-negative bacterial sepsis or an adverse drug reaction. Aside from the common misdiagnoses listed, cases of TSS have been misdiagnosed as an astoundingly wide range of other diseases. However, by obtaining a careful history and physical examination in combination with appropriate laboratory tests, one can usually distinguish between TSS and other illnesses.

THERAPY

All patients should be examined carefully for sites of possible *S. aureus* infection, such as cutaneous and subcutaneous focal lesions. Surgical wounds, if present, should receive special attention. Most cases of postoperative TSS occur in the absence of obvious local signs of infection of the surgical wound, despite cultural documentation of the presence of *S. aureus*. Thus, any surgical wound, even if grossly uninfected, should be closely examined and probably explored. Any focal infection, such as an abscess, should be adequately drained. A careful pelvic examination should be performed on all female patients; any foreign bodies in the vagina, such as tampons, diaphragms, or contraceptive sponges, should be removed and cultured. Care should be taken to avoid leaving any fragments of tampons or contraceptive sponges in the vagina. Cultures of blood, the oropharynx, the vagina, and any focal lesions should be obtained. Some clinicians have recommended saline or povidone-iodine irrigation of any wound present or douching of the vagina on the possibility that this may remove organisms and preformed toxins not yet absorbed; this is of unproven benefit, but unlikely to be harmful.

The therapy of TSS is primarily supportive. The first priority is hemodynamic stability. Patients can have prodigious fluid requirements during the first 24 to 48 hours of their illness, sometimes in the range of 10 to 20 L per day. Initially, attempts should be made to treat hypotension with intravenous crystalloid, such as normal saline, rather than pressors because relative volume depletion is usually present. Vasopressor therapy should be used only if fluid replacement alone fails to achieve adequate blood pressure and urine output.

Moderately to severely ill patients with TSS should be treated intially in an intensive care unit or other setting where they can be monitored closely. Good urine output should be maintained (greater than 25 ml per hour), and careful attention should be paid to records of fluid input and output, since fluid overload commonly occurs. In severely ill patients, monitoring of the central venous pressure, pulmonary capillary wedge pressure, and ar-

TABLE 2 Differential Diagnosis of Toxic Shock Syndrome

All Patients	*Infants*	*Postpartum Women*	*Women of Reproductive Age*
Scarlet fever	Kawasaki syndrome	Endometritis	Pelvic inflammatory disease
Drug reaction	Staphylococcal scalded-skin syndrome	Septic pelvic thrombophlebitis	
Sepsis		Septic abortion	
Appendicitis			
Leptospirosis			
Viral illness with exanthem (measles, etc.)			
Rocky Mountain spotted fever			

terial pressure may be required for optimal management.

Although antimicrobial therapy has not been shown to affect the course of the acute illness, it has been shown to reduce the frequency of recurrent episodes. All patients suspected of having TSS should be treated with parenteral antimicrobial therapy effective against *S. aureus*, such as a penicillinase-resistant penicillin (e.g., nafcillin 1 g IV every 4 hours) or, if penicillin-allergic, with a cephalosporin that has antistaphylococcal activity or with vancomycin. In addition, if gram-negative sepsis cannot be ruled out, the addition of an aminoglycoside until blood culture results are available may be prudent. Parenteral antimicrobial therapy should be continued until the patient is stable and afebrile. The benefit of additional oral antimicrobial therapy after this time is unproven, but many physicians use oral therapy to complete a 10 to 14-day course of treatment.

Although commonly used, high-dose corticosteroid therapy is of unproved benefit in TSS. On the basis of evidence from a retrospective analysis of a limited number of cases, some experts recommend giving methylprednisolone (10 to 20 mg per kg every 6 to 8 hours) for the first 2 to 3 days of illness to patients who are hypotensive; such therapy should be considered for critically ill patients, but is probably unnecessary for most patients.

The outpatient treatment of suspected mild cases of TSS is an unexplored area. Removal of any intravaginal foreign bodies, maintenance of good fluid intake, and administration of oral antibiotics effective against *S. aureus* would be reasonable therapy for patients with mild illness, but there is no published information on this point, and the efficacy of oral antibiotics in eradicating *S. aureus* from the vagina is unknown.

PREVENTION

It is unclear why there has been a recent upsurge in the number of cases of TSS. Until more is understood about the nature of the disease and its relationship to menstruation and tampons, patient education remains the mainstay of prevention. Women need to be aware of the symptoms of TSS and, at the first sign of any of these symtoms, should remove tampons and seek medical assistance.

The risk of developing menstrual TSS, even among tampon users, is low. Women who have not had TSS and who wish to reduce that already-low risk even further can do so by not using tampons. For women who wish to continue using tampons, evidence suggests that they can partially reduce their risk of developing menstrual TSS by using tampons intermittently with napkins or pads and/or by using tampons of the lowest absorbency compatible with their needs. There is no evidence to suggest that more frequent changing of tampons will prevent TSS.

Women who have had menstrual TSS are at risk of having recurrent episodes with subsequent menstrual periods. They should be advised not to use tampons. Women who receive effective antistaphylococcal therapy and who do not resume tampon use have the lowest risk of recurrences (approximately 5% or less).

The value of vaginal cultures in defining those at risk of developing a first episode of TSS is unknown. There is, at present, no indication for performing such cultures for healthy women. The value of follow-up vaginal cultures in women who have had TSS is also unknown. Similarly, although the level of serum antibodies against TSST-1 can be measured, the use of this test to screen women cannot be recommended at this time.

INFECTION ASSOCIATED WITH HEMATOLOGIC MALIGNANCY

KENNETH H. MAYER, M.D.
STEPHEN H. ZINNER, M.D.

DIAGNOSTIC CONSIDERATIONS

Improvements in the care of patients with malignancy range from blood component replacement therapy and bone marrow transplantation to new, intensive chemotherapeutic multidrug protocols. However, patients with hematologic malignancies often die from infection. The frequency of infectious complications in these patients is due to several factors; (*1*) the intrinsic immunosuppression of the underlying process; (*2*) intensive cancer chemotherapy; and (*3*) the increased survival time of patients successfully treated with these regimens.

Certain malignancies and treatments are associated wtih a high likelihood of specific infectious problems (Table 1). For example, *Listeria monocytogenes* is more likely to be implicated in meningitis in patients with lymphomas than in patients with leukemias. The likely pathogens that infect these patients are often a function of specific defects in host defense mechanisms that are associated with the underlying disease (Table 2). Nonetheless, an empiric therapeutic approach based on the probabilities of a specific infection must be tempered by the clinical awareness of the complicated histories of these patients.

For example, a patient with acute myelocytic leukemia may be predisposed to bacterial infection at the time of induction of chemotherapy because of a lack of functional granulocytes but then, after remission, specific cytotoxic chemotherapy and corticosteroids may predispose to infections associated with impaired cellular and humoral immunity.

Integrity of the skin and mucosa is critical to host defense in patients with malignancies. The tissue disruption caused by direct extension or metastasis is more often a problem for patients with solid tumors, but mucosal lesions are not uncommon in patients with leukemias. Nosocomial infections are abetted by procedures that violate the normal barriers, such as the placement of intravenous and urinary catheters or endotracheal tubes, as well as by hyperalimentation and decubitus ulcers. Bacterial pathogens, particularly staphylococci that colonize the skin or aerobic gram-negative bacilli in the gut are the most frequent causes of nosocomial infection.

Polymorphonuclear leukocytes are the most important cellular defense against bacterial and fungal infections. The incidence of infection increases in linear fashion as the neutrophil count falls to fewer than 1,000 cells per cubic millimeter, and infection occurs in more than 50 percent of patients once the white blood cell count has fallen to less than 500 cells per cubic millimeter.

In patients with malignancy, neutropenia may be due to neoplastic infiltration of the bone marrow or to the use of cytostatic agents and marrow irradiation. The underlying illness, as well as cytotoxic chemotherapy, corticosteroids, and radiation, may impair neutrophil function, as may the hypophosphatemia occasionally seen with intravenous hyperalimentation.

Neutropenic patients frequently develop fever. Although temperature elevations may be due to the underlying disease process, several studies have reported that bacteremia is present in approximately 20 percent of these febrile episodes and that other microbiologically documented infections account for another 20 percent. Proven infections and probable infections occur in an additional 40 percent of these patients. Thus, in the majority of neutropenic patients, the presence of fever indicates the presence of infection.

The major pathogens responsible for infection in febrile neutropenic patients include *Staphylococcus aureus, Staphylococcus epidermidis, Pseudomonas aeruginosa, Escherichia coli,* and *Klebsiella pneumoniae.* The presence of fever (higher than 38.5 °C) justifies the

TABLE 1 Bacterial Pathogens and Hematologic Malignancies

Pathogen	*Acute Leukemia (ALL, AML)*	*Chronic Lymphocytic Leukemia*	*Hodgkin's and Other Lymphomas*	*Multiple Myeloma*
Staphylococci	+	0	+	+
Pneumococci	0	+	+	++
Listeria	0	0	++	0
Enterobacteriaceae	++	+	++	++
Pseudomonas	++	0	+	+
Salmonella	+	0	++	0
Anaerobes	0	0	+	0
M. tuberculosis	+	0	+	0
Nocardia	+	+	++	0

Note: 0 = no specific association; + = definite association; + + = frequent association.

TABLE 2 Defects in Host Defenses in Patients with Hematologic Malignancies

	Humoral Immunity	*Cell-Mediated Immunity*	*Granulocyte Number or Function*	*Mechanical Barriers*
Neoplasms*				
Acute myelocytic leukemia	0	+	++	+
Chronic myelocytic leukemia	0	0	0	0
Acute lymphocytic leukemia	0	+	++	+
Chronic lymphocytic leukemia	++	+	0	0
Multiple myeloma	++	0	0	0
Hodgkin's disease: stage I	0	0	0	0
stage II-IV	0	++	0	0
Non-Hodgkin's lymphoma	0	++	0	+
Therapy				
Radiation	0	0	+	+
Steroids	0	++	+	0
Cytotoxic	+	+	++	+
Other factors				
Malnutrition	+	+	0	0
Surgery	0	+	0	++
Hyperalimentation	0	0	+	++
Foreign bodies (e.g., IV lines, catheters)	0	0	0	++

Note: 0=no specific association; +=definite association; ++=frequent association.
* Defects at time of diagnosis, before intervention.

empiric use of antibiotics appropriately selected for activity against these organisms (see below and Table 3).

Intact humoral immunity is important for the production of antibodies that potentiate bacterial phagocytosis. Deficits in this limb of the immune response are seen commonly in multiple myeloma and the lymphomas. Splenic infiltration with malignant cells and splenectomy for staging of the disease result in impaired production of opsonizing antibodies, a factor that may predispose to overwhelming infection with *S. pneumoniae, Hemophilus influenzae*, and other encapsulated bacteria. Cytotoxic chemotherapy as well as the malnutrition associated with malignancy may also impair antibody synthesis.

Lymphocytes and macrophages are critical for appropriate immune responses to challenge intracellular organisms—including viruses and protozoa—and intracellular bacteria such as *Salmonella* species, mycobacteria, and *Listeria monocytogenes*. Impairment of cellular immunity occurs in patients with lymphoreticular malignancies and those who receive corticosteroid therapy.

SIGNS AND SYMPTOMS OF INFECTION

Many of the usual hallmarks of infection are not present in these compromised patients. Some malignant processes may themselves mimic infection. Some patients with malignancies may not be febrile when infected; this is especially so in elderly patients.

A careful history and physical examination are critical to establish prompt and appropriate diagnosis of infection even though some or all of the usual clinical signs

TABLE 3 Useful Antibiotic Combinations for Empiric Therapy of Febrile Neutropenic Patients

1.	A Penicillin	*or*	A Cephalosporin	*or*	A Carbapenem	*plus*	An Aminoglycoside
	Carbenicillin 30 g/day Ticarcillin 18 g/day Timentin 18 g/day Azlocillin 18 g/day Piperacillin 18 g/day Mezlocillin 18 g/day		Cefazolin 6 g/day Cefotaxime 6–12 g/day Ceftizoxime 6–12 g/day Moxalactam 6–12 g/day Cefoperazone 4–6 g/day Ceftazidime* 6–12 g/day		Imipenem* 4 g/day		Amikacin 15 mg/kg/day Gentamicin 5 mg/kg/day Tobramycin 5 mg/kg/day Netilmicin 5 mg/kg/day
				or	A Monobactam Aztreonam 4–8 g/day		
2.	*or* Double Beta-Lactam Combinations (in doses noted above)						
	Piperacillin Mezlocillin Azlocillin Ticarcillin	*plus*	Moxalactam or Ceftazidime*				

Note: Choice of regimen should be based on local susceptibility data.
* May be useful as a single agent in patients with moderate or predictably short-term granulocytopenia.

of infection such as warmth, tenderness, swelling, or erythema might be lacking. Similarly, patients with pneumonia and severe neutropenia may not demonstrate a pulmonary infiltrate on chest roentgenogram until several days after the onset of the infection. Also, iatrogenic foci such as indwelling venous and urinary catheters may be responsible for bacteremia with a minimal local response.

Alimentary tract symptoms of painful perioral ulcerations, enteritis, or proctalgia may indicate the presence of infection with mouth or gut flora and the attendant risk of bacteremia. Rectal fissures and perirectal abscesses may be present with minimal symptoms or clinical findings. Dysphagia should prompt a search for candidal or herpetic esophagitis.

Although some pathogens have predilections for certain sites, the specific infecting organism often cannot be predicted. The depression of host immunity in these patients is such that proper management mandates appropriate cultures and prompt empiric therapy. Occult diagnostic clues may be present in the retina, skin, sinuses, lymph nodes, rectum, and pelvis.

Pulmonary infiltrates in these patients are a special problem, since it is often impossible to make an etiologic diagnosis from the nonspecific signs and symptoms. These patients may be febrile, tachypneic, and hypoxic and usually need prompt diagnosis and therapy. Several organisms may be present simultaneously, including *Pneumocystis carinii*, cytomegalovirus, *Nocardia asteroides, Aspergillus* species, and/or *Candida* species, necessitating prompt bronchoscopy or other invasive procedures for biopsy and culture, although concomitant thrombocytopenia may make such diagnostic procedures hazardous.

Neutropenic patients with profound (fewer than 100 granulocytes per cubic millimeter) and persistent granulocytopenia are at particular risk of gram-negative rod bacteremia. This complication is especially likely when high fever, low platelet count and hypotension are present, although fever alone may indicate bacteremia with these organisms. Because of the high mortality associated with gram-negative rod bacteremia in neutropenic patients, treatment with appropriate antibiotics should be initiated empirically and promptly.

THERAPEUTIC APPROACH

The febrile neutropenic patient represents a particular clinical challenge: the antibiotics selected should provide adequate bactericidal activity against the many different possible pathogens. Cultures of blood, urine, and cerebrospinal fluid (if indicated) should be obtained promptly. Any other obvious foci, such as pus from any inflamed site, swab of an inflamed pharynx, purulent sputum, or drainage fluid should be examined microscopically and cultured.

In the absence of a noninfectious cause of fever such as transfusions or a fever-producing drug, antibiotics should be started immediately. A wide range of antibiotics is available for use as empiric therapy in febrile neutropenic patients. Although single, broad-spectrum antibiotics have been advocated by some, patients with profound and persistent granulocytopenia should be treated with a combination of antibiotics.

Several combinations available can be used in empiric therapy of febrile neutropenic patients (see Table 3). These combinations should provide high serum bactericidal activity and be synergistic in their activity against the common infecting organisms. There is no single drug combination of choice. We recommend the use of a beta-lactam agent (e.g., azlocillin,mezlocillin, or piperacillin) plus an aminoglycoside (e.g., amikacin or other). Local antibiotic susceptibility patterns should determine the precise choice. Double beta-lactam combinations, such as piperacillin or azlocillin plus moxalactam, have been used with some success and these regimens avoid aminoglycoside-associated nephrotoxicity and ototoxicity. All of these drugs should be administered intravenously at their maximal dosage.

The precise choice of the aminoglycoside utilized depends on the local antibiotic susceptibility patterns. Gentamicin, tobramycin, or netilmicin are closely equivalent where aminoglycoside resistance is not common. Since amikacin is less likely to be inactivated by bacterial enzymes than other drugs, it is preferable in institutions with significant aminoglycoside resistance. Aminoglycosides are rapidly bactericidal and are active against most aerobic gram-negative bacilli, including *P. aeruginosa*.

The choice of beta-lactam drug in combination therapy is somewhat wider with the availability of extended-spectrum penicillins (carbenicillin, ticarcillin, azlocillin, mezlocillin, piperacillin), the monobactams (aztreonam), and the newer cephalosporins (cefotaxime, cefoperazone, moxalactam, ceftizoxime, ceftazidime) and carbapenems (imipenem). Timentin, a combination of ticarcillin and the beta-lactamase inhibitor clavulanic acid, may also be useful in this setting.

Most studies comparing various antibiotic combinations have shown equivalent efficacy in febrile neutropenic patients, with response rates approaching 80 percent. Poorer prognosis is likely in profoundly neutropenic patients, especially if infected with organisms susceptible to only one agent in the combination.

A recent multi-institution international study has reported that azlocillin plus amikacin was more effective in single gram-negative rod bacteremia than was cefotaxime plus amikacin when the infecting organisms were sensitive to both drugs in the combination. Azlocillin plus amikacin was also more effective than ticarcillin plus amikacin against ticarcillin-resistant organisms.

Once antibiotics have been instituted empirically, they should be continued for 4 days before reevaluating therapy (Fig. 1). If the patient defervesces, whether or not an organism has been identified, therapy should be continued for an additional 5 to 7 days or until the granulocyte count has exceeded 500 cells per cubic millimeter (this policy remains somewhat controversial). If the patient remains febrile with a microbiologically documented infection, antibiotics may need to be added or changed,

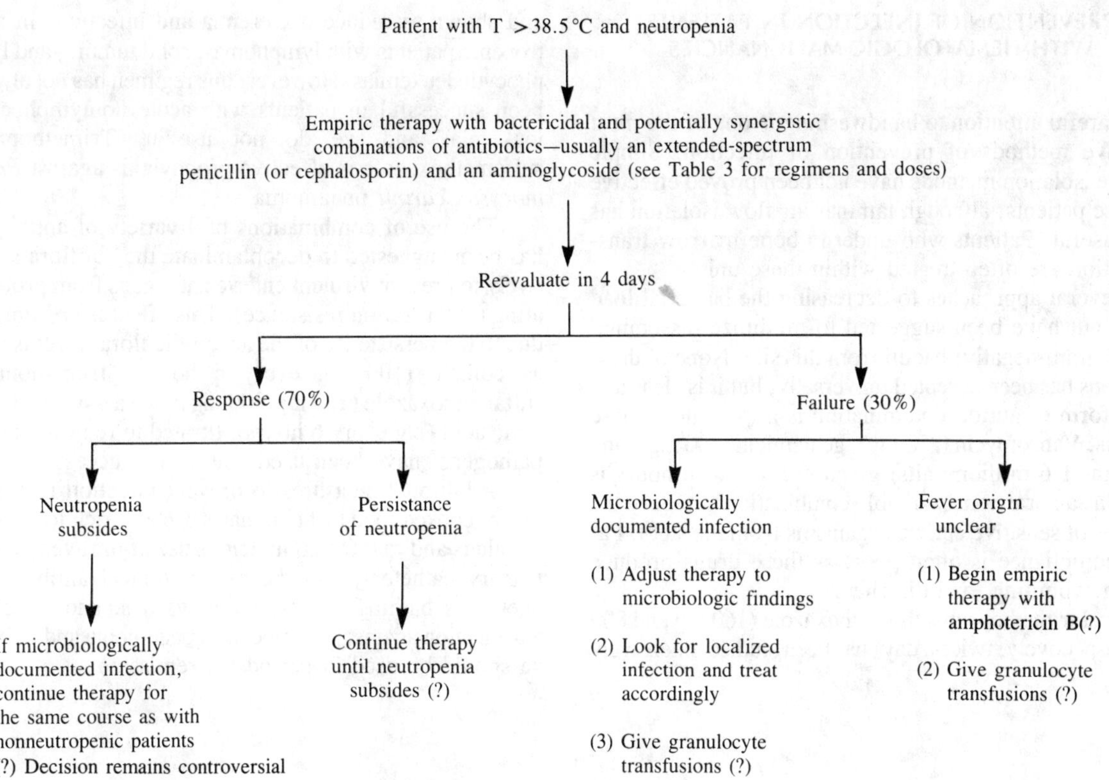

Figure 1 Algorithm for the management of febrile, neutropenic patients with hematologic malignancies.

localized infections should be sought and drained, and consideration should be given to granulocyte transfusions.

The patient who remains febrile with a presumed but undiagnosed infection is at high risk of fungal infection. Neutropenic patients who succumb to infection have a high frequency of autopsy-proved disseminated fungal infection. Therefore, although it has not been definitively proved, empiric antifungal therapy with amphotericin B should be considered in neutropenic patients with persistent fever (about 4 days) of unknown origin.

Candida and *Aspergillus* infections are the commonest fungal infections in patients with hematologic malignancies. Diagnosis is often difficult and may require biopsy of infected tissue (lung, esophagus, liver). Serologic diagnosis is not always possible, but new techniques for detecting circulating fungal antigens are being introduced. Cryptococcal meningitis is not uncommon in patients with lymphomas and requires examination of cerebrospinal fluid to find the organism on smear (India ink or Gram stain) or in culture. Cryptococcal antigen can be detected in CSF, blood, or urine.

Amphotericin B remains the drug of choice for disseminated fungal infections in the neutropenic patient. It is given intravenously in large volumes of dextrose and water at a dose of 0.7 to 1.0 mg per kilogram per day. We usually begin therapy with a test dose of 1 mg, followed by 5- to 10-mg increments daily or larger increments (e.g., 20 mg) every other day, if tolerated by the patient. 5-Fluorocytosine is useful in combination with amphotericin B in the treatment of cryptococcal meningitis and some candidal infections and allows lower doses of the latter drug. Although useful in localized candidal infections, ketoconazole has not proved useful in disseminated candidal infections or in aspergillus or mucor infections.

Viral infections may cause serious morbidity in patients with hematologic malignancies. Varicella-zoster virus and herpes simplex virus may produce local or disseminated infection. Acyclovir (Zovirax) is useful in decreasing the time required for healing and in decreasing viral shedding. It may prevent dissemination to vital organs. Adenosine arabinoside (Vidarabine) is also useful. Disseminated cytomegaloviral (CMV) and Epstein-Barr viral infections are more refractory to therapy, although interferon has been used with some success in patients with CMV infection.

Specific therapy is necessary for optimal control of infections due to protozoa. *Pneumocystis carinii* pneumonia is treated with trimethoprim-sulfamethoxazole intravenously (20 mg per kilogram per day trimethoprim; 100 mg per kilogram per day sulfamethoxazole) or with pentamidine isethionate (4 mg of base per kilogram per day). *Toxoplasma gondii* meningoencephalitis is best treated with pyrimethamine (25 mg per day after 100 mg loading dose) and sulfamethoxazole (4 to 6 g per day, depending on size of patient and severity of infection).

PREVENTION OF INFECTION IN PATIENTS WITH HEMATOLOGIC MALIGNANCIES

Careful attention to handwashing is one of the most effective methods of prevention of infection. Simple reverse isolation methods have not been proved effective in these patients, although laminar air flow isolation has been useful. Patients who undergo bone marrow transplantation are often treated within these units.

Several approaches to decreasing the bacterial load in the gut have been suggested to minimize dissemination of gram-negative bacilli from this site. None of these regimens has been accepted universally, but it is clear that some form of gut decontamination is important in these patients. Vancomycin (250 mg), gentamicin (200 mg), and nystatin (1.6 million units) given every 4 to 6 hours is useful as an oral nonabsorbable combination to reduce the number of sensitive enteric organisms from the stool. Patient compliance is often poor, as these drugs produce nausea, vomiting, and diarrhea.

Oral trimethoprim-sulfamethoxazole (160 mg and 800 mg, respectively, twice a day) has been studied extensively and shown to reduce bacteremia and infections in neutropenic patients with lymphomas, solid tumors, and lymphocytic leukemias. However, this regimen has not always been successful in patients with acute nonlymphocytic leukemias and we do not use it. Trimethoprim-sulfamethoxazole is effective prophylaxis against *Pneumocystis carinii* pneumonia.

The use of combinations of a variety of antibiotics has been suggested to decontaminate the gut flora selectively to prevent virulent enteric pathogens from proliferating (colonization resistance). This effect is presumably due to the persistence of the anaerobic flora. Agents such as colistin (100 mg every 6 hours), trimethoprim-sulfamethoxazole (160 mg/800 mg twice a day), and nalidixic acid (2 g every 6 hours), titrated to remove enteric pathogens, have been used with some success.

Additional measures to prevent infection include a diet of cooked food that eliminates bacteria-rich foods such as salads and raw fruits, judicious use of intravenous and urinary catheters, and the use of topical antibacterial agents as bathing agents, mouthwashes, and douches. Vaccination against pneumococcal pneumonia and influenza should be used in periods of remission.

SOLID TUMORS—ASSOCIATED INFECTION

GERALD P. BODEY, M.D.

Although it is recognized that infection is a common complication in patients with hematologic malignancies, it is not generally appreciated that infection is the proximate cause of death in 50 percent of patients with solid tumors. The discovery of curative chemotherapy for some malignancies has led to the use of more intensive regimens. Consequently, the frequency of infection is increasing in these patients. The spectrum of infection is also changing; some organisms that had been associated with infection in patients with hematologic malignancies are now causing infections in patients with solid tumors.

CONSIDERATIONS IN EVALUATING FEBRILE CANCER PATIENTS

Patients with solid tumors who develop fever fall into one of the following three categories: patients with neutropenia or other impaired host defense mechanisms, patients who are acutely ill and have an obvious site of infection, and patients with prolonged fever and no obvious site of infection. Table 1 lists important factors that must be considered when evaluating the cancer patient who presents with fever. By considering these factors, the physician is able to place the patient into the appropriate category.

Neutropenia is a common factor predisposing to infections, although solid tumors seldom cause neutropenia except when they involve the bone marrow. However, many patients are treated with myelosuppressive antitumor agents. Indeed, the use of chemotherapy as an adjuvant to surgery or radiation is gaining increasing acceptance as more effective regimens are discovered. Since the neutrophil is a primary defense against invasion and dissemination of infection, the neutropenic patient is at high risk of developing infection. Both the frequency and severity of infection are related to the degree and duration of neutropenia. Other deficiencies in host defense mechanisms are more often associated with hematologic malignancies. Nevertheless, deficiencies in cellular immunity and immunoglobulin production may result from cancer chemotherapy, malnutrition, or advanced malignant disease.

The type and stage of malignancy impact on the risk of infectious complications. Bronchogenic carcinoma frequently causes bronchial obstruction leading to pneumonia. Since this malignancy is particularly associated with smoking, many patients also have bronchitis and emphy-

TABLE 1 Factors to Consider in Assessing Fever in Cancer Patients

Duration of fever
Neutrophil count
Type of malignancy
Type of antitumor therapy
Administration of adrenal corticosteroids
Other deficient host-defense mechanisms
Presence of foreign body
Hospital- or community-acquired fever
Assessment of patient's condition

sema. Gynecologic cancers are often treated with radiotherapy, which may lead to infectious complications in the abdomen and pelvis. Large, ulcerated breast tumors may not be resectable and become superinfected.

In addition to causing myelosuppression and immunosuppression, antitumor agents have other effects that may predispose to fever and infection. Drugs such as adriamycin, nitrogen mustard, and vincristine are sclerosing agents and cause thrombophlebitis. Busulfan, mitomycin C, and methotrexate may cause pulmonary infiltrates that resemble an infection. Adrenal corticosteroids are often administered as specific or supportive therapy. They are used to reduce intracranial pressure in patients with primary or metastatic brain tumors. Unfortunately, they adversely affect many host defenses against all types of infection.

The management of malignant disease often requires the insertion of foreign bodies. Patients with genitourinary tumors may require urinary catheters, splints, or external drainage. Patients with central nervous system tumors may require ventricular shunts or Ommaya reservoirs for therapy. Vascular catheters are frequently inserted to facilitate the administration of chemotherapeutic agents or nutritional supplements.

Pneumonia and bacteremia are the predominant infections in patients with solid tumors. However, specific predisposing factors associated with certain tumors may be of critical importance. For example, pneumonia is especially prevalent among patients with head and neck or lung cancers. Abdominal or pelvic abscesses are frequent in patients with gynecologic malignancies, especially if they have received radiotherapy. Since the neutrophil is the primary defense against dissemination of infection, bacteremia is especially common among these patients. Superinfection of necrotic breast tumors is a serious problem and may serve as a focus for dissemination when the patient develops neutropenia following chemotherapy. Most cases of meningitis not associated with prosthetic devices occurring in patients with solid tumors are associated with head and neck malignancies or surgical procedures.

Taking into consideration those predisposing factors applicable to the patient helps the physician to focus on those organisms most likely to cause infection (Table 2). Unfortunately, this is not an infallible guide and broad-spectrum coverage must be provided in most instances if the infecting organism has not been identified at the onset of therapy. However, the application of this knowledge will ensure adequate antibiotic coverage against the likeliest infecting organisms. For example, if a patient is neutropenic, the likeliest causes of infection are gram-negative bacilli and *Staphylococcus aureus*. If the patient also has an indwelling intravenous catheter, *Staphylococcus epidermidis* and other skin organisms may be the cause. Pseudomonas infection is especially frequent among neutropenic patients. Patients with prolonged neutropenia are susceptible to fungal infection, especially if they have prior bacterial infection or have received adrenal corticosteroid therapy.

It is important to differentiate between nosocomial and community-acquired infection, since the causative organisms are likely to be different. However, since cancer patients require repeated hospitalizations their infections may be caused by nosocomial pathogens even if onset occurs when the patient is at home. For example, only 19 percent of 410 cases of pseudomonas bacteremia in cancer patients developed when the patients were in the community. However, 34 percent of these latter patients had been discharged from the hospital within the preceding 2-week period. Hence, patients may become colonized while in the hospital, but develop infection after they have returned home.

TABLE 2 Organisms Likely to Cause Infection Related to Predisposing Factors

Factor	*Organisms*
Neutropenia	*P. aeruginosa*, other gram-negative bacilli, *S. aureus*, fungi
Hospital-acquired	*P. aeruginosa, S. aureus*, other gram-negative bacilli
Lung, head, and neck cancer	*M. tuberculosis*, bacterial pneumonia, and lung abscess
Gastrointestinal, gynecologic cancer	Polymicrobial bacteremia, mixed aerobic and anaerobic abscesses
Parenteral hyperalimentation	*Candida, Torulopsis*
Intravenous catheters	*S. epidermidis, S. aureus, Acinetobacter*, skin organisms, gram-negative bacilli
Ventricular catheters, Ommaya shunts	*S. epidermidis, S. aureus*, gram-negative bacilli
Adrenal corticosteroids	*Candida, Aspergillus*
Impaired cellular immunity	*Listeria, M. tuberculosis, Cryptococcus, Nocardia*

Although certain organisms are most apt to cause infection, it is important to recognize that these patients may become infected by an extensive array of organisms, especially if they are treated with chemotherapy. Cryptococcal meningitis and disseminated nocardiosis have been found in patients with carcinoma of the breast. Cytomegaloviral infection and legionella pneumonia have occurred in patients with lung cancer and disseminated candidiasis in patients with gynecologic malignancies. *Clostridium difficile* colitis has been described in patients who received cancer chemotherapy but no antibiotics. Hence, one must be aware of the wide variety of possible infecting organisms when approaching the diagnosis and therapy of these patients.

MANAGEMENT OF FEBRILE CANCER PATIENTS

Patients with Neutropenia

The principles that should be applied in the management of febrile neutropenic patients are listed in Table 3. Patients who are neutropenic require immediate attention

TABLE 3 Principles Governing the Treatment of Fever in Patients with Neutropenia

Classic signs and symptoms of infection are often absent; thus, many patients have "fever of unknown origin"
Untreated infection can disseminate rapidly and terminate fatally; hence, antibiotic therapy must be instituted promptly
Majority of acute infections are caused by gram-negative bacilli
Organisms generally considered nonpathogenic can cause serious infection in these patients
Initial antibiotic selection should be influenced by susceptibility patterns within the hospital
A single antibiotic is unlikely to provide optimal coverage
Some antibiotics are suboptimal in neutropenic patients
Schedule of antibiotic administration may be of importance

and prompt antibiotic therapy. The patient should be given a careful physical examination, but it is important to recognize that the classic signs and symptoms of infection are frequently absent in neutropenic patients. Judgement alone is not a reliable prognosticator for the presence of infection in these patients. In one study, infection was found to be present in 28 percent of patients who were initially considered by the examining physician to have fever due to noninfectious causes.

Since untreated infection disseminates rapidly and may be fatal, these patients require prompt antibiotic therapy. Appropriate cultures should be performed immediately, but other diagnostic procedures should be delayed until antibiotic therapy is initiated. In the absence of localized signs of infection, significant fever is a temperature of 101 °F (38.5 °C) if not associated with the administration of pyrogenic substances such as blood transfusions or immunotherapy. If the patient does not appear acutely ill, it is appropriate to collect the necessary specimens for cultures and observe the patient for a few hours. However, if fever persists after 2 to 3 hours, a second blood sample should be collected, and antibiotic therapy should be instituted. Patients who have developed fever after administration of pyrogenic substances should also be considered for antibiotic therapy if they do not begin to defervesce after several hours.

In general, beta-lactam antibiotics are preferred for the treatment of infections in neutropenic patients. If the organism is susceptible, these antibiotics are effective even in patients with severe neutropenia. They are relatively nontoxic and can be administered at high doses to ensure adequate serum concentrations. Other proven effective antibiotics in neutropenic patients are vancomycin and the combination trimethoprim-sulfamethoxazole. Unfortunately, although the aminoglycosides have a broad spectrum of activity against most gram-negative bacilli, they are much less effective in neutropenic patients and should not be relied upon as single agents. Furthermore, neutropenic patients have repeated infections and often require prolonged antibiotic therapy, both factors that increase the likelihood of aminoglycoside-induced nephrotoxicity.

At the present time, no single antibiotic provides adequate coverage alone as initial therapy in neutropenic patients. The combination of an antipseudomonal penicillin (ticarcillin, 4 g over 2 hours every 4 hours; piperacillin, 3 g over 2 hours every 4 hours) and an aminoglycoside (gentamicin or tobramycin, 5 mg per kilogram per day, or amikacin, 15 mg per kilogram per day in divided doses every 6 to 8 hours) is usually chosen. However, equally acceptable regimens include a broad-spectrum cephalosporin (cefoperazone, 2 to 3 g every 6 to 8 hours or moxalactam, 2 g every 4 hours) plus an aminoglycoside, an antipseudomonal penicillin plus trimethoprim-sulfamethoxazole, or an antipseudomonal penicillin plus a broad-spectrum cephalosporin. Patients who receive cefoperazone or moxalactam should also be given vitamin K routinely, especially if they have thrombocytopenia. Therapy should subsequently be altered on the basis of the results of cultures from the site of infection. If the infection is believed to be related to an intravascular catheter, vancomycin (500 mg every 6 hours) provides reliable coverage against all of the gram-positive organisms likely to cause these infections. If abdominal symptoms are present, anaerobic coverage should be included.

Patients with Normal or Elevated Neutrophil Counts

Patients with normal or elevated neutrophil counts can be divided into two categories on the basis of the duration of fever and the physical examination (Fig. 1). If the patient has fever of short duration, appears to be acutely ill, or has leukocytosis or an apparent site of infection, appropriate cultures should be performed expeditiously, and the patient should be treated with antibiotics. Table 4 lists some of the possible antibiotic regimens based upon the site of infection. It is recognized that some of these regimens have not been widely utilized, but they are appropriate in these patients when consideration is given to those organisms most likely causing the infection. Every effort should be made to relieve obstruction or provide adequate drainage of abscesses, since these types of infection are not likely to resolve with antibiotics alone.

If the patient has a normal neutrophil count (or, occasionally, leukocytosis), does not appear ill, and has had fever for several weeks, there is a good possibility that the fever is tumor-induced. Fever is especially likely to occur in patients with hepatoma, renal cell carcinoma, and some sarcomas. Although the mechanism for most tumor-related fever remains unknown, it may be due to tissue necrosis or tumor emboli. Intermittent fever may be caused by antitumor agents such as arabinosylcytosine and bleomycin. Fever is usually intermittent because therapy is usually administered in short courses at several-week intervals. It must be remembered that prolonged fever may be due to chronic infections such as tuberculosis, histoplasmosis, or cytomegaloviral infection, and occasional patients have occult abscesses. A detailed description of the work-up of these patients is beyond the scope of this chapter, but would depend upon a careful history and physical examination. Antibiotic therapy should not be given on an empiric basis to most of these patients.

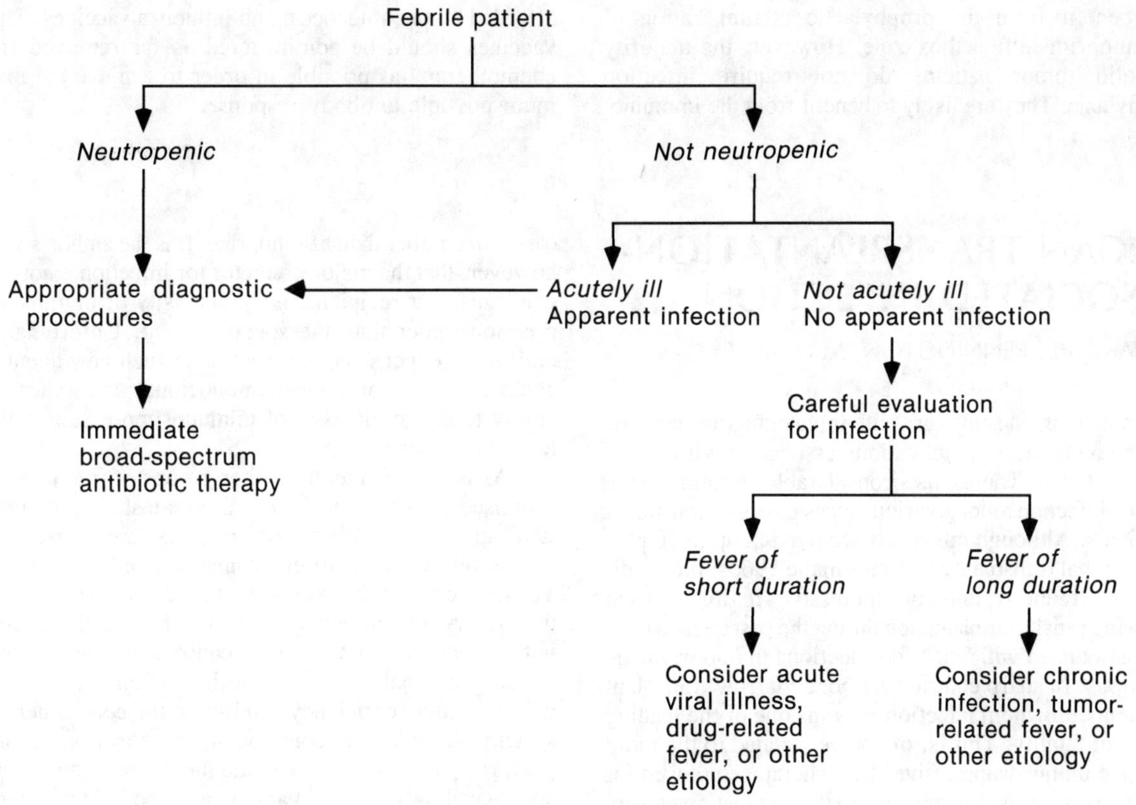

Figure 1 Approach to the febrile cancer patient.

TABLE 4 Initial Antibiotic Combination for Patients with Adequate Neutrophils Based Upon Site of Infection

Site (type)	*Antibiotic Combination*	*Predominant Organisms*
Catheter-related	Antistaphylococcal penicillin* plus aminoglycoside‡	*S. aureus, S. epidermidis,* JK diphtheroids, gram-negative bacilli
Skin and soft tissue	Antistaphylococcal penicillin* or cephalosporin† plus aminoglycoside‡	*S. aureus,* gram-negative bacilli
Pneumonia	Broad-spectrum penicillin or cephalosporin† plus aminoglycoside‡	Usually gram-negative bacilli, including *P. aeruginosa*
Aspiration pneumonia	Penicillin G or clindamycin plus aminoglycoside‡	Mouth flora, anaerobes, gram-negative bacilli
Abdominal or pelvic	Clindamycin or metronidazole plus aminoglycoside‡ or cephalosporin† or trimethoprim-sulfamethoxazole	Multiple organisms
Meningitis	Cefotaxime, moxalactam, or trimethoprim-sulfamethoxazole plus vancomycin or antistaphylococcal penicillin,* if catheter-related	*S. epidermidis, S. aureus,* gram-negative bacilli

* We believe that oxacillin or nafacillin are most appropriate. Vancomycin should be substituted in hospitals where there is a high frequency of infections caused by other gram-positive organisms.

† In immunosuppressed patients we prefer broad-spectrum cephalosporins (cefotaxime, ceftizoxime, cefoperazone, moxalactam) unless in vitro susceptibility testing indicates that the less expensive cephalosporins are as active.

‡ We believe that for routine use gentamicin, tobramycin, amikacin, and netilmicin are equivalent, unless in vitro susceptibility testing indicates otherwise.

PREVENTION OF INFECTION

Antibiotic prophylaxis has become an accepted practice for patients with acute leukemia. However, its role in patients with solid tumors is more controversial. Most of the latter patients do not experience severe or prolonged neutropenia; hence, their risk of infection is not very great. There are some patients who develop repeated infection whenever their neutrophil count decreases because they have, for example, persistent localized infection or chronic bronchitis or obstruction. Many of these patients will benefit from the prophylactic administration of trimethoprim-sulfamethoxazole. However, the majority of solid tumor patients do not require infection prophylaxis. They are likely to benefit from the immunity afforded by pneumococcal and influenza vaccines. These vaccines should be administered as far removed from chemotherapy as possible in order to achieve the maximum possible antibody response.

ORGAN TRANSPLANTATION-ASSOCIATED INFECTION

JAMES E. PENNINGTON, M.D.

Infections, in some cases life-threatening, remain one of the commonest complications associated with organ transplantation. There exists considerable variation in the risk for infection among various types of organ transplant recipients. Although infections occurred in up to 70 percent of renal transplant recipients in the 1960s, the modified and reduced immunosuppressive regimens used following renal transplantation during the past decade have been associated with marked reductions in opportunistic infections. In sharp contrast are bone marrow transplant recipients, in whom infection remains one of the leading causes of fatality. This is, of course, related to the more intensive immunosuppressive chemotherapy employed for bone marrow transplantation and to the fact that myelosuppression is commoner among these patients. Although less common, heart, heart-lung, and liver transplantation procedures are increasing in frequency. The immunosuppressing regimens used for these patients are somewhat more intensive than those used for renal transplant recipients. It is not surprising, therefore, that infectious complications continue to be a relatively common problem among this latter group of patients.

Regardless of which organ is transplanted, the major goal of immunosuppressing regimens is to impair normal function of the lymphocyte-directed cellular immune system. Accordingly, opportunistic infections, for which cell-mediated immune protection is essential, occur with particular frequency among organ transplant recipients. Members of the herpesvirus group, especially cytomegalovirus (CMV), herpes simplex, and Epstein-Barr virus (EBV), are quite common. In addition, Listeria, Nocardia, *Pneumocystis carinii*, Cryptococcus, and *Legionella* species are notable for their frequency.

Somewhat overlooked, however, are the more mundane, yet extremely common, bacterial pathogens causing urinary tract and skin infections. In one recent report, 98 percent of all infections occurring in renal transplantation patients during the first 6 months after transplantation were bacterial in etiology. Nearly one-half of these infections originated in the urinary tract, and no fatalities were reported.

Finally, there have been efforts to correlate frequency and types of infection with specific immunosuppressive agents. For example, an increased risk of *Pneumocystis carinii* pneumonia has been described recently among renal transplant recipients treated with cyclosporine rather than azathioprine. It is the author's view, however, that the major predictor for infection among organ transplant recipients is the intensity of immunosuppression rather than the specific agent. Unfortunately, until more experience is gained with such new agents as cyclosporine or anti-T-cell monoclonal antibodies, the ability to gauge intensity of immunosuppression will be less than precise.

As is common among other groups of immunocompromised patients, the organs at greatest risk for infection among transplantation patients are those most extensively exposed to environmental microorganisms. Thus, mucocutaneous surfaces, the respiratory tract, and the urinary tract are the organs most frequently involved with infection. Somewhat in contrast to patients with hematologic malignancies, but like patients with the acquired immunodeficiency syndrome, the central nervous system is a relatively common site of infection in transplant recipients. Finally, hepatic functional abnormalities are exceedingly common among all types of transplantation patients. Deciphering infectious versus noninfectious etiologies (e.g., azathioprine hepatitis, graft-versus-host disease, veno-occlusive disease, radiation hepatitis) for hepatic dysfunction is exceedingly difficult. Confounding this difficulty is the apparent frequency among transplant recipients of non-A, non-B hepatitis, for which diagnostic serology does not yet exist.

TEMPORAL PATTERN OF INFECTIONS

Renal Transplant Recipients

A temporal pattern exists for infectious complications among renal transplant recipients (Table 1). During the early postoperative period, surgical wound infections, urinary tract infections associated with bladder catheterization, and mucocutaneous herpes simplex infections due to reactivation of endogenous virus are most frequent. Thirty days after transplantation, cytomegaloviral infections of the lung, liver, and bone marrow become the predominant infectious disease. *Pneumocystis carinii* pneumonia also may occur during this period. It is also during this period that rejection-associated fever is most frequent. Differentiation of rejection fever from occult infection may be quite difficult. Recent evidence suggests that occult Epstein-Barr viral infection also may account for cryptic fever during this period. Although the first 3 to 4 months after transplantation is the time of greatest risk for infection, later infections may occur. Cryptococcal pneumonia and meningitis, herpes zoster, and severe

TABLE 1 Temporal Patterns of Infection in Renal Transplantation Patients

Time (days) After Transplant	*Usual Infections*
1–30	Herpes simplex (mucocutaneous) Bacteria (urinary tract, surgical wound IV sites)
30–90	Cytomegalovirus (lung, liver, marrow) *Candida* (mucocutaneous, esophagus, urinary tract) *Pneumocystis* (lungs) *Nocardia* (lungs, brain) *Legionella* species (lungs) *Aspergillus* (lungs, CNS) *Mycobacteria* (lungs, CNS) *Listeria* (CNS) Epstein-Barr virus (liver, occult fever)
>90	*Cryptococcus* (lungs, CNS) Mycobacteria (lungs, CNS) Pneumococcus (lungs, bacteremia)

pneumococcal infections are notable for their late occurrence.

Bone Marrow Transplant Recipients

The first 4 months following transplantation is the period of highest risk for infection for marrow recipients (Table 2). The greatest difficulties often occur during the period in which marrow recipients are intensely myelosuppressed. This is generally the initial 20 to 40 days after the transplantation. The clinical approach to fever during this period resembles closely that described for febrile neutropenic patients with hematologic malignancies. Thus, empiric antibiotics are used routinely for fever and are designed to offer coverage for aerobic gram-negative bacilli. Suspicion of skin- or intravascular-cannula-related sepsis also requires coverage for *Staphylococcus aureus* and *Staphylococcus epidermidis*. In persistently febrile neutropenic patients who do not respond to empiric antibacterial agents, an empiric trial of amphotericin B may be warranted. Mucocutaneous herpes simplex is another common problem during this early posttransplantation period. Intravenous acyclovir is useful in treating such patients. Furthermore, recent investigations suggest that intravenous or oral acyclovir may be useful as prophylaxis against early herpes simplex infections in marrow recipients. Since this approach also appears to retard the development of antiherpes immunity, and since these are as yet investigational, indications for acyclovir prophylaxis cannot be routinely recommended at this time.

The later phase of infections among marrow recipients is remarkable for the high incidence of life-threatening cytomegaloviral pneumonias. To date, there is no specific therapy for CMV infection. DHPG (2′-NDG) is an investigational agent closely related to acyclovir that shows some promise in treating CMV. Also, investigational studies suggest that CMV antisera may be effective as prophylaxis in seronegative patients. At present, however, severe CMV pneumonias are one of the most serious problems among marrow transplant recipients. The routine use of prophylactic trimethoprim-sulfamethoxazole among marrow recipients has greatly reduced the incidence of *Pneumocystis carinii* pneumonias. There is presently no U.S. Food and Drug Administration indication for gamma globulin prophylaxis in these patients.

TABLE 2 Temporal Patterns of Infection in Bone Marrow Transplantation Patients

Time (days) After Transplant	*Usual Infections*
1–30	Gram-negative bacilli (blood, lungs, skin) *Staphylococcus aureus* and *Staphylococcus epidermidis* (blood, skin) Herpes simplex (mucocutaneous, esophagus, trachea, lungs) *Candida* (mucocutaneous, esophagus, disseminated)
30–90*	*Aspergillus* (lungs) *Candida* (as above) Cytomegalovirus (lungs, disseminated)
>90	Herpes zoster (skin, disseminated)

* *Pneumocystis carinii* pneumonia is rarely encountered if patients receive prophylactic TMP/SMZ.

Other Transplant Groups

By and large, heart and liver transplant recipients most closely resemble renal transplant recipients in the types and times of infectious complications. Naturally, the specific surgical procedures involved increase the incidence of thoracic and pulmonary infections (heart) or intra-abdominal infections (liver) among these patients. Although some have reported a particularly high incidence of nocardial and mycobacterial infections among heart transplant recipients, this experience may be regional.

CLINICAL APPROACH TO INFECTIONS

The diagnostic, therapeutic, and prophylactic approaches for the usual infectious diseases encountered among transplantation patients are presented in Table 3. In Figures 1 and 2, management schemes for two common clinical infectious syndromes (fever with no source and fever with new lung infiltrate) are presented. It should be noted that in Figure 2 an alternative to the early invasive diagnostic procedure (i.e., empiric antibiotic trial) is listed. My strong preference, however, is to obtain a diagnostic specimen (lung biopsy or bronchoscopic lavage specimen) as early as possible (within 24 to 36 hours) in these patients, regardless of the infiltrate pattern. This approach will provide critically important information to guide therapy and will circumvent the common situation in which a patient fails the initial empiric treatment, but by that time has clinically deteriorated and is no longer a surgical, or even bronchoscopic, candidate. As far as

TABLE 3 Diagnosis, Treatment, and Prophylaxis of Specific Infections in Transplantation Patients

Type of Infection	*Usual Sites*	*Diagnostic Procedures*	*Treatment*	*Prophylaxis*
Bacterial				
Usual (e.g., staphylococci, streptococci, gram-negative bacilli)	Urine Skin Lungs Blood	Cultures and Gram stains of appropriate specimens	Indicated antibiotics	Oral TMP/SMZ (1 single-strength tablet daily) for patients with recurrent urinary tract infections ''Pneumococcal vaccine''
Legionella species	Lungs	Culture on charcoal yeast extract medium (sputum, transtracheal aspirate, lung biopsy, blood) Direct fluorescent antibody stains (sputum, tracheal aspirate, lung tissue) Indirect fluorescent antibody titers	Erythromycin, either 1 g IV, q6h or 500 mg PO QID (plus rifampin, 600 mg/day, if needed, on the basis of severity of illness)	None
Listeria monocytogenes	CNS Blood	Gram stains, cultures	Ampicillin IV, 2–3 g (depending on severity of illness) q4h (plus gentamicin if blood culture is positive); duration of treatment: until positive response	None
Viral				
Cytomegalovirus	Lungs Liver Retina	Complement fixation titer Culture of urine, buffy coat, lung tissue Monoclonal antibody stain of lung tissue (frozen sections) DNA hybridization of lung tissue specimen	None currently available (DHPG, investigational)	CMV antisera for seronegative bone marrow recipients (investigational) Alpha-interferon in renal transplant recipients (investigational)
Herpes simplex	Skin Mucosa CNS Lungs	Tzanck preparations (not specific for simplex) Cultures of lesions or tissues Immunofluorescent staining	Acyclovir, 6 mg/kg IV, q8h for 5 days; topical may be effective in renal transplant patients. Oral useful in mildly immunosuppressed patients (investigational)	Intravenous or oral acyclovir in bone marrow recipients (investigational)
Herpes zoster	Skin Lungs Liver	Tzanck preparations (not specific for zoster) Cultures of lesions or tissues Immunofluorescent staining	Acyclovir, 12 mg/kg IV, q8h for 5 days (reduce in patients with renal impairment)	None
Epstein-Barr virus	Liver	Serology only	None currently available	Alpha-interferon in renal transplant recipients (investigational)
Hepatitis B virus	Liver	Serology only	None currently available	Vaccine not used routinely
Fungal				
Cryptococcus	Lungs CNS Skin	Latex agglutination for antigen (serum and CSF) Cultures, India ink (CSF), cytology (CSF)	Amphotericin B 0.3 mg/kg/day plus 5-fluorocytosine (5-FC) 150 mg/kg/day (reduce 5-FC for renal insufficiency)	None
Candida	Skin Mucosa Urinary tract Blood	Cultures, gram-stained smears (Serum candida antigen, investigational)	Mucocutaneous infections: ketoconazole, 200–600 mg (depending on severity of infection) orally per day in a single dose Urinary tract: bladder irrigation with amphotericin B 50 mg/day, if catheter is in place. Oral 5-FC, 50–100 mg/kg/day (depending on severity of infection) in 4 divided doses if not catheterized; *note:* ketoconazole is not well excreted in urine Systemic infection: amphotericin B 0.6 mg/kg/day	Nystatin (oral); ketoconazole 200–400 mg/day (depending on degree of immunosuppression)
Aspergillus	Lungs CNS	Cultures, histology	Amphotericin B 0.6 mg/kg/day	None
Nocardia	Lungs CNS Skin	Cultures, acid-fast stains, Gram stains	Sulfadiazine 8–12 g/day (depending on severity of infection) in 4 divided doses; often required for several months	None

TABLE 3 Diagnosis, Treatment, and Prophylaxis of Specific Infections in Transplantation Patients (Continued)

Type of Infection	*Usual Sites*	*Diagnostic Procedures*	*Treatment*	*Prophylaxis*
Mycobacteria				
M. tuberculosis	Lungs CNS	Cultures, acid-fast stains	INH 300 mg/day plus rifampin 600 mg/day plus ethambutol 15 mg/kg/day (see other sections)	INH 300 mg daily for known positive skin reactors, indefinitely
M. avium-M. intracellulare	Lungs Marrow	Cultures, acid-fast stains	Ansamycin plus clofazamine (both investigational but can be obtained) (sensitivities of other agents, unpredictable, and must be carefully monitored)	None
Parasitic				
Pneumocystis carinii	Lungs	Lung biopsy	TMP/SMZ IV (20 mg/kg/day of TMP component; reduce for renal failure) Switch to pentamidine 4 mg/kg/day IM if no response after 4 days of TMP/SMZ	TMP/SMZ double-strength tablet (160 mg TMP and 800 mg SMZ) twice per day
Toxoplasma gondii	Brain Liver Lungs	Indirect immunofluorescent antibody (IgM)	Pyrimethamine 25 mg every other day to 50 mg/day every day plus sulfadiazine 6–8 g/day (depending on severity of infection) plus folinic acid 10 mg/day	None

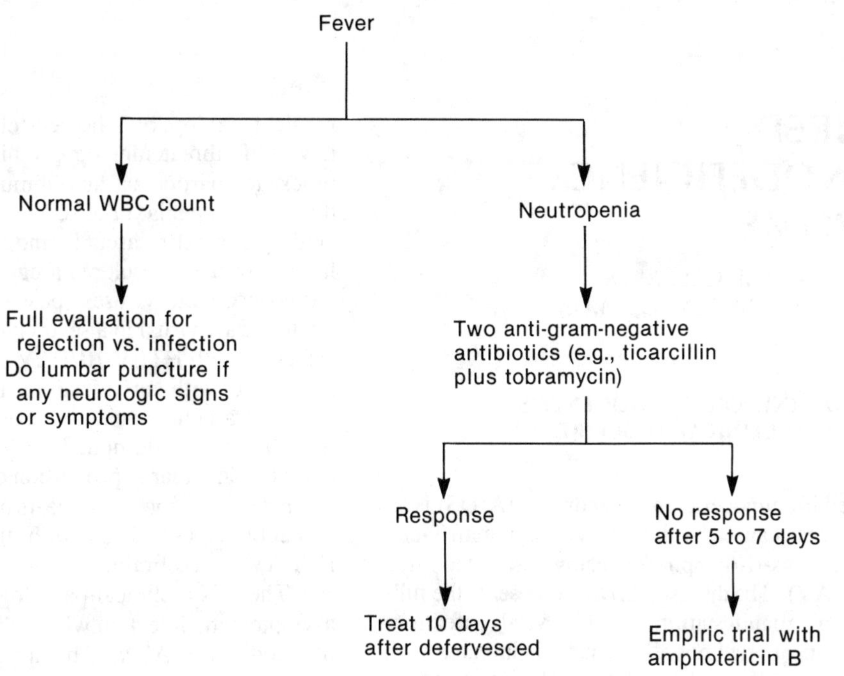

Figure 1 Fever with no apparent source and negative blood cultures

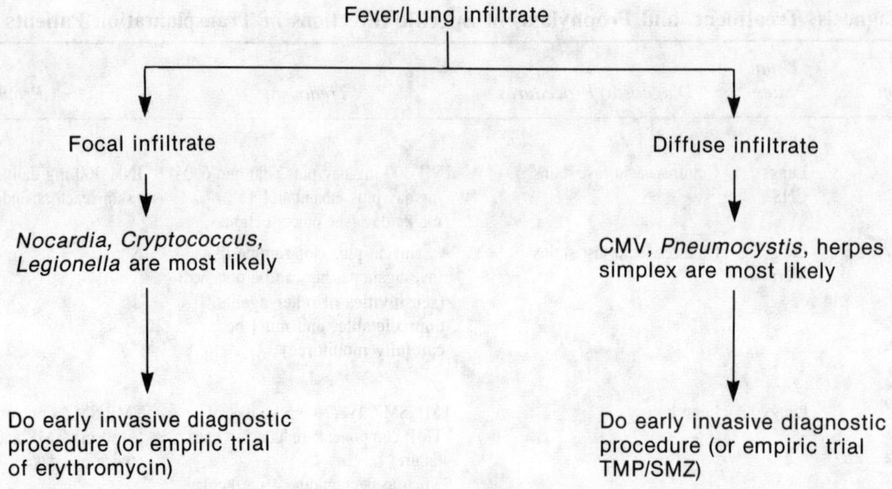

Figure 2 Fever and new lung infiltrate in transplantation patient without purulent sputum and with normal white cell counts. If patient is neutropenic, then gram-negative bacillary pneumonia or invasive aspergillus infection (both present with focal patterns) are also possibilities.

which invasive diagnostic procedure to use, this decision must be individualized. The following factors influence this choice: (1) Tempo of illness. For rapidly advancing pneumonia, only one chance is likely. Thus, open lung biopsy is the procedure of choice (fewest false-negatives). For less acute processes, fiberoptic bronchoscopic biopsy (yield around 50%) can be used first, then followed by open lung biopsy if no diagnosis is obtained. (2) Type of lesion. Peripheral cavitary lesions are particularly amenable to transthoracic thin-needle aspirates, and diffuse infiltrates are particularly poor lesions to approach with this procedure. (3) Bleeding status. For uremic or thrombocytopenic patients, open lung biopsy provides the best hemostasis. (4) Local expertise and experience.

ACQUIRED IMMUNODEFICIENCY SYNDROME

NEAL H. STEIGBIGEL, M.D.
GERALD H. FRIEDLAND, M.D.

DEFINITION, PATHOGENESIS, AND CLINICAL DESCRIPTION

Acquired immunodeficiency syndrome (AIDS) is an infectious disease caused by the retrovirus, human T-cell lymphotropic virus-III/lymphadenopathy-associated virus (HTLV-III/LAV). The disease, AIDS, represents the full-blown clinical manifestation of this viral infection; however, it appears that not all individuals infected with HTLV-III/LAV will develop AIDS. AIDS is primarily defined by the clinical criteria listed in Table 1. These clinical manifestations are largely the result of the lymphotropism of the virus for the T-helper-cell, resulting in dysfunction and premature death of a cell central to the immune system. The grave immune deficiency that results from loss of T-helper-cell function leads to a variety of life-threatening opportunistic infections and sometimes to particular autoimmune disorders, such as thrombocytopenia, or to several types of malignancy (including Kaposi's sarcoma and B-cell lymphomas). The latter may be the result of unregulated replication of potentially oncogenic viruses (possibly cytomegalovirus and Epstein-Barr virus) in a severely immunosuppressed host. Infection with HTLV-III/LAV per se may sometimes be associated with an infectious mononucleosis-like syndrome or aseptic meningitis several weeks after presumed inoculation. In addition, HTLV-III/LAV is particularly neurotropic. A large proportion of patients with AIDS develop dementia months to years after initial infection. This dementia is associated with the presence of HTLV-III/LAV in the brain.

There is a clinical-pathological continuum between asymptomatic infection with HTLV-III/LAV and the full-blown disease, AIDS. The latter must currently be considered an ultimately fatal condition with death caused by major opportunistic infections, malignancy, or inanition within 1 year in about 50 percent and within 2 years in about 80 percent of patients. Intermediate clinical manifestations of the infection include chronic generalized lymphadenopathy (nodes 1 cm or more in size in at

TABLE 1 Case Definition of AIDS

Standard definition: The presence of a disease at least moderately indicative of underlying cellular immunodeficiency occurring in a previously healthy individual without a known cause for immunodeficiency; these diseases include

Opportunistic infections

Protozoal or helminthic
- *Pneumocystis carinii* pneumonia
- Toxoplasmosis (CNS or pulmonary)
- Cryptosporidiosis (causing diarrhea >1 month)
- Strongyloidiasis (pulmonary or disseminated)

Fungal
- Esophageal candidiasis
- Cryptococcosis (CNS or disseminated)

Bacterial
- "Atypical" mycobacteriosis (disseminated)

Viral
- Cytomegaloviral infection (pulmonary, GI, or CNS)
- Herpes simplex (mucocutaneous persisting >1 month)
- Progressive multifocal leukoencephalopathy

Malignancies
- Kaposi's sarcoma in persons <60 years
- Lymphoma limited to brain

Supplementary definition (utilizes results of testing for serum antibodies or culture of HTLV-III/LAV)

In the absence of the above diseases, any of the following is considered indicative of AIDS if the patient has a positive serologic test or virologic documentation of HTLV-III/LAV infection
- Disseminated histoplasmosis
- Isosporiasis (causing diarrhea >1 month)
- Bronchial or pulmonary candidiasis
- Non-Hodgkin's lymphoma of high grade pathologic type and of B-cell or unknown immunologic phenotype
- Kaposi's sarcoma in patients 60 years of age or older

In the absence of opportunistic infection, a histologically confirmed diagnosis of chronic lymphoid interstitial pneumonia in a child under 13 years of age will be considered as indicating AIDS unless tests for HTLV-III/LAV are negative

Patients will be excluded from case definition if they have a negative result on testing for serum antibody to HTLV-III/LAV, have no other type of HTLV-III/LAV test with a positive result, and do not have a low number of T-helper lymphocytes or a low ratio of T-helper to T-suppressor lymphocytes

Note: Modified from CDC surveillance definition. MMWR 1982; 31:507–514 and MMWR 1985; 34:373–375.

least two extrainguinal areas) (lymphadenopathy syndrome, LAS) and a complex (AIDS-related complex, ARC) that may include chronic lymphadenopathy, fever, weight loss, and unexplained oropharyngeal candidiasis. Unexplained oral candidiasis is defined as that which occurs in individuals who have not received antibiotics within 1 month or corticosteroid treatment and who do not have an apparent condition, such as diabetes mellitus, known to be associated with candidiasis. When the manifestations progress to include a particular major opportunistic infection or other conditions listed in Table 1, the condition is defined as AIDS (with the grave prognosis already noted). About 5 to 10 percent of individuals in high-risk groups who have evidence of infection (as indicated by the presence of serum antibodies to HTLV-III/LAV) followed for 2 to 3 years have developed AIDS and 20 to 25 percent, ARC. About 15 to 20 percent of individuals with ARC followed over 2 to 3 years have developed AIDS. High-risk individuals who manifest unexplained oral candidiasis have a particularly high rate of developing AIDS.

EPIDEMIOLOGY

Transmission of this retroviral infection appears to require the inoculation of infected body fluids, particularly blood or semen. Therefore, intimate contact between an infected individual and a susceptible person is required for transmission. HTLV-III/LAV can be present in saliva and tears, but there has as yet been no evidence that these fluids play a role in transmission of infection. Therefore, those at high risk for the infection as well as the disease have been sexually active male homosexuals, needle-sharing intravenous drug abusers, recipients of blood transfusions or hemophiliacs, infants born of mothers at high risk, and heterosexual partners of those in high-risk groups. There is as yet no evidence that casual contact with infected individuals may transmit HTLV-III/LAV infection or disease. The incubation period ranges from months to several years. The disease may be transmitted by individuals infected with HTLV-III/LAV who are asymptomatic. Laboratory tests with high sensitivity and specificity have been developed for detecting serum antibodies to HTLV-III/LAV. The vast majority of individuals with tests confirmed as demonstrating such antibodies have been shown to carry viable HTLV-III/LAV in their blood, regardless of their clinical status. They are, therefore, potentially infectious. Individuals in high-risk groups who do not demonstrate serum antibodies will only occasionally harbor HTLV-III/LAV in their blood.

ASSOCIATED LABORATORY FINDINGS IN PATIENTS WITH AIDS

In addition to the presence of HTLV-III/LAV as well as viral-specific antibodies in the blood, the following laboratory abnormalities are usually found in patients with AIDS: leukopenia, lymphopenia, polyclonal increase in immunoglobulins—especially of the IgG and IgA classes—decreased numbers of T-helper lymphocytes, decreased ratio of T-helper to T-suppressor lymphocytes, and cutaneous anergy to antigens of the delayed hypersensitivity type. AIDS patients often have a mild to moderate anemia and sometimes have thrombocytopenia.

MANAGEMENT OF OPPORTUNISTIC INFECTIONS IN PATIENTS WITH AIDS

As yet there is no specific effective therapy for AIDS per se. Antiviral therapy directed at HTLV-III/LAV may become available in the future. Such antiviral agents will probably need to penetrate the central nervous system,

TABLE 2 Therapy of Opportunistic Infections in AIDS

Organ System and Infection	*Drug*	*Usual Dose and Route in Adults*	*Duration of Therapy**	*Comments*
Skin, mucous membranes				
Herpes simplex	Acyclovir	200–400 mg PO q4–6h†	7 days	Repeat with recurrences
		or		
		5 mg/kg IV q8h†	7 days	
Severe or disseminated herpes zoster	Acyclovir	200–800 mg PO q4–6h†	7 days	
		or		
		5 mg/kg IV q8h†	7 days	
Pulmonary				
Pneumocystis carinii pneumonia	Trimethoprim (TMP)/ sulfamethoxazole (SMZ)	5 mg/kg TMP/ 25 mg/kg SMZ IV q6h†	21 days	After treatment consider initiating suppressive therapy with either TMP/SMZ one double-strength tablet BID twice weekly, or Fansidar (sulfadoxine and pyrimethamine) one tablet weekly
	or			
	Pentamidine isethionate	4 mg/kg/day slowly IV (over 1h) or IM	21 days	
Gastrointestinal				
Oropharyngeal candidiasis	Ketoconazole	200 mg PO daily		Treatment usually required indefinitely
	or			
	Nystatin oral suspension	5 ml "swish and swallow" q4–6h		
	or			
	Clotrimazole troches	One troche 5 × daily		
Candida esophagitis	Ketoconazole	200 mg PO daily or BID		Treatment with ketoconazole usually required indefinitely
	or			
	Amphotericin B	0.6 mg/kg IV daily†	10 days	
Cryptosporidiosis	Spiramycin (?)‡	1 g PO q6h	14 days	Spiramycin therapy of questionable efficacy; opiates and hyperalimentation are palliative

Neurologic				
Toxoplasma gondii encephalitis	Pyrimethamine *and* Trisulfapyrimidines *and*	75 mg PO on first day, then 25 mg PO daily 1.0–1.5 g PO q6h		Continue indefinitely because of high relapse rate
	Folinic acid	10 mg PO daily		Folinic acid prevents bone marrow depression from pyrimethamine
Cryptococcal meningitis or other forms of dissemination	Amphotericin B *or*	0.5–0.6 mg/kg IV daily†	Administer total of about 2 g over about 8 weeks	High relapse rate suggests the initiation of suppressive therapy, 25 mg IV twice weekly, after initial therapy
	Amphotericin B *and* Flucytosine	0.3–0.4 mg/kg IV daily† 35 mg/kg PO QID†	6 weeks	Flucytosine often poorly tolerated and should generally not be used in renal failure without determination of blood levels
Systemic infections				
Disseminated *M. avium-M. intracellulare* infection	Isoniazid *plus* Ansamycin‖ plus Clofazamine# plus Ethambutol	300 mg PO daily; 150 mg PO daily; 200 mg PO daily; 15 mg/kg PO daily	Indefinite	Therapy of questionable benefit;§ duration of therapy uncertain
Disseminated cytomegaloviral infection	DHPG** *or* BW B759U**	2.5–5 mg/kg IV q8h†; 2.5 mg/kg IV q8h†	14 days; 14 days	Investigational drugs; efficacy under study

* Duration of therapy is not clearly established.
† Dose should be modified with renal insufficiency.
‡ Available as Rovamycin from Poulenc in Canada.
§ Efficacy currently under investigation.
‖ Available from the Centers for Disease Control, Atlanta, Georgia.
\# Available from Ciba-Geigy Pharmaceuticals Company, Summit, New Jersey.
** Investigational acyclic nucleotides available as DHPG (from Syntex, Inc., Palo Alta, California) or as BW B759U (from Burroughs Wellcome, Research, Triangle Park, North Carolina).

which often harbors HTLV-III/LAV. Antiviral therapy will likely require prolonged or even life-long administration. Specific antiviral therapy may need to be combined with agents directed at repairing the immune defects of AIDS. However, no agent has yet been established as an effective immunomodulating agent in AIDS.

In the meantime, our therapy for AIDS is palliative, but it often prolongs life with some reasonable quality. This therapy consists of important supportive measures and specific and effective therapy for the opportunistic infections and, in some cases, for the malignancies that are part of the natural history of this illness.

Most of the opportunistic infections developing in patients with AIDS are caused by ubiquitous organisms of "low virulence," which are known to establish latent infections in normal individuals. These endogenous pathogens become activated to produce disease when there is severe depression of cell-mediated immunity. Following effective treatment of such infections in AIDS, there tends to be a high relapse rate, probably associated with reactivation of residual organisms that cannot be entirely eliminated by either the treatment or the poor cellular defense mechanisms in these patients. True reinfection is also a possibility. Therefore, antimicrobial therapy of such infections must often be prolonged and relapse may be diminished by the use of long-term (indefinite) suppressive therapy following the initial, intensive treatment period. The symptoms, signs, and laboratory abnormalities of these infections—especially when manifest in the lungs and central nervous system—can be too nonspecific to allow an accurate diagnosis unless biopsy and culture of abnormal tissue are undertaken. This principle cannot be overemphasized for proper management of these patients. Our treatment regimens for these infections are outlined in Table 2.

In addition to the infections due to low-virulence organisms (*Pneumocystis carinii, Mycobacterium avium–Mycobacterium intracellulare*, herpes simplex virus, *Toxoplasma gondii, Cryptococcus neoformans*, cytomegalovirus, *Cryptosporidium*) we have also observed life-threatening infections caused by classic virulent pyogenic bacteria (especially, *Streptococcus pneumoniae, Hemophilus influenzae* type b, *Staphylococcus aureus*, and *Salmonella* species) in some AIDS patients.

The commonly encountered opportunistic infections in patients with AIDS often present with characteristic clinical pictures, although etiologic diagnosis should be confirmed with appropriate laboratory or biopsy studies. *P. carinii* pneumonia is the commonest major opportunistic infecton in patients with AIDS and is often the first to occur. Dyspnea and nonproductive cough are characteristic symptoms, often associated wth interstitial pulmonary infiltrates. Diagnosis should be established by bronchoscopy with transbronchial biopsy or examintion of material obtained by bronchial lavage. When the chest roentgenogram is not characteristic, justification for the biopsy may be established by demonstrating either a substantial decrease in arterial oxygen tension with exercise or diffuse uptake of gallium by lung scan. Rapid assessment of biopsy material for *P. carinii* may be obtained by examination of "touch preps" of biopsy material stained by the Giemsa method.

Cytomegaloviral infections are often manifest as chorioretinitis, pneumonitis (sometimes together with *P. carinii*), esophagitis, enteritis, colitis (often showing ulcerated mucosa with characteristic intranuclear and intracytoplasmic inclusions of epithelial cells) or adrenal gland involvement (sometimes with adrenal insufficiency). Herpes simplex infections are often prolonged and severe, with painful ulcerations of the oropharynx, genitalia, perianal region, and rectum.

M. avium–M. intracellulare infections are frequent and associated with the presence of organisms in the blood, liver, spleen, and bone marrow. Noncaseating granuloma may be found in the liver (often with high levels of serum alkaline phosphatase) or bone marrow. The contribution of this infection to morbidity (fever, inanition) and mortality in these patients is difficult to assess, as multiple opportunistic infections are often present simultaneously. Pulmonary tuberculosis and occasionally disseminated tuberculosis may be encountered. As yet, the duration of treatment for tuberculosis in patients with AIDS is uncertain.

Cryptosporidium may produce enteritis with prolonged, profuse, and debilitating diarrhea. Infections due to *Cryptosporidium*, herpes simplex, and cytomegalovirus are more frequent in patients with AIDS who are male homosexuals compared with those in the heterosexual, intravenous drug-abuser group.

Toxoplasmosis of the central nervous system in patients with AIDS commonly presents as mass lesions in the brain (well-visualized on CT scan, especially in conjunction with use of contrast dye) producing seizures, focal neurologic signs, and altered consciousness. Serologic testing is often not helpful in diagnosis, but brain biopsy utilizing proper staining techniques usually establishes the etiology.

Cryptococcal meningitis also occurs frequently and is usually associated with headaches, nausea and vomiting, and changes in mental status and vision. In these patients the diagnosis is most efficiently made by assaying for the cryptococcal antigen in the cerebrospinal fluid by the latex agglutination technique. Other forms of cryptococcal dissemination are encountered, including involvement of lungs, bone marrow, and spleen. Other neurologic syndromes noted in patients with AIDS include frequent ataxia and progressive dementia, probably due to HTLV-III/LAV infection of brain; and progressive multifocal leukoencephalopathy, a demyelinating disorder characterized by focal weakness, seizures, and changes in mental status and caused by certain strains of papovavirus for which there is no established therapy.

Oropharyngeal candidiasis occurs very frequently in patients with AIDS. Candida infection may involve the esophagus, with resulting dysphagia. Endoscopy readily establishes the diagnosis.

Patients with AIDS often demonstrate adverse reactions to drugs. This is particularly encountered in the treatment of *P. carinii* pneumonia. About two-thirds of AIDS patients treated with trimethoprim-sulfamethoxazole

(TMP/SMZ) for this infection will develop rash, leukopenia, or other side effects. Pentamidine therapy is often complicated by hypoglycemia, hyperglycemia, and nephrotoxicity. Both drugs are about equally effective,and there appears to be no advantage to combination therapy that might increase side effects. TMP/SMZ is usually used first; if there is no clinical improvement in 5 to 7 days, pentamidine is substituted. When pentamidine is used because of adverse effects from the use of TMP/SMZ, the clinical response to the former is often satisfactory. However, when the switch is made because of inadequate clinical improvement with TMP/SMZ therapy, the mortality despite pentamidine therapy is very high. Respiratory support is often needed for these patients, but those who require endotracheal intubation have a high mortality, reflecting the far-advanced stage of their respiratory infection and poor host defenses. Recurrence of *Pneumocystis* pneumonia is noted in 20 to 25 percent of AIDS patients. For this reason, the duration of the treatment with TMP/SMZ or pentamidine has not yet been clearly established. Although not yet proved as efficacious by controlled trials, we suggest that indefinite suppression of residual *P. carinii* infection be attempted after initial treatment by the continued use of TMP/SMZ or Fansidar (sulfadoxine and pyrimethamine) in patients who can tolerate these drugs (Table 2).

SUPPORTIVE THERAPY

Appropriate supportive therapy can significantly increase the quality of life of patients with AIDS. Treatment of pain with analgesics and of diarrhea with opiates is often indicated. Maintenance of reasonable nutrition through dietary counseling and high protein, high caloric supplementation is helpful. Emotional support, financial aid, and the provision of medical and personal services and entitlements are essential for the patient with AIDS. These services generally must be facilitated by trained social workers, mental health workers, and also by referral to community groups offering support services. Well-supervised group therapy can provide critical emotional support to selected patients. Finally, avoidance of lifestyle practices that might result in acquisition of new infections should be encouraged.

A discussion of the management of the malignant tumors that occur in AIDS is beyond the scope of this article. However, it should be mentioned that the clinical manifestations of disseminated Kaposi's sarcoma that occur in these patients may mimic those of certain opportunistic infections when there is involvement of lymph nodes, lungs, or gastrointestinal tract by the tumor. Regarding therapy, the use of recombinant alpha-interferon has been associated with temporary remission of Kaposi's sarcoma in some AIDS patients. Local radiation of tumor masses is occasionally indicated.

PREVENTION OF AIDS

The development of a safe and effective vaccine for HTLV-III/LAV infection is a long-range goal. For the present, advice to the general population must focus on sensible behavior modification, namely, warnings concerning the dangers of intravenous drug abuse (particularly needle sharing and the use of unsterile equipment) and promiscuous sexual behavior are indicated. The use of condoms might limit the transmission of infection during sexual intercourse, but is as yet of unproven efficacy. Sexual partners who are in high-risk groups for development of AIDS are a potential danger for HTLV-III/LAV transmission. These include prostitutes, who are often intravenous drug abusers. A number of practices should diminish the frequency of AIDS developing in blood transfusion recipients and hemophiliacs. These include the screening of blood for HTLV-III/LAV antibodies at blood banks (begun in 1985); the continued policy of requesting that high-risk individuals not donate blood; and the development of new practices to inactivate any potentially contaminating HTLV-III/LAV in certain blood fraction products.

Individuals who are already infected with HTLV-III/LAV must be carefully counseled. The ultimate prognosis for an asymptomatic infected individual is unknown. Discussions need to be supportive and compassionate, but also forthright concerning the potential for transmission of infection to sexual partners or, in the case of intravenous drug abusers, to potential needle sharers. Infected individuals must not donate blood, other body fluids, or organs for transplantation.

Finally, neither health care workers (except possibly for rare victims of needle-sticks) nor household contacts of AIDS patients (except for their sexual partners or children born of infected mothers) appear to be at increased risk for developing HTLV-III/LAV infection. Reassurance to these groups will help in the care of patients with AIDS.

INFECTION OTHER THAN AIDS IN HOMOSEXUAL MEN

THOMAS C. QUINN, M.D.

The recognition of the acquired immunodeficiency syndrome (AIDS) as a sexually transmitted disease primarily among homosexual men focused attention on the health care problems of the gay community. Compared with heterosexual men, homosexual men experience greater prevalence rates of gonorrhoea, syphilis, anal warts, hepatitis B infection, and cytomegaloviral infection. Certain enteric diseases, including giardiasis, amebiasis, shigellosis, campylobacteriosis, and salmonellosis, are also endemic and sexually transmitted among homosexual men. The other sexually transmitted infections such as herpes, chlamydial infections, genital warts, chancroid, lymphogranuloma venereum, and granuloma inguinale also occur frequently among homosexual men. In contrast to heterosexuals, homosexuals have many of these infections in nongenital sites such as the mouth, pharynx, intestine, and anorectum. Indeed, many of these infections—hepatitis A, hepatitis B, cytomegalovirus, and secondary syphilis—present with systemic signs of disease.

Because of the magnitude and complexity of these problems and the potential for transmission to other individuals, physicians and public health officials need to be aware of the epidemiology, etiology, and clinical manifestations of these infections. Although the immunosuppresive effects of these infections are not fully realized, indirectly they may have an effect on increasing susceptibility to the etiologic agent of AIDS, HTLV-III.

EPIDEMIOLOGY

There are several factors responsible for the high prevalence rates of these infections. Homosexuality per se is not a major risk factor, but, rather, the promiscuous life style that is practiced by many homosexual men is a predominant factor. A moderately sexually active man not uncommonly has relations with 100 or more men per year. Anonymity of sexual contact exacerbates the risk and complicates contact tracing and prevention of reinfection.

Asymptomatic carriage of sexually transmitted pathogens is a common problem among homosexual men. Urethral, pharyngeal, and anorectal asymptomatic infection with *Neisseria gonorrhoeae, Chlamydia, Treponema,* and enteric organisms—such as *Campylobacter, Entamoeba histolytica* and *Giardia*—occur frequently and must be sought. This carriage state represents a human reservoir of the infection, and this state plus promiscuity are primarily responsible for the continued transmission of these pathogens.

Another major risk factor for increased infection among homosexual men is the frequent practice of sexual activity allowing for infection in nongenital sites, such as anal intercourse, anilingus, and fellatio following anal intercourse. These practices are primarily responsible for the transmission of eneteric pathogens, including hepatitis viruses, in this population. Anorectal infections with the conventional venereal pathogens is caused by rectal intercourse. The role of fomite transmission, such as may occur with the shared use of unsterilized equipment for rectal douching and colonic irrigation in gay houses, remains unknown, although an outbreak of amebiasis has been traced to such use of unsterile equipment.

SCREENING EXAMINATION

Certain sociologic factors must be taken into consideration when obtaining a history from a sexually active homosexual. Preference of sexual partners, number of sexual partners, types of sexual practices, illness of sexual partners, and the past history of sexually transmitted diseases must be assessed and incorporated into the medical evaluation of each patient. A medical history should attempt to differentiate between clinical syndromes that might suggest one or more etiologic infectious agents, since homosexual men are frequently exposed to multiple pathogens.

After the sexual and medical history is obtained, a detailed physical examination with anoscopy should be performed on all high-risk patients. Since many of these individuals are at high risk for AIDS as well as other sexually transmitted pathogens, the physical examination must be complete and include examination of the skin, lymph nodes, oral cavity, abdomen, genitalia—for urethral discharge or genital ulcers—and a complete inspection of the perianal area and anal canal, including digital rectal examination and anoscopy.

Initial screening tests for symptomatic homosexual men should include a urethral and rectal Gram stain for the evaluation of polymorphonuclear leukocytes (PMNs) and intracellular gram-negative cocci indicating infection with *N. gonorrhoeae* Serologic tests for syphilis, darkfield examination, and Tzanck preparation of any external ulcerations should be performed to rule out syphilis and herpes simplex viral infection. Routine cultures of the pharynx, urethra, and rectum for *N. gonorrhoeae* should be performed. At this point, if any of the screening tests are positive, specific therapy may be instituted (Table 1) and sexual contacts examined for the presence of each particular infection. I recommend a rectal Gram stain for all homosexual men whether symptomatic or not. If symptoms persist following treatment, or if the aforementioned screening tests are negative, more extensive examination and cultures should be performed, including sigmoidoscopy, rectal biopsy, lymph node aspiration, or skin biopsy, as indicated.

TABLE 1 Treatment of Sexually Transmitted Diseases Commonly Seen In Homosexual Men

Specific Infection	*Recommended Treatment*	*Alternative*
Neisseria gonorrhoeae		
Rectal or urethral infection	APPG* 4.8 million units IM plus probenecid 1.0 g PO	Spectinomycin 2.0 g IM
Pharyngeal infection	APPG* 4.8 million units IM plus probenecid 1.0 g PO	Trimethoprim-sulfamethoxazole (80 mg/400 mg) nine tabs PO daily for 5 days
Chlamydia trachomatis		
Non-LGV serovars	Tetracycline 500 mg PO 4 times a day for 7 days	Erythromycin 500 mg PO 4 times a day for 7 days
LGV serovars	Tetracycline 500 mg PO 4 times a day for 21 days	Erythromycin 500 mg PO 4 times a day for 21 days
Treponema pallidum† 1′, 2′ early latent (<1 yr)	Benzathine penicillin G 2.4 million units IM	Tetracycline 500 mg PO 4 times a day for 15 days
Herpes simplex virus	Acyclovir ointment 5% 6 times a day for 7 days	Supportive therapy
Hemophilus ducreyi (chancroid)	Erythromycin 500 mg PO 4 times a day for 14 days	Trimethoprim-sulfamethoxazole double strength tab (160 mg/800 mg) 2 times a day for 14 days
C. granulomatous (donovanosis)	Tetracycline 500 mg PO 4 times a day for 14–21 days	Ampicillin 500 mg PO 4 times a day for 14–21 days, depending on response
Condyloma accuminata	Podophyllin 25% to lesion every other day	Cryotherapy Surgery
Scabies, pediculosis	Lindane (1%) lotion or shampoo	

* APPG=aqueous procaine penicillin G.
** See elsewhere in this volume for a discussion on treatment of latent and neurosyphilis.

URETHRITIS

The etiology of urethritis differs in homosexual and heterosexual men; gonococcal urethritis is more frequent than nongonococcal urethritis (NGU) in homosexual men, whereas heterosexual men have predominantly NGU. In addition, although 40 percent of heterosexual men with NGU have *Chlamydia trachomatis* urethral infection, only 10 to 20 percent of homosexual men with NGU have *Chlamydia* present. *Chlamydia* is also the major cause of postgonococcal urethritis (PGU) in heterosexual men, whereas *Chlamydia* is rarely present among homosexual men with PGU. Indeed, the etiology of NGU and PGU in gay men is unknown at present, but pathogens other than *N. gonorrhoeae* and *Chlamydia* that should be included in the differential diagnosis include *Ureaplasma urealyticum, Trichomonas*, herpes simplex virus, and *N. meningitidis*.

Gonococcal urethritis is usually symptomatic, with asymtomatic urethral infection occurring in less than 5 percent of infected individuals. However, asymptomatic infections accumulate in the population and therefore may account for a higher proportion of cases in a prevalence survey. In contrast, pharyngeal and anorectal infection is frequently asymptomatic in more than 50 percent of cases. The incubation period is 2 to 5 days after contact, and the symptoms may vary from a thin mucoid discharge to grossly purulent discharge in the case of urethral infection. Meatal irritation, dysuria, and frequency are common complaints. If symptoms are ignored or the infection is only partially treated, it can persist in an asymptomatic or moderately symptomatic state, and can eventually spread to produce complications, including epididymitis, prostatitis, and, rarely, disseminated gonococcal infection (DGI). NGU is also frequently symptomatic, although the symptoms are usually milder than those observed in gonococcal urethritis. The discharge is not as purulent, and there may be only a slight mucoid discharge. Other symptoms include dysuria and pruritus. Epididymitis is a complication of untreated NGU.

The diagnosis of gonococcal urethritis is established by the demonstration of gram-negative diplococci within neutrophils in a Gram stain of the urethral discharge. This diagnosis is then confirmed by the isolation of *N. gonorrhoeae* by culture. The diagnosis of NGU is made when five or more leukocytes per 1,000× magnification are present on Gram stain of the urethra and no gram-negative diplococci are present within the PMNs.

Treatment should be instituted on the basis of the gram-stained urethral smear. Gonococcal urethritis is treated with 4.8 million units of aqueous procaine penicillin G, preceded by 1 g probenecid. Tetracycline, 500 mg orally four times per day for 7 days, is recommended for the treatment of NGU. Persistence of symptoms following treatment usually represents reinfection, antibiotic resistance in the case of penicillinase-producing *N. gonorrhoeae*, poor patient compliance in the case of oral antibiotics, or the emergence of postgonococcal urethritis (PGU). Reinfection is ascertained by history and the failure to treat sexual partners. Penicillinase-producing *N. gonorrhoeae* is confirmed in the laboratory, and treatment consists of spectinomycin, 2 g intramuscularly. Like NGU, PGU is less frequent in homosexual men than in heterosexual men. Cultures for *Chlamydia* and *Ureaplasma*, etiologic agents of PGU, are not routinely available. Empiric therapy, which is usually successful, consists of tetracycline, 500 mg four times per day orally.

ANOGENITAL SKIN LESIONS

Anogenital skin lesions may be classified as ulcerative or nonulcerative. The etiology and incidence of ulcerative lesions vary greatly in different parts of the world and among different populations. Ulcerative lesions most commonly seen in homosexual men include herpes simplex viral infection, syphilis, and less frequently, lymphogranuloma venereum (LGV), chancroid, and donovanosis (granuloma inguinale). Nonulcerative lesions include condyloma accuminata, condyloma lata of secondary syphilis, scabies, genital warts, and molluscum contagiosum. Other sexually transmitted infections may manifest systemically as dermatologic lesions, and these include secondary syphilis, hepatitis, disseminated cytomegalovirus, and disseminated gonococcal infections.

The occurrence of syphilis in homosexual men is responsible for more than 50 percent of all the reported cases in the United States. Although the manifestations of syphilis are the same in homosexual men as in heterosexual men and women, anal and oral chancres are more common in homosexual men and frequently missed by the physician. Since primary chancres are not frequently detected in homosexual men, the lesions of secondary syphilis, such as condyloma lata, maculopapular rash, proctitis, or rectal masses, are frequently identified as the common manifestations of syphilis in homosexual men. Consequently, in order to identify syphilis at an earlier stage in this population, frequent serologic testing for syphilis should be performed in all homosexually active men every 6 months. The other clinical manifestations, diagnosis and treatment of syphilis are discussed in more detail elsewhere in this volume.

Herpes simplex viral infections also occur commonly in homosexual men. Vesicular lesions are usually apparent on the genitalia, the perianal area, and in the oral cavity. The primary infection is usually accompanied by fewer than 10 to 20 vesicles and, sometimes, by a single, painful, shallow ulcer known as herpetic chancre. Urethral infection may present with dysuria and a urethral discharge. The vesicles are present for 3 to 5 days before rupturing to form small, nonindurated ulcers. The primary infection may be accompanied by inguinal pain, lymphadenopathy, and constitutional symptoms such as fever, malaise, and headache. Recurrent attacks occur in about two-thirds of all cases and are usually restricted to a small area for a shorter period of time (10 days).

Diagnosis of herpes simplex viral infection is made by demonstration of the characteristic multinucleated giant cell on a Tzanck smear. The diagnosis is confirmed by isolation of the virus in culture. Treatment has typically been supportive, consisting of analgesics, sitz baths, and stool softeners in the case of anorectal herpes. Recently, acyclovir, an antiherpes drug, has been developed for the treatment of primary herpes infection and is available in intravenous, ointment, and oral forms. Although acyclovir may be beneficial in primary herpes, it does not appear to be significantly effective in recurrent disease, except when taken orally as suppressive therapy. Other aspects of diagnosis and treatment of herpes infection are described in more detail elsewhere in this volume.

Genital ulcers may be secondary to lymphogranuloma venereum (LGV), due to an invasive serovar of *C. trachomatis*. After an incubation period of 1 to 3 weeks, a small painless ulceration may appear at the site of inoculation. This heals spontaneously within several days and is followed by prominent inguinal lymphadenopathy. The adenopathy is unilateral in two-thirds of cases and bilateral in the remainder. These nodes progressively enlarge over a month and eventually become fluctuant and are frequently referred to as bubos. If therapy is delayed, the overlying skin becomes inflamed, and draining fistulas may appear. Systemic symptoms of fever, myalgias, and malaise are common. Late complications, such as anorectal strictures or ulcerative colitis, may occur in neglected cases.

The diagnosis of LGV is dependent on the ability to culture the virus from the infected site. LGV infection can also be confirmed by the demonstration of systemic antibodies to LGV at a titer of greater than 1:256; this will differentiate between LGV and non-LGV infections. Tetracycline is the treatment of choice, 500 mg orally four times a day for 3 weeks. Fluctuant bubos in LGV should be aspirated as needed to prevent spontaneous rupture. As with other STDs, examination and treatment of sexual partners is indicated.

Chancroid, caused by *Hemophilus ducreyi*, causes small painful ulcerations. These ulcerations are usually associated with unilateral, tender, fluctuant inguinal adenopathy. Differential diagnosis includes herpes, primary syphilis, granuloma inguinale, and LGV. The diagnosis is made by culturing the edge of the ulcer or lymph node aspirate on supplemented chocolate agar. Treatment of choice is trimethoprim-sulfamethoxazole, one double-strength table twice daily for 10 days or until the ulcer and lymphadenopathy resolve. Alternative treatment is erythromycin, 500 mg orally four times daily. Fluctuant nodes should be aspirated as needed in order to minimize the risk of spontaneous rupture.

Granuloma inguinale or donovanosis is an infection due to *Calymmatobacterium granulomatis*. Most cases of donovanosis in the United States have been identified in homosexual men. After 1 to 4 weeks of incubation, a beefy, granulomatous ulcer with elevated borders develops in the genitalia or anorectal area. Lymphadenopathy is uncommon, but the surrounding induration can extend into the inguinal area, resulting in an "pseudobubo." The lesion resembles squamous cell carcinoma, which may also complicate long-standing cases, emphasizing the need for biopsy in uncertain cases. Diagnosis is made by a Wright or Giemsa stain of the scraping of the ulcer bed. The presence of blue-black bipolar-staining bacilli in the cytoplasm of large mononuclear cells is diagnostic. The treatment is tetracycline, 500 mg four times daily until the lesion has healed completely. For treatment failures, ampicillin 500 mg four times daily, streptomycin 1.0 g twice daily, gentamicin 1 mg per kilogram twice daily, or chloramphenicol, 500 mg four times daily, have all been advocated.

Condyloma accuminata or anogenital warts are caused by human papilloma viruses. These pink or brown cauliflower-like lesions appear on the glans penis, perineum, and anorectal regions. The lesions may be mildly pruritic, but otherwise cause few symptoms. The highly infectious condyloma accuminata of secondary syphilis need to be differentiated from these warts; this is accomplished by performing darkfield microscopy for spirochetes and on the basis of the flat characteristic appearance of the warts. Therapy varies according to the site of involvement. For external genital and perianal warts, an application of 25 percent podophyllin in compound tincture of benzoin is advocated. For anorectal or oral warts, cryotherapy, electrocauterization or surgery is recommended.

Molluscum contagiosum presents as a flesh-colored, 2 to 5 mm, frequently umbilicated papule; it is caused by a pox virus. A cheesy material can often be expressed from the center of the lesion, and multiple lesions are common. Diagnosis is made by the clinical appearance, which is highly suggestive. Confirmation can be obtained by biopsy or examination of the expressed caseous material, which reveals molluscum bodies (basophilic cytoplasmic inclusions filled with the virium). Treatment consists of removal of the caseous center by pressure after nicking the center with a scalpel or needle. Spontaneous resolution occurs in most cases. Podophyllin 20 percent compound or cryotherapy with liquid nitrogen can be used in resistant cases.

Ectoparasites such as lice (pediculosis) and mites (scabies) are seen more frequently in heterosexuals than in homosexuals. The primary symptom of pediculosis is itching, primarily in the genital area, although any hairy part of the body can be involved. Close examination of the infected area show nits attached one-half to 1 inch from the base of the hair shaft. Scabies is often characterized by pruritis, which is typically worse at night. The lesions are symetric and consist of pathognomonic burrows made by the female. The burrows vary from 1 mm to 10 mm in length and are commonly seen in men in interdigital web spaces of the hand, wrist, elbow, beltline, penis, and scrotum. Gamma benzene hexochloride (lindane) is the treatment of choice for both infections. The medication for pediculosis is applied as a shampoo that can be washed off in 4 minutes. For scabies, a 1 percent lotion or cream is applied to the body from the neck down and washed off the next day. A single application is usually effective for scabies, whereas a second application 1 week later may be necessary for pediculosis.

HEPATITIS

Hepatitis A or B can be sexually transmitted and are frequent infections seen in homosexual men. The risk of developing hepatitis B infection has been shown to exceed 20 percent annually among seronegative homosexual men attending clinics for sexually transmitted diseases. It is estimated that the annual infection rate for hepatitis A is comparable to that observed for hepatitis B infection. Other infections commonly seen in homosexual men that may also manifest as hepatitis include cytomegaloviral infection, Epstein-Barr viral infection, and secondary syphilis. Indeed, more than 95 percent of homosexual men will become seropositive for cytomegalovirus and Epstein-Barr virus. The clinical spectrum of acute hepatitis in homosexual men is similar to that seen in any other group of healthy individuals and ranges from totally asymptomatic and anicteric (50%) to icteric, symptomatic disease (45%) and to severe fulminant disease (5%). The clinical presentation and diagnosis of viral hepatitis is discussed in greater detail in a separate chapter.

Immune serum globulin is recommended for any persons reporting sexual contact within the prior 2 weeks with an individual having a known case of hepatitis A and for persons reporting contact with viral hepatitis of unknown etiology. Immune serum globulin has been shown to be effective in preventing overt hepatitis A viral infection in 80 to 90 percent of persons treated either before or within 2 weeks of intimate contact. The dose is 0.02 ml per kilogram intramuscularly. Presently, there are no studies that demonstrate the efficacy of immune serum globulin prophylaxis in the prevention of non-A, non-B hepatitis in sexual contacts of recently infected homosexual men. When there has been sexual contact with an individual with recent hepatitis B infection, hyperimmune hepatitis B immune globulin (HBIg) is recommended, 0.06 ml per kilogram intramuscularly, as soon after exposure as possible. The dose should be repeated in 1 month.

Hepatitis B vaccine (Merck Sharp & Dohme; Heptavax B vaccine) has recently been developed and is effective in providing a high rate of protection (at least 92%) in persons receiving three vaccinations of 20 μg (1 ml) each over a 6-month period. Due to the high rate of hepatitis B infection, vaccination is recommended for all seronegative homosexual men and sexual contacts of recently infected individuals. In general, if sexual contact has occurred with a person with evidence of a recent hepatitis B infection, the sexual contact should be given passive prophylaxis with HBIg, followed by a vaccination with Heptavax B. These individuals need to be counseled that they still may acquire the disease and that they should refrain from sexual activity until they are HBsAg-negative and HBsAB-positive by serotesting.

INTESTINAL INFECTIONS

Due to the sexual practices that involve fecal or rectal contamination (anilingus, anal intercourse, or fellatio following anal intercourse), homosexual men are particularly susceptible to sexually transmitted gastrointestinal infections. Although many of these infections are polymicrobial and asymptomatic, a systematic approach to diagnosis that incorporates sexual history, symptoms and findings on physical examination, anoscopy, mucosal biopsy, and screening tests should guide the clinician in the selection of specific diagnostic tests and appropriate antimicrobial therapy. A flow chart is shown in Figure 1 that outlines the steps required in the evaluation of a homosexual man with intestinal symptoms.

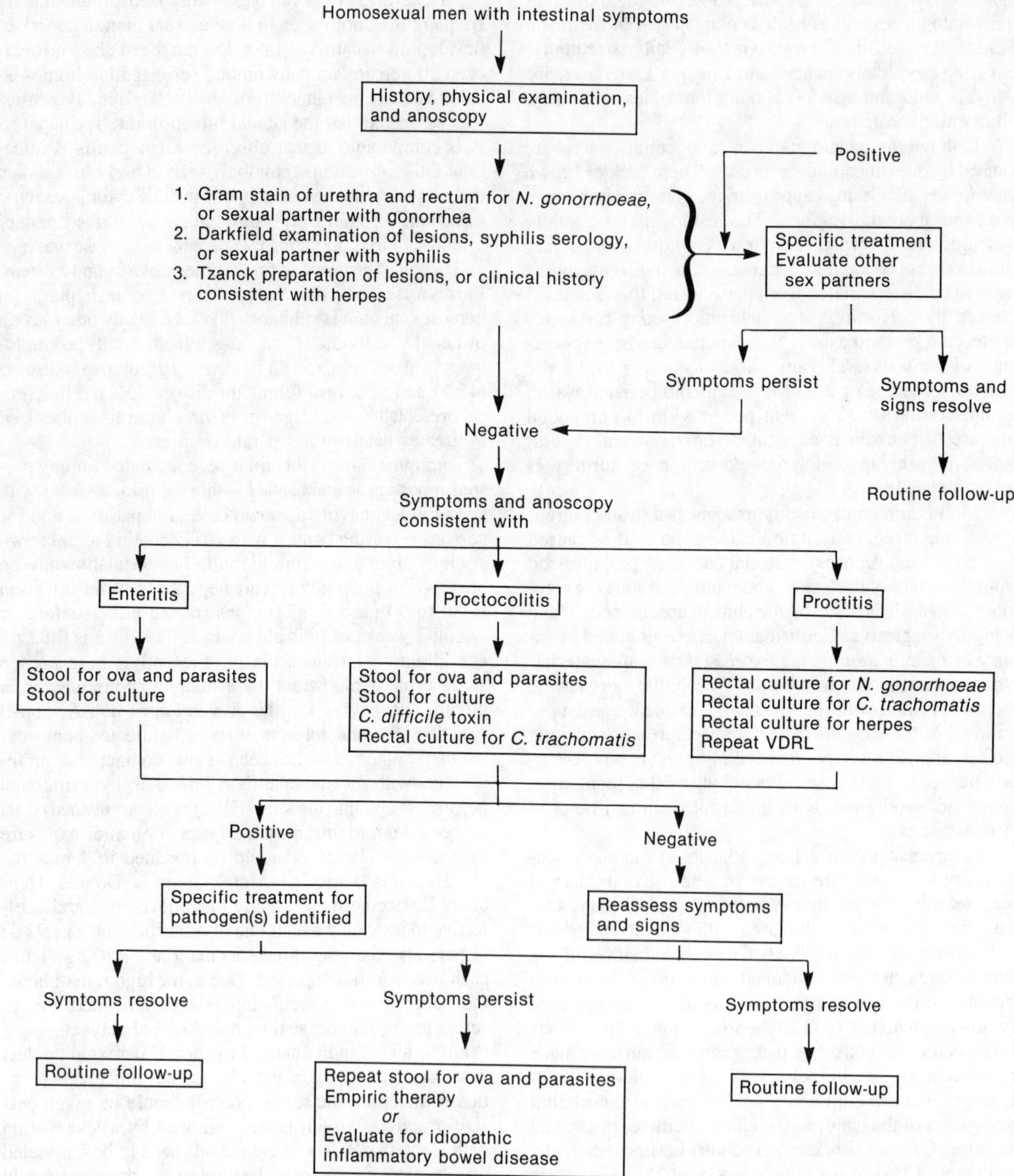

Figure 1 Evaluation of homosexual men with intestinal or anorectal symptoms

If the patient is asymptomatic, he should be carefully screened by culture and serologic tests for rectal and pharyngeal gonorrhea and syphilis. About two-thirds of persons with rectal or pharyngeal gonorrhea will be asymptomatic, whereas others will have symptoms consisting of mild proctitis or pharyngitis, respectively. In the case of pharyngeal infection, symptoms can include a sore throat, and on oral examination, the pharynx may appear erythematous or completely normal. In the case of rectal infection, symptoms may include constipation, anorectal discomfort, tenesmus, and a mucopurulent discharge. On anoscopy, the mucosa may appear normal or slightly erythematous in the distal 5 to 10 cm of the rectum. Complications such as fistula formation, perirectal abscess, rectal stricture, and disseminated gonococcal infection have been reported. Diagnosis is based on the identification of intracellular gram-negative diplococci within polymorphonuclear leukocytes on Gram stain of the pharyngeal or rectal mucosa, particularly in symptomatic individuals, and diagnosis is confirmed by culture of *N. gonorrhoeae*. The sensitivity of Gram stain compared with culture is about 50 percent in infections of the rectum or pharynx. Treatment of both rectal and pharyngeal gonorrhea is presented in Table 1.

Anorectal or oral syphilis is commonly asymptomatic and presents as a painless chancre. Darkfield examination is often inadequate since nonpathogenic treponemes are often present within the gastrointestinal tract and may be misdiagnosed for *Treponema pallidum*. Therefore, diagnosis is frequently dependent on the demonstration of seropositivity. A further discussion on diagnosis and treatment of syphilis is presented elsewhere in this volume.

In homosexual men with gastrointestinal symptoms, the presence of anorectal pain and a mucopurulent or bloody discharge suggests proctitis or proctocolitis. Proctitis is commonly associated with tenesmus and constipation, whereas proctocolitis is more often associated with diarrhea. In both, anoscopy usually shows the presence of friability, mucus, and pus, which should be sampled for microbiologic studies and Gram stain. Most cases of proctitis are due to *N. gonorrhoeae*, herpes simplex virus, *C. trachomatis*, or primary or secondary syphilis. Rectal infection with *Chlamydia* is indistinguishable from rectal gonorrhea. Symptoms are often absent or mild. Infection with *C. trachomatis* of the LGV serovar is more pathogenic and often associated with systemic symptoms. Rectal involvement may be characterized by severe anorectal pain, bloody mucopurulent discharge, and tenesmus. LGV infection of the rectum may present as acute ulcerative proctocolitis with evidence of granuloma formation on biopsy specimens. Sigmoidoscopy often reveals diffuse friability in the rectum, with discrete ulcerations occasionally extending to the descending colon. Strictures and fistulas may be prominent, and these can often be misdiagnosed clinically for Crohn's disease or carcinoma of the rectum. Diagnosis of chlamydial proctitis or proctocolitis is made by isolation of *C. trachomatis* in culture. The new rapid diagnostic tests for *C. trachomatis* have not been very helpful for detecting rectal infection. Treatment for chlamydial infection consists of tetracycline, 500 mg four times a day orally for 1 week for non-LGV infections and up to 3 to 4 weeks for LGV infections, depending on response.

Herpes infection in homosexual men can often involve the rectum, the perianal area, the oral cavity, and/or the pharynx. Symptoms of anorectal herpes include localized pain, constipation, rectal discharge, hematochezia, fever, chills, malaise, and headache. Neurologic symptoms include paresthesias, dysesthesias, neuralgia, difficulty with micturition, impotence, and severe constipation. Diagnosis of anorectal HSV infection is based on the clinical appearance of herpetic vesicles or ulcerations—interally, externally, or both—and on the recovery of herpes in culture. Treatment is supportive with use of analgesics, sitz baths, and stool softeners. Acyclovir has not been adequately tested for the treatment of anorectal herpes.

Proctocolitis or colitis reflects more extensive inflammation involving the rectum and colon and is usually caused by enteric pathogens such as *Campylobacter, Shigella, Salmonella, E. histolytica,* and *C. trachomatis* of the LGV serovar. A history of recent antibiotic use should suggest evaluation for *Clostridium difficile* infection. Treatment regimens are outlined in Table 2 for infections with these pathogens.

The occurrence of diarrhea and abdominal bloating or cramping, without anorectal symptoms, in association with normal anoscopy and sigmoidoscopy, is consistent with inflammation of the small intestine or enteritis. In homosexual men, enteritis limited to the small intestine is often attributable to *Giardia lamblia*, but *Campylobacter, Shigella, E. histolytica,* and *Cryptosporidium* can produce enterocolitis with or without lesions involving the distal colon or rectum. Diagnosis of these pathogens is made by a stool culture for enteric pathogens and stool examination for ova and parasites. Therapeutic options for proctocolitis and enteritis are varied and will be influenced by the cause (bacterial or protozoan), by local differences in the prevalence of enteric pathogens, by the patterns of antimicrobial susceptibility of these pathogens, and by the availability of timely microbiologic diagnostic support.

The etiologic diagnosis of proctitis, proctocolitis, and enteritis in homosexual men is compounded by the frequency of mixed infections. It is not uncommon that a homosexual man with one infection will later be found to have additional pathogens present. Symptoms will frequently persist despite adequate treatment of a documented infection. Reinfection, poor compliance, antimicrobial resistance, or the presence of multiple infections may be responsible for persistence of symptoms. Therefore, repeat evaluations or empiric therapy based on signs and symptoms of clinical syndrome may be warranted. Since all of the agents discussed above are sexually transmitted, appropriate treatment of sexual partners is indicated to prevent reinfection and to reduce community spread of these pathogens. Homosexually active men should also be counseled that oral-anal sex with multiple male part-

TABLE 2 Treatment of Enteric Infections Commonly Seen in Homosexual Men

Specific Infection	*Recommended Treatment*	*Alternative*
Entamoeba histolytica	Metronidazole 750 mg PO 3 times a day for 10 days	Diiodohydroxyquine 650 mg PO 3 times a day for 20 days
Giardia lamblia	Metronidazole 250 mg PO 3 times a day for 7 days	Quinacrine hydrochloride 100 mg PO 3 times a day for 7 days
Shigella species	Trimethoprim-sulfamethoxazole (160 mg/800 mg) PO twice a day for 7 days	Ampicillin 500 mg PO 4 times a day for 7 days
Campylobacter species	Erythromycin 500 mg PO 4 times a day for 7 days	Tetracycline 500 mg PO 4 times a day for 7 days
Salmonella species	Antibiotics not recommended except for severe, bacteremic cases	Chloramphenicol 500 mg IV q6h for 10 days; ampicillin 1 g IV q4h for 10 days; trimethoprim-sulfamethoxazole 2 tabs q12h for 10 days (these are therapeutically equivalent regimens)
Cryptosporidium species	Supportive, fluid therapy; spiramycin* 1.0 g PO 4 times a day	
Isospora belli	Supportive, fluid therapy; spiramycin* 1.0 g PO 4 times a day	

* Cryptosporidia and isospora infections do not require treatment in immunocompetent patients. Spiramycin recommended for infections in AIDS patients only. Treat until there is a response and then for an additional week.

ners is associated with a high risk of intestinal infection. Furthermore, the presence of intestinal rectal symptoms should lead to medical consultation and cessation of sexual contact until a specific diagnosis is made, therapy is given, and cure is documented.

INFECTION FOLLOWING BURN INJURY

RONALD G. TOMPKINS, M.D., Sc.D.
JOHN F. BURKE, M.D.

Infection of the burn wound is still the major cause of complications and death in thermally injured patients. To prevent the sequelae of wound infection, the best approach is to prevent wound infection. The problem is a large, open wound of necrotic tissue and the decreased host resistance that results from serious thermal trauma. Basic science and clinical studies have shown that decreased host resistance after burn injury is more important in determining the seriousness of infection than is the virulence of the causative bacterium. Factors resulting in decreased host resistance should be minimized. Necrotic tissue must be removed and wounds, closed. Secondary derangements in physiology and metabolism leading to caloric and protein starvation must be corrected. Treatment in regard to prevention of infection may be summarized as follows: 1. Promptly excise the necrotic tissue of the burn injury and immediately close the wound with skin grafts. 2. Maintain the patient in a controlled, isolated environment such as a bacterial-controlled nursing unit (BCNU) to protect the wound from cross-contamination. 3. Apply topical antibacterial agents such as 0.5 percent silver nitrate solution, 10 percent mafenide acetate cream (Sulfamylon), or silver sulfadiazine cream to reduce bacterial colonization of the burn wound. 4. Routine antibiotics given with the idea of avoiding burn wound infection do not prevent that infection. These antibiotics only lead to an emergence of bacterial strains that are resistant to that particular antibiotic. Prophylactic antibiotics with the intention of preventing burn wound infection should not be given. There are, however, several clinical states in which antibiotics may be used effectively for prevention. One of these clinical states occurs immediately after injury when host defense is seriously reduced. During this time, penicillin is given specifically to prevent beta-hemolytic streptococcal infection for a 3-day period, which begins immediately after the injury. A second clinical state occurs because of the high incidence of bacteremia during excision of colonized burn eschar. During these periods, antibiotics should be given and should be selected on the basis of sensitivities of the bacteria that are actually growing in the burn wound. These preventive perioperative antibiotics are started immediately before the operative period and stopped after the patient returns physiologically to normal, which is usually within 24 hours after operation.

TOPICAL WOUND CARE

Before application of a topical agent, all grease, oil, loose skin, burned clothing, and other contaminants are removed, and a thick layer of wide-mesh gauze dressing is placed on the wound and saturated with 0.5 percent silver nitrate. A 0.5 percent silver nitrate solution not only markedly decreases bacterial growth on the burn wound, but also minimizes water evaporation and may be used for donor sites and newly grafted areas as well as the burn wound. Silver nitrate is not used in the perineum or on the face because of the mechanical problems of application. Dressings are soaked with 0.5 percent silver nitrate solution every 2 hours to maintain a 0.5 percent concentration at the wound surface. A lesser concentration is not bacteriostatic and a greater concentration damages viable skin. Dressings are changed daily. The other two topical agents frequently used are sulfamylon and silver sulfadiazine. They are supplied in cream form and are applied directly to the burn wound after the initial removal of wound contaminants. They are reapplied twice daily. Care must be taken to remove previous sulfamylon or silver sulfadiazine before a fresh layer is applied. Sulfamylon easily penetrates eschar and is systemically absorbed and excreted by the kidney. Since sulfamylon is a carbonic-anhydrase inhibitor, metabolic acidosis may develop in the presence of renal or respiratory failure. Allergic reactions and hemolysis in patients deficient in glucose-6-phosphate dehydrogenase (G6PD) may develop for both sulfamylon and silver sulfadiazine. An unusual reaction of methemoglobinemia results when nitrates are reduced by wound bacteria such as certain *Escherichia coli* and *Klebsiella*.

PREVENTIVE ANTIBIOTICS

Antibiotics supplement the patient's natural ability to ward off infection. The use of antibiotics for indiscriminate periods in a general attempt to avoid infection is an ineffective approach that may result in alterations in the normal flora, allergic reactions, and wound colonization by resistant bacterial strains. Antibiotics are used for two general indications: established infection and prevention of infection during periods of reduced host resistance. There are two periods of reduced host resistance seen in thermally injured patients. The first occurs immediately after burns and the second occurs perioperatively during manipulation of contaminated burn eschar. Penicillin G (1.2 million units per day intravenously) or penicillin V (1 g per day orally) is given for 3 days after the burn injury in all cases of serious second-degree and all third-degree burns for the prevention of beta-hemolytic streptococcal cellulitis. In the case of penicillin allergy, erythromycin (2 g per day intravenously or orally) is administered. Active immunization against *Clostridium tetani* with adult-type adsorbed tetanus and diphtheria toxoids (0.5 ml intramuscularly) is given in all cases of serious burn injury unless clear documentation of recent immunization (within 1 year) exists. Passive immunization with human tetanus immunoglobulin TIG(H) (250 to 500 units, intramuscularly) is given at a separate site if the wound is extensive or grossly contaminated or if the state of tetanus immunity is unknown.

Antibiotics are administered immediately prior to the operation, during the operative procedure, and in the immediate postoperative period until normal cardiovascular hemodynamics are reestablished (usually within 24 hours) and other normal physiologic signs are present. The antibiotic given is chosen on the basis of previous burn wound cultural results and sensitivities of the organisms. If these are unavailable, general antimicrobial coverage for both gram-positive cocci and gram-negative rods is recommended. Preventive intravenous antibiotics for the commonly encountered *Staphylococcus aureus* are nafcillin (8 g per day) or, alternatively, with penicillin allergy, vancomycin 1 g per 12 hours in adults or 50 mg per kilogram per day in children. For purposes of prevention, these are seldom administered for more than 24 hours. The common gram-negative rod bacteria encountered are *Pseudomonas aeruginosa, E. coli, Enterobacter, Klebsiella, Acinetobacter*, and *Proteus*. The recommended intravenously administered aminoglycoside is either gentamicin or tobramycin (1.5 mg per kilogram per day), the choice of which depends on bacterial sensitivities. We reserve tobramycin for settings where laboratory results prior to surgery indicate resistance to gentamicin. Both vancomycin and aminoglycoside serum levels should be obtained when these antibiotics are continued for more than 72 hours.

ESTABLISHED INFECTION

Identification of invasive infection requiring antibiotics is difficult because burn wounds are rarely sterile, and it is difficult to distinguish between wound colonization and wound invasion on the basis of wound bacteriology alone. Some indications for antibiotic treatment in burn patients include the following: 1. Deterioration of the patient's overall clinical condition together with a considerable increase in the number of bacteria cultured from the wound (from scant or moderate growth to abundant growth). 2. Signs or symptoms of bacteremia with or without positive blood cultures. 3. Less specific findings of sepsis such as isolated cardiovascular failure, altered mental alertness, hypothermia, spiking fevers, or ileus.

The causative organism can usually be determined by referring to the recent surveillance cultures of the burn wound, urine, and respiratory tract secretions. In large thermal injuries, surveillance cultures should be taken of body fluids on a regular basis, at least weekly. Often the last strain cultured from the burn wound is the strain responsible for the invasive infection. More definitive information can be obtained from blood cultures, which should be obtained at the first clinical indication of invasive infection. The concept of quantitative burn wound cultures is not practical for routine burn care. In assessing methods giving evidence on wound invasion, the highest correlation of all with invasive burn wound infection is histologic evidence of bacterial invasion of viable tissue at the base of the wound. The biopsy of the wound should be subjected to grinding and bacterial quantitation as well as histology. This is not usually practical in the routine clinical setting.

Gram-negative bacteria, especially *E. coli, Klebsiella*, and *Enterobacter*, are most often responsible for invasive infection. These organisms are best managed on the basis of sensitivity testing. When the involved pathogen cannot be identified, both an aminoglycoside and a penicillinase-resistant penicillin should be given for wide-spectrum coverage until more specific antibiotic therapy can be administered. Treatment can be initiated with the same antibiotics and dosages recommended in the previous section. For life-threatening infection, the treatment of pseudomonas infection is often enhanced with carbenicillin (30 g per day). In patients with large, open wounds—especially children—drug leakage from the wound complicates accurate therapy that anticipates serum levels based on body size. Actual serum levels obtained by peak and trough levels must be used for accurate therapy.

Treatment of infection in thermally injured patients differs little from the treatment of infection in other patients except the resistance to infection is seriously depressed because of the extent of the unrepaired injury.

INFECTION FOLLOWING TRAUMA

ELLIOT GOLDSTEIN, M.D.
EILEEN MURPHY, M.D.

Traumatic injuries are invariably subject to infection due to contamination by exogenous microorganisms or the introduction of endogenous flora into previously sterile sites. In general, the likelihood of posttraumatic infection depends on the injury and its extent. For example, injuries of an extremity resulting in open fractures with embedded skin flora and foreign materials or abdominal wounds that penetrate the intestinal tract are more prone to infection than injuries in which the integument and intestine remain intact. Since the internist and general practitioner most often treat these infections and those complicating soft tissue and head injuries as well, the following discussion confines itself to posttraumatic infections of these four sites.

GENERAL PRINCIPLES

Recognition of the role of exogenous and endogenous microorganisms, foreign material, and devitalized tissue in initiating posttraumatic infection has resulted in a few general principles for prophylaxis. The wound is first washed free of bacteria with saline rather than antibiotic solutions. Saline is chosen because comparative studies have shown that irrigation with antibiotics adds little to perioperative prophylaxis when parenteral therapy is also administered. Moreover, irrigation with antibiotics may increase the likelihood of colonization with resistant bacteria. Devitalized tissue is then debrided under sterile conditions. After debridement, drains are inserted to prevent blood and tissue fluids from accumulating in dependent wound spaces. If the wound is clean and fluid accumulation is unlikely, drains are contraindicated since they allow bacterial colonization, thereby increasing the possibility of infection.

Since all injuries, even minor ones, pose the threat of tetanus, every patient is considered for prophylaxis with tetanus toxoid, using the combined tetanus and diphtheria preparation. This decision is determined by the patient's immunization history. Patients who have received a primary immunization series of three injections and who have not had a booster injection in 10 years are given adsorbed tetanus toxoid. Five years is the deciding interval for severe injuries likely to be contaminated by clostridial spores. Patients with minor injuries in whom immunization is uncertain are treated with tetanus toxoid; if the injury is considered one of high risk, 500 units of human tetanus immune globulin is given with the toxoid.

SPECIFIC INJURIES

Abdomen

Infection that occurs in 10 to 15 percent of patients is the major complication of abdominal trauma. Puncture of the gastrointestinal tract produced by gunshots, knives, or other causes permit gastrointestinal contents to leak into the peritoneum. Since large numbers of aerobic and anaerobic bacteria populate the gastrointestinal tract, the spill provokes mixed infections with these bacteria. Coincident with their occurrence in the gastrointestinal tract, the gram-negative enteric aerobes, *Escherichia coli, Klebsiella* species, and *Enterobacter* species, and the gram-negative anaerobe, *Bacteroides fragilis*, are frequent causes for infection. Failure to eradicate gastrointestinal bacteria from the soiled peritoneum in the perioperative period results in posttraumatic abdominal infections and abscess formation.

The diagnosis of abdominal infection, which was formerly a formidable clinical challenge, has been made considerably easier by advances in technology. No longer is the diagnosis limited to the interpretation of tenuous findings of hiccups, abdominal tenderness, rebound, and ileus in a patient with fever and an elevated white blood cell count. Approximately 80 percent of abdominal abscesses are identifiable by ultrasonography, which can be performed at the bedside and, for this reason, is our initial diagnostic choice. Computerized tomography offers greater sensitivity and specificity than ultrasound, but because this procedure requires transportation to the radiology department, it is less suitable for critically ill patients. Computerized tomography is recommended for patients who tolerate transfer to radiology and the procedure is of particular value in cases where ultrasonography provides inconclusive information. Scintigraphy with indium 111–labeled leukocytes also accurately detects abdominal infections, but because the technique requires a waiting period of 24 hours before the scintiscans are evaluated, its use is limited to cases in which the diagnosis is in doubt despite evaluation by ultrasonography and computerized tomography. Nuclear magnetic resonance, the newest method for detecting intra-abdominal infection may prove to be the most accurate technique. However, at present, comparative studies defining the place of this diagnostic method are not available. Scintigraphy with gallium-67 is no longer considered of value in diagnosing abdominal abscesses because of its lesser accuracy. Additional clues to the presence of an abdominal infection are blood cultures containing commonly found abdominal pathogens and physiologic evidence suggesting sepsis, e.g., an unexplained anion gap of more than 20 mEq per liter, diminished systemic vascular resistance of less than 800 dynes sec cm^{-5}, or unexplained hypotension.

The management of a patient with abdominal trauma begins at surgery where hemostatis is effected, devitalized tissue and foreign materials are removed, damaged tissue is repaired, the wound area is cleansed, and tetanus prophylaxis is ensured. The risk of posttraumatic infection is reduced by instituting antibiotic therapy with cefoxitin (100 mg per kilogram per day intravenously in divided doses at 6-hour intervals), a cephalosporin that is efficacious against the commonly encountered gram-negative enteric and anaerobic bacteria, or gentamicin (5.0 mg per kilogram per day intravenously in divided doses at 8-hour intervals) and clindamycin (30 mg per kilogram per day intravenously in divided doses at 6-hour intervals). The newer third-generation cephalosporins and other combinations such as gentamicin and metronidazole may be equally as efficacious in reducing the risk of posttraumatic abdominal infection. Our own preference is to use cefoxitin (100 mg per kilogram per day in 6-hour divided doses initially), as this agent provides efficacious therapy with lesser toxicity and expense. Despite the above measures, abdominal infections occur in approximately 20 percent of patients with intestinal perforations due to abdominal trauma. The clinician must be constantly aware of this possibility in patients with persistent low-grade fever and unexplained abdominal tenderness. We cannot overemphasize the importance of early diagnosis of abdominal infections in minimizing morbidity and mortality. Once diagnosed, abscesses or collections of pus are drained percutaneously by use of ultrasonic or computerized tomographic guidance or at laparotomy. Our preference is to choose ultrasound for cases in which the abscesses are clearly defined and the drainage path avoids viscera. When more than one abscess is present or the possibility of undetected infection exists, laparotomy is recommended. Infected materials are removed and cultured using Penrose drains or sump drains attached to a vacuum pump. The antibiotic regimen is reevaluated, and agents are chosen on the basis of new cultural and sensitivity results. While awaiting these results, the previously mentioned regimen of gentamicin plus clindamycin is chosen. The duration of antibiotic therapy depends on the patient's course, which is monitored clinically and with repeated imaging procedures. In general, parenteral antibiotics are continued for up to one week after apparent clinical cure.

Spleen

Splenectomy following abdominal trauma presents special problems in regard to infection. First, a small percentage of patients develop subphrenic abscesses postoperatively. This incidence is increased in cases with associated bowel perforations, and it is reported that open drainage also enhances this incidence. When necessary, drainage is performed with a closed system using suction. Antimicrobial agents, either cefoxitin, ceftizoxime, cefotaxime, or gentamicin and clindamycin are administered throughout the operative and immediate postoperative period (24 hours) in uncomplicated cases without bowel perforations. Cefoxitin is our choice in this situation because of the increased vulnerability of splenectomized patients to infection with encapsulated microorganisms. Chemotherapy is continued for longer periods in complicated cases or ones with bowel perforations. Second, because the spleen serves to filter bacteria, septicemia is inordinately common in the postsplenectomy period, particularly in young children. These infections are due to encapsulated bacteria (pneumococcus, *Hemophilus influenzae, E. coli*) and are frequently fulminant, resulting in rapid death. Because septicemia can be overwhelming in this patient population, treatment with large doses of ampicillin, 200 mg per kilogram per day in divided doses at 4-hour intervals, and gentamicin, 5 mg per kilogram per day in divided doses at 8-hour intervals, is instituted at the first signs of sepsis. Third, patients who are splenectomized and receive multiple blood transfusions are prone to serious infections with cytomegalovirus. This illness, for which there is no treatment, is characterized by persistent fever, interstital pneumonitis, and the presence of atypical lymphocytes. Definitive diagnosis depends on the identification of typical owl's eye cells in pulmonary lavage fluids or culture of the virus from lavage fluids or urine.

The risk of fulminant septicemia in the years following splenectomy was first recognized in children, but is now also known to occur, albeit at a lower incidence, in adults. Although overwhelming septicemia can occur at any time, the risk is highest in the first two years following splenectomy. The pneumococcus is responsible for approximately one-half of the cases, with other encapsulated bacteria accounting for the remainder. We vaccinate all patients with pneumococcal vaccine to minimize this risk. Children are also vaccinated with meningococcal vaccine types A and C. In addition, children younger than 5 years of age receive oral penicillin VK (100,000 units per kilogram per day in twice daily doses to a maximum of 1.6 million units) as chemoprophylaxis. We also recommend chemoprophylaxis with oral penicillin VK (20,000 units per kilogram per day in twice daily doses) for adults during the first 2 years following splenectomy even though the virtue of this prophylaxis is unproved. Patients who have had splenectomies are advised to seek prompt medical attention for respiratory illnesses or fever.

Bone

Traumatic injuries that result in open fractures should be regarded as contaminated and likely to become infected. For this reason, many physicians add cephalosporins or aminoglycosides to irrigating fluids. We do not recommend this practice because its effectiveness is unproved and because locally administered antibiotics may promote superinfection with resistant bacteria. Debridement is of major importance and, unless the surgeon is certain about its adequacy, the wound is left open. Cultures obtained prior to completing the surgical procedure are used to guide antimicrobial therapy in the postoperative period. *S. aureus* and *Staphylococcus epidermidis* and the gram-negative bacilli (*E. coli, Enterobacter* species, *Klebsiella* species, and *Pseudomonas* species) are most often implicated in posttraumatic osteomyelitis. Anaerobes are less common pathogens, but recent studies suggest that they cause infection sufficiently often to warrant culturing for them. *Nocardia* and fungi are infrequent causes of infection.

Since infection is a common complication of severe fractures, systemic antibiotics are routinely administered prior to surgery and in the postoperative period. Cefazolin, at a dosage of 100 mg per kilogram per day given intravenously at 6-hour intervals, provides effective therapy for most staphylococci and gram-negative bacilli. Whether cephalosporins (cefoxitin, ceftizoxime, or cefotaxime), which have additional activity against anaerobic bacteria, are better choices is an unsettled question. Combinations of an aminoglycoside, usually gentamicin with clindamycin, are also useful in the initial treatment of severely contaminated fractures. Because the combination is more toxic and of unproven advantage to the cephalosporins, we prefer the cephalosporins even in severe injuries. Also, we consider the differences that exist in the ability of antibiotics to penetrate bone to be of unproven clinical importance, and, therefore, this information is not used in deciding therapy. The duration of therapy is unpredictable, as it depends on the rate of wound healing. If the wound remains uninfected and heals appropriately, antibiotic therapy is discontinued prior to secondary closure. Wounds that become infected are recultured and antimicrobial therapy is chosen on the basis of these in vitro bacterial sensitivity results.

Two potential causes for the persistence of posttraumatic infections of bone are unremoved sequestra and infected fixation devices. Sequestra, which are sometimes identifiable radiologically as opaque foreign bodies, serve as niduses for infection, often producing sinus tracts. Cure of these low-grade infections requires aspiration of the sinus tract, removal of the sequestra, and the application of antimicrobial therapy. Antimicrobial therapy is based on cultures from the sequestra and not the sinus tract. Infected fixation devices pose a therapeutic dilemma. As a rule, cure is unlikely as long as the device is present. However, since alignment of the fracture is critical for future functional use, we leave infected devices in place until the fracture is stable or the alignment can be maintained by external fixation. During this period, antibiotics are used to suppress the smoldering infection. It is important to emphasize the need to remove the infected rod, plate, or screw as soon as the fracture is stable since these infections result in osteomyelitis, sequestra formation, and wound breakdown. Posttraumatic bone infections due to less common microorganisms like *Actinomyces, Nocardia*, or fungi are treated with penicillin (*Actinomyces*), trimethoprim-sulfamethoxazole (*Nocardia*), or amphotericin B (fungi) according to the schedules recommended in the chapters pertaining to these infections.

Soft Tissue

Posttraumatic injuries of soft tissue are cleansed and treated with antibiotics in the aforementioned manner except for cases complicated by a gas-associated myonecrosis or cellulitis. These latter infections, which are classified clinically as gas gangrene, anaerobic cellulitis, and necrotising fasciitis, follow contamination of an inadequately debrided wound by enzyme, toxin, and gas-producing bacteria (*Clostridium perfringens* and *septicum*, anaerobic streptococci, *Bacteroides* species, *E. coli, Enterobacter* species, *Klebsiella* species). Once within devitalized tissue, these microorganisms grow luxuriantly, rapidly destroying contiguous tissues. Because of their fulminant nature, these infections are medical emergencies requiring prompt diagnosis and therapy. Diagnosis is suspected when crepitus is noted clinically or when a radiograph shows subcutaneous gas in an area of cellulitis. Such findings mandate immediate surgical exploration to determine the extent of tissue destruction and to identify the pathogens by Gram stain and culture. Infections due to *Clostridia* species in which myonecrosis is present are debrided of dead muscle and fascia. Although we are invariably reluctant to recommend amputation, experience has taught us that the procedure is warranted if uncertainty exists regarding the viability of unexcised tissues. Clostridial infections are treated with 2 million units of penicillin administered intravenously at 3-hour intervals. Except for *B. fragilis* infections, infections due to nonclostridial anaerobic bacteria are treated in a similar manner. It is worth noting that these infections tend to be confined to fascia and to be less severe than clostridial infections; as such, they usually require less extensive surgery. Infections due to *Bacteroides* species are treated with cefoxitin or metronidazole rather than penicillin because of the tendency of these anaerobes to manifest penicilln resistance. Infections with gram-negative Enterobacteriaceae are treated initially with cefoxitin, ceftizoxime, or cefotaxime, and these agents are continued unless in vitro sensitivity testing indicates greater susceptibility to an aminoglycoside. If available, treatment with a hyperbaric oxygen chamber is helpful in retarding tissue necrosis. Polyvalent gas gangrene antitoxins are no longer used because they did not prove to be effective.

Central Nervous System

Although head injuries are common, infection of the central nervous system is infrequent because of the protection afforded by the skull and dura mater. For infection to occur, these barriers must be breached, permitting bacteria to enter the central nervous system. Fractures producing fistulae are those involving the frontal and ethmoid sinuses, the cribiform plate, and the temporal bone. Fractures that result in cerebrospinal fluid rhinorrhea and otorrhea are suspected in patients with severe paranasal injuries, bilateral orbital hematomas, mastoid bruising, or hemotympaneum. The site of the fistula is often evident from the radiologic position of the fracture. However, small fractures may elude radiologic detection, and in some cases, the diagnosis is very difficult. In these instances, ^{99}Tc-labeled albumin or fluorescein dyes are injected intrathecally, and the fistula is identified by scintiphotos showing radioisotope leaking from the anterior fossa or by demonstrating dye in small gauze packs placed within the nasal cavity. When the leakage is large, clinically evident excesses of clear nasal fluid can be shown to be cerebrospinal fluid by demonstrating high concentrations of glucose. The origin of lesser discharges is exceedingly difficult to prove since the dextrostix method, which is commonly used to detect small amounts of cerebrospinal fluid, can be falsely positive because of the glucose content of nasal mucus.

The risk of bacterial meningitis in patients with a dural tear is estimated to be 5 to 25 percent. Meningitis is most likely in the first 2 weeks following trauma, but it can occur at any time as long as the leak is present. Patients with persistent or intermittent rhinorrhea are also prone to recurrent episodes of meningitis. A cerebrospinal fluid fistula should be suspected in all patients who develop meningitis immediately following head trauma, who have had severe head trauma in the past, or who have had meningitis previously. The pneumococcus causes approximately 80 percent of posttraumatic meningitis. *H. influenzae* and *Neisseria meningitidis* are other important causes. Staphylococci and gram-negative bacilli infrequently cause posttraumatic meningitis. When these bacteria cause meningitis, it is usually as a result of contiguous bone and soft tissue infection in patients with large cranial defects or penetrating wounds.

The initial management of a head injury is the same as that for other soft tissue and bone injuries, namely wound cleansing, debridement, and the application of parenteral antibiotics, usually cephalosporins or penicillins. Whether chemotherapy is warranted is uncertain as its efficacy has never been documented. However, analogy with injuries at other sites suggests that chemotherapy with a cephalosporin is likely to minimize posttraumatic bone and soft tissue infections. Prevention of meningitis in patients with a cerebrospinal fluid leak with either cephalosporin or penicillin is, however, unlikely to be successful because neither agent effectively penetrates into cerebrospinal fluid in the absence of inflammation and neither reliably eliminates the pneumococcus from the nasopharynx. Because of these considerations, our practice is to treat patients with extensive head trauma with cefazolin, but not to use cephalosporins or penicillins as chemoprophylaxis in patients with closed fractures and cerebrospinal fluid leaks. Such patients are observed for meningitis and treated promptly with large doses of penicillin (12 to 20 million units per day) at the first signs of cerebral infection.

Most tears of the dura heal spontaneously within 1 or 2 weeks following injury, obviating the need for surgical repair. Indications for surgery are persistence of the leak and the occurrence of meningitis. Cerebrospinal fluid otorrhea usually ceases spontaneously; operative repair is seldom required.

Infection of the brain after a compound fracture of the cranium more often results in brain abscess than meningitis. Brain tissue is relatively resistant to infection and in cases receiving early neurosurgical care, posttraumatic brain abscesses are uncommon. Such abscesses are usually due to contamination with *S. aureus*, gram-negative bacilli, and anaerobes. Since the injured area of brain is undoubtedly contaminated, parenteral antibiotics such as cefazolin or nafcillin (150 mg per kilogram per day in divided doses at 4-hour intervals) plus penicillin (8 million units per day in divided doses at 6-hour intervals) or metronidazole (30 mg per kilogram per day

TABLE 1 Antibiotic choices in Treatment of Posttraumatic Infection

Site	*Antibiotic*	*Dosage*
Abdomen	Clindamycin	30 mg/kg/day q8h
	plus	
	Gentamicin	5 mg/kg/day q8h
Spleen	Ampicillin	200 mg/kg/day q6h
	plus	
	Gentamicin	5 mg/kg/day q8h
Bone	Cefazolin	100 mg/kg/day q6h
Soft tissue		
Aerobic	Cefazolin	100 mg/kg/day q6h
Gas gangrene	Penicillin G	16 million units/day q3h
Head	Cefazolin	150 mg/kg/day q4h
	plus	
	Metronidazole	30 mg/kg/day q6h

Note: Selections apply for cases in which antimicrobial sensitivity test results are either not available or support these choices. Other factors such as renal failure, penicillin hypersensitivity, or availability of aminoglycoside assays should be considered before applying these recommendations.

in divided doses at 6-hour intervals) are administered perioperatively, and treatment is continued as long as infection seems likely. Our preference is cefazolin plus metronidazole as this combination has utility against many gram-negative bacilli and virtually all anaerobes of importance. The role of newer cephalosporins like cefotaxime, ceftizoxime, or moxalactam, which traverse the blood brain barrier and have broad prophylactic activity against gram-positive cocci, gram negative bacilli, and anaerobes is unknown. Future studies may show that these agents provide better prophylaxis than the aforementioned agents but, at present, such data are not available. Abscesses that develop despite therapy are drained and treated with antibiotics on the basis of cultural results according to the regimens detailed in the chapter on *Localized Infection of the Central Nervous System.*

ANIMAL BITE INFECTION

ELLIE J. C. GOLDSTEIN, M.D.

One out of every two Americans will in their lifetimes be bitten by a domestic or a wild animal or by another human. Bite wounds account for approximately 1 percent of all emergency department visits. A careful history and physical examination is essential to the treatment of these wounds.

DOG AND CAT BITES

One to two million persons are bitten by dogs and 300,000 to 400,000, by cats yearly in the United States. Most of these wounds are trivial in nature and do not require medical attention. The patients who present for medical attention are in two distinct categories:

1. Patients who present less than 8 hours after injury usually do so for care of tear wounds and avulsions and/or because of the fear of rabies or tetanus. Established infection is rarely present.
2. Patients who present more than 8 to 12 hours after injury most often have established infection.

A careful history of the type of animal involved, whether the attack was provoked or unprovoked (petting a stray or even a neighbor's dog should be considered a provoked attack), behavior of the biting animal, geographic location, and time of the attack should be obtained. Many counties require the treating physician to report all bite wounds to the local health department.

The wound should be diagramed on the chart to note its size, depth, and location in relation to bones and joints as well as scratches and puncture sites. The presence or absence of swelling and ecchymoses due to crush injury should be noted. Assessment of tendon, muscular, and sensory functions of the involved area is important.

Wound Care

Bleeding should be controlled. If the patient presents less than 8 hours after injury and the wound is not infected, a culture need not be obtained. If infection is already established, closed wounds should be opened and eschars removed to drain pus or focal abscesses and to obtain specimens for cultures. The wound should be copiously irrigated. Puncture wounds may be irrigated by entering in the plane of the puncture with an 18-gauge needle attached to a 20-ml syringe. Irrigation reduces the bacterial inoculum and helps prevent infection if it is not already established. Foreign bodies should be removed, and necrotic tissue and nonviable skin tags should be cautiously debrided. Some physicians even debride puncture wounds. Facial wounds or those likely to cause disfiguring scars should be debrided cautiously, if at all, and should be seen by a plastic surgeon.

Infected wounds should remain open. There are no scientific data as to whether the early-presenting noninfected wounds may be closed primarily or require closure by delayed primary or secondary intention. Facial wounds are usually closed primarily.

Elevation of the affected part (daytime in a sling and nighttime with pillows for the first 2 to 3 days following injury) is essential to decrease swelling and to assure proper therapy for the infection. The lack of elevation is one of the most frequent reasons for poor or slow healing and even progression of infection. Immobilization with a bulky dressing or plaster splint is advisable, especially when the hand is involved.

Antibiotics

The role of antibiotics in patients who present less than 8 hours after injury remains controversial. However, studies from our laboratory show that 68 to 82 percent of these wounds yielded potential aerobic and/or anaerobic pathogens. Although most studies have focused on the isolation of *Pasteurella multocida*, our studies show *P. multocida* to be present in only 21 percent of both infected and noninfected dog bite wounds, but in 40 to 60 percent of cat bite wounds. Other oral bacteria, such as alpha streptococci, beta streptococci, *Staphylococcus* species, *EF-4* (CDC alpha-numeric designation), nonfragilis *Bacteroides* species, *Fusobacterium* species, and anaerobic gram-positive cocci are also frequently isolated from dog and cat bite wounds.

The bacteria isolated from these early presenting wounds are similar to those cultured from later-presenting infected wounds. Consequently, all bite wounds not trivial in nature should be considered contaminated and treated with antibiotics. Penicillin V is active against *P. multocida* and most of the other aerobic and anaerobic bacteria isolated from these wounds. Penicillin V (phenoxymethyl penicillin), 500 mg orally four times per day for 10 days should be given to patients who are clinically infected. If the patient presents less than 8 hours following injury and does not have clinical signs of infection, 5 days of therapy should be given. Ampicillin (500 mg by mouth four times a day) may be used as an alternative agent. If *Staphylococcus aureus* is suspected, as from Gram stain, dicloxacillin (a penicillinase-resistant penicillin), 500 mg orally four times a day should be given in addition to penicillin V. We have recently compared the activity of amoxacillin/clavulanic acid (Augmentin) to penicillin with and without dicloxacillin and found them to be equally effective. Amoxicillin/clavulanic acid may be used as an agent of second choice. Patients less than 130 pounds should be given 250 mg orally three times per day and those more than 130 pounds, 500 mg by mouth three times per day for the same durations as outlined above. Loose stools are a frequent adverse effect, but rarely cause alteration of therapy.

Penicillinase-resistant penicillins (such as dicloxacillin when used alone), oral cephalosporins (such as cephalexin, cephradine, and cefadroxil) and clindamycin are less effective than penicillin V and should not be used as empiric therapy. Tetracycline (500 mg orally four times per day) is a good alternative agent in the penicillin-allergic patient, but cannot be used in pregnant women or children who are still forming teeth. Erythromycin (500 mg orally four times per day) may be used as a third-line agent, but may be ineffective against 50 percent of *P. multocida* isolates. Therapeutic failures are frequent, especially in cat bite wounds where P. multocida is a frequent pathogen.

Infection usually presents as cellulitis in proximity to the wound. A gray, malodorous discharge may be present, but lymphangitis and systemic symptoms are infrequent. However, tenosynovitis, septic arthritis, osteomyelitis, bacteremia, and even meningitis may occur. Animals should not be allowed to lick open wounds because secondary infection and bacteremia due to their oral flora (e.g., *P. multocida, DF-2*) may occur, especially in the compromised host.

If a patient presents more than 12 to 24 hours after injury and does not show clinical signs of infection, the patient should be watched but antibiotics may be withheld. Infected patients usually have mild to moderate infection due to the oral aerobic and anaerobic bacteria of the biting animal. Most patients can be managed as outpatients and given oral antimicrobial therapy. Careful follow-up either by examination or telephone is essential. Patients who require hospitalization include those with severe infection, infection that has advanced one joint above the wound, patients with joint or bone involvement, septic arthritis, noncompliant patients or those who have failed outpatient therapy.

One must always consider the possibility of plague, tularemia, and cat-scratch disease in unusual cases.

Tetanus

Tetanus toxoid (0.5 ml intramuscularly) should be administered to patients without a booster within 5 years. A primary course should be given to unimmunized individuals.

Plague

Plague, due to *Pasteurella pestis*, is associated with direct animal contact and usually occurs, therefore, in veterinarians and animal handlers (see chapter on *Plague*). People usually become infected from flea bites, but direct animal contact, such as a domestic cat bite or even scratch, may cause disease. There is an incubation period of 2 to 6 days, and systemic symptoms and lymphadenopathy are frequent. Hospitalization and isolation are required. Diagnosis is by culture or by a fourfold antibody response. Streptomycin (30 mg per kilogram per day in divided doses) or tetracycline (30 to 50 mg per kilogram per day) should be given. Chemoprophylaxis for close contacts is recommended.

Tularemia

Tularemia is due to *Francisella tularensis*, a gram-negative coccobacillus that grows poorly on routine culture media. It causes high fever, chills, and malaise. Human infection usually follows tick bite, but may be associated with direct animal contact with rabbits and sometimes cats (see chapter on *Tularemia*). Most patients present with ulceroglandular disease, but tularemia may manifest as oculoglandular or pulmonic disease. Diagnosis is often made by a fourfold rise in antibody titers. Isolation of the organism may be successful if the specimen is cultured on cysteine blood agar, glucose blood agar, or thioglycollate broth containing cysteine. Streptomycin (15 to 20 mg per kilogram per day intramuscularly for 10 days) is the drug of choice for all forms of tularemia. Tetracycline, 500 mg orally four times per day for 14 days, is a second-choice agent since relapse may be more frequent. Relapses are not infrequent and may be retreated with the same drug as they are usually not due to the development of resistance.

Cat Scratch Disease

Cat scratch disease develops 3 to 30 days after exposure and is usually manifested as tender, regional (axilla, 65%; cervical, 25%) adenopathy often associated wth fever and malaise. When a patient presents with cervical adenopathy, cat scratch disease should be considered. In young women this should be considered in the differential diagnosis of Hodgkin's disease. Although the cause of cat scratch disease remains unknown, a fastidious gram-negative rod has been isolated from the lymph nodes of some patients. Some reports have suggested *Rothia denticarisa*, a gram-positive bacterium as the pathogen. The disease usually pursues a benign course with the resolution of adenopathy in 6 to 8 weeks. Occasional cases may persist up to one year. There is no specific therapy available.

RAT BITE FEVER

Rat bite fever (RBF) is a single designation for two diseases that are caused by either *Streptobacillus moniliformis*, a pleomorphic gram-negative rod, or *Spirillum minor*, a spirochete. Most cases are secondary to a rat bite, including bites by laboratory rats, but exposure to other domestic and wild animals may result in disease. Raw milk has also acted as a vector.

RBF due to *S. moniliformis* has an incubation period of 3 to 10 days. The original rat bite wound is often healed before the onset of the illness. Disease usually begins with a rigor and a high fever followed by headache, vomiting, myalgias, and regional adenopathy. Arthralgias and arthritis with effusion may occur. There is an associated rash that may be maculopapular or petechial and appears on the palms and soles. If untreated, the fever may persist or relapse and be associated with a 10 percent mortality.

Diagnosis may be by culture of the organism using special media supplemented with 20 percent rabbit or horse serum incubated in carbon dioxide. Often a false-positive test for syphilis develops and may lead to misdiagnosis. Treatment with procaine penicillin G, 600,000 units intramuscularly twice a day for 14 days, is usually curative. Tetracycline, 500 mg orally four times per day, or streptomycin, 7.5 mg per kilogram twice a day intramuscularly should be used in the penicillin-allergic patient or as second-choice therapy.

RBF due to *S. minor* has an incubation period of 1 to 3 weeks, but also begins as an acute febrile illness with high fever, rigors, and myalgias. Infection due to *S. minor* may be differentiated from that due to *S. moniliformis* if the original bite wound reappears at the onset of illness. This form produces fewer joint symptoms. Diagnosis is by darkfield examination of patient specimens or animal inoculation. Procaine penicillin G, 600,000 units intramuscularly twice a day for 10 days is usually curative. Tetracycline, 500 mg orally four times per day, and streptomycin, 7.5 mg per kilogram intramuscularly twice a day, are effective alternative agents.

OTHER ANIMAL BITES

Patients may be bitten by a variety of other domestic and wild animals. The therapy of these wounds should follow the general guidelines of bite wound care as outlined in the prior section. There are no studies on the bacteriology of these exotic wounds, and, therefore, antimicrobial therapy should be based on an individual case basis. Rabies is a major concern in wild animal bites (see Rabies section, below).

Monkey Bites

Monkey bites may be particularly serious and develop bacterial infection. In addition, Old World monkeys may transmit simian herpesvirus B to humans. A vesicular lesion may develop at the site of the bite, and progressive and fatal illness may occur. Fever, adenopathy, confusion, and paralysis may occur. Diagnosis is by viral isolation or a fourfold rise in antibody titers. No specific therapy exists and supportive care is warranted.

Seal Finger

Seal finger is a cutaneous painful infection occurring in fish cleaners, aquarium workers, veterinarians, and others exposed to seals. It may be associated with arthritis of nearby joints. No etiologic agent has been identified but the infection responds to tetracycline, 500 mg orally four times per day for 10 days. Penicillin V is not effective. Prompt treatment is necessary because amputation can be a consequence of late or inadequate treatment.

Erysipelothrix

Erysipelothrix rhusiopathia is a gram-positive rod that produces cellulitis in persons handling saltwater fish, shellfish, as well as meat and poulty products. Approximately 1 week after exposure, a red violaceous lesion occurs at the site of a cut or abrasion, usually on the hands. As the infection advances, one may note raised borders and central clearing. Diagnosis is by culture of a biopsy specimen from the advancing edge of the lesion. Arthritis may occasionally complicate the course. Therapy with wound care, as previously noted, and penicillin, 500 mg orally four times per day for 10 days is curative.

RABIES

Domestic

In 1982, the Centers for Disease Control reported 6,212 cases of rabies in animals (Table 1) with the following distribution: skunks, 50 percent; raccoons, 19 percent; bats, 16 percent; cattle, 5 percent; foxes, 3.5 percent; cats, 3 percent; dogs, 2 percent; other domestic animals, 1 percent; and other wild animals 0.6 percent. Rodents, including squirrels and rabbits, are rarely rabid. This represented a 13 percent decline compared with 1981, mostly due to a reduction in rabies in skunks. However, there was a marked increase in rabies in raccoons, reflecting a spreading outbreak in the mid-Atlantic states. The decision to treat a bite patient for rabies depends on the type of biting animal and local data about the rabies reservoir.

Rabies may also be acquired by inhalation, as in cave explorers, by laboratory accident and by corneal transplantation. Despite the frequency of rabies in wild and domestic animals, only one or two cases of human rabies are reported in the United States annually.

Foreign

Any animal bite acquired outside the United States should be considered suspect, especially if from an area known to have an endemic focus, such as Latin America, Africa, or Asia (except Japan and Taiwan). Travelers should be warned to avoid contact with local animals. If an extended stay is planned in an area with a high rate of endemic rabies, then pre-exposure prophylaxis should be considered.

Clinical Disease

Rabid animals begin to secrete virus from several days (dogs and cats) to 6 months or a year (bats and atypical cases) before the onset of symptoms. Viral secretion is episodic and may be absent during the symptomatic period. The human incubation period is usually from 18 to 60 days after exposure, but may be up to 1 year. Individuals with head and neck wounds may have a shorter incubation period.

Rabies begins with a nonspecific prodrome lasting 2 to 10 days and consisting of fever, malaise, fatigue, headache, and anorexia. Patients may also have diarrhea, irritability, insomnia, sore throat, and, in 50 percent of cases, paresthesias at the wound site. The acute neurologic period is often accompanied by episodic hyperactivity, hallucinations, seizures, nuchal rigidity, and eventual paralysis, coma, and death.

Diagnosis is by viral isolation (difficult after neutralizing antibody appears), demonstration of Negri bodies by immunofluorescence in infected (brain) tissue or by antibody titers. Domestic dogs and cats are usually observed for 10 days for signs of rabies. Ferral dogs and cats and wild animals are usually killed and brain specimens (especially the hippocampus and cerebellum) are checked for Negri bodies.

Therapy

Table 2 summarizes the current guidelines of the Immunization Practices Advisory Committee (ACIP) guidelines for rabies immunization. The human diploid cell vaccine (HDCV) is an inactivated viral vaccine of fixed virus grown in human diploid cell culture. HDCV has replaced the duck embryo vaccine and has fewer and less serious adverse effects. Allergic reactions are rare. Rabies immune globulin (RIG) is a gamma globulin concentrate obtained from the plasma of immunized human donors. This has replaced equine rabies antiserum.

Preexposure Prophylaxis; Postexposure Prophylaxis in Immunized Persons

Preexposure prophylaxis is warranted for veterinarians, virologists and laboratory personnel with potential contact, spelunkers, and people visiting or living in a highly endemic area abroad, especially if distant from medical care. Only HDCV is given as a 0.1 ml intramuscular (deltoid) injection on day 0, 7, and 21 or 28. Boosters of 0.1 ml HDCV are given at least every 2 years. Although almost all recipients develop antibody titers, they can not rely upon this for protection from rabies if bitten. After exposure they should receive doses of 0.1 ml HDCV on day 0 and day 3.

Postexposure Prophylaxis

Postexposure prophylaxis in unimmunized individuals should begin as soon as possible after injury. HDCV is given on day 0, 3, 7, 14, and 28. In addition, RIG (40 IU per kilogram or 18 IU per pound) should be given on day 0. Most recipients develop antibodies, but this response may be blocked by steroids or immunosuppressive medications.

There have only been three known human survivors of rabies and therapy appears to be ineffective. Interferon therapy has been attempted, but it has not been effective. The complications of rabies are multisystem events, and patients require specific and supportive care.

Information can be obtained from local health departments, the Centers for Disease Control, Atlanta, Georgia (404-329-3085, daytime; or 1-404-329-3888, nighttime) or the Merieux Institute, Inc., Lyons, France (in the United States, 800-327-2842).

SNAKE BITES

It is estimated that 45,000 persons are bitten by snakes in the United States each year: 8,000 are due to venomous snakes and result in 7,000 cases of envenomization. Of the 115 species of snakes found in the United States, only 20 are poisonous and belong to the vipers (rattlesnakes, copperheads, and cottonmouths or water moccasins), which cause 98 percent of the bites, or to the coral snake family (see Fig. 1). Maine, Hawaii, and Alaska have no indigenous venomous snakes. Although in many locales it is illegal to keep pet poisonous snakes, more than 50 percent of victims are bitten by their own pet or a snake they are handling.

Identify, if possible, the species of snake involved, its size, and the circumstances of the bite. Blood pressure and other vital signs should be monitored frequently. The location of the fang marks should be noted as well as the presence of edema, ecchymoses, muscle fascicu-

TABLE 1 RABIES—Reported Cases in Animals, by Area and Species of Animal, United States, 1982

		Domestic				Wild				
Area	*Total*	*Cattle*	*Cats*	*Dogs*	*Other Domestic*	*Skunks*	*Raccoons*	*Bats*	*Foxes*	*Other Wild*
United States	6,212	296	207	145	80	3,088	1,156	977	220	43
New England	38	-	-	-	2	-	-	20	16	-
Maine	21	-	-	-	2	-	-	3	16	-
N.H.	1	-	-	-	-	-	-	1	-	-
Vt.	2	-	-	-	-	-	-	2	-	-
Mass.	9	-	-	-	-	-	-	9	-	-
R.I.	-	-	-	-	-	-	-	-	-	-
Conn.	5	-	-	-	-	-	-	5	-	-
Mid. Atlantic	204	13	1	7	-	37	27	82	35	2
N.Y.	113	12	1	2	-	21	1	41	35	-
N.J.	16	-	-	-	-	-	-	16	-	-
Pa.	75	1	-	5	-	16	26	25	-	2
E.N. Central	651	47	26	29	9	458	6	63	10	3
Ohio	81	3	-	3	1	55	-	14	2	3
Ind.	76	1	1	2	2	60	-	10	-	-
Ill.	294	17	15	9	3	218	2	26	4	-
Mich.	7	4	-	-	-	1	-	2	-	-
Wis.	193	22	10	15	3	124	4	11	4	-
W.N. Central	1,209	167	84	42	28	831	6	38	7	6
Minn.	224	32	15	11	4	150	1	9	1	1
Iowa	377	77	38	10	11	227	2	7	2	3
Mo.	123	7	2	6	1	97	-	10	-	-
N. Dak.	97	16	7	3	2	64	-	2	3	-
S. Dak.	115	18	11	4	4	75	2	1	-	-
Nebr.	126	13	4	4	2	101	-	2	-	-
Kans.	147	4	7	4	4	117	1	7	1	2
S. Atlantic	1,392	2	28	12	-	126	1,061	120	32	11
Del.	2	-	-	-	-	-	-	2	-	-
Md.	153	1	-	-	-	14	118	17	2	1
D.C.	5	-	-	-	-	-	5	-	-	-

Va.	745	1	9	2	-	59	646	9	12	7
W. Va.	62	-	-	-	-	8	43	10	-	1
N.C.	66	-	-	-	-	26	-	38	2	-
S.C.	66	-	12	3	-	-	35	13	3	-
Ga.	213	-	6	5	-	17	163	13	7	2
Fla.	80	-	1	2	-	2	51	18	6	-
E.S. Central	649	6	5	13	7	444	48	104	21	1
Ky.	134	3	2	8	7	97	-	9	7	1
Tenn.	356	2	-	3	-	323	1	16	11	-
Ala.	146	1	3	2	-	24	47	66	3	-
Miss.	13	-	-	-	-	-	-	13	-	-
W.S. Central	1,162	51	58	32	30	812	4	155	14	6
Ark.	157	4	2	4	-	126	-	19	2	-
La.	32	-	2	-	-	20	-	10	-	-
Okla.	189	23	14	6	3	136	-	6	-	1
Tex.	784	24	40	22	27	530	4	120	12	5
Mountain	288	6	1	2	2	86	-	184	4	3
Mont.	97	5	-	1	-	56	-	32	1	2
Idaho	11	-	-	-	-	-	-	11	-	-
Wyo.	27	-	-	-	-	2	-	25	-	-
Colo.	47	-	-	-	-	-	-	47	-	-
N. Mex.	22	-	-	1	-	8	-	13	-	-
Ariz.	60	1	1	-	2	20	-	32	3	1
Utah	18	-	-	-	-	-	-	18	-	-
Nev.	6	-	-	-	-	-	-	6	-	-
Pacific	619	4	4	8	2	294	4	211	81	11
Wash.	8	-	-	-	-	-	-	8	-	-
Oreg.	5	-	-	-	-	-	-	5	-	-
Calif.	517	4	4	1	2	294	4	198	9	1
Alaska	89	-	-	7	-	-	-	-	72	10
Hawaii	-	-	-	-	-	-	-	-	-	-
Guam	-	-	-	-	-	-	-	-	-	-
P.R.	66	-	2	8	4	-	-	-	-	52
V.I.	-	-	-	-	-	-	-	-	-	-

From: Annual summary, 1982. MMWR 31:1983.

TABLE 2A Rabies Postexposure Prophylaxis Guide—July 1984

The following recommendations are only a guide. In applying them, take into account the animal species involved, the circumstances of the bite or other exposure, the vaccination status of the animal, and presence of rabies in the region. Local or state public health officials should be consulted if questions arise about the need for rabies prophylaxis.

Animal Species	*Condition of Animal at Time of Attack*	*Treatment of Exposed Person**
Domestic		
Dog and Cat	Healthy and available for 10 days of observation	None, unless animal develops rabies†
	Rabid or suspected rabid	RIG§ and HDCV
	Unknown (escaped)	Consult public health officials. If treatment is indicated, give RIG§ and HDCV
Wild		
Skunk, bat, fox, coyote raccoon, bobcat, and other carnivores	Regard as rabid unless proven negative by laboratory tests¶	RIG§ and HDCV
Other		
Livestock, rodents, and lagomorphs (rabbits and hares)	Consider individually. Local and state public health officials should be consulted on questions about the need for rabies prophylaxis. Bites of squirrels, hamsters, guinea pigs, gerbils, chipmunks, rats, mice, other rodents, rabbits, and hares almost never call for antirabies prophylaxis.	

TABLE 2B Criteria for Preexposure Immunization

Risk Category	*Nature of Risk*	*Typical Populations*	*Preexposure Regimen*
Continuous	Virus present continuously, often in high concentrations. Aerosol, mucous membrane, bite, or nonbite exposure possible. Specific exposures may go unrecognized.	Rabies research lab workers.* Rabies biologics production workers	Primary preexposure immunization course. Serology every 6 months. Booster immunization when antibody titer falls below acceptable level.*
Frequent	Exposure usually episodic, with source recognized, but exposure may also be unrecognized. Aerosol, mucous membrane, bite, or nonbite exposure.	Rabies diagnostic lab workers,* spelunkers, veterinarians, and animal control and wildlife workers in rabies epizootic areas.	Primary preexposure immunization course. Booster immunization or serology every 2 years†
Infrequent (greater than population-at-large)	Exposure nearly always episodic with source recognized. Mucous membrane, bite, or nonbite exposure.	Veterinarians and animal control and wildlife workers in areas of low rabies endemicity. Certain travelers to foreign rabies epizootic areas. Veterinary students.	Primary preexposure immunization course. No routine booster immunization or serology.
Rare (population-at-large)	Exposure always episodic, mucous membrane, or bite with source recognized.	U.S. population-at-large, including individuals in rabies-epizootic areas.	No preexposure immunization.

* *All bites and wounds should immediately be thoroughly cleansed with soap and water.* If antirabies treatment is indicated, both rabies immune globulin (RIG) and human diploid cell rabies vaccine (HDCV) should be given as soon as possible, *regardless* of the interval from exposure. Local reactions to vaccines are common and do not contraindicate continuing treatment. Discontinue vaccine if fluorescent-antibody tests of the animal are negative.

† During the usual holding period of 10 days, begin treatment with RIG and HDCV at first sign of rabies in a dog or cat that has bitten someone. The symptomatic animal should be killed immediately and tested.

§ If RIG is not available, use antirabies serum, equine (ARS). Do not use more than the recommended dosage.

¶ The animal should be killed and tested as soon as possible. Holding for observation is not recommended.

Reprinted from MMWR 33:393–408, 1984.

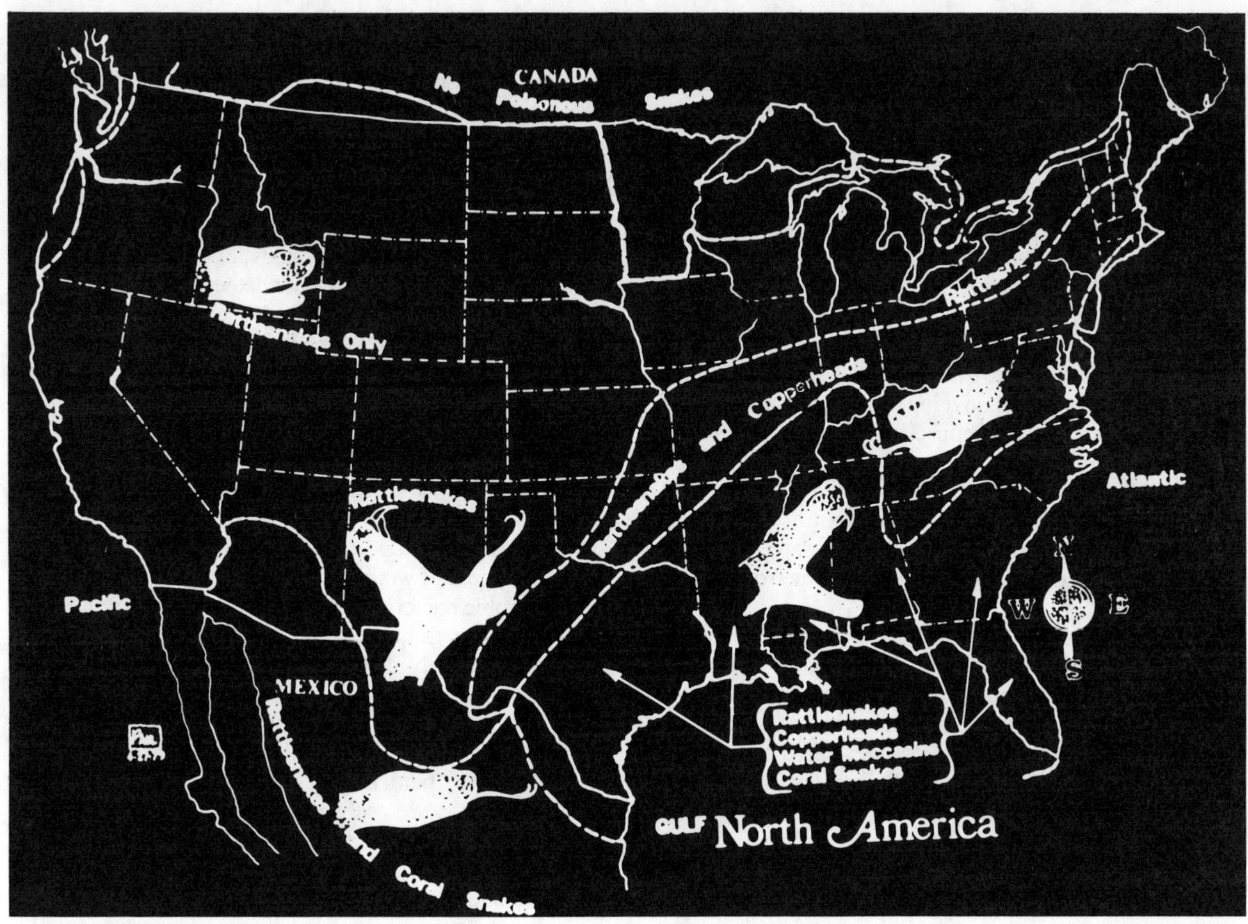

Figure 1 Distribution of poisonous snakes in the United States.

lations, and bleeding. Patients should be asked about paresthesias, especially periorally. Before antivenin is used, blood should be drawn for complete blood count, platelet count, protime, partial thromboplastin time, fibrin split products, fibrinogen level, blood type and cross match for 4 units of blood, electrolytes, creatinine, and BUN. Urine analysis should be done. The leading edge of edema should be marked with a pen and the circumference of the injured extremity measured at two known points. Remarking the leading edge of swelling and remeasurement should be done at appropriate intervals and recorded on a flow sheet.

The severity of envenomization is graded for both adults and children as follows:

Grade	*Signs*	*Antivenin*
0	No local or systemic symptoms	None
Mild	Local swelling only	5 vials
Moderate	Progressive swelling; systemic symptoms; laboratory changes	10 vials
Severe	Marked local reaction; progressive edema; severe systemic symptoms; severe laboratory changes	15 vials

Antivenin is prepared from horse serum and skin testing should be performed prior to initiation of therapy. Antivenin is difficult to dissolve. Fifty milliliters of antivenin (5 vials) may be mixed with 150 to 200 ml of normal saline and given intravenously. The first 10 ml should be administered slowly (½ hour), but may need to be titrated according to the individual patient. If a reaction occurs, withhold therapy and give the patient 50 mg of benadryl or 0.2 to 0.5 ml of epinephrine (depending upon body weight), awaiting response prior to the slow resumption of therapy. Reactions may include decrease in blood pressure; anaphylaxis; apprehension; flushing; itching; urticaria; facial, tongue, and pharyngeal edema; cough; dyspnea; cyanosis; and vomiting. The initial dose can be given over 30 minutes to 2 hours. It is often slightly quicker (10 to 20 minutes) when given by slow intravenous push.

If there is severe envenomization two intravenous access lines should be started. Measure the level of progression of edema every 15 to 30 minutes. If there is progression of edema 30 minutes after the initial antivenin dose, persistant fasciculations, or oral paresthesias, repeated doses of 5 to 15 vials of antivenin may be given every hour until symptoms are controlled. Fasciotomies are rarely required and adequacy of capillary filling and tissue pressures may be measured. The role of hypothermia remains controversial.

Tetanus toxoid (0.5 ml intramuscularly) should be given in patients requiring a booster. Oxygen may be given if needed. Patients may be allowed to drink simple fluids. Transfusion should be given only for blood loss. Type and cross matches drawn after the administration of antivenin may have problems with matching reactions. Plasma expanders, such as plasmanate and hetastarch—not crystalloid solutions such as dextrose and water or normal saline—may be given for hypotension. The affected area should be maintained in a position of function, with splinting if required. Antimicrobial agents are given only if signs of infection develop or if there has been self therapy in the field. The empiric antimicrobial agent used should cover both aerobic and anaerobic bacteria as found in the snake mouth. Specific therapy should be given when cultural data are returned. We use cefoxitin, 1 to 2 g intravenously every 4 hours as empiric therapy. Alternative choices include other cephalosporins, metronidazole, and ampicillin.

Most patients require only several days of hospitalization. The swelling should begin to resolve within 24 to 48 hours of cessation of antivenin therapy.

Information regarding the treatment of venomous snake bites may be obtained from local zoos and poison control centers. The Oklahoma Poison Control Center (405-271-5454) may be contacted about the availability of rare antivenins.

The greater the amount of antivenin used, the more likely the patient is to develop serum sickness 5 to 30 days after therapy. Serum sickness may be manifested as rash, arthralgias, fever, glomerulonephritis, or other antigen-antibody disease. It may be managed with careful monitoring and short-course steroid therapy, such as 40 mg prednisone daily for 5 days to two weeks. If the longer course is required then tapering dosage may be necessary.

HUMAN BITES

Human bites comprise actual bite wounds and clenched-fist injuries. No estimates of their frequency exist. Most are due to fights, but they may be seen as part of the battered child syndrome, in hospital personnel, or as a result of a self-inflicted wound or even a "love-nip." Human bites are more prone to infection than animal bites. These injuries are often mistakenly considered innocuous by many physicians.

Occlusional Human Bite Wounds

Human bites may occur in any part of the body, but are frequently on the proximal phalanx of the long finger of the dominant hand. Complications include cellulitis, tenosynovitis, osteomyelitis, septic arthritis, and amputation. Scarlet fever, hepatitis B, actinomycosis, tuberculosis, and syphilis have been transmitted from human bites.

The propensity to infection is determined, in part, by the depth of the wound, extent of crush injury, the exact compartments entered, and the oral bacteria inoculated. General wound care should be performed as outlined previously. Specimens for cultures should be obtained prior to therapy. Roentgenograms should be taken either for baseline comparison or to rule out osteomyelitis when the bite wound is near a bone. Lavage, elevation, and immobilization are essential. Wounds, except perhaps those to the face, should be left open whether infected or uninfected. Closure by delayed primary or secondary intention is recommended. Wounds to the face are usually closed and often seen by a plastic surgeon. If scarring is of concern, either because of the location of the wound such as on the face, on other exposed areas, or due to the severity of the wound, then a plastic surgeon should be consulted.

Staphylococcus aureus, previously considered the most frequent and important pathogen, is present in only 20 to 30 percent of wounds. Fifty percent of wounds yield oral anaerobic bacteria. The alpha-hemolytic streptococci are the most frequently isolated organism. Other organisms commonly isolated from these wounds include *Eikenella corrodens* and *Hemophilus* species. Rarely are penicillin- (or ampicillin-) resistant gram-negative rods isolated from these wounds. Although *S. aureus* may be susceptible to penicillinase-resistant penicillins and cephalosporins, some oral anaerobic bacteria are relatively resistant, and *E. corrodens* is resistant to them and also to clindamycin. Consequently, antimicrobial therapy should be both penicillin V (500 mg orally four times per day) plus dicloxacillin, a penicillinase-resistant penicillin (500 mg orally four times per day) or a cephalosporin such as cephalexin (500 mg orally four times per day). Infected wounds should be treated for a minimum of 10 days and uninfected, early-presenting (< 8 hours after injury) wounds for 5 days. When intravenous antibiotics are required, many newer beta-lactam antibiotics such as moxalactam, cefoperazone, cefotaxime, and ceftizoxime are active against *E. corrodens*, but may have poorer activity against *S. aureus*. Cefoxitin, 1 to 2 g every 4 hours intravenously, for moderate and severe infections that require intravenous therapy should be used. Amoxacillin/clavulanic acid, 500 mg orally three times per day appears to be effective therapy for those wounds amenable to oral outpatient therapy.

Clenched-Fist Injuries

Clenched-fist injuries (CFIs) are the most serious of all bite wounds. They occur when a person delivers a forceful blow with a clenched fist to another's mouth. The resulting laceration may be small (less than 5 mm), but may inoculate bacteria into the subcutaneous tissue and the joint space. When the fist is later relaxed, the inoculated bacteria may travel to deeper tissues. An occasional blow may sever or lacerate a tendon or cause a fracture. The third and fourth metacarpophalyngeal (MCP) joints of the dominant hand are most often involved. Most patients wait 4 to 12 hours after the onset of clinical infection before seeking medical therapy. They awaken or note pain and a proximally spreading swelling of the affected hand, with or without a purulent discharge. Once infected, all CFI patients should be hospitalized and treated aggressively.

The hand should be examined by someone familiar with hand surgery. Examination of the wound, and joint if necessary, under bloodless conditions may be required to determine the extent of injury and involvement. This may be done with regional anaesthesia and tourniquet control. Debridement, copious irrigation, and drainage are essential. The integrity of the joint capsule should be assessed.

Aerobic and anaerobic cultures should be performed. Roentgenograms should be obtained prior to splinting. A plaster splint, from the fingers to the elbow, should be applied for immobilization. A second film should be obtained 10 to 14 days later to rule out osteomyelitis. The hand must be kept elevated.

Empiric antimicrobial therapy should include both a penicillin, 3 million units every 4 hours intravenously, and oxacillin, a penicillinase-resistant penicillin, 2 g intravenously every 4 hours, or as a single drug alternative, cefoxitin, 2 g intravenously every 4 hours. This covers most potential pathogens such as *S. aureus* (25% of wounds), *E. corrodens* (25%), and anaerobic bacteria (55%). Specific therapy should be instituted when culture results return. If one fails to take into account the susceptibility pattern of *E. corrodens* when selecting empiric therapy, there may be a higher rate of complications and residual disability due to insidious and progressive infection. Duration of therapy should be on an individual basis, but not be less than 7 days. In severely infected patients, 14 days of therapy is required. If the joint capsule is found to be intact or the patient presents prior to the development of infection, treatment may be with a shorter course of therapy (5 days) and even on an outpatient basis. The appropriate situation for treating patients with clenched-fist injuries as outpatients is infrequent. If possible, penicillin V (500 mg orally four times per day) plus dicloxacillin (500 mg orally four times per day) should be used as empiric therapy. Careful follow-up at 24 to 48 hours is indicated, but most such patients fail to show up for such appointments.

Secondary complications such as osteomyelitis, septic arthritis, tendon necrosis, and collar-button abscess are frequent. If osteomyelitis occurs, 6 weeks of intravenous therapy followed by 1 to 3 months of oral therapy is indicated. Abscesses require surgical drainage. A significant minority of patients require secondary debridement of tissue and/or necrotic bone. There is a high incidence of residual disability, such as stiff joints and hands.

RESPIRATORY TRACT INFECTIONS

OTITIS MEDIA

GEORGE VAN HARE, M.D.
PAUL A. SHURIN, M.D.

Acute otitis media is one of the commonest and most troublesome of pediatric illnesses, and every practitioner who deals with children can expect to encounter the disease or its complications frequently. Disease of the middle ear may account for as many as one-third of all visits to pediatricians. The presence of symptoms and signs of illness (fever, irritability, otalgia, anorexia, vomiting) in addition to the presence of fluid in the middle ear is generally used to identify episodes of acute otitis media.

Clinicians should, however, be aware that otitis media may present without symptoms. Persistence of middle ear effusion for a period of weeks or months is the commonest sequel of acute otitis media; persistent or chronic disease must be defined by serial examinations scheduled to detect effusions without regard to the presence of symptoms. Chronic middle ear disease is a frequent cause of conductive hearing loss and delay in language acquisition. Furthermore, recent information indicates that middle ear effusions may be present before 2 months of age in many children. Those with onset in the first months of life have the greatest risk for chronic and recurrent disease and for developmental sequelae of otitis media. Accurate diagnosis and careful, close follow-up are essential in children with acute otitis media and persistent middle ear effusion.

DIAGNOSIS

Otoscopy

Acute otitis media is defined as the presence of fluid in the middle ear. Currently, standard diagnosis is by pneumatic otoscopy. The most sensitive otoscopic sign of middle ear effusion is the reduction or loss of tympanic membrane mobility with positive and negative pressure insufflation. These changes are best appreciated when an otoscope with a tight-fitting or sealed lens and speculum is used. During the examination, the speculum should completely occlude the ear canal. For effective use of pneumatic otoscopy, examiners need to develop skill in identifying subtle changes in tympanic membrane mobility and appearance.

Tympanocentesis

Tympanocentesis and culture of middle ear fluid provide objective diagnosis, identification of causative bacterial agents, and testing for antibiotic susceptibility. The procedure can easily be learned by any interested physician. Thus, tympanocentesis may be applied whenever the microbiologic information would be clinically helpful. The procedure will also provide prompt relief of pain in children with severe otalgia caused by otitis media.

Tympanocentesis is clearly indicated in a few circumstances. In infants younger than 6 weeks of age—particularly those younger than 3 weeks of age—with otitis media, enteric gram-negative organisms or staphylococci, which may not be susceptible to the usual oral antimicrobial agents, may be isolated. Immunocompromised children should also have tympanocentesis if otitis media is diagnosed. Children who do not respond symptomatically to initial antimicrobial therapy may be infected with resistant organisms. Finally, those with mastoiditis or other suppurative complications should have diagnostic tympanocentesis. The procedure is performed by inserting an 18- or 20-gauge spinal needle attached to a syringe or suction trap through the inferior portion of the drum and aspirating. If no fluid appears in the syringe, there may still be middle ear fluid in the needle; a small amount of broth should be drawn into the syringe through the needle and then cultured.

Tympanometry

The development of tympanometry for objective identification of middle ear effusion is a significant advance in the diagnosis of otitis media. A tympanogram is obtained by inserting a small probe with an airtight seal into the external canal. The pressure in the canal is varied while a tone is presented and tympanic membrane compliance (or other acoustic properties of the tympanic membrane-middle ear system) is measured. A normal result is a peak in tympanic membrane compliance at approximately atmospheric pressure, whereas patients with middle ear effusion will have poor compliance with no peak, producing a "flat" tympanogram.

Tympanometry provides objective detection of middle ear effusion and can be used to supplement otoscopic examination. An effective application of tympanometry would be in the follow-up of children with otitis media. If normal tympanograms are obtained, the clinician has strong evidence that the middle ear effusions have resolved. Although tympanometry appears to be potentially accurate at all ages, special instrumentation and diagnostic standards are needed for infants younger than 7 months of age. Tympanograms are most helpful in difficult-to-examine patients (e.g., those with narrow or tortuous canals) or when there is uncertainty in the diagnosis. They may be difficult to obtain in uncooperative children.

PATHOGENESIS AND MICROBIOLOGY

The pathogenesis of otitis media is not completely understood. There is much evidence, however, that the disease is related to dysfunction of the eustachian tube, which, in turn, may be secondary to viral upper respiratory tract infections or to physiologic, anatomic, or genetic factors. Bacterial agents, however, play a prominent role in otitis media, and treatment is currently directed at eradication of these organisms from the middle ear. Table 1 lists the predominant organisms that are isolated from middle ear effusions. *Streptococcus pneumoniae* is the commonest with nontypable *Hemophilus influenzae*, second. The recent occurrence of beta-lactamase production (and, consequently, ampicillin resistance) in strains of *H. influenzae* has resulted in the reevaluation of initial therapy for otitis media. The proportion of *H. influenzae* strains that are ampicillin resistant varies between 5 and 20 percent in different geographic areas. Thus, with *H. influenzae* causing 20 percent of episodes of otitis media, resistant strains of *H. influenzae* are involved in 1 to 4 percent of all cases of acute otitis media. Several groups have noted an increase in the rate of isolation of *Branhamella catarrhalis* in the last several years. This organism currently accounts for 14 percent of cases in Cleveland and, in 75 percent of these, is resistant to ampicillin.

In infants younger than 6 weeks of age, the same respiratory pathogens are the most frequent agents of otitis media. However, approximately 15 percent of cases are caused by such diverse bacteria as *Escherichia coli, Klebsiella, Staphylococcus aureus*, and group B streptococci.

Mycoplasma pneumoniae and *Chlamydia trachomatis* are rarely isolated from middle ear fluid and are not important causes of otitis media. Respiratory viruses, especially respiratory syncitial virus, are associated with the occurrence of otitis media in children and may predispose to bacterial infection of the middle ear.

ANTIMICROBIAL TREATMENT

The treatment of acute otitis media is directed against the bacterial pathogens that are the most likely cause of the infection. When choosing an antibiotic for use in treatment, the physician should consider the child's age, clinical presentation, and history of prior reactions to antibiotics. In uncomplicated cases of acute otitis media, the drug of choice is amoxicillin (Table 2 and Fig. 1). However, for children who are particularly susceptible to severe or disseminated infection, the initial choice should be an antibiotic effective against the common drug-resistant agents, e.g., Augmentin (amoxicillin-clavulanic acid), trimethoprim-sulfamethoxazole (TMP/SMZ), or erythromycin-sulfisoxazole (these are listed in our order of preference). Examples of these high-risk patients include children younger than 2 years of age who present with high fever and those with underlying disease. The physician should consider culturing the middle ear exudate, blood, and other potential sites of infection in these patients.

Treatment failure, although unusual, does occur in some cases. Failure of treatment may be diagnosed in the child with persistence of middle ear effusion and of symptoms such as fever, ear pain, and irritability. For these children, alternative antibiotics may be required (Table 2): these are Augmentin (amoxicillin-clavulanic acid), TMP/SMZ, erythromycin-sulfisoxazole, and cefaclor in order of preference. It should be noted that several studies have indicated that the currently recommended dose of 40 mg per kilogram per day of cefaclor is inadequate in the treatment of otitis media. We currently recommend the use of a higher dose, 60 mg per kilogram per day.

TABLE 1 Occurrence and Antibiotic Resistance of Bacterial Agents of Acute Otitis Media

		Frequency of Resistance to Antimicrobial Drugs				
Organism	*Number of Cases (%)**	*Ampicillin*	*Cefaclor*	*Amox-CA*	*TMP/SMZ*	*Erythro-Sulfa*
Streptococcus pneumoniae	107 (30%)	Infrequent	S	S	S	S
Hemophilus influenzae	77 (21%)	15%	S	S	Infrequent	S
Branhamella catarrhalis	50 (14%)	75%	S	S	S	S
No bacterial pathogen	124 (35%)	--	--	--	--	--

Note: S = sensitive, Amox = amoxicillin, CA = clavulanic acid, TMP/SMZ = trimethoprim-sulfamethoxazole, Erythro-Sulfa = erythromycin-sulfisoxazole.
* Data are from 358 patients at Cleveland Metropolitan General Hospital, 1979–1984.

TABLE 2 Oral Antibiotic Therapy for Acute Otitis Media

Amoxicillin	
Recommended dose:	30–50 mg/kg/day, divided, q8h (there is no evidence that 50 mg/kg/day is more effective than 30 mg/kg/day)
Advantages:	serious side effects very rare; inexpensive
Disadvantages:	not active against beta-lactamase-producing *H. influenzae* and *B. catarrhalis*
Trimethoprim-sulfamethoxazole	
Recommended dose:	8 mg TMP and 40 mg SMZ /kg/day, divided, q12h
Advantages	twice-daily dosing may improve compliance; active in vitro against ampicillin-resistant *H. influenzae*; highly effective in clinical trials; inexpensive
Disadvantages:	serious sulfonamide reactions may occur, including myelo-suppression and Stevens-Johnson syndrome
Cefaclor	
Recommended dose:	60 mg/kg/day, divided, q8h (dose approved by the FDA is 40 mg/kg/day; this dose has been inadequate in some clinical trials)
Advantages:	active in vitro against ampicillin-resistant *H. influenzae*; serious reactions are rare
Disadvantages:	expensive; serum-sickness-like reactions may occur, especially if repeated courses are given; high rate of persistent middle ear infection during therapy
Erythromycin-sulfisoxazole	
Recommended dose:	50 mg erythromycin acid and 150 mg sulfisoxazole/kg/day, divided, q6h
Advantages:	active in vitro against beta-lactamase-producing *H. influenzae* and *B. catarrhalis*; effective in clinical trials
Disadvantages:	qid dosing is inconvenient; serious sulfonamide reactions may occur, including myelosuppression and Stevens-Johnson syndrome
Amoxicillin–clavulanic acid	
Recommended dose:	40 mg amoxicillin/kg/day, divided, q8h
Advantages:	clavulanic acid confers resistance to beta-lactamase, so the combination is active in vitro against beta-lactamase-producing *H. influenzae* and *B. catarrhalis*; effective in clinical trials
Disadvantages:	expensive

CLINICAL COURSE AND FOLLOW-UP

Although symptoms of otitis media usually abate after a course of appropriate antibiotics, patients may have persistent middle ear effusion that can last several months. Persistent effusion following acute otitis media is seen in 50 percent of infants 1 month after initial presentation, in 20 percent after 2 months, and in 10 percent after 3 months. These effusions are often associated with conductive hearing loss that may interfere with normal development of speech and language. Evaluation one month after diagnosis of the acute episode is important to identify those children with persistent middle ear disease. Children with demonstrated hearing loss and persistent middle ear effusion should be referred to an otolaryngologist if these findings persist longer than 2 to 3 months or are associated with possibly related functional deficits, such as language delay or poor school performance.

TYMPANOSTOMY TUBES

The placement of tympanostomy tubes is indicated in several circumstances. A child with a 3-month history of persistent middle ear effusion should be considered for drainage of the effusion and insertion of tympanostomy tubes, particularly if there is conductive hearing loss. If a child has a persistently retracted tympanic membrane with negative middle ear pressure but no effusion, tympanostomy tubes are usually indicated, particularly if the child also suffers from otalgia, tinnitis, vertigo, or conductive hearing loss. Finally, many otolaryngologists recommend the placement of tubes for the prevention of recurrent otitis media. There are, however, no adequate trials comparing this approach with antimicrobial prophylaxis.

DECONGESTANT-ANTIHISTAMINE COMBINATIONS

Physicians have frequently prescribed combinations of decongestants and antihistamines as part of the therapy for middle ear disease. Although pseudoephedrine hydrochloride has been shown experimentally to reduce nasal airway resistance, clinical trials of the drug in middle ear disease have not been encouraging. A recent trial of pseudoephedrine hydrochloride plus chlorpheniramine maleate showed no difference between this combination and placebo treatment with respect to the rate of resolution of the effusion. Adverse effects such as sedation, irritability, and anorexia were reported significantly more often in the group taking the decongestant-antihistamine combination. We cannot recommend the use of these drugs for the purpose of promoting resolution of persistent middle ear effusion. The common practice of long-term treatment of persistent middle ear effusion with these agents is to be condemned.

ANTIMICROBIAL DRUG PROPHYLAXIS

Several clinical trials have demonstrated that long-term antimicrobial prophylaxis for selected patients can significantly lower the attack rate of otitis media. Con-

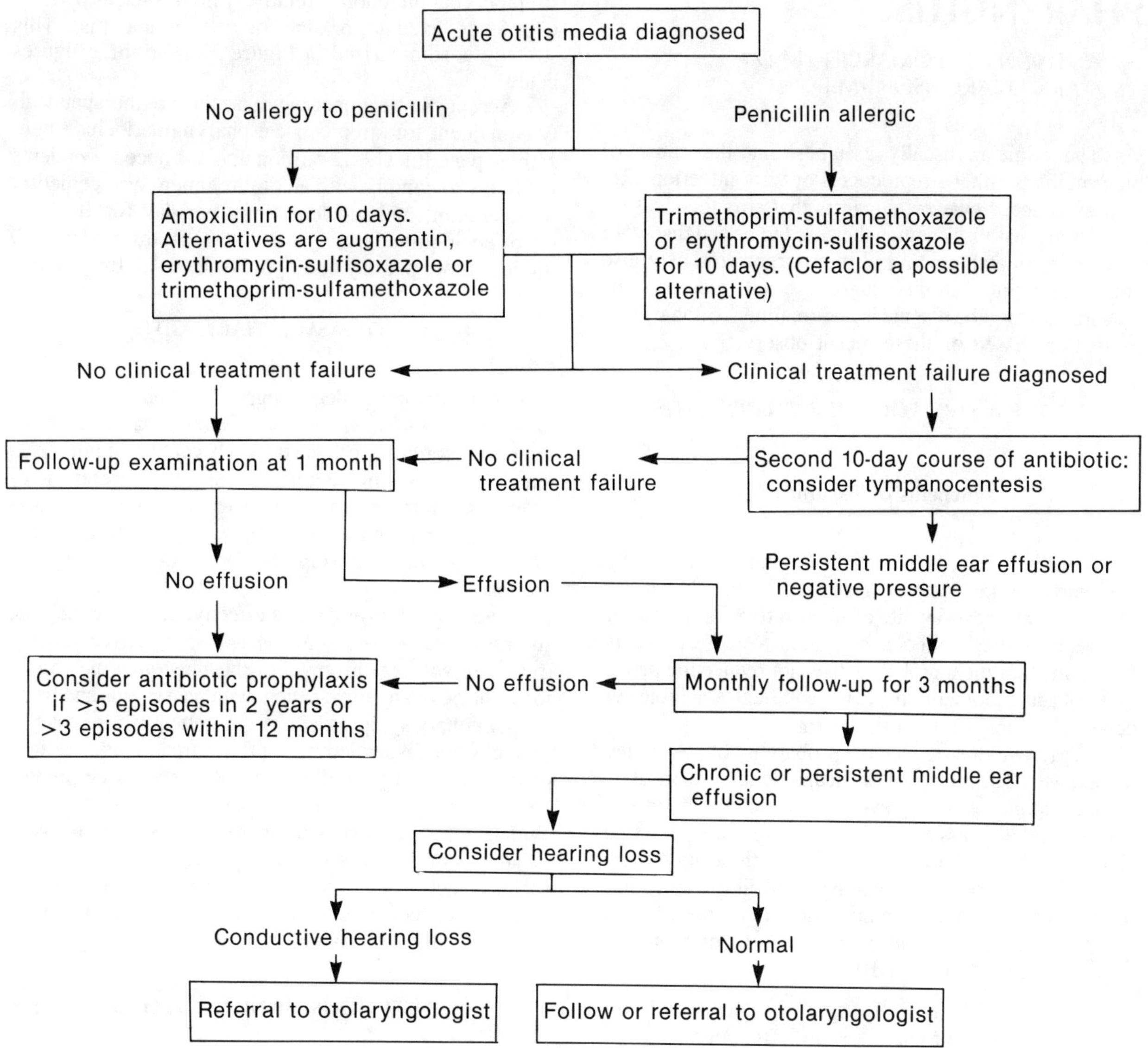

Figure 1 Medical treatment of otitis media.

sidering the morbidity associated with frequent episodes of acute otitis media as well as the problem of persistent middle ear effusion and conductive hearing loss, we recommend drug prophylaxis for children with more than five documented episodes of acute otitis media within 2 years or three episodes within 1 year. Sulfisoxazole prophylaxis has been effective in clinical trials. The dose of sulfisoxazole is approximately 75 mg per kilogram per day given in two divided doses. Administration can be continued for three months or longer. Amoxicillin, 15 to 20 mg per kilogram once daily, may be used as an alternative to prophylaxis with sulfonamides.

PNEUMOCOCCAL VACCINE

Pneumococcal polysaccharide vaccine has been investigated as prophylaxis against otitis media in three separate trials. Although the vaccine was effective in decreasing infection with the pneumococcal serotypes present in the vaccine, there was no reduction of the total number of cases of otitis media seen in the vaccinated children. Furthermore, the currently available vaccine is not adequately immunogenic during the first two years of life. Pneumococcal vaccine, then, is not recommended for prophylaxis against otitis media in normal children.

PHARYNGITIS

ANTHONY L. KOMAROFF, M.D.
MARK D. ARONSON, M.D.

The clinician usually assumes that the cause of pharyngitis is either streptococcal or viral infection. Recent evidence, however, suggests that streptococcal infections are less virulent than they used to be and that other potentially treatable nonviral microorganisms may also cause pharyngitis. In this chapter we will present some new ideas about the diagnosis and treatment of pharyngitis that are based on these recent observations.

GROUP A STREPTOCOCCAL PHARYNGITIS

Benefits of Treatment

Treatment speeds the relief of symptoms if it is begun early in the illness. Treatment probably further reduces an already low rate of suppurative complications and reduces the likelihood of spread to close contacts. However, treatment probably does not reduce the probability of acute glomerulonephritis, although available evidence is inconclusive on this point.

Treatment does reduce the probability of acute rheumatic fever. The incidence of rheumatic fever in most developed countries is, however, exponentially lower than it was even 30 years ago, when some of the most extensive clinical studies were conducted. In the United States in the 1980s, we estimate that the probability of an attack of acute rheumatic fever in an adult with untreated streptococcal pharyngitis (and no past history of rheumatic fever) is less than one in 10,000.

Strategy for Diagnosis and Treatment

The often-recommended strategy of culturing every patient with pharyngitis and treating the culture-positive patients incurs two risks. On one hand, the culture result may be falsely positive (the patient may be a streptococcal carrier and not actually infected) in 30 to 60 percent of cases. Giving treatment can thus subject the patient to the risks of adverse reactions to medication without any benefit from treatment. On the other hand, because of the delay in obtaining the result of the throat culture and the fact that the culture can be falsely negative, treatment (and its expected benefits) can be delayed or denied.

For these reasons, instead of the traditional strategy, we favor one that individualizes diagnosis and treatment decisions. We recommend obtaining a specimen for culture from any patient who is at special risk for streptococcal infection (for example, patients with a past history of acute rheumatic fever, schoolaged children, including teenagers, or young adults) or from any patient in whom clinical findings suggest that the probability of streptococcal infection is relatively high (such as patients with fever, exudate, or anterior cervical adenitis). This strategy is summarized in Figure 3 of the three figures below.

Acceptable treatment regimens that are therapeutically equivalent for streptococcal pharyngitis include benzathine pencillin G, 1.2 million unis IM once for patients not likely to comply with an oral regimen; oral penicillin V potassium, 250 mg four times per day for 10 days; or for penicillin-allergic patients, oral erythromycin, 250 mg four times per day or 500 mg twice a day for 10 days.

MYCOPLASMA PHARYNGITIS

Accumulating evidence suggests that pharyngitis from infection with *Mycoplasma pneumoniae* may be as common as or commoner than streptococcal pharyngitis, particularly in young adults. Also, the presence of bronchopulmonary symptoms (such as cough or wheezing) along with pharyngitis, suggests pharyngitis due to *M. pneumoniae*. Unfortunately, no rapid diagnostic tests are available.

Because erythromycin is effective in eradicating the streptococcus, as well as *M. pneumoniae*, we recommend treatment with erythromycin, 250 mg four times a day for 10 days, of any toxic patient with pharyngitis and bronchopulmonary symptoms or of any patient whose pharyngitis has not responded promptly to treatment after four or more days of penicillin therapy. It should be pointed out, however, that this recommendation is not based on evidence that erythromycin is efficacious in such cases; no studies of this question have yet been conducted. The various enteric-coated forms of erythromycin may be less likely to produce gastrointestinal side effects, but 1 g per day is usually well tolerated in adults.

INFECTIOUS MONONUCLEOSIS

Pharyngitis often occurs with infectious mononucleosis. It may be worth making the diagnosis of infectious mononucleosis (as contrasted with other forms of viral pharyngitis) in order to alert the patient to symptoms suggesting complications, particularly ruptured spleen and upper airway obstruction.

Heterophil antibody is found in approximately 2 to 6 percent of patients younger than the age of 40 years seeking care for pharyngitis, but is extremely uncommon in patients over 40 years of age. Most cases of pharyngitis associated with a positive heterophil antibody are mild and may not have the charactersitic hematologic findings (lymphocytosis with greater than 10% atypical lymphocytes) or the full-blown clinical picture of infectious mononucleosis.

We recommend obtaining a differential white blood cell count and a heterophil test in patients with any one of the physical examination findings shown in Figure 2, because the presence of these findings greatly raises the probability of infectious mononucleosis. Rapid differen-

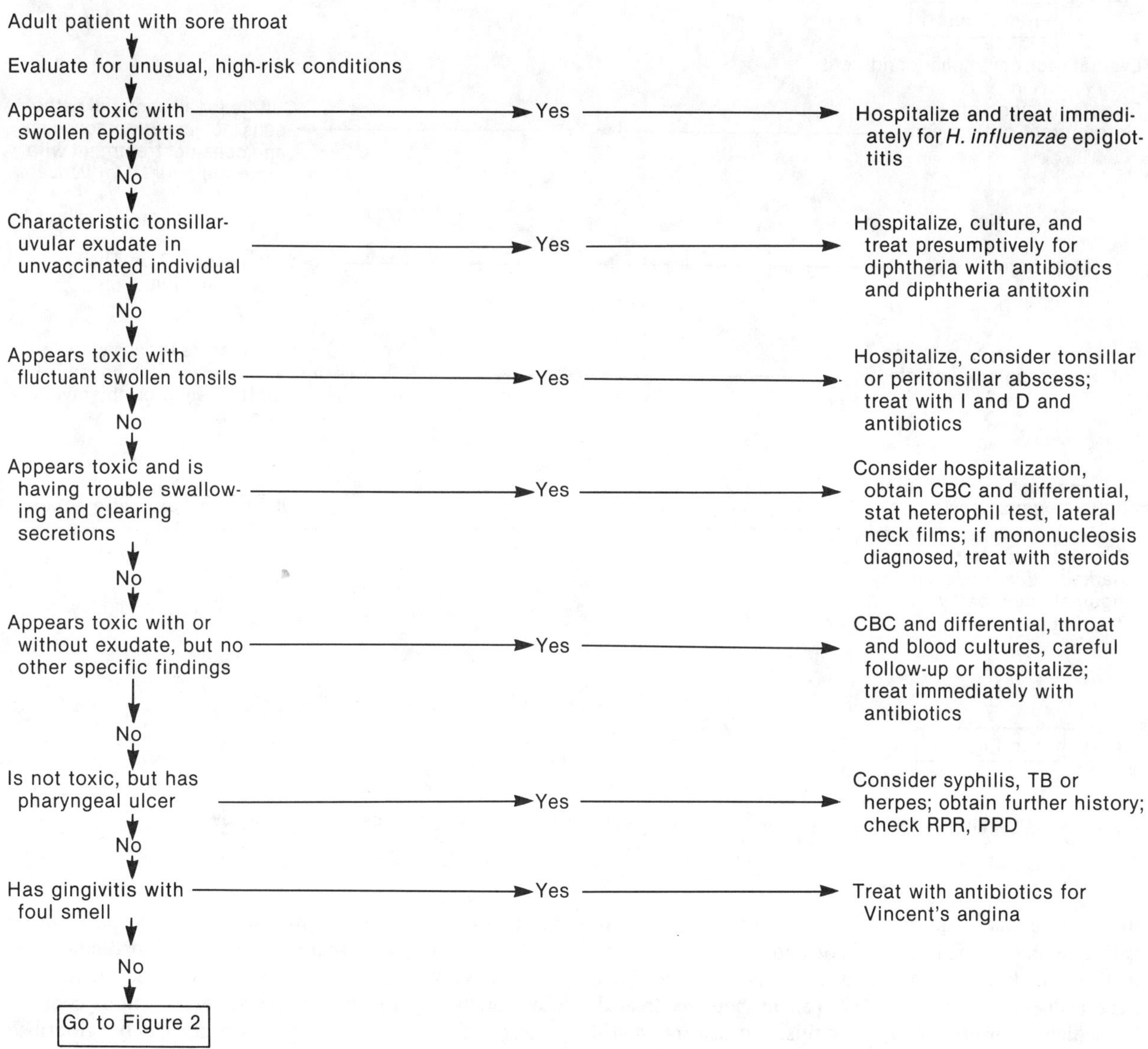

Figure 1 Algorithm describing an evaluation for unusual or high-risk conditions. The designation *toxic* refers to findings such as high fever, prostration, tachycardia, and thready pulse.

tial slide tests (spot tests) for heterophil antibody have largely replaced the traditional Paul-Bunnell heterophil test. One instance in which the Paul-Bunnell test is superior to the spot test is in a patient with a definite or possible past history of infectious mononucleosis in whom the spot test is more likely to be falsely positive. The characteristic hematologic and serologic abnormalities of infectious mononucleosis often occur within 1 week of the onset of symptoms in the majority of patients, but either of these may be absent in a patient or may not appear until 2 or 3 weeks after onset.

OTHER CAUSES OF PHARYNGITIS

Pharyngeal gonorrhea, although usually an asymptomatic infection, may be the cause of pharyngitis in 1 percent of patients seeking care. It should always be suspected—and pharyngeal cultures on Thayer-Martin medium obtained—when the patient is known or thought to be a male homosexual. Obtaining cultures on Thayer-Martin medium might also be wise for patients with intercurrent symptoms of genitourinary infection, with rectal sores or pain, or with persistent pharyngitis.

We recommend cultures on appropriate media for meningococci or *Corynebacterium diphtheriae* when a known epidemic raises the possibility of these otherwise rare pharyngeal pathogens. A diphtheritic membrane may be absent in cases of diphtheria, and a pseudomembrane may be seen in infectious mononucleosis and illnesses other than diphtheria. Nevertheless, an apparent membrane, especially when covering the uvula or soft palate, should be cultured for *C. diphtheriae*.

A swollen, red epiglottis indicates epiglottitis. This condition, rare in adults, is a medical emergency. Sore

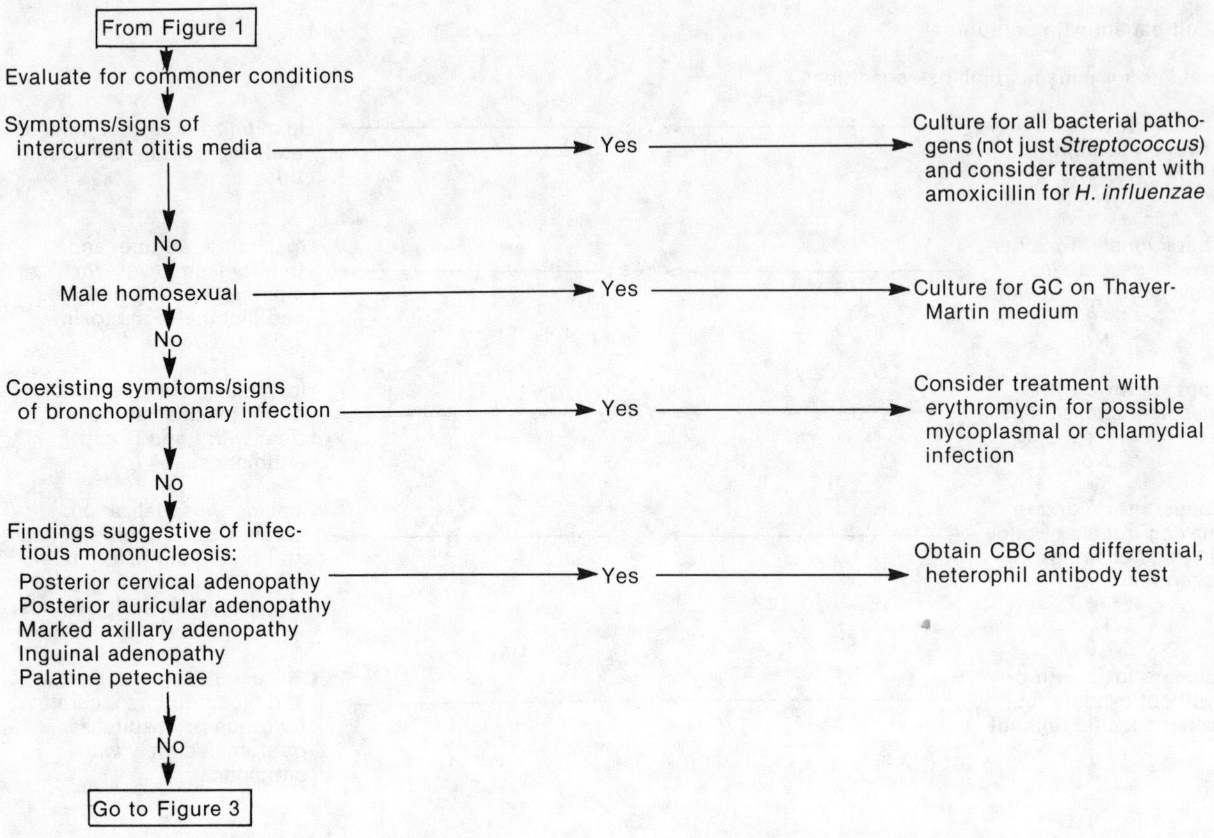

Figure 2 Algorithm describing an evaluation of more common nonstreptococcal causes of pharyngitis.

throat, hoarseness, and stridor, along with direct visualization of an inflamed epiglottis on depression of the tongue, are the key symptoms and signs. Lateral neck films may be diagnostically useful. The patient should be treated immediately for presumed epiglottitis; because *Hemophilus influenzae* is the usual pathogen, chloramphenicol, 1 g IV every 6 hours, is an appropriate antibacterial agent. The patient should be kept under constant observation for respiratory obstruction, a life-threatening event. Manipulation of the epiglottis by a swab or an endoscope may provoke laryngeal spasm and should be avoided. *Hemophilus influenzae* may also be a cause of pharyngitis, sometimes with concurrent otitis media. When the patient has concurrent otitis media, a throat culture for all bacterial pathogens (not just beta-hemolytic streptococci) should be obtained. When the throat culture demonstrates a heavy and predominant growth of *H. influenzae*, appropriate treatment should be initiated: ampicillin or amoxicillin, 500 mg every 6 hours.

Several viruses cause pharyngitis. Perhaps the commonest are the respiratory viruses (influenza virus, parainfluenza virus, adenovirus, respiratory syncytial virus, rhinovirus, coronavirus, and enterovirus). Patients with primary type II herpes simplex infection frequently have pharyngitis in association with their genital lesions. Type I herpes simplex virus may also cause pharyngitis, but the data on this association are not conclusive. An important cause of pharyngitis and stomatitis, particularly in the summer, is herpangina, a viral syndrome caused primarily by coxsackievirus A. No specific therapy exists for these viral infections, but preparations containing hydrogen peroxide in a glycerin base can be prescribed to relieve symptoms.

Recent evidence suggests that pharyngitis may sometimes be caused by non-group A streptococci and *Chlamydia trachomatis*. Confirmation of the etiologic role of these organisms and the implications for treatment await further studies. There is little evidence that the staphylococci are pharyngeal pathogens.

Notable gingivitis in association with pharyngeal inflammation suggests Vincent's angina, a mixed infection with a spirochete and fusiform gram-negative bacillus that responds to penicillin therapy. A single pharyngeal ulcer is most often caused by a fusobacterium infection. However, such an ulcer can be a primary chancre or a tuberculous granuloma; serologic testing for syphilis and an evaluation for tuberculosis should be undertaken. Several ulcers, especially in association with a rash, may represent secondary syphilis and should lead to serologic testing. Unilateral tonsillar swelling, if fluctuant, suggests a peritonsillar abscess requiring incision and drainage; on rare occasions, a hard, nonfluctuant, unilateral tonsillar mass may be a carcinoma or lymphoma. In patients with a sore throat and a prominent headache, the possibility

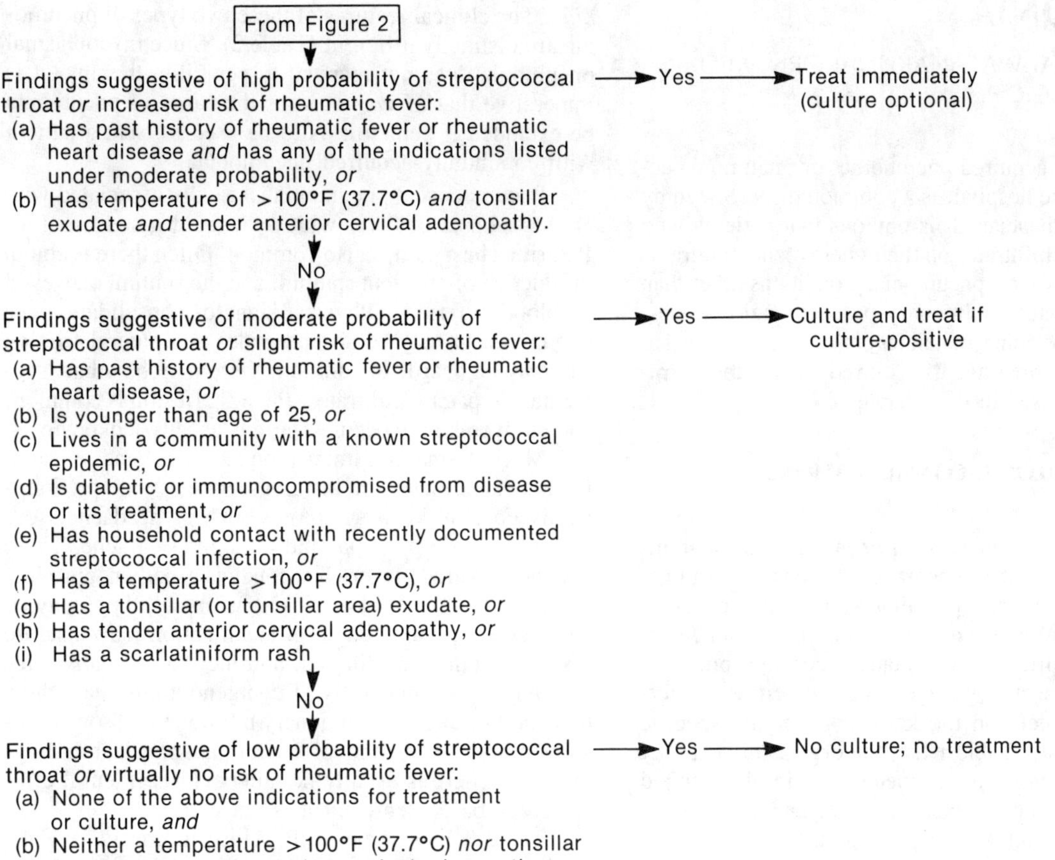

Figure 3 Algorithm describing an evaluation of the probability of group A streptococcal pharyngitis and the risk of developing acute rheumatic fever. Immediate treatment is preferred for those individuals whose throat culture results will not be complete for 9 days into the illness, since treatment after that time has not been shown to be protective against rheumatic fever.

of meningitis must be considered. Patients with acute leukemia may present with pharyngitis and, characteristically, have a foul, necrotic exudate.

The evaluation of patients for these unusual, high-risk conditions is summarized in Figure 1. Figures 1, 2, and 3 describe a sequential consideration of (1) the unusual or high-risk condition; (2) the more common forms of nonstreptococcal pharyngitis; and (3) an evaluation of possible group A streptococcal pharyngitis and the risk of acute rheumatic fever.

FOLLOW-UP ISSUES

In a patient with a throat culture positive for group A *Streptococcus*, a sore throat unresponsive to penicillin for 1 week suggests several possibilities: poor compliance with the penicillin regimen, mycoplasmal pharyngitis, infectious mononucleosis, gonococcal pharyngitis, or, possibly, other forms of nonviral pharyngitis. Cervical adenopathy should remit within 1 month in streptococcal pharyngitis and within 2 months in infectious mononucleosis; failure to remit suggests lymphoma, leukemia, granulomatous diseases, or a malignant neoplasm of the head, neck, or chest. Contacts of patients with streptococcal pharyngitis who become symptomatic or asymptomatic living mates of those patients who are at high risk for infection (for example, those with a past history of acute rheumatic fever or indigent people living in crowded conditions) should have cultures performed and be treated if the culture is positive.

COMMUNITY-ACQUIRED PNEUMONIA

CHATRCHAI WATANAKUNAKORN, M.D., F.A.C.P., F.C.C.P.

Community-acquired pneumonia, or pneumonia acquired outside the hospital, is a common disease seen by the practicing physician. It is obvious that patients who have pulmonary infiltrates on their chest roentgenograms do not necessarily have pneumonia. Conditions other than infections may cause pulmonary parenchymal diseases. Only the diagnosis and management of pneumonia that is caused by infectious agents acquired outside the hospital will be discussed in this chapter.

ETIOLOGIC CONSIDERATIONS

Historically, pneumonia has been classified anatomically according to the appearance of roentgenograms: lobal pneumonia, bronchopneumonia, interstitial pneumonia, and others. With the advent of antimicrobial agents, it is more appropriate for clinicians to consider pneumonia in terms of the etiologic agent, because effective therapy depends largely on the knowledge of the specific infecting organism. Table 1 lists the organisms that may cause community-acquired pneumonia in the United States. The list is not an exhaustive one and does not include bacteria, fungi, viruses, and parasites that are unlikely to cause pneumonia in adults and that are acquired outside the hospital in the United States. When pneumonia develops in patients in nursing homes or in patients who have had recent hospitalization, it should be considered hospital-acquired pneumonia.

TABLE 1 Organisms That May Cause Community-Acquired Pneumonia

Common bacteria
- *Streptococcus pneumoniae*
- *Mycoplasma pneumoniae*

Less common bacteria
- *Hemophilus influenzae*
- *Legionella pneumophila*
- Mixed aerobic-anaerobic bacteria (aspiration pneumonia)
- *Staphylococcus aureus*
- *Klebsiella pneumoniae*
- *Mycobacterium tuberculosis*
- Other mycobacteria

Other important organisms (list is not exhaustive)
- Influenza virus
- Adenovirus
- Varicella virus
- Measles virus
- *Histoplasma capsulatum*
- *Blastomyces dermatitidis*
- *Coccidiodes immitis*
- *Cryptococcus neoformans*
- *Chlamydia psittaci*
- *Coxiella burnetii*
- *Pneumocystis carinii*

The two most common types of pneumonia are caused by *Streptococcus pneumoniae* and *Mycoplasma pneumoniae*. The clinical features of these two types of pneumonia are distinctly different (Table 2). Since mycoplasmal pneumonia does not respond to penicillin therapy, it is imperative that *Mycoplasma* as the cause of pneumonia be excluded if penicillin is to be used to treat a patient with community-acquired pneumonia.

Pneumococcal pneumonia is usually associated with an acute onset of fever with or without a sudden chill. Pleuritic chest pain is also common. Often there is cough productive of purulent sputum, and the sputum may even be bloody or rusty. Physical signs of consolidation are common, but may be absent. Rales and pleural friction rub may be heard. In addition, there may be lobar, segmental, or patchy infiltrates. Pleural effusion is common, and empyema may occur. There is usually leukocytosis.

Mycoplasmal pneumonia, on the other hand, is usually associated with an insidious onset, with predominantly constitutional symptoms such as headache, sore throat, malaise, myalgia, and sometimes earache. There may be low-grade fever. The cough is usually nonproductive and may be ''hacking.'' Occasionally, there may be some clear sputum. Physical examination may disclose rash and bullous myringitis, and there are usually rales unilaterally or bilaterally. Roentgenograms may show unilateral or bilateral pulmonary infiltrates and sometimes show more extensive involvement than physical findings indicate. There is usually no leukocytosis. Pleural effusion may be present, but it is not common.

Table 3 lists some useful clues in considering the etiology of community-acquired pneumonia. *Hemophilus influenzae* has increasingly been shown to cause pneumonia in adults, usually in patients with chronic obstructive lung disease who smoke. Onset is usually acute, as in pneumococcal pneumonia, and there may be unilateral or bilateral lung involvement.

Community-acquired pneumonia caused by *Klebsiella pneumoniae* is not common and usually develops in alcoholics. The patient with Klebsiella pneumonia is usually toxic with high fever, and sputum is purulent.

Mixed aerobic-anaerobic (aspiration) pneumonia is more common in alcoholics, in patients with seizure disorders, and in patients with swallowing disorders. These patients usually have poor dental hygiene. The fever is generally high, and the patient looks toxic. Sputum production is usually copious, purulent, and foul-smelling. Roentgenograms of the chest may disclose abscess formation.

Staphylococcus aureus pneumonia is uncommon. It may present as a superinfection in patients who have influenza pneumonia with sudden onset of high fever and purulent sputum. More commonly, it occurs in intravenous drug abusers as a result of septic pulmonary emboli from tricuspid valve endocarditis. It typically presents with high fever, chills, dyspnea, tachypnea, tachycardia, and pleuritic chest pain. There may be scanty sputum production that may also be bloody. Chest films usually show multiple patchy infiltrates with or without cavities. Blood cultures invariably yield *S. aureus*.

TABLE 2 Clinical Features Differentiating Pneumococcal Pneumonia and Mycoplasmal Pneumonia

Features	*Pneumococcal Pneumonia*	*Mycoplasmal Pneumonia*
Onset of symptoms	Acute; fever, often with a sudden chill	Insidious, low-grade fever
Cough	Productive of purulent, sometimes rusty, sputum	Nonproductive, hacking cough, sometimes minimally productive of clear sputum
Other symptoms	Pleuritic chest pain	Headache, sore throat, malaise, myalgia, earache
Physical findings	Rales, signs of consolidation, pleural friction rub	Rash, bullous myringitis, rales, rhonchi often bilateral
Leukocytosis	Present	Absent
Chest roentgenogram	Often lobar or segmental, pleural effusion common	Patchy, may be bilateral, may have pleural effusion
Sputum Gram stain	Polymorphonuclear leukocytes and gram-positive diplococci	If available, few polymorphonuclear leukocytes and no bacteria
Diagnostic work-up	Blood culture, sputum Gram stain and culture	Cold agglutinins, complement-fixing antibodies (acute and convalescent)
Response to penicillin	Yes	No
Response to erythromycin	Yes	Yes

Pneumonia caused by *Legionella pneumophila* has increasingly been diagnosed in patients who acquire pneumonia in the community. Cases of this type of pneumonia occur in a sporadic manner, but a history of exposure to dust at a construction site may be a helpful clue to *Legionella* as the cause. The onset is usually abrupt with high temperature. Mental confusion, abdominal pain, and diarrhea are common symptoms. There is usually scanty mucoid sputum with many pus cells and no organism on Gram stain. Chest roentgenograms may show lobar distribution early, progressing bilaterally. Analysis of arterial blood gas shows severe hypoxemia. There is mild leukocytosis. There may be hyperbilirubinemia with elevated levels of transaminases. Elevated levels of serum creatinine phosphokinase, myoglobinuria, hematuria, and renal failure may be found. If the diagnosis is not made and the patient is given beta-lactam and/or aminoglycoside antibiotics, the clinical condition will deteriorate, sometimes very rapidly.

Pulmonary tuberculosis is uncommon in the United States. However, it should be suspected when patients, especially the elderly, are not responding to appropriate antibiotic therapy for bacterial pneumonia. Other species of *Mycobacterium* may also cause pulmonary infiltrates, usually of a subacute or chronic nature.

Influenza virus may cause hemorrhagic pneumonia in some patients during an influenza epidemic. Adenovirus pneumonia is uncommon, occurring mostly in people housed in closed quarters, such as armed forces recruits. Varicella pneumonia may occur as a serious com-

TABLE 3 Useful Clues in the Etiology of Community-Acquired Pneumonia

Clues	*Etiology To Be Considered*
Sudden onset of high fever with one chill	Pneumococcus
Sore throat, headache, malaise, earache, hacking cough	Mycoplasma
Chronic obstructive pulmonary disease	Pneumococcus, *Hemophilus influenzae*
Alcoholics	Pneumococcus, *Klebsiella*, mixed aerobic-anaerobic (aspiration)
Seizure disorder, bad dental hygiene	Mixed aerobic-anaerobic (aspiration)
Copious, foul-smelling sputum	Mixed aerobic-anaerobic (aspiration)
Purulent sputum, leukocytosis	Bacterial pneumonia
Intravenous drug abuser	*Staphylococcus aureus*
Mental confusion, high fever, diarrhea, abnormal hepatic function, unresponsive to beta-lactam drugs	*Legionella pneumophila*
Contact with parakeet, parrot, working in turkey processing plant	*Chlamydia psittaci*
Not responding to appropriate antibiotic therapy	*Mycobacterium tuberculosis*, fungi
Male homosexual	*Pneumocystis carinii*
Severe hypoxia	*L. pneumophila, P. carinii*

plication in some adults with chicken pox. The measles virus may also cause pneumonia in adults with clinical measles.

Histoplasma capsulatum seldom causes acute pneumonia except when a large number of spores are inhaled, usually in a unique setting, e.g., cleaning chicken coops, demolishing old barns. Dyspnea, low-grade temperature, and nonproductive cough are usual symptoms. The areas endemic for histoplasmosis in the United States are along the Ohio and Mississippi rivers. *Blastomyces dermatitidis* may cause pulmonary infections with or without cutaneous lesions. If cutaneous lesions are present, diagnosis can easily be made by a potassium hydroxide preparation and culture of pus from these lesions. However, the diagnosis may not be obvious if there are no cutaneous lesions. The areas endemic for blastomycosis are similar to those for histoplasmosis. Coccidioidomycosis should be considered if a patient has a history of travel to the southwestern United States. *Cryptococcus neoformans* may cause symptomatic pulmonary infection in patients who have a history of taking corticosteroids or have Hodgkin's disease or diabetes mellitus.

Psittacosis and Q fever should be considered in the differential diagnosis of atypical pneumonia. *Chlamydia psittaci* may be transmitted from parakeets, parrots, and turkeys to humans, causing pneumonia. *Coxiella burnetii* can be found in materials from contaminated cows in this country, especially in California. Inhalation of *C. burnetii* can cause pneumonitis.

Recently, acquired immunodeficiency syndrome (AIDS) has been reported in male homosexuals and, to a lesser extent, in intravenous drug abusers and hemophiliacs. *Pneumocystis carinii* pneumonia may be the initial presenting problem in AIDS patients. The pneumonia is usually bilateral and diffused. Lung biopsy is usually required for diagnosis.

DIAGNOSTIC CONSIDERATIONS

A detailed history is imperative in the diagnosis of community-acquired pneumonia. Most patients will have pneumonia due to pneumococcus or mycoplasma. Table 2 lists the important differential features of pneumococcal pneumonia and mycoplasmal pneumonia. There are also other clues listed in Table 3 that may be helpful in considering other causes of pneumonia. Table 4 lists the laboratory methods of diagnosis of major pathogens causing community-acquired pneumonia.

Beside chest roentgenography, Gram stain and culture of sputum are the most important laboratory procedures in the diagnosis of bacterial pneumonia. A good sputum specimen from deep cough is essential. In general, a good sputum sample should contain at least 25 neutrophils and fewer than 20 epithelial cells per high-power field. For a diagnosis of bacterial pneumonia, bacteria of a predominant type should be seen on the Gram stain. If the Gram stain shows many leukocytes and mixtures of different types of bacteria, a mixed aerobic-anaerobic aspiration penumonia should be suspected. Two to three blood cultures should be obtained, since some patients with bacterial pneumonia will have bacteremia. If the blood cultures are positive, the etiology of the pneumonia is further confirmed.

The diagnosis of mycoplasmal pneumonia is based mainly on clinical features. Although *Mycoplasma pneumoniae* can be cultured from sputum specimens, many patients do not have productive sputum. Furthermore, most clinical microbiology laboratories are not capable of doing mycoplasmal cultures. The diagnosis of mycoplasmal pneumonia can be confirmed by serology, i.e., a fourfold rise in complement-fixing antibody to *Mycoplasma pneumoniae*. Cold-agglutinin antibody is a nonspecific test, but a high titer in a patient who has clinical features of mycoplasmal pneumonia supports the clinical diagnosis.

Legionella pneumonia should be diagnosed and therapy started on clinical grounds. Some laboratories are equipped to do *Legionella* immunofluorescent antibody stain of sputum and also sputum culture for *Legionella*. Otherwise, the diagnosis can be confirmed by a fourfold rise of indirect fluorescent antibody.

Acid-fast stain of sputum is a rapid method for the diagnosis of mycobacterial infection, which should be confirmed by sputum cultures for mycobacteria; a PPD skin test should be done. Potassium hydroxide preparation and fungal cultures should be done in the diagnosis of deep fungal infection; serial serology may be helpful. Viral pneumonia can be diagnosed by sputum culture for virus and serial serology. Psittacosis and Q fever should be diagnosed by serology. *Pneumocystis carinii* pneumonia is usually diagnosed by methenamine-silver stain of a lung biopsy specimen.

TABLE 4 Diagnostic Methods for Community-Acquired Pneumonia

Etiologic Agents	*Diagnostic Methods*
Pyogenic bacteria	Blood cultures Sputum Gram stain Sputum culture
Mycoplasma pneumoniae	Serology
Legionella pneumophila	Sputum culture for *Legionella* Sputum immunofluorescence stain Serology
Mycobacteria	Sputum acid-fast stain Sputum culture for mycobacteria PPD skin test
Virus	Sputum culture for virus Serology
Fungus	Sputum culture for fungus Potassium hydroxide preparation of sputum Serology
Chlamydia psittaci	Serology
Coxiella burnetii	Serology
Pneumocystis carinii	Methenamine-silver stain of lung specimen

TABLE 5 Antimicrobial Therapy for Community-Acquired Pneumonia

Etiologic Agent	*Drugs of First Choice*	*Alternative Drugs*
Streptococcus pneumoniae	Penicillin G 600,000 units IV q6h *or* Penicillin V 500 mg PO q6h (mild cases)	Erythromycin 500 mg IV, *or* PO q6h (penicillin allergy)
Mycoplasma pneumoniae	Erythromycin 500 mg PO q6h	Tetracycline 500 mg PO q6h
Hemophilus influenzae	Ampicillin 1–2 g IV q4h	Cefuroxime 750–1,500 mg IV q8h (resistant strain) *or* Tetracycline 250 mg IV q6h (penicillin allergy)
Mixed aerobic-anaerobic (aspiration)	Penicillin G 1 million units IV q4h	Clindamycin 300–600 mg IV q6h (penicillin allergy or no response to penicillin)
Staphylococcus aureus	Nafcillin 1–2 g IV q4h *or* Cefazolin 1–2 g IV q8h *or* Penicillin 5 million units IV q6h (if organism is sensitive)	Vancomycin 500 mg IV q6h or 1 g IV q12h (first choice drug if organism is methicillin-resistant)
Klebsiella pneumoniae	Cefazolin 2 g IV q8h	Gentamicin 1.7 mg/kg IV q8h (penicillin allergy or resistant organism)
Legionella pneumophila	Erythromycin 0.5–1 g IV q6h	
Chlamydia psittaci	Tetracycline 500 mg PO q6h	
Coxiella burnetii	Tetracycline 500 mg PO q6h	
Pneumocystis carinii	TMP/SMZ 20 mg/kg of TMP plus 100 mg/kg of SMZ IV per day in 4 divided doses	Pentamidine (iethionate 4 mg/kg per day given in one dose IV or IM)

THERAPEUTIC CONSIDERATIONS

Specific antimicrobial therapy depends on the infecting agent or on the most likely infecting agent based on clincial features. Table 5 lists the antimicrobial drugs of choice and alternative drugs for infecting agents most likely to cause community-acquired pneumonia.

Parenteral penicillin G is the drug of choice, and oral penicillin V may be used in mild cases of pneumococcal pneumonia. If a patient is allergic to penicillin, erythromycin is a good alternative drug. Mycoplasmal pneumonia may be treated with either erythromycin or tetracycline. In a patient whose clinical features are not definitive for either pneumococcal or mycoplasmal pneumonia, erythromycin is the preferred drug, since it is effective against both types of pneumonia.

The drug of choice for *Hemophilus influenzae* pneumonia is ampicillin. If the infecting strain is resistant to ampicillin, cefuroxime, a new second-generation cephalosporin, may be used. In patients with severe penicillin allergy, tetracycline may be used. Nafcillin or cefazolin are the drugs of choice for *Staphylococcus aureus* pneumonia. Penicillin G should be used if the infecting strain is sensitive to it. If the infecting strain is resistant to methicillin and therefore resistant to all beta-lactam antibiotics, or if a patient has a severe penicillin allergy, vancomycin should be used.

For pneumonia caused by *Klebsiella pneumoniae*, cefazolin is the drug of choice. If the organism is resistant to cefazolin, or if the patient has a severe penicillin allergy, gentamicin is a good alternative drug. Some authorities suggest the combination of cefazolin and gentamicin for the treatment of klebsiella pneumonia, but there is no good clinical study showing better results than those obtained with a single drug. The new second- and third-generation cephalosporins (cefamandole, cefuroxime, cefonicid, ceforanide, cefoxitin, cefotaxime, moxalactam, cefoperazone, ceftizoxime, ceftriaxone, ceftazidime) may be used if the infecting strain is resistant to cefazolin.

For aspiration pneumonia that is caused by mixed

aerobic-anaerobic bacteria, penicillin G is the drug of choice. Clindamycin is a good alternative drug in patients who are allergic to penicillin or who fail to respond to penicillin G.

The drug of choice for the treatment of pneumonia caused by *Legionella pneumophila* is erythromycin. Although some authorities empirically add rifampin to erythromycin for patients who are seriously ill, there has been no clinical study to show that this is beneficial. For psittacosis and Q fever, tetracycline is the drug of choice.

Trimethoprim-sulfamethoxazole (TMP/SMZ) is the drug of choice for the treatment of *Pneumocystis carinii* pneumonia. Unfortunately, many patients with AIDS cannot tolerate TMP/SMZ because of severe adverse drug reactions. Pentamidine is the alternative drug. Pentamidine administration is associated with multiple side-effects and toxicities, e.g., phlebitis, sterile abscess with intramuscular injection, hypoglycemia, leukopenia, renal toxicity, hepatic toxicity.

HOSPITAL-ACQUIRED PNEUMONIA

BARNEY S. GRAHAM, M.D.
WILLIAM SCHAFFNER, M.D.

Pneumonia accounts for 15 percent of all nosocomial infections; only nosocomial urinary tract infections and surgical wound infections occur more frequently, 40 percent and 21 percent, respectively. Hospital-acquired pneumonias, however, are responsible for 60 percent of all deaths due to nosocomial infections and, per episode, are more costly than urinary tract or surgical wound infections.

Establishing a specific diagnosis in patients with hospital-acquired pneumonia is difficult. Many processes are clinically and roentgenographically indistinguishable from pneumonia. These include pulmonary emboli, chemical pneumonitis, neoplastic infiltrates, cardiogenic and noncardiogenic pulmonary edema, pulmonary hemorrhage, postoperative atelectasis, drug hypersensitivity reactions, graft-versus-host disease, rheumatologic disorders, and radiation pneumonitis. Thus, in hospitalized patients with new pulmonary infiltrates—especially in the presence of purulent sputum, fever, and leukocytosis—one often must empirically treat several processes simultaneously. The initial choice of antimicrobial agents will be determined by the hospital's nosocomial flora, the patient's underlying disease, and recent diagnostic or therapeutic interventions. After empiric therapy has begun, a series of diagnostic steps can be undertaken that may result in a simpler, more specific therapeutic regimen.

INFECTIOUS RESPIRATORY HAZARDS DURING HOSPITALIZATION

In the hospital, a patient may be exposed to a variety of respiratory tract pathogens and other hazards that can predispose to pneumonia. Less than 2 percent of normal adults have persistent oropharyngeal colonization by gram-negative aerobic organisms. In contrast, hospitalized patients who are moderately or seriously ill have a prevalence of oropharyngeal colonization with gram-negative bacilli of up to 70 percent. Patients with respiratory disease and those who are bedridden or moribund have the highest rate of colonization. Such colonization of the oropharynx by gram-negative bacilli is an important prelude to nosocomial pneumonia. In one study, pneumonia occurred in 23 percent of colonized patients, but in only 3 percent of noncolonized patients. The source of the colonizing bacteria has not been well defined. The patient's endogenous bowel flora has been suggested as a source as well as the contaminated hospital milieu, including inhalational therapy equipment and the hands of hospital personnel. Furthermore, under the pressure of widespread antimicrobial use in hospitals, the colonizing gram-negative bacilli are not only more prevalent, but more resistant, and other bacterial organisms not ordinarily considered to be respiratory pathogens, such as enterococci, have been recognized to cause pneumonia.

Oropharyngeal carriage of *Staphylococcus aureus* also occurs frequently in hospitalized patients, thus influencing the choice of antimicrobial therapy, especially in nosocomial aspiration pneumonia.

Legionella pneumophila has been found to be an important cause of nosocomial pneumonia in some institutions. The frequency of *L. pneumophila* as a nosocomial pathogen in hospitals where it is endemic can be as high as 35 percent. Even more startling is that in one hospital, where legionellosis had not previously been recognized, prospective evaluation revealed that 14 percent of nosocomial pneumonias were caused by this agent. Autopsy studies have revealed that *L. pneumophila* may be responsible for up to 6 percent of fatal nosocomial pneumonias in some institutions.

Although much less appreciated, viral agents may be present in the hospital environment and pose a risk of pneumonia to some patients. These include influenza A and B viruses in the elderly and chronically ill, respiratory syncytial virus in infants and the elderly, adenovirus in infants, and herpesviruses in immunocompromised hosts.

Tuberculosis can also be a nosocomial infection. Infants, the elderly, and hospital employees are at particular risk. The infection is ordinarily spread via aerosolized droplets, but contaminated instruments have, rarely, been a vehicle of transmission.

AN APPROACH TO MANAGING THE PATIENT

Recommendations for managing various infections usually begin with the premise that a diagnosis has been made and a pathogen has been identified. Reaching this stage in the management of an infectious illness, however, is a most difficult task. We would like to address the problem of how to treat the patient before a specific diagnosis is made and how to make a specific diagnosis after treatment has been started. In the debilitated, hospitalized patient, pneumonic processes are rarely diagnosed immediately. Sputum is often difficult to obtain, and, when obtained, Gram-stained sputum requires a more complex interpretation in hospital-acquired than in community-acquired pneumonia. Because of the nature of the patients who acquire pneumonia in the hospital, decisions to do invasive diagnostic procedures are belabored, and the procedures are often delayed. These factors plus the already-precarious condition of the host demand that an empiric antimicrobial regimen be instituted concurrent with the diagnostic work-up. The choice of empiric antimicrobial agents can determine the mortality due to the illness and must be based on the physician's personal experience as well as the local, and reported experience with the infectious process.

We have created a conceptual framework for several types of patients prone to hospital-acquired pneumonias that will assist the clinician in formulating empiric antimicrobial regimens (Table 1). The diagnosis and prevention of nosocomial pneumonia will be discussed briefly in following sections; Tables 2 and 3 provide a list of recommended therapeutic regimens for pneumonias caused by specific pathogens.

Several new third-generation cephalosporins have become available and are changing the management of many infectious processes. Some have improved activity against *Pseudomonas aeruginosa* (cefoperazone, ceftazidime, imipenem, aztreonam), the resistant Enterobacteriaceae (cefotaxime, moxalactam, cefoperazone, ceftizoxime, ceftazidime, imipenem, aztreonam), and *Bacteroides fragilis* (cefotaxime, moxalactam, ceftazidime, ceftriaxone, ceftizoxime, imipenem, aztreonam). Some have long half-lives, which allow less frequent dosing (ceftriaxone). Despite these assets, we feel that there are very limited indications for their use. The only specific indications for a third-generation cephalosporin are when a blood isolate proves to be sensitive only to that agent or when a person has both gram-negative bacillary pneumonia and meningitis. The best use of third-generation cephalosporins might be in empiric antimicrobial regimens. Although they are not included in our first-line therapy, it is appropriate to use them in patients who are likely to have *P. aeruginosa* or resistant Enterobacteriaceae causing the pneumonia. They are especially useful in a patient with penicillin allergy or renal insufficiency. In neutropenic or immunosuppressed patients, addition of an aminoglycoside to the empiric regimen, is still prudent.

Aspiration

The pathogenesis of hospital-acquired pneumonia involves either aspiration of oropharyngeal pathogens, blood-borne pathogens, or inhaled pathogens. Aspiration is by far the most important factor in the development of hospital-acquired pneumonia and should be a primary consideration in each of the patient groups mentioned subsequently. Aspiration is a universal phenomenon. Normal persons have repeatedly been demonstrated to aspirate during sleep. In a single night of observation, aspiration was documented to occur in more than 45 percent of normal individuals and in more than 70 percent of patients with a depressed sensorium.

The factors that increase the frequency of aspiration include alcoholic stupor and any of a multitude of other conditions that alter consciousness, chronic sinusitis with purulent nasopharyngeal drainage, esophageal disorders, neurologic disorders affecting the swallowing mechanism, topical anesthetics in the airway, restrictive lung disease, advanced age, instrumentation of the airway or esophagus, tracheoesophageal fistula, and gastrointestinal obstruction.

Aspiration pneumonia has a complex pathogenesis including infection, chemical pneumonitis, and airway obstruction by foreign bodies. The microbiology of aspiration pneumonia is a reflection of the oropharyngeal flora, which will include gram-negative bacilli, *S. aureus*, and penicillin-resistant anaerobes in the hospitalized patient. In a patient without other complicating factors, a regimen of clindamycin and an aminoglycoside would have good activity against these organisms.

Impaired Immunity

The lung is ordinarily protected from infection by a complex series of mechanical systems as well as by local and systemic and humoral and cell-mediated immune mechanisms. Rather than review pulmonary defense mechanisms in general, special considerations for certain groups of individuals are reviewed with regard to their susceptibility to hospital-acquired pneumonia.

NOSOCOMIAL PNEUMONIA

The Elderly

Although senescence of both cell-mediated and humoral immunity has been documented in the elderly, no correlation with the nature of oropharyngeal colonization or risk of pneumonia has been shown. Rather, underlying disease and exposure to other risk factors seem to play a greater role in determining the likelihood that an elderly person will develop pneumonia.

TABLE 1 Relative Importance of Pathogens in the Causation of Nosocomial Pneumonia Relative to a Patient's Underlying Condition

*Pathogen**	*Advanced Age*	*Alcoholism*	*Chronic Lung Disease*	*Postoperative*	*Burns*	*Mechanical Ventilation*	*Organ Transplantation*		*Neutropenia*	*Immunosuppressive Drugs Including Corticosteroids*	*Inhalational Devices*	*Prolonged Hospitalization or Recent Antimicrobial Therapy*
							Renal	*Bone Marrow*				
Gram-positive cocci												
Streptococcus pneumoniae (pneumococcus)	+++	+++	+++	++	++	++	++	++	++	+++	++	++
Streptococcus faecalis (enterococcus)	++	+	+	+	+	0	+	+	+	+	0	++
Staphylococcus aureus	+++	+++	+++	+++	+++	++	+++	+++	+++	+++	++	+++
Gram-negative bacilli												
Escherichia coli	+++	+++	+++	+++	+++	+++	+++	+++	+++	+++	+++	+++
Klebsiella pneumoniae	+++	+++	+++	+++	+++	+++	+++	+++	+++	+++	+++	+++
Other Enterobacteriaceae	++	++	++	++	+++	++	++	+++	+++	++	+++	+++
Pseudomonas aeruginosa	++	++	++	++	+++	++	++	+++	+++	++	+++	+++
Other	+	+	+	+	++	+	++	++	++	++	++	++
Anaerobic bacteria												
Bacteroides fragilis	+++	+++	+++	++	++	++	++	++	++	++	0	++
Other	+	+	+	+	+	+	+	+	+	+	0	+
Legionella species												
Legionella pneumophila	++	++	++	+	+	+	++	++	++	++	+	++
Other	+	+	+	+	+	+	+	+	+	+	0	+
Mycobacteria												
Mycobacterium tuberculosis	+	+	+	0	0	0	++	++	+	++	+	+
Other	0	0	0	0	0	0	+	+	0	+	0	0

Fungi and higher bacteria												
Candida albicans or *Torulopsis glabrata*	+	+	+	+ +	+ +	+	+ +	+ +	+ +	+ +	0	+ +
Cryptococcus neoformans	0	0	0	0	0	0	+ +	+	+	+ +	0	0
Aspergillus fumigatus	0	0	0	0	0	0	+ +	+ +	+ +	+ +	0	0
Nocardia asteroides	0	0	0	0	0	0	+ +	+	+	+ +	0	0
Other	0	0	0	0	0	0	+	+	+	+	0	0
Viruses												
Herpes simplex	0	0	0	+	+ +	+ +	+	+ +	+	+	0	0
Herpes varicella-zoster	+	+	0	0	0	0	+	+	+	+	0	0
Cytomegalovirus	0	0	0	+	0	0	+ + +	+ + +	+ +	+ +	0	0
Influenza A (in wintertime epidemics)	+ +	+ +	+ +	+	+	+	+	+	+	+	0	+
Respiratory syncytial virus (in wintertime epidemics)	+ +	+ +	+ +	0	0	+	+	+	+	+	0	0
Other	+	+	+	+	+	+	+	+	+	+	0	+
Protozoa												
Pneumocystis carinii	0	0	0	0	+	0	+ +	+ +	+ +	+ +	0	0
Toxoplasma gondii	0	0	0	0	+	0	+	+	+	+	0	0
Helminths												
Strongyloides stercoralis	0	0	0	0	0	0	+ +	+	0	+	0	0
Other	0	0	0	0	0	0	+	0	0	+	0	0

Note: This table represents the personal experience of the authors and may not fully apply to other institutions. Symbols used: + + + = the organism should absolutely be covered in initial empiric regimen, if effective therapy is available; + + = the organism should not be covered with initial therapy unless there is tangible evidence that it may be involved (however, it should be covered if clinical deterioration occurs and a diagnosis is not in hand); + = the organism is rarely a cause of nosocomial pneumonia in these hosts and should only be considered in unusual cases; 0 = the organism should not be a consideration.

* *Mycoplasma*, *Chlamydia*, and *Rickettsia* are not common considerations in nosocomial pneumonia.

Mechanical barriers to pulmonary infection become less effective as a person ages. Oropharyngeal colonization with gram-negative bacilli is increased in the elderly, probably as a consequence of an alteration in mucosal defense, which ordinarily impairs the adherence of bacteria. Epiglottal dysfunction and impaired cough reflex are also more likely to be present in the elderly patient, resulting in more frequent and larger amounts of oropharyngeal aspiration. Normally, mucociliary clearance is responsible for the removal of up to 20 percent of lung bacteria, but in the elderly this function is impaired, making the lung more susceptible to the challenge of oropharyngeal aspiration. The combination of these factors not only increases the likelihood of pneumonia in the elderly patient, but makes the likelihood of a multiorganism infection much greater.

Elderly hospitalized patients with pneumonia should, therefore, be considered in light of their underlying conditions and recent events (i.e., surgical procedures, instrumentation, or documented bacteremia or infection at another site), as well as the fact that they have a high risk of oropharyngeal aspiration.

One must also be aware of seasonal factors. There is a fairly regular winter increase in mortality due to pneumonia that has been attributed to influenza. Elderly persons seem to be especially susceptible to influenza viruses and have a higher fatality rate. Most of this excess mortality is caused by influenza A. Wintertime hospital epidemics affecting the elderly population have been reported not only for influenza A, but also occasionally for influenza B and respiratory syncytial virus. If an unvaccinated elderly person is admitted to the hospital in the midst of a nosocomial influenza epidemic, that person should be treated prophylactically with amantadine, 100 mg twice daily. If pneumonia occurs in this setting in a patient not already receiving amantadine, then amantadine, 100 mg twice daily, should be added to the treatment regimen.

Alcoholics

Alcoholics have long been recognized to be more susceptible to pneumonia than the general population. They have a high risk of aspiration, even after entry into the hospital. Furthermore, they can experience leukopenia, and their granulocyte function can be impaired for up to 2 weeks after abstaining from alcohol.

Gram-negative bacilli and pneumococci are the organisms at which therapy should be directed in the alcoholic who develops new or worsening pneumonia in the hospital. The prevalence of oropharyngeal colonization with gram-negative bacilli is high among alcoholics, with *Klebsiella pneumoniae* and *Escherichia coli* being the two most prominent pathogens.

One must also be alert to the possibility of mixed infection in this population, especially when the chest roentgenogram shows pulmonary necrosis. The presence of the pneumococcus in sputum or even in the blood does not preclude a coinfection with anaerobes, *S. aureus*, or *K. pneumoniae*.

TABLE 2 Specific Antimicrobial Therapy for Nosocomial Pneumonia

Pathogen	*Ideal Therapy*	*Alternative Therapy*
Gram-positive cocci		
Streptococcus pneumoniae (pneumococcus)	Penicillin	Erythromycin
Streptococcus faecalis (enterococcus)	Ampicillin	Vancomycin
*Staphylococcus aureus**	Nafcillin	Cephalothin
Gram-negative bacilli		
*Escherichia coli**	Ampicillin	Cefazolin
*Klebsiella pneumoniae**	Cefazolin and gentamicin	Based on sensitivities
Other Enterobacteriaceae*	Based on sensitivities	---
*Pseudomonas aeruginosa**	Ticarcillin or piperacillin and an aminoglycoside	Based on sensitivities
Other*	Based on sensitivities	---
Anaerobic bacteria		
Bacteroides fragilis	Clindamycin	Metronidazole
Other	Penicillin	Clindamycin
Legionella species		
Legionella pneumophila†	Erythromycin	---
Other	Erythromycin	---
Mycobacteria		
Mycobacterium tuberculosis	Isoniazid and ethambutol	Isoniazid and rifampin
Fungi and higher bacteria		
Candida albicans or *Torulopsis glabrata*	Amphotericin B	---
Cryptococcus neoformans	Amphotericin B + flucytosine	---
Aspergillus fumigatus	Amphotericin B	---
Nocardia asteroides	Trimethoprim-sulfamethoxazole	---
Viruses		
Herpes simplex	Acyclovir‡	---
Herpes varicella-zoster	Acyclovir‡	---
Cytomegalovirus	---	---
Influenza A	Amantadine	---
Respiratory syncytial virus	---	---
Protozoa		
Pneumocystis carinii	Trimethoprim-sulfamethoxazole	Pentamidine
Toxoplasma gondii	Pyrimethamine	Sulfadiazine
Helminths		
Strongyloides stercoralis	Thiabendazole	---

Note: Dosages for each antimicrobial agent can be found in Table 3.
* Staphylococcal and gram-negative bacillary pneumonias are usually treated for 14 days.
† Legionellosis requires 3 weeks of therapy to prevent relapse.
‡ Acyclovir has not been proved effective or ineffective in herpes virus pneumonias.

Patients with Malignancies

Aside from aspiration-caused pneumonia, most hospital-acquired pneumonia in patients with malignancy occurs in the setting of neutropenia. Although these patients are prone to develop pneumonia from a broad spectrum of organisms because of their underlying neoplasm and its systemic effects, hospital-acquired pneumonias are almost always related to myelosuppressive or immunosuppressive therapy or invasive procedures.

TABLE 3 Antimicrobial Dosages for Adults with Hospital-Acquired Pneumonia and Normal Renal Function

Agent	*Dose*	*Route*	*Interval (hours)*
Acyclovir	5 mg/kg	IV	8
Amantadine	100 mg	PO	12
Amikacin	5 mg/kg	IV	12*
Amphotericin B			
(for *Candida*)	0.2 mg/kg	IV	24
(for cryptococcosis)	0.3 mg/kg	IV	24
(for aspergillosis)	0.7 mg/kg	IV	24
Ampicillin	2 g	IV	4
Cefazolin	2 g	IV	6
Cefotaxime	2 g	IV	6
Cephalothin	2 g	IV	4
Clindamycin	600 mg	IV	6
Erythromycin	1 g	IV	6
Ethambutol	15 mg/kg	PO	24
Flucytosine	25 mg/kg	PO	6
Gentamicin	1 mg/kg	IV	8*
Isoniazid	300 mg	PO	24
Metronidazole	500 mg	IV	6
Nafcillin	2 g	IV	4
Penicillin G	3×10^6 units	IV	4
Pentamidine	4 mg/kg	IM	24
Piperacillin	3 g	IV	4
Pyrimethamine	25 mg	PO	24
Rifampin	600 mg	PO	24
Sulfadiazine	50 mg/kg	IV	12†
Thiabendazole	25 mg/kg	PO	12
Ticarcillin	3 g	IV	4
Tobramycin	1 mg/kg	IV	8*
Trimethoprim-sulfamethoxazole			
(for pneumocystosis)	0.5 amp/10 kg	IV	6‡
Vancomycin	1 g	IV	12

* Requires a loading dose of 1.5 times the estimated routine dose. Peak and trough serum levels should be measured to adjust dosage.
† Requires loading dose of 75 mg/kg
‡ One amp of trimethoprim-sulfamethoxazole contains 80 mg of trimethoprim and 400 mg of sulfamethoxazole.

Neutropenic Patients

As in other infections in the neutropenic patient, the gram-negative bacilli *P. aeruginosa*, *K. pneumoniae*, and *E. coli* predominate. These patients not only experience fulminant infections and an extremely high mortality, but the usual clues to diagnosis of pneumonia are often absent. Although the patients usually have fever and pulmonary infiltrates there is a decreased frequency of cough, sputum production, and purulent sputum as judged by Gram stain. Indeed, the scarcity of polymorphonuclear leukocytes in sputum makes it imperative that clinicians notify the microbiology laboratory that the patient is neutropenic. Many laboratories screen sputum specimens to determine whether they contain leukocytes and discard specimens with few neutrophils unless otherwise advised.

Empiric therapy in this group of patients is critical. Pneumonia is often associated with bacteremia and is rapidly fatal without antimicrobial therapy. Several regimens have been found to be equally effective, but in most studies the response rate in neutropenic patients with pneumonia has not exceeded 50 percent. When faced with a febrile neutropenic patient with new pulmonary infiltrates or effusions, our practice is to initiate therapy with ticarcillin, cefazolin, and an aminoglycoside. This regimen includes at least two drugs with activity against the three major gram-negative pathogens as well as against *S. aureus*. The aminoglycoside chosen is usually tobramycin unless the patient is known to have had a tobramycin- or gentamicin-resistant organism in the past or is already receiving one of those two drugs, in which case amikacin is used. Also, in those hospitals with a known gentamicin-resistant nosocomial flora, amikacin is chosen.

After 48 hours, when the initial culture results are known and the patient's clinical course has been observed, a decision is made to modify the antimicrobial regimen. Unless *K. pneumoniae* or *S. aureus* has been identified as the pathogen, cefazolin is discontinued to avoid the slightly greater risk of nephrotoxicity when a cephalosporin and aminoglycoside are administered concurrently. If a specific pathogen is identified, the regimen is modified accordingly. If a pathogen is not identified, which is often the case, ticarcillin and the aminoglycoside are continued until the neutropenia has resolved or a more specific diagnosis is made.

If the neutropenic patient develops pulmonary infiltrates, fungal pneumonia is a consideration from the outset, especially if the patient is already receiving antimicrobial agents. *Candida albicans* is the commonest fungal invader, and if its presence can be documented on mucous membranes as thrush or if there is evidence of its dissemination in the skin or the eye, amphotericin B should be initiated. A dose of 0.2 mg per kilogram per day is sufficient to treat candidal pneumonia and should be continued for 10 to 14 days or longer if the neutropenia has not resolved.

Aspergillus fumigatus is perhaps the most important fungal respiratory pathogen in the neutropenic patient. Aspergillus pneumonia is such a common complication of prolonged neutropenia in our institution that we advocate an aggressive approach to its empiric treatment. Therapy requires a high dose of amphotericin B, at least 0.7 mg per kilogram per day. If the febrile neutropenic patient has nodular pulmonary infiltrates or if pleuritic chest pain is a prominent feature of the illness, amphotericin B is part of the initial empiric regimen. If the patient with localized or diffuse pulmonary infiltrates has not responded clinically to empiric antibacterial therapy within 48 to 72 hours, amphotericin B is empirically added to the regimen. Successful therapy of aspergillus pneumonia in the setting of malignancy is dependent on early therapy, and, in our institution, the aggressive empiric approach has notably reduced the morbid consequences of this disease (Fig. 1).

Other fungal, protozoal, viral, and bacterial respiratory pathogens are recognized to complicate the course of neutropenic patients. *Pneumocystis carinii* is perhaps the commonest of these. If the chest roentgenogram shows a characteristic sunburst appearance with diffuse interstitial pulmonary infiltrates emanating from the hila, empiric therapy with trimethoprim-sulfamethoxazole is warranted. However, the roentgenographic appearance of

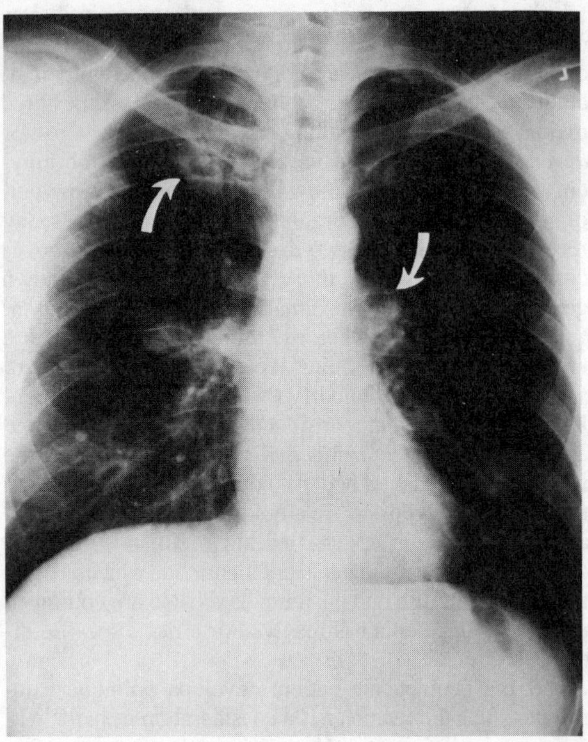

Figure 1 A 49-year-old man received high-dose cytosine arabinoside and daunomycin as consolidation therapy for acute myelomonocytic leukemia. On the eighth day of neutropenia, he became febrile and was treated with ticarcillin, tobramycin, and cefazolin. He remained febrile for 6 days before amphotericin B was begun because of the appearance of scattered pulmonary infiltrates on the roentgenogram. He promptly defervesced. The neutropenia resolved 4 days later, at which time the pulmonary lesions were cavitated (arrows), creating a pathognemonic appearance on chest roentgenogram for pulmonary aspergillosis. He was treated with a total of 750 mg of amphotericin B and did well until his leukemia relapsed 4 years later.

pneumocystis pneumonia may be very subtle and can even be unilateral or lobar. In the absence of a specific diagnosis in a neutropenic patient with pneumonia who is not responding to antibacterial and antifungal therapy, it is reasonable to institute empiric therapy with trimethoprim-sulfamethoxazole at a dose adequate to treat pneumocystosis (Table 2).

Legionella species are a growing concern as respiratory pathogens in neutropenic patients and provide few clinical clues to suggest their presence. The timing and consideration for administering empiric intravenous erythromycin for this infection are much the same as for the use of trimethoprim-sulfamethoxazole in the empiric treatment of pneumocystosis. Certain hospitals have documented high rates of endemic nosocomial legionellosis. In those institutions, intravenous erythromycin is often included in the initial antimicrobial regimen.

Organ Transplant Recipients

Pulmonary infiltrates in the hospitalized patient who has undergone organ transplantation are a special problem. Renal transplant recipients and allogeneic bone marrow transplant recipients will be discussed separately. The patient who has undergone autologous bone marrow transplantation should be given the same considerations as neutropenic patients, and the management of patients with other organ transplants (heart, lung, and liver) can be extrapolated from the following recommendations.

Renal Transplant Recipients

After renal transplantation, a patient can develop pneumonia from a disturbingly broad gamut of microbial pathogens. These patients, like other hospitalized patients, are prone to develop hospital-acquired pneumonia caused by gram-negative bacilli and *S. aureus*. This type of pneumonia usually occurs in patients who are admitted for graft rejection, have become debilitated from the progression of their underlying illness, or are already being treated for one pulmonary infection and develop a bacterial superinfection. The chest roentgenogram usually shows a focal process, and the patient usually has an abrupt onset of illness.

A more common situation in the period 1 to 4 months after transplantation is the subacute or insidious onset of fever and malaise, followed by the development of cough and the appearance of diffuse or multifocal infiltrates on chest roentgenogram. This syndrome is most often due to cytomegalovirus (Fig. 2).

Before the cumulative dose of corticosteroids given to renal transplant recipients was reduced, *A. fumigatus* was also a common cause of pneumonia. In our institution we have also seen *P. carinii, Cryptococcus neoformans, Blastomyces dermatitidis, Histoplasma capsulatum, Mycobacterium tuberculosis*, and *Strongyloides stercoralis* causing this syndrome. Other organisms including *Candida* species, *Mycobacterium* species, *Nocardia asteroides*, herpes simplex virus, and Epstein-Barr virus are potential pathogens. Most of these processes represent reactivated infections brought on by immunosuppressive therapy.

Empiric antimicrobial therapy with cefazolin and gentamicin is appropriate for the hospitalized renal transplant patient with the abrupt onset of fever and localized pulmonary infiltrate. In the patient already receiving antimicrobial therapy who develops a respiratory tract superinfection, ticarcillin plus tobramycin or amikacin would be better choices, since *P. aeruginosa* becomes a prominent concern.

In the patient with multifocal or diffuse pulmonary infiltrates, it is obvious that a simple empiric antimicrobial regimen cannot be constructed that has reasonable activity against all of the potential etiologic agents. Although these patients are often quite ill, the emergency use of antimicrobial agents is not as crucial as it is for neutropenic patients or debilitated patients with gram-negative or

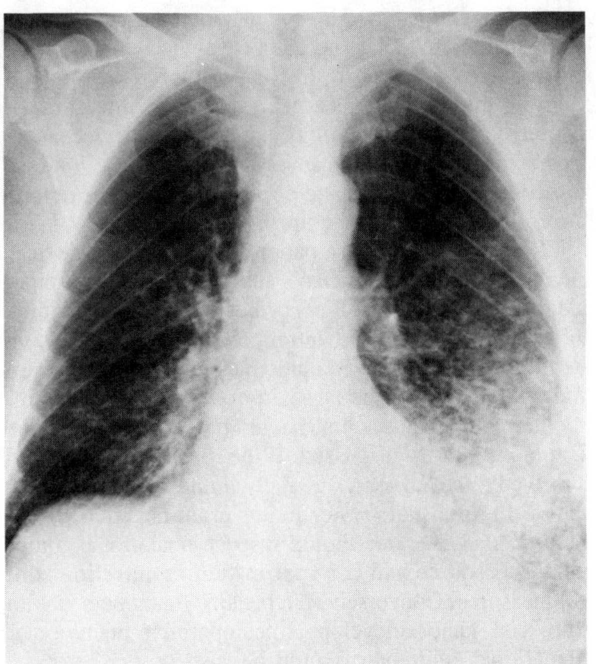

Figure 2 A 58-year-old man was hospitalized for chronic graft rejection 3 months after a cadaveric renal transplantation. After shortness of breath and hemoptysis developed, a chest roentgenogram revealed diffuse interstitial infiltrates with an appearance of alveolar filling in the left lower lobe. Cytologic examination of bronchial washings revealed the diagnostic intranuclear inclusions of cytomegalovirus. A reduction in his doses of prednisone and azothioprine resulted in renal graft rejection, but the cytomegalovirus pneumonia resolved.

staphylococcal pneumonia. Instead, the speed with which a specific etiologic diagnosis is made is a better determinant of outcome. These patients do not have as high an incidence of thrombocytopenia as do patients with chemotherapy-induced neutropenia, so bleeding complications from invasive diagnostic procedures are less common. We advocate an aggressive diagnostic approach in these patients that will provide a specific diagnosis within 5 days from the onset of illness. This often requires open lung biopsy, which will be discussed subsequently.

Allogeneic Bone Marrow Transplant Recipients. More than 50 percent of allogeneic bone marrow transplantations are complicated by pneumonia. Because of their prolonged neutropenia, those patients who develop pneumonia should receive initial treatment as described previously (Neutropenic Patients). However, like patients who have undergone renal transplantation, they are susceptible to the full spectrum of microbial invaders and have a greater predilection for opportunistic, nonbacterial respiratory infections that any other patient group. The problem is further complicated by the high frequency of idiopathic pneumonia in these patients, which can range up to 35 percent. The onset of nonbacterial pneumonia peaks in the second month after transplantation and is insidious in nature. It is more likely to occur in patients who have received the bone marrow transplantation for leukemia than for aplastic anemia, and among leukemics, it is likelier to occur in patients in relapse than in those in remission at the time of transplantation. The severity of graft-versus-host disease is also correlated with the frequency of pneumonia.

Although cytomegaloviral and idiopathic pneumonia are the most frequent types of pneumonia in these patients, *P. carinii* and viral pathogens, including herpes simplex virus, varicella-zoster, Epstein-Barr virus, and adenovirus, are recognized causes of pneumonia.

There is no drug with documented efficacy against any of these organisms in the lung except *P. carinii* which is susceptible to trimethoprim-sulfamethoxazole or pentamidine. In patients with thrombocytopenia who are at high risk of having bleeding complications, it is therefore reasonable to add trimethoprim-sulfamethoxazole to the empiric antibacterial and antifungal regimen without proceeding to invasive diagnostic procedures. However, there is good reason to believe that acyclovir would be efficacious against herpes simplex and varicella-zoster pneumonias, and new analogues of acyclovir are showing promise in the treatment of cytomegaloviral pneumonia. Hence, it may not be long before the same aggressive diagnostic approach recommended for renal transplant patients with pneumonia will be suggested for the patient who has received an allogeneic bone marrow transplant, despite the higher risk of procedural complications.

Postoperative Patients

Postoperative pneumonia is estimated to cause 10 percent of surgical mortality. The onset of fever and production of purulent sputum usually occurs within 5 days of the operative procedure and is almost uniformly related to aspiration of oropharyngeal or gastric contents.

Several risk factors have been identified that can help the clinician predict who will develop postoperative pneumonia. These include the site of operative procedure (thoracic and upper abdominal procedures result in more postoperative pneumonia than does lower abdominal surgery), duration of surgery, underlying condition of the patient (the elderly, patients with pulmonary disease, those with poor nutritional status, and patients with a high score by the classification of the American Society of Anesthesiologists have an increased risk of pneumonia), and the length of preoperative hospital stay. The young, nonsmoking patient who is fit, has a normal serum albumin, and undergoes a lower abdominal surgical procedure of short duration has a negligible risk of pneumonia.

The organisms responsible for postoperative pneumonia are a reflection of the oropharyngeal flora and include the gram-negative aerobes, *S. aureus*, and a variety of anaerobes—some of which are penicillin-resistant. Initial empiric therapy with cefazolin and gentamicin is appropriate. If the patient has had an obvious aspiration event or if the surgery performed was a complicated intra-abdominal procedure with a risk of peritonitis or anaerobic sepsis, clindamycin should be added to the regimen. In the complicated, postoperative intubated patient receiving multiple antimicrobial agents in the surgical intensive care unit, the emergence of pulmonary superinfection caused by resistant Enterobacteriaceae, *P. aeruginosa*, enterococci, and *Candida* species should be a prime consideration. Empiric therapy in this group of patients should include ticarcillin in combination with tobramycin or amikacin; if mucocutaneous candidiasis or candiduria is present, low-dose amphotericin B (0.2 mg per kilogram per day) should be added until the specific agents causing the pneumonia are determined.

INHALATIONAL DEVICES

Contaminated inhalational devices have been associated with both endemic and epidemic cases of hospital-acquired pneumonia. In recent years, rigorous infection control practices have considerably diminished this risk. The source of the etiologic pathogen can usually be traced to a water-containing reservoir in the equipment. Epidemics have been associated with contaminated intermittent positive-pressure breathing machines, humidifiers, mechanical ventilators, nebulizers, inhalational medications, and even Wright's spirometers. The organsims responsible for these pneumonias are invariably gram-negative water-liking aerobes. The most prominent of these pathogens have been *Serratia marcescens* and *Pseudomonas* species. Other possible offenders include *Legionella* species, *K. pneumoniae, Aerobacter* species, *Achromobacter* species, *Alcaligenes* species, and *Acinetobacter* species. The patients incurring pneumonia by this route obviously have serious underlying illnesses and are already at risk for hospital-acquired pneumonia. Many of these infections are, in fact, superinfections of a preexisting pneumonitis. The same devices and organisms continue to cause a low endemic rate of nosocomial pneumonias and occasional epidemics despite currently recommended control measures.

Recent exposure of a patient to inhalational devices should increase the physician's anticipation that a hospital-acquired pneumonia will occur but will rarely affect the choice of initial empiric antimicrobial therapy. Only in the midst of a recognized epidemic should the initial antimicrobial regimen be targeted at a specific organism. In other circumstances, one should base the choice on the factors previously discussed. If the respiratory pathogen is proved to be *S. marcescens, Pseudomonas cepacia*, or one of the unusual, water-liking gram-negative bacilli mentioned above, one should suspect inhalational equipment as a source and consider instituting infection control measures. Conversely, if a healthy young person with a few risk factors develops a postoperative pneumonia, inhalational equipment should be suspect.

BRONCHOSCOPY

Pneumonia following bronchoscopy is rare, occurring with a frequency of less than 1.0 percent. When a patient develops a lower respiratory tract infection following bronchoscopy, the causative pathogens will usually represent the oropharyngeal flora (Fig. 3).

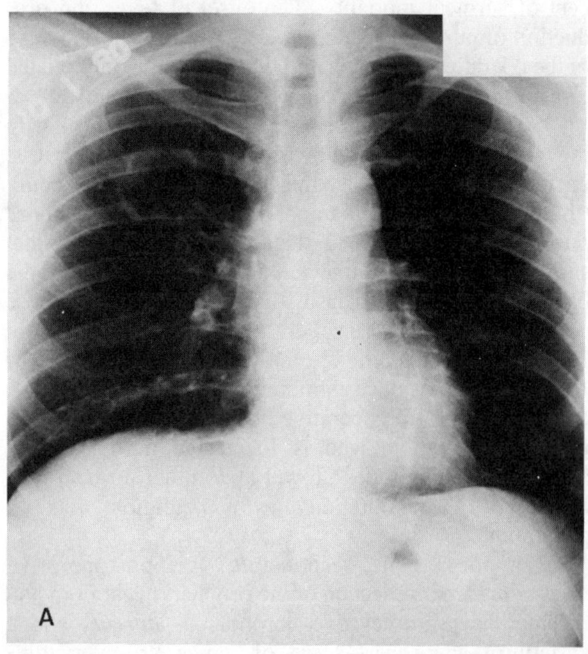

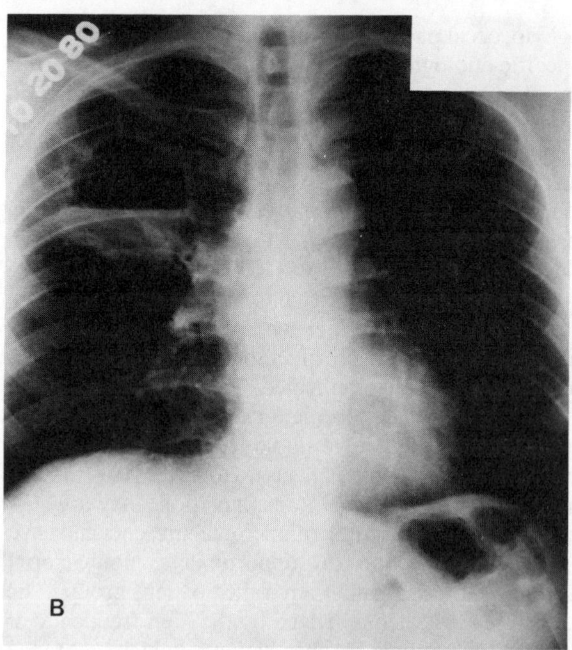

Figure 3 A 65-year-old diabetic man was admitted with a right upper-lobe cavitary lesion on chest roentgenogram that was due to blastomycosis (Fig. 3A). Nine days after transbronchial biopsies of the lesion via bronchoscopy, his temperature rose, chest pain developed, and an air-fluid level within the cavity became apparent (Fig. 3B). Percutaneous needle aspiration yielded a pure growth of *Eikenella corrodens*, which is part of the normal human oral flora and which was evidently introduced into the lower respiratory tract at the time of bronchoscopy.

TABLE 4 Prevention of Hospital-Acquired Aspiration Pneumonia

Be aware of the problem
Avoid the use of medications (including anesthesia) that depress consciousness
Avoid instrumentation of the airway
Use nasogastric tubes sparingly and, when used, choose the smallest, softest tube appropriate for the intended purpose
Use feeding gastrostomies, jejunostomies, or IV catheters for nutrition of patients with recurrent aspiration
Maintain good oral hygiene
Avoid feeding patients who are in a supine or recumbent position; rather, keep them upright
Avoid the use of oral anesthetics, dentures, extremely hot or cold substances, or other agents that impair the sensitivity of the oropharynx and thereby disturb deglutition
Avoid conditions that delay gastric emptying, including unpalatable food, low gastric pH, hyperosmolar or large-volume meals, meals with high fat content, and drugs with anticholinergic activity
Disallow food intake for 8 hours before induction of general anesthesia or other procedures that might induce vomiting

It is distinctly unusual for a contaminated instrument or solution to be the cause of postbronchoscopic pneumonia; however, an outbreak of *S. marcescens* pneumonia has been reported, and transmission of tuberculosis via fiberoptic bronchoscopy has also been recognized.

Bronchoscopy has been the occasional source of pseudoepidemics. *Trichosporon* species, *Penicillium* species, *Pasturella multocida, P. cepacia*, and *Mycobacterium gordonae* have all been reported to cause such an occurrence by contaminating bronchoscopy equipment or solutions. Although these organisms did not result in clinical illness, there were clusters of patients with culture-positive bronchial washings or false-positive acid-fast smears.

DIAGNOSIS

The diagnosis of hospital-acquired pneumonia is much more difficult than that of community-acquired pneumonia. Examination of the chest roentgenogram provides helpful clues, but rarely secures the identity of the etiologic agent. A focal pulmonary infiltrate on chest roentgenogram in a hospitalized patient with an acute febrile illness implies a bacterial process. A caveat, however, is that in immunosuppressed patients aspergillosis, cryptococcosis, nocardiosis, and even herpes simplex virus can cause focal pulmonary processes. Diffuse pulmonary infiltrates are rarely of bacterial origin and are more likely to represent viral, protozoal, fungal, or mycobacterial infections. However, many patients with diffuse pulmonary disease acquire bacterial superinfections, and in the early stages of an overwhelming bacterial bronchopneumonia or aspiration pneumonia, the roentgenographic appearance may be diffuse. Some patterns seen on chest roentgenograms are highly suggestive of a particular pathogen and include the patchy, pleural-based infiltrates of aspergillosis that become nodular, then cavitate, leaving a cresent of air on the inner rim; the linear infiltrates caused by *P. carinii* that seem to grow out from the hilum in a butterfly-like pattern; and the miliary pattern that is characteristic of tuberculosis and also may be seen in blastomycosis and histoplasmosis. When a necrotizing pneumonitis is suggested by the chest roentgenogram, the possibility of mixed infections, *K. pneumoniae* or other gram-negative bacilli, and anaerobic organisms should be remembered. Images seen on chest roentgenograms can help to modify the empiric antimicrobial regimens but should not be the final step in the diagnostic evaluation.

At least 7 percent of patients with nosocomial pneumonia have documented bacteremia, and up to 15 percent of all nosocomial bacteremias can be attributed to a pneumonia. Not only does a positive blood culture provide diagnosis of a specific organism, but it defines a group of patients with an extremely high mortality. It is, therefore, important to include blood cultures as part of the routine diagnostic evaluation of hospital-acquired pneumonia. Examination of smears and cultures of pleural fluid, urine, skin lesions, and other involved sites can also provide useful information. When the patient appears to have an overwhelming bacterial infection, Wright-stained buffy coat smears may also aid in the diagnosis.

Serologic studies are rarely useful in the acute management of patients with hospital-acquired pneumonia. They are not interpretable until a convalescent serum is available and can often be confusing, especially in the cases of fungal and herpesviral serology. There are, as always, exceptions. Serologic methods are

TABLE 5 Modification of Hospital- or Health-Care-Provider-Induced Risk Factors for Hospital-Acquired Pneumonia

Design hospital ventilation systems with proper airflow and filtration
Use appropriate isolation procedures for hospitalized persons with transmissable diseases
Demand frequent handwashing among hospital personnel
Decrease length of hospital stay
Avoid the use of nonessential antimicrobial agents
Use the lowest possible dose of corticosteroid or other immunosuppressive agent
Use the minimum length and depth of anesthesia
Avoid the use of endotracheal and tracheostomy tubes
Shorten operative procedures
Reduce preoperative hospital stay
Properly clean bronchoscopy equipment and decontaminate it with glutaraldehyde or ethylene oxide gas sterilization
Be aware of respiratory viral epidemics in the community and, when they occur, consider the use of masks on symptomatic patients and personnel, reduction of the frequency of visitation, and administration of oral amantidine, 100 mg twice daily, for patients at high risk
Encourage yearly influenza vaccination of hospital personnel

still the most commonly employed means of diagnosing legionellosis. Also, the serum cryptococcal antigen test can rapidly provide the diagnosis of cryptococcal pneumonia.

Sputum examination has been the cornerstone of diagnosis in patients with pneumonia for more than a century. If done properly, it can yield spectacular diagnostic rewards. The most critical step is the sputum collection. This should be a physician-supervised event, since the accuracy of the test depends entirely on obtaining a bit of purulence from the lower respiratory tract. If the patient is unable to cough, nasotracheal suction or aerosolized-saline induction of sputum with chest percussion is often fruitful. Once obtained, the densest, most purulent portion of the specimen should be smeared on a glass slide and gram-stained. One should look for a field under the oil immersion objective that contains polymorphonuclear leukocytes to the exclusion of epithelial cells. If a predominant organism is present, it should influence the initial antimicrobial regimen. In the hospitalized patient with pneumonia, it is expected that the oropharynx will be heavily colonized with gram-negative bacilli. This will make the sputum Gram stain hard to interpret, but should not preclude doing the test.

Other tests on the sputum should be performed in some settings. Carbolfuchsin can be used to detect acid-fast organisms. The addition of 10 percent potassium hydroxide to fresh sputum that is heated over a flame for an instant and then examined under a coverslip can reveal yeast or fungal elements. A Wright's or giemsa stain can reveal *H. capsulatum* within macrophages. In the cytology laboratory, a routine Papanicolaou's stain is useful for the detection of *Blastomyces dermatitidis*; stains such as periodic acid-Schiff, methenamine silver, and mucicarmine provide even greater contrast for the visualization of fungi and protozoa. Toluidine blue has been reported to demonstrate *P. carinii* in pulmonary secretions.

The use of monoclonal antibodies with the fluorescent antibody technique is revolutionizing the ability to make rapid diagnoses. Fluorescent antibody techniques are available now for the rapid detection of *L. pneumophila* and respiratory syncytial virus in respiratory tract secretions, and this method will soon be applied to many other respiratory pathogens.

There is a large literature on the usefulness and safety of transtracheal aspiration to obtain diagnostic specimens from the patient with pneumonia. In our institution, however, this technique is not used. Rather, we rely on bronchoscopy.

Flexible fiberoptic bronchoscopy is seldom needed in the diagnosis of hospital-acquired pneumonia in the nonimmunosuppressed host. Most such patients with an acute focal nosocomial pneumonia will have a diagnosis made from sputum examination, blood culture, or other noninvasive means, or will have responded to the institution of empiric antimicrobial therapy prior to the time that bronchoscopy would be considered. In some cases, however, there will be a need for a definitive pathogen-specific diagnosis. Patients with necrotizing pneumonitis, those with possible bronchial obstruction from foreign bodies or carcinoma, and those who have not shown clinical improvement within 72 hours after the initiation of empiric treatment would all be candidates for bronchoscopy.

In the immunosuppressed patient who develops a focal or diffuse pneumonia, bronchoscopy should be considered immediately unless a specific diagnosis is in hand. These patients are, in general, more fragile, less likely to respond to empiric treatment, and can quickly develop coagulopathies or severe hypoxia that might preclude the chance to safely perform bronchoscopy. In addition, because the spectrum of pathogens affecting these patients is so broad, establishment of a specific diagnosis is critical to the selection of appropriate therapy.

There are several ways of collecting specimens through the bronchoscope to diagnose pulmonary infections. The methods used will depend on which infections are suspected and host factors such as the degree of hypoxemia and the presence of nonreversible coagulopathies. Simple aspiration of lung secretions through the bronchoscope is rarely sufficient to make a reliable diagnosis. The tip of the bronchoscope is contaminated with the same heavily colonized oropharyngeal secretions that make the interpretation of sputum smears and cultures so difficult. The use of a double-lumen, telescoping-cannula brush catheter with a distal polyethylene glycol occlusion to collect the lower respiratory secretions will produce more reliable specimens. The specificity of culture results from specimens obtained with the protected catheter brush can be further enhanced by doing Gram stains and quantitative cultures.

Bronchial brushing can increase the diagnostic yield in cytologic preparations for patients with cytomegaloviral, herpes simplex viral, or *P. carinii* pneumonia. Although bacterial cultures obtained with the unprotected brush are difficult to interpret, the recovery of *Nocardia* is reportedly increased when this technique is used, and *Nocardia* should always be considered a pathogen.

Even more than the technique of bronchial brushing, transbronchial biopsies can increase the diagnostic yield of bronchoscopy. This procedure seems to be especially useful for invasive fungal, protozoal, viral, and granulomatous infections. The use of this technique for the diagnosis of hospital-acquired pneumonia is, therefore,

TABLE 6 Modification of Intrinsic Host Risk Factors for Hospital-Acquired Pneumonia

- Recognize underlying lung disease and optimize its treatment
- Do not allow smoking in the hospital
- Improve nutrition
- Maximize arterial pO_2
- Reduce pulmonary edema
- Optimize total blood volume
- Educate patients preoperatively about postoperative respiratory exercises, including coughing, deep breathing, incentive spirometry, and chest physiotherapy
- Use the influenza and pneumococcal vaccines in the appropriate patients

TABLE 7 Minimizing the Infectious Hazards of Inhalational Devices

Avoid violating the lower airways with instruments or aerosols
Discontinue ventilatory support as soon as possible
Clean and dry in-line nebulizers or inhalational equipment between each patient use
Change nebulizers and tubing on mechanical ventilators every 24 hours (clean them, decontaminate with 0.25% acetic acid rinse, and let dry before reuse)
Condensed fluid in ventilation tubing should never be drained retrograde, but should be emptied into an external receptacle
Suctioning and other procedures that transgress the intubated airway should be done using aseptic technique and sterile equipment
Respirometers should have single-use disposable extension pieces or be sterilized between each patient use
Hand-powered resuscitation bags should be sterilized before use on other patients

most practical for those immunosuppressed patients who are likely to have these types of opportunistic infections.

Many of the patients with pneumonia in whom bronchoscopy will be considered will be thrombocytopenic or have a prolonged bleeding time for some other reason. Both bronchial brushing and transbronchial biopsy are hazardous in this setting. One solution to this dilemma is bronchoalveolar lavage. This is distinct from bronchial washings in which only a small amount of saline is introduced into a segmental bronchus, then aspirated for stains and cultures. Bronchoalveolar lavage is performed by passing the bronchoscope to the point of occlusion into a subsegmental bronchus. Normal saline in 30-ml aliquots is then used to lavage the involved subsegment, followed by aspiration of the fluid. Up to a total of 200 ml of saline is used, but the lavage is discontinued if, after each instillation, aspiration of more than 50 ml or less than 15 ml occurs. The lavage fluid is pooled and divided in two parts. One is used for direct smears, stains, and cultures. The other is mixed with an equal volume of alcohol, subjected to cytocentrifugation, smeared, and stained with Papanicolaou's and other appropriate cytologic stains. This technique is almost as sensitive as transbronchial biopsy, yet poses an insignificant risk of hemorrhage.

Transthoracic needle aspiration, although useful for some malignant and infectious pulmonary disorders, is not productive in the diagnosis of hospital-acquired pneumonia. Most hospitalized patients with pneumonia are receiving empiric antimicrobial treatment prior to the time this procedure would be done, which markedly reduces its sensitivity. The procedure is frought with the problems of pneumothorax and hemorrhage, and only a small amount of material can be obtained for cytologic examination. For these reasons, when bronchoscopy has failed, we usually proceed directly to open lung biopsy if there is an urgent need to make a diagnosis in the patient with hospital-acquired pneumonia.

As noted above, most patients with hospital-acquired pneumonia will have a clinical response to empiric treatment or have a diagnosis established by noninvasive means long before the diagnostic step of bronchoscopy is reached. Even fewer will require open lung biopsy. This procedure is reserved primarily for immunosuppressed patients and only occasionally is needed for a nonimmunosuppressed patient with a diffuse pneumonitis. The procedure-related mortality is less than that for transbronchial biopsy. The diagnostic rate in patients with pneumonia is well over 90 percent compared with approximately 70 percent for bronchoscopy with transbronchial biopsy. In patients with thrombocytopenia, which includes most patients with chemotherapy-induced neutropenia and those who have undergone bone marrow transplantation, open lung biopsy is preferable to transbronchial biopsy or brushing. Although we tend to rely on empiric therapy in these patients because of their high risk of procedural complications, if the patient is not clinically responding to empiric therapy and bronchoalveolar lavage is nondiagnostic, open lung biopsy is performed. In contrast, the renal transplant patients, who less often have coagulopathies, should be given a more aggressive diagnostic evaluation with less emphasis on empiric therapy. If the results of bronchoscopy with transbronchial biopsy are nondiagnostic, we think that these patients should have open lung biopsy performed immediately.

PREVENTION

The ultimate goal in the management of hospital-acquired pneumonia should be prevention. Diagnosis is extremely difficult; treatment is often unsuccessful; and both are very costly. The preventive measures center around eliminating or reducing the risk factors already discussed. They are considered in four categories: prevention of aspiration, modification of intrinsic host risk factors, modification of hospital or health-care-provider-induced risk factors, and precautions for the use of inhalational equipment. The recommendations are listed in Tables 3 through 6. More specific and detailed recommendations can be found in references available on request from the authors.

Finally, it has been shown that nearly 50 percent of patients with pneumococcal pneumonia had been hospitalized within the previous 5 years. Patients with nosocomial pneumonia have proved themselves to be susceptible to respiratory pathogens. We feel that they should be included in the group of high-risk patients who should receive pneumococcal vaccine before leaving the hospital.

PLEURAL EFFUSION AND EMPYEMA

MAURICE A. MUFSON, M.D.

Invasion of the pleural space by fluid (pleural effusion) and pus (empyema) as a complication of infection occurs in 40 to 50 percent of bacterial pneumonias, but much less often in mycoplasmal or viral pneumonias. It occurs with varying frequency in other infections such as pulmonary tuberculosis and fungal infections, in noninfectious conditions including carcinoma of the lung, cirrhosis, congestive heart failure, pancreatitis, and in collagen-vascular diseases (Fig. 1). The initial step in the diagnosis and treatment of pleural effusion is to decide whether fluid invasion is a transudate associated with a noninfectious disease, an exudate complicating pneumonia (a parapneumonic effusion) or other infection, or an empyema (frankly purulent pleural fluid). Early recognition and therapeutic intervention are essential to achieve complete resolution of parapneumonic effusions and empyemas.

ETIOLOGY

Pleural effusions accompanying pneumonia develop most commonly in the course of bacterial pneumonias—mainly those due to *Staphylococcus aureus*, pneumococcus (*Streptococcus pneumoniae*), *Haemophilus influenzae*, hemolytic streptococci, anaerobic bacteria, and gram-negative bacteria—as well as in pulmonary tuberculosis. Pleural effusion, but not empyema, occurs occasionally in *Mycoplasma pneumoniae*, but rarely in viral pneumonias. The predominant bacterial pathogens of empyema are *S. aureus* and various gram-negative bacteria, such as *Klebsiella*, Enterobacteriaceae, *Pseudomonas*, and the anaerobic bacteria.

DIAGNOSIS

Physical examination and the upright chest radiograph can detect accumulations of fluid in the pleural space of at least 300 to 500 ml. The characteristic physical findings of pleural effusion and empyema are decreased chest wall expansion; diminished, markedly decreased, or absent breath sounds and a flat percussion note; and, in the presence of large amounts of pleural fluid, a contralateral mediastinal shift. Fever, rapid respirations, shallow breathing, and involuntary or voluntary splinting of the affected side of the chest accompany parapneumonic effusions and empyema. Large effusions can be detected by physical examination alone. Small pleural effusions may be overlooked, however, without the aid of radiographic examination. If the patient is asymptomatic and an effusion is suspected to be small, further diagnostic tests would not be warranted to confirm its presence. However, if the patient has symptoms, e.g., fever, malaise, for which no other cause is apparent, then a thorough diagnostic work-up should follow. Small effusions may be recognized by comparing radiographs (lateral and anterior-posterior films) of the chest that are taken upright with the lateral decubitus radiograph with the affected lung inferiorly. Small effusions should be suspected when the costophrenic angle is blunted or one hemidiaphragm is obscured. However, when an effusion or empyema is loculated, little, if any, change occurs in its configuration in the lateral decubitus position. Small or loculated effusions may need to be confirmed by diagnostic thoracentesis, by ultrasound, or by computed tomography.

A diagnostic thoracentesis should be done in all cases and 50 to 100 ml withdrawn. The tests usually done on pleural fluid include determination of lactic dehydrogenase (LDH), total protein, glucose, and pH; culture for bacteria and other microorganisms as appropriate; Gram stain of smear; total white blood cell and differential counts; a total red blood cell count; and, when available, determination of adenosine deaminase (ADA). The selection of tests should appropriately reflect the list of diagnostic possibilities. Exudative pleural effusions contain high levels of LDH, usually greater than 200 IU (or a level more than 60% of the serum LDH level), total protein values of at least 50 percent of the serum protein (usually 3.0 g per 100 ml or greater in the effusion), glucose levels of less than 60 mg per 100 ml, pH less than 7.30, and a total white blood cell count of more than 1,000 to 2,000 per cubic centimeter. Polymorphonuclear leukocytes predominate in parapneumonic effusions of bacterial origin, and lymphocytes, in tuberculous effusions. The combination of an ADA value of more than 40 IU per liter and a polymorphonuclear leukocyte exudate strongly suggests a parapneumonic effusion. When pulmonary tuberculosis is suspected, a pleural biopsy should be done for identification of the organism by histologic examination and culture. Grossly bloody effusions, however, are unusual as part of infections and usually indicate malignant neoplasma, pulmonary infarction, or trauma to the chest.

TREATMENT

The basic approach to the treatment of parapneumonic pleural effusions and empyema involves therapy directed both at eradication of the infection and removal of the accumulated fluid. The appropriate choice of antibiotics demands that the infecting organism be identified. In the treatment of parapneumonic effusions (except those caused by *Mycoplasmae pneumoniae*), antibiotics should be used intravenously and in adequate doses. The selection of antibiotics for the treatment of parapneumonic effusions and empyema follows these guidelines: for *S. pneumoniae* and hemolytic streptococci, aqueous penicillin (2.4 to 6.0 million units daily in divided doses IV), ampicillin (200 to 400 mg per kilogram per day IV), or for the penicillin-allergic patient, vancomycin (0.5 g every 6 hours IV); for *S. aureus*, penicillin for appropriately sensitive strains—otherwise, nafcillin (2 g every 4 hours IV; for

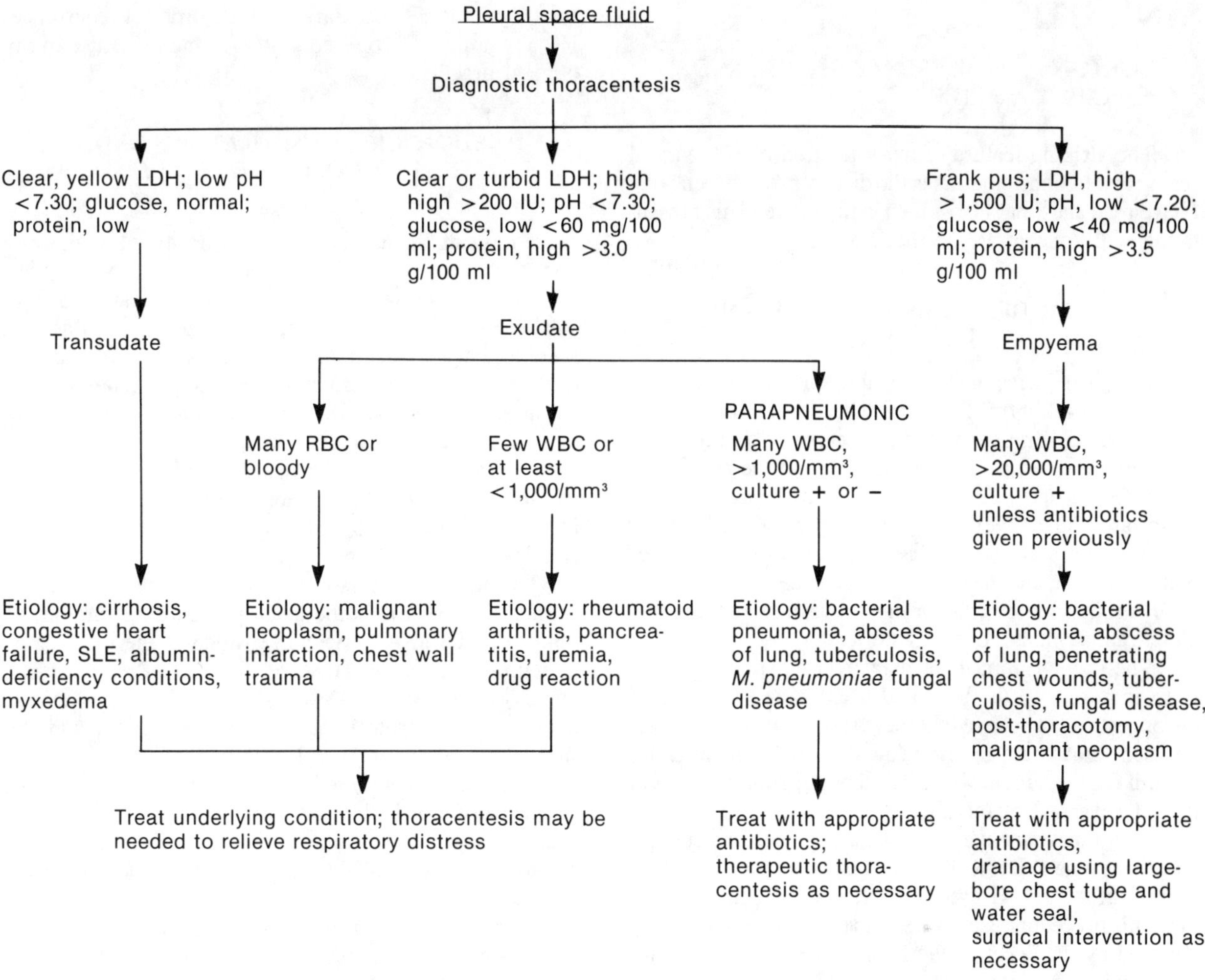

Figure 1 Evaluation, common etiologies, and management of pleural effusion and empyema.

H. influenzae, chloramphenicol (50 mg per kilogram per day IV); for anaerobic bacteria (except *Bacteroides fragilis*), penicillin G; for *B. fragilis*, clindamycin (300 to 900 mg every 6 hours IV); for gram-negative bacteria, tobramycin (3 to 5 mg per kilogram per day in divided doses IV) alone or in combination with pipercillin, especially for *Pseudomonas* species (3.0 g every 4 hours IV); and for *Mycoplasma pneumoniae*, erythromycin (1 g every 6 hours PO).

Parapneumonic effusions usually clear without drainage procedures. However, a few of these patients may require one or more therapeutic thoracenteses. When the fluid has a pH of less than 7.00 and/or a glucose level below 40 mg per 100 ml, consideration should be given to immediate closed-tube thoracostomy. Complicated parapneumonic effusions and empyema require complete drainage using a large-bore thoracostomy tube. The tube is positioned in the most dependent portion and connected to underwater-seal drainage with continuous suction. As the volume of drainage diminishes to less than 50 ml daily or ceases, the chest tube is gradually withdrawn. Adhesions or a "lung peel" require surgical intervention. When the lung does not reexpand or when a "pleural peel" forms, thoracotomy and a decortication procedure must be performed. Such procedures are necessary in relatively few cases of empyema.

SINUSITIS

BURTON A. WAISBREN, B.S., M.S., M.D,
F.A.C.P., F.A.S.I.D.

The striking feature of my reflection of 30 years of seeing and treating sinusitis is the dichotomy between what I have read and what I have seen in my office. This presentation will concentrate on the latter.

INITIAL DIAGNOSIS AND TREATMENT

Lucy Freeman, in an enjoyable book entitled *Flight from Fear* (delightful for those who do not suffer from sinus trouble), emphasized many years ago that hostility is an important cause of sinus trouble. At the first interview, facing up to this possibility with the patient is as important a maneuver as any other. It may take months of psychiatric care to achieve acceptance on the part of both the patient and the doctor that sinusitis is a psychiatric problem; this etiologic factor must always be kept in mind and attempts made to deal with it.

The second immediate maneuver for the physician is to inquire into the use, and usually the overuse, of decongestants. I believe that these should seldom, if ever, be used. However, the first few days without them are painful for the patient who gives them up, and the patient must be warned of this fact.

The third maneuver is saline lavage performed with an ear syringe filled with warm saline (a pinch of salt in a glass of water). If used three times a day for several days this procedure usually heals the mucosa that has been battered by the decongestant, allows its swelling to subside, and, most important, allows drainage to begin.

Fourth, the patients should be taught to breathe steam after each lavage, perhaps by putting a towel over the head, bending over the wash basin, and turning on hot water while inhaling the steam. They then may find it advantageous to put hot moist towels over the face for 10–15 minutes.

This approach to sinus complaints will, in my experience, resolve the great majority of such problems providing the patient can be made to acknowledge psychological as well as the addictive aspects of the nasal decongestants. However, when the problem is recurrent, I often add tetracycline, 500 mg three times a day for 4 days, to the steam lavage and instruct the patient to start the entire program as soon as the congestion, headache, and sore face that signal an attack of sinus trouble begin. Tetracycline is not indicated if the patient is hypersensitive to it or if the organism is resistant; in the latter case the choice of antibiotic should be based on the results of in vitro studies.

With the knowledge that this five-pronged approach will solve the vast majority of sinus problems, let us consider the type of case that might drive a physician to a reference book of this sort. What pathologic processes or deficiencies can lead to chronic recurrent sinusitis? These will be listed in the order in which they should be ruled out, but not necessarily in their order of recurrence. Here, again, the proposed system is the one I use in my clinical practice.

ETIOLOGIC CONSIDERATIONS AND DIAGNOSTIC WORK-UP

Culturing the nasal secretions is rarely of help, since one rarely cultures known pathogens. The one exception to this is when a pure culture of coagulase-positive staphylococci is obtained on repeated cultures. In this case specific, intense treatment of the staphylococcus is in order. I never use a single agent to treat a serious staphylococcal infection because when this organism is recalcitrant or in an inaccessible place, one ought to try to attack it not only at its cell membranes, but at its ribosomal apparatus as well. For this, oxacillin and lincomycin, given in divided doses of 1.5 g per day for 10 days, are an easily tolerated and safe regimen.

Quantitative immunoglobulins should be studied next. Intractable sinusitis is the usual presenting symptom of immunoglobulin A deficiency, which is the most common immunodeficiency disease. The lack of secretory immunoglobulin A (IgA) causes inability of mucous membranes to protect themselves adequately, and the sinuses are particularly vulnerable.

A second immunologic deficiency disease that might be the cause, particularly of staphylococcal sinusities, is Job's disease, which should be ruled out by an IgE determination and, if available, a polymorphonuclear movement study.

A third immune disease to be sought in difficult cases is granulomatous disease of children, or even adults, in which case tests of polymorphonuclear function show abnormalities. In the case of either Job's disease or granulomatous disease, treatment of the sinusitis depends on control of the underlying immune deficiency with long-term antibiotic and immunomodulation therapy.

Roentgenograms of the sinuses are indicated in all cases of intractable sinusitis, and they occasionally reveal cysts, tumors, or other indications for surgery. However, any type of surgical intervention in sinusitis, whether local lavage or the notorious Caldwell-Luc operation, is usually counterproductive.

Bone scans, on the other hand, are often useful, since they may reveal osteomyelitis of the temporal or maxillary bones, in which case intensive, long-term treatment for this disease is indicated. By the same token, indium scans are helpful because they may reveal a drainable abscess requiring surgery.

A nasal smear may often be helpful in formulating a therapeutic program for sinusitis. If the smear reveals only eosinophils, one would tend to be more aggressive in searching for an allergic cause for the disease.

Additional features of the patient's history to be considered on the initial contact are history of aspirin sensitivity; presence of nasal polyps, bronchitis, asthma, smoking, recurrent boils, recurrent pneumonia; and in this day and age, life style.

Nasal polyps are not an unusual accompaniment to chronic sinusitis and must always be considered. As an internist I have never been able to get a good look into the nasal cavity and suggest that this should be done by an expert. When one finds nasal polyps, aspirin sensitivity should be considered. The patient may have to give up aspirin entirely and even may need to search out a salicylate-free diet. When one finds polyps, asthma often is a factor as well and, in fact, may be the problem that needs the most attention. The treatment of nasal polyps with beclomethasone nasal spray 42 μg per metered spray has been a major development in the control of this condition, and since it has been used the necessity for "scooping out' nasal polyps at frequent intervals seems to have decreased.

OTHER ETIOLOGIES

When one arrives at the point where hostility, drainage, moderate antibiotic use, nasal polyps, aspirin sensitivity, asthma, and immune deficiency have been considered and treated or ruled out, five other possibilities must be considered if symptoms persist. These are fungal infection, bronchiectasis, cystic fibrosis, a tumor, or mixed bacterial infection with anaerobes.

Although one should try to obtain an accurate culture of the sinus secretions, it is often necessary to treat empirically with a combination of antibiotics that will destroy anaerobes and attack resistant bacteria at more than one metabolic site. For this I suggest a combination of chloramphenicol 2 grams per day, lincomycin 1.5 grams per day, and Flagyl 1 gram per day with 10 ml of gamma globulin given as a potentiator. Others may desire to use more conservative and traditional antibiotic combinations.

When one orders cultures for fungi, it should always be remembered that *Actinomyces* is an anaerobic fungus and that blastomycosis is usually best diagnosed by biopsy. Of course, mucomycosis must always be considered as a cause of chronic invading sinusitis in diabetic patients. Blastomycosis and mucomycosis respond to amphotericin B total dose of 1.5 grams; a daily dose of 5 to 20 mg can be increased from 5 mg per day by 5-mg increments to 20 mg per day, provided the patient's blood urea nitrogen level does not become elevated. This is continued until the patient gets a total dose of 1.5 grams. Of course, penicillin is the drug of choice for actinomycosis. Penicillin G 10 million units IV per day for 1 month will cure actinomycosis. It can be given on an outpatient basis via a subclavian catheter left in place. Treatment should be prolonged in these cases for at least a month.

The diagnosis of cystic fibrosis, even in young adults, or of bronchiectasis should be relatively easy if one thinks of them.

Tumors of the sinuses are not rare and they should always be sought in problem cases. The computed tomographic scan will prove a valuable tool when it is added to the more traditional roentgenograms and bone scans. Wegener's granulomatosis is the most common tumor of the sinuses, but the literature abounds with case reports of neoplasms of various other types. The tissue diagnosis in these cases will direct treatment.

Finally, in addition to the immunologic work-up mentioned in the beginning of this paper, in today's society the advent of intractable sinusitis is not infrequently the first manifestation of an acquired immune deficiency (AIDS). As is becoming well known, AIDS is best diagnosed by the test for HTV-III and by T-cell subsets, which should show a deficiency of helper T-cells. Beta-2-microglobulin, for some reason, is also markedly elevated in this disease.

BRONCHITIS

SANFORD CHODOSH, M.D.

CHRONIC BRONCHITIS

The morbidity and premature mortality associated with chronic bronchitis account for the significant societal and economic importance of this disease. Decreasing this impact is dependent on the proper recognition of the disease and utilization of appropriate therapy. Although chronic bronchitis is not solely related to infection, the treatment of the frequently occurring bacterial bronchial infections appears to be a major factor in the course of the disease.

Definition

The definition of chronic bronchitis is based on the clinical symptoms of chronic productive cough on most days for at least three months of the year for two successive years. The diagnosis should not be accepted until other causes of these symptoms have been excluded, for example, asthma, tuberculosis, carcinoma of the lung, cystic fibrosis, congestive heart failure, and pulmonary mycoses.

Epidemiology

More than 30 percent of cigarette-smoking Americans have the symptoms of chronic bronchitis, but nonsmokers also have the disease. It is a common disease throughout the world, being most prevalent in adults, with a small male-to-female predominance. Cigarette smoking is the predominant factor associated with chronic bronchitis, but exposure to air pollution, bronchopulmonary infections, inhalation of occupational dusts and fumes, and allergic respiratory disease are commonly noted historical antecedents.

Pathophysiology

The two basic underlying characteristics of the pathophysiology appear to be the vagal-stimulating and cellular toxic responses of the bronchial tissues to the various stimuli. The cholinergic action of the vagal stimulation effects an increase of the bronchomotor tone of the bronchial smooth muscle, which results in a narrowing of the bronchial airways. Hypersecretion of mucoproteins by the bronchial submucosal mucous glands and the mucosal goblet cells is also partially a cholinergic effect and leads to hypertrophy and hyperplasia of these tissues. Excessive intralumenal secretions contribute to the bronchial obstruction. Many of the toxic stimuli cause injury and death of bronchial mucosal cells, which may lead to shallow mucosal ulceration. Ciliary activity is markedly impaired and, when combined with the increased secretions, leads to a breakdown of the essential clearance of foreign substances by the mucociliary escalator. Toxic agents consequently have prolonged contact with the bronchial tissues. The result of this acute tissue damage is a classic inflammatory response in which the polymorphonuclear neutrophil is prominent. Macrophages will predominate when the areas recovering from injury outnumber areas with new acute damage. The exudate that results from the inflammatory response mixes with the mucinous secretions and, when coughed out, is the sputum that is characteristic of chronic bronchitis. Microscopic evaluation of this sputum will reveal a predominance of neutrophils or macrophages, depending on the acuteness of the inflammatory process, less than 3 percent eosinophils, and about 10 percent small, degenerated bronchial epithelial cells.

The bacteria most commonly associated with infectious exacerbations in the chronic bronchitic are *Hemophilus influenzae* and *Streptococcus pneumoniae*. Although less common, *Neisseria* species can account for 5 to 10 percent of acute exacerbations. Gram-negative enterics are rarely etiologic in nonhospitalized bronchitics, and staphylococci are virtually never seen in such patients. Besides its role in acute infections, *H. influenzae* also indolently infects the bronchial mucosa and likely serves as a chronic intrinsic stimulus and a nidus for subsequent acute bacterial exacerbations.

Clinical Manifestations

The symptoms and signs of many chronic bronchitics never extend beyond chronic cough and sputum production, and most patients accept these symptoms as being normal. Airways obstruction may be measured early in the course of the disease, long before shortness of breath is clinically noted. The demonstration of airways obstruction is not diagnostic of chronic bronchitis, but physiologic measurements help in the periodic assessment of the severity of the disease.

Recurrent bronchopulmonary infections are common. The frequency of occurrence of acute bronchitis and pneumonia varies considerably among bronchitics, and individual patterns can be altered by therapeutic interventions. Acute exacerbations in chronic bronchitis are characterized clinically by increases of cough frequency and severity, increased production of a more purulent sputum, chest congestion and discomfort, increased dyspnea and wheezing, malaise, feverishness, and chilliness. It is not necessary for all of these symptoms and signs to be present. This complex of symptoms is not pathognomic of a bacterial etiology and can occur with acute exacerbations due to viral infection, secretion clearance problems, exposure to inhalant toxins, or even asthma.

The specific etiology can be determined by examination of the sputum. The sputum criteria for a bacterial etiology are an increase of neutrophilic inflammation and the presence of significant numbers of bacteria on Gram stain. Neutrophil increase is manifested by a combination of increases of sputum volume, the percentage of sputum cells that are neutrophils, and the concentration of cells in the specimen. When baseline numbers or percentgage of neutrophils are not known, it is necessary to depend on history, e.g., the patient reports increased raising of sputum. The common bacteria seen in these exacerbations are small, gram-negative, pleomorphic, coccobacillary bacteria consistent with *H. influenzae*, gram-positive diplococci consistent with *S. pneumoniae* gram-negative kidney-shaped diplococci consistent with *Neisseria* species, or a mixture of these. Table 1 gives the mean numbers of bacteria per oil-immersion field in the sputum Gram stains of stable chronic bronchitics. An increase is significant when the numbers of bacteria exceed three standard deviations from these mean values. By these criteria for bacterial infection, only 50 percent of several thousand acute exacerbations observed in a large population of patients with chronic bronchial disease were associated with bacterial infection. The sputum cellular and microbiologic characteristics of nonbacterial exacerbations lack evidence of the combined increases of neutrophilic inflammation and bacterial populations.

TABLE 1 Numbers of Bacteria per Gram Stain Oil-Immersion Field in Clinically Stable Chronic Bronchitics

	Number of Bacteria	
	Mean	*Mean + 3 SD*
Hemophilus influenzae-like	1.3	11.4
Streptococcus pneumoniae-like	1.9	7.7
Neisseria-like	0.9	17.4

Bacteriologic cultures, drug sensitivity testing, or colony counts are rarely helpful in chronic bronchitis and can actually provide misleading and delayed information as compared with the prompt results available from Gram stain.

Pathogenic bacteria are frequently isolated from chronic bronchitics when no other evidence of infection is present. Peripheral blood leukocytosis and fever are infrequently associated with acute bacterial exacerbations of chronic bronchitis. If these are present, the possibility of pneumonitis should be considered. A small percentage of chronic bronchitics have frequent exacerbations of bronchial bacterial infection despite adequate treatment of each acute episode. Bronchiectasis or other bronchial pathology should be suspected in such patients.

Treatment

General Management

The management of acute bacterial exacerbations is easier if the chronic bronchitic is already on a good regimen of background therapy. This should include control of inhalants, e.g., cigarette smoke, air pollutants, marijuana, or occupational dusts and fumes, management of secretions, and treatment of airways obstruction. If background therapy is not in place, it may be necessary to institute these measures concomitant with the antimicrobial therapy. Chronic bronchitic smokers must be told repetitively to stop, and those who do stop need support to continue abstinence. Active cigarette smokers take longer to clear bronchial infections than do nonsmokers or ex-smokers. Exposure to other toxic inhalants should also be decreased as much as possible. These simple measures usually result in marked alleviation, if not complete disappearance, of bronchitic symptoms.

Patients who continue to have chronic productive cough usually will benefit from measures aimed at improving the clearance of secretion. Hydration is the cornerstone of secretion management. The regular oral ingestion of extra nonalcoholic fluids is essential. In colder climates, winter heating reduces the relative humidity and results in thicker secretions that are more difficult to clear. This problem can be greatly relieved if humidification is provided during the heating season. When this is done, many expected ''winter colds' fail to materialize. Expectorant therapy should be tried in those bronchitics who persist with cough and secretion problems. Subjective benefit is often noted when adequate dosages are employed: either 300 to 600 mg of guaifenesin and/or 10 to 30 drops of saturated solution of potassium iodide four times a day. Occasional patients with resistant secretion problems may benefit from aerosolized mucolytic therapy provided as nebulized acetylcysteine inhaled three to four times a day (3-4 ml of a 10 percent solution). My preference is to give the higher doses, then back down as the patient begins to respond. Physiotherapy aimed at loosening secretions is indicated when other measures are not sufficiently effective. All of these measures may be needed concurrently in acutely ill, hospitalized patients, whereas the vast majority of outpatients can be managed with only hydration and expectorants.

Chronic bronchitics who have exertional dyspnea or more than moderate airways obstruction on pulmonary function testing should be treated with continuous theophylline therapy. Sufficient theophylline should be given to attain a therapeutic blood level (10 to 20 μg per ml). The precise mechanism of action in chronic bronchitis is not clear, but most patients report subjective improvement of exercise ability with theophylline therapy. True bronchodilator therapy for chronic bronchitics is possible with the use of anticholinergic agents, e.g., ipratropium bromide or glycopyrrolate, but these are not yet approved for use in the United States.

Antimicrobial therapy

Prompt and adequate antimicrobial therapy for the bronchial infections that occur in chronic bronchitis is essential. Double-blinded and crossover studies demonstrate that treatment with antimicrobial agents with fair activity against *H. influenzae* (e.g., cefaclor) result in a high rate of treatment failures as compared with agents with good activity (e.g., doxycycline). The goal of treatment of acute bacterial exacerbations is to decrease the overall morbidity of chronic bronchitis by prompt reversal of the acute infectious process, providing the longest period free of acute exacerbations and minimizing troublesome adverse effects (Table 2). Most antimicrobial agents with satisfactory in vitro activities against *H. influenzae, S. pneumoniae*, and *Neisseria* species are also clinically efficacious. Microorganisms resistant to some of these drugs have been reported with increasing frequency in some geographic locations, but the expected correlation between in vitro resistance and clinical outcome is not always evident.

It is important to treat all documented episodes of acute bacterial bronchitis, since it is not possible to predict the course that the infection will take. Prompt treatment shortens the period of morbidity. The antimicrobial doses should lean toward the top of the recommended range, and the minimal duration of therapy should be 10 to 14 days. Occasional patients require longer therapy. Experience from a series of blinded and controlled studies indicates that prompt reversal of the acute process will occur in well over 85 percent of exacerbations treated with oral ampicillin, bacampicillin, amoxacillin, tetracycline, doxycycline, or trimethoprim-sulfamethoxazole. However, there are significant differences among these in regard to the posttreatment infection-free period and the nature of side effects. Table 2 details daily dosages for a number of these agents.

The drug of choice is still ampicillin, which is efficient and economical. However, penicillin allergy limits its use, and the need to ingest drug on an empty stomach affects compliance. Most patients note some gastrointestinal adverse effects, but this does not usually interfere with completion of the prescribed course. Bacampicillin,

TABLE 2 Oral Antimicrobial Agents for Acute Bacterial Bronchitis in Chronic Bronchitics

	Dosage Schedule	Percentage of Treatment Failures*	Infection-Free Period†
Ampicillin	0.5–1.0 g QID	12.7	1.00
Bacampicillin	800 mg BID	15.8	1.01
Amoxicillin	0.5–1.0 g TID	9.5	0.86
Doxycycline	100 mg BID	14.5	0.85
Minocycline	100 mg BID	23.8	0.72
Tetracycline	0.5 g QID	--	--
Trimethoprim/sulfamethoxazole	2–3 tablets BID‡	19.0	0.51
Methacycline	300 mg BID	21.1	0.46
Erythromycin§	0.5 g QID	--	--
Cephalexin§	0.5 g QID	35.3	0.31
Cefaclor§	250 mg TID	70.0	0.31
Penicillin V Potassium§	0.5 g QID		

Note: Drugs are listed in order of choice. Where doses are expressed as ranges, determination of dose should be made on the basis of severity of infection. This author prefers to start with high doses.

* From double-blinded crossover studies. Defined as failure to respond within the 2-week treatment period or rebound infection within 2 weeks after treatment.

† From double-blinded crossover studies. Ratios calculated relative to ampicillin, with which the infection-free periods varied from 117 to 302 days.

‡ 80 mg TMP and 400 mg SMZ per tablet.

§ Recommended only when better-choice antimicrobial agents cannot be used.

which converts to active ampicillin after gastrointestinal absorption, is as effective as ampicillin. Advantages over ampicillin are twice-a-day dosing without regard to meals, almost total absorption, very high blood levels, and fewer gastrointestinal adverse effects. The cost of the drug is its major drawback. Amoxicillin does not provide as long an infection-free period as ampicillin.

When ampicillin is contraindicated, one of the synthetic tetracyclines should be the drug of choice. Regular tetracycline presents a problem of compliance even at the minimum dose of 0.5 g four times per day. Doxycycline and minocycline are comparable in efficacy, require only twice-a-day dosing without regard to meals, and have fewer compliance-restricting effects. Trimethoprim-sulfamethoxazole is an acceptable choice if ampicillin or tetracyclines cannot be utilized. However, it has a much shorter infection-free period (Table 2). Cefaclor, cephalexin, and erythromycin should only be considered if the use of all of the other agents are contraindicated. These antimicrobial agents are associated with a high incidence of treatment failure and early reinfection.

Parenteral therapy is indicated when the patient either is sufficiently ill to be hospitalized, is not responding to therapy, or therapy involves agents not administered orally. The agent chosen should be active against the predominant organism(s) observed on Gram stain. It is not necessary to treat against all organisms recovered on sputum culture. Ordinarily, ampicillin (6 g per day) is appropriate. If the patient is penicillin allergic or the organism is resistant to ampicillin, the alternatives are a parenteral tetracycline such as doxycycline, 200 to 400 mg per day (dose depending on the severity of infection); a cephalosporin such as cefazolin, 3 g per day, or cefuroxime, 750 mg to 1.5 g every 8 hours (depending on the severity of infection and whether coverage for *H. influenzae* is necessary); or chloramphenicol, 2 to 4 g per day (I prefer to start with 4 g and decrease the dose as the patient responds to therapy because of chloramphenicol's toxicity).

A small subgroup of chronic bronchitics will have frequent infectious exacerbations despite adequate response to each course of antimicrobial drugs. Long-term antimicrobial therapy is usually beneficial in these special cases, and the dose required to prevent break-through infection has to be determined for each patient. The duration of therapy required to alter the pattern of recrudescence may vary from 3 months to as long as the lifetime of the bronchitic.

Prevention

Bronchitics should be instructed to avoid conditions that could make them more susceptible to bacterial exacerbations. Useful measures are avoidance of circumstances that may expose them to viral respiratory infections, maintenance of good secretion clearance, bronchodilator therapy, and yearly immunization with influenza vaccine. A single immunization with polyvalent pneumococcal vaccine is recommended, although efficacy in these patients has not been demonstrated. The routine chronic use of antimicrobial agents to prevent infections is not recommended. Extensive anecdotal experience suggests that optimizing the background therapy and the intensive treatment of each acute bacterial exacerbation do reduce the frequency of occurrence and duration of subsequent bronchial infections.

ACUTE BRONCHITIS

Definition

Acute bronchitis is an inflammatory process of the bronchi that is acute in onset and self-limited. Cough, often productive of small amounts of sputum, is the prominent respiratory symptom. Acute bronchitis is usually preceded by or associated with upper respiratory involvement, which may be manifested by coryza, pharyngitis, laryngitis, and headache.

Epidemiology

The etiology of acute bronchitis is either infectious or irritative. Acute bronchitis due to inhalation of toxic fumes, dusts, smoke, or fire is easily identified historically. The commonest infectious causes of acute bronchitis are respiratory viruses such as influenza, adenoviruses, rhinoviruses, cornaviruses, and parainfluenza viruses. Although commoner in winter months in temperate climates, outbreaks may occur at any time or place if the conditions for a high rate of infectivity exist. *Mycoplasma pneumoniae* is a less common etiology than viruses, but should be considered during epidemic-like outbreaks. A primary bacterial etiology without underlying chronic pulmonary disease is common.

Pathophysiology

The pathology in acute viral bronchitis is remarkably similar to that seen in bronchial asthma and is characterized by edematous and hyperemic bronchial mucosa and increased mucus secretion. The airways are generally more reactive to inhaled irritants, again simulating asthma. Intracellular inclusion bodies in the bronchial epithelial cells and areas of denuded epithelium can be seen. The inflammatory cellular response is usually neutrophilic, although a monocytic response has been reported in mycoplasmal infection.

Differential Diagnosis

In young children, acute viral bronchitis may be confused with asthma. The absence of any evidence of atopic disease should exclude asthma. It is important to differentiate viral from bacterial acute bronchitis. With the latter, the duration of symptoms is often longer, and a sputum Gram stain will quickly resolve the problem. Pneumonia may be associated with acute bronchitis and should be suspected in patients who are sicker, have pleuritic pain, and have fever and leukocytosis.

Treatment

Acute viral bronchitis is generally treated symptomatically by the patient without contact with the medical care system. This therapy should consist of hydration, rest, aspirin, expectorants, and antitussive agents. Oral fluids should be increased and humidification of the air is often soothing. Guaifenesin in doses of 100 to 300 mg every 4 hours is useful when secretion clearance is a problem. Standard doses of aspirin alleviate some of the systemic symptoms associated with the acute bronchitis. Antitussive agents are indicated when coughing interferes with normal activities and simple measures (cough drops, simple syrup, expectorants) have failed. Dextromethorphan, 15 to 30 mg, codeine, 15 to 30 mg, or one of the codeine derivatives may be needed to control cough. The higher doses of both expectorant and antitussives are indicated for the more troublesome symptoms. If the symptoms of airways obstruction are troublesome, the temporary use of bronchodilator therapy should be considered. Antibiotics are not indicated for acute viral bronchitis. When *M. pneumoniae* infection is suspected, a tetracycline or erythromycin may be indicated. However, most cases will resolve spontaneously without such treatment.

Bacterial infection should be considered when symptoms of acute bronchitis last beyond a week. The diagnosis should be confirmed by Gram stain of the sputum. The presence of purulent sputum indicates inadequate secretion clearance and is not pathognomic for a bacterial etiology. When bacterial infection is documented, treatment for 7 days with a tetracycline or ampicillin is indicated (see comments in Chronic Bronchitis section).

Prevention

Individuals who have frequent recurrences of acute bronchitis should be suspected of having some underlying chronic lung disease. Identification of such disease and subsequent treatment will often reduce the incidence and severity of the recurrent attacks. In patients with clinically significant cardiopulmonary disease, annual immunization with influenza vaccine is recommended, as is the routine immunization of children with pertussis vaccine.

LUNG ABSCESS

RICHARD D. MEYER, M.D.

Lung abscess is defined as pulmonary parenchymal suppuration with a single or multiple area(s) of necrosis leading to cavity formation, frequently accompanied by an air-fluid level. A size of 2 cm or more on chest radiograph, the usual diagnostic screening method, has been suggested as an arbitrary dividing point; the presence of multiple cavities of less than 2 cm primarily within one pulmonary segment or lobe—generally in patients who are markedly ill—has been called necrotizing pneumonia. Both conditions are part of a spectrum of infection that frequently originates as pneumonitis, primarily from anaerobic bacteria as etiologic agents, and chest radiographs in both necrotizing pneumonitis and lung abscess frequently show parenchymal infiltrates associated with and surrounding cavitation.

The vast majority of lung abscesses are termed primary and involve anaerobic bacteria that have gained access to pulmonary parenchymal tissue by aspiration. Secondary lung abscesses follow an associated condition such as localized obstruction (e.g., carcinoma, foreign body), systemic infection (e.g., *Staphylococcus aureus* tricuspid valvular endocarditis and septic pulmonary emboli), or immunosuppression from an underlying disorder or chemotherapy predisposing to infection.

PREDISPOSING FACTORS AND PATHOGENESIS

Aspiration of oropharyngeal secretions is the major predisposing factor; it can be found in more than 75 percent of patients and probably occurs in an even greater percentage, including the otherwise normal patients who present with a lung abscess. The commonest causes of suspected aspiration are altered consciousness from, in general order of occurrence, alcoholism (acute or chronic), cerebrovascular accidents, drug overdose or abuse, general anesthesia, seizure disorder, and miscellaneous conditions (e.g., head trauma, diabetic coma). Other factors are presence of periodontal disease which is found in substantially more than one-half of patients in some series, dysphagia from neurologic or esophageal dysfunction, and, in fewer patients, recent dental surgery, vomiting or presence of a nasogastric tube. Factors predisposing a secondary lung abscess include bronchial obstruction from carcinoma, bronchiectasis, lung cysts, bullous emphysema, and pulmonary infarction.

The dependent pulmonary segments in a patient lying on his back or side are the apical segments of the lower lobes and the posterior segments of the upper lobes, respectively. The most commonly affected area following aspiration is the posterior segment of the right upper lobe. The lower lobes are more involved following aspiration in the upright or semi-upright position. However, virtually any segment of any pulmonary lobe may be involved.

Coughing, ciliary action, and the actions of polymorphonuclear leukocytes and alveolar macrophages constitute some of the local host defenses to the aspirated material containing bacteria. Foreign bodies and gastric acidity pose additional threats to the patient in aspiration. Failure of host defenses leads to a pneumonitis, which then may result in lung abscess and, in about one-third of cases, an associated empyema. The usual interval for cavity formation on radiographs is approximately 1 week.

BACTERIOLOGY

Meticulous studies implicate anaerobic bacteria in more than 90 percent of cases of primary lung abscess, and anaerobes are recovered alone in about one-third of total cases. The usual number of anaerobic isolates was two to three per case in earlier studies, but in other recent studies, a mean of six per case has been recovered. The commonest isolates are *Fusobacterium nucleatum, Bacteroides melaninogenicus, Peptostreptococcus* species, *Peptococcus* species, *Bacteroides* species other than *Bacteroides fragilis*, microaerophilic streptococci, and other organisms. *B. fragilis*, which is regularly resistant to penicillin G, is found in about 5 percent of cases, but the emergence of beta-lactamase-mediated penicillin resistance has also been documented in other isolates of anaerobes. These resistant isolates from this anatomic area include *B. melaninogenicus* as well as other isolates in the *Bacteroides melaninogenicus*–Bacteroides asachrolyticus group; less commonly found are isolates of *Bacteroides ureolyticus* and members of the *Bacteroides ruminocola* group.

The most frequently isolated aerobes are *S. aureus, Klebsiella pneumoniae*, and other enteric gram-negative bacilli. The frequently nosocomial source of these and many other aerobes is obvious. Less commonly found are *Hemophilus influenzae, Pseudomonas aeruginosa,* and *Streptococcus pneumoniae* type III. *Legionella pneumophilia* as a sole agent causes lung abscess probably only in immunosuppressed patients, particularly those receiving corticosteroids.

CLINICAL MANIFESTATIONS

The usual course is subacute; at presentation the mean duration of symptoms (low-grade fever, productive cough, and malaise) is 12 days. The course may be longer and more indolent in many patients; in those, weight loss and anemia may be found. Physical examination reveals signs of a localized pneumonia; it may also reveal evidence of a predisposing condition and a pleural effusion.

DIAGNOSIS

Radiographs are the cornerstone of diagnosis. Thoracic computerized tomography (CT) is usually not necessary but may be more sensitive than plain radiographs. Culture sources for bacteriologic confirmation are limited. Expectorated sputum should not be examined for anaerobes because it is always contaminated with the anaerobic flora of the mouth. Bronchoscopy using a shielded catheter (an uncomfortable procedure not always reliable for cultures) or transtracheal aspirate (a potentially risky procedure) are required to obtain suitable specimens. It must be emphasized that although bacteriologic results and results of susceptibility tests are becoming more important in guiding management of certain lung abscesses, most patients who are only mildly or moderately ill with community-acquired typical lung abscess can be treated without any bacteriologic monitoring. If specimens are obtained for bacteriologic studies, they should be obtained before any antibiotic therapy. An exception occurs in a patient on therapy with significant clinical deterioration. Pleural fluid (empyema), which occurs in about one-third of patients with lung abscess is a source of easily obtainable material for culture and susceptibility testing. Thoracentesis should be almost invariably performed before consideration of transtracheal aspiration or bronchoscopy.

Indications for procedures other than thoracentesis are more controversial. These procedures must be performed by experienced individuals. Transtracheal aspiration specimens are suitable for anaerobic and aerobic cultures. Moreover, the procedure is not without discomfort or risk of complications and cannot be performed in uncooperative patients and in presence of uncorrectable bleeding diathesis or severe hypoxia. Fiberoptic bronchoscopy is frequently performed to rule out obstruction, and cultures are obtained then; however, they are unsuitable for culture because of upper airway contamination, adulteration with antibacterial topical anesthetics, and the fact that in common practice they are performed after a few days of antibiotic therapy. The exact role of bronchoscopy with semiquantitative cultures obtained with a shielded apparatus, such as the BFW brush (Medi-tech; Watertown, Massachusetts) remains to be shown. The role of percutaneous transthoracic needle aspiration is also under evaluation. Generally, it is most suitable for peripheral lesions; there is a risk of creating a bronchopleural fistula from entering a pulmonary cavity.

Blood cultures are rarely positive except in cases of secondary lung abscess. Tuberculosis, nocardiosis, infected lung cysts, bullous emphysema, and other conditions must be excluded. Malignancy as a cause of secondary lung abscess is another major concern in certain patients.

THERAPY

Prolonged antimicrobial treatment is the cornerstone of therapy. The choice of agent can be based on expected pathogens and patterns of susceptibility. Penicillin G has been the established drug of choice for therapy of primary lung abscess (doses given below). Reservations about its universal use in the nonallergic affected patient primarily center about two types of observations. The first are in vitro studies that document beta-lactamase-positive anaerobic isolates of the previously mentioned species in about 15 percent of recently carefully studied cases. Nonetheless, many such patients do respond to penicillin G therapy, a fact suggesting that only the majority of isolates need be susceptible in many patients. The second are clinical observations that (1) in occasional but dramatic examples, there are clinical failures of penicillin G therapy alone, followed by prompt response to the addition of metronidazole or substitution of clindamycin; and (2) the results of a comparative study of penicillin G given at a dose of 6 million units per day versus clindamycin, 1.8 g per day, that favored use of clindamycin (although some have commented that they would have preferred a higher dose of penicillin G). Clindamycin and metronidazole remain active against most of the implicated isolates resistant to penicillin G. Clindamycin may not be active against some peptostreptococci, fusobacteria, and nonperfringens clostridia. Metronidazole is not active against microaerophilic streptococci and actinomyces and thus cannot be used as single-agent therapy. For patients who are mildly to moderately ill, penicillin G can initially be given intravenously at a dosage of 10 to 18 million units per day (dose depending on condition of patient and severity of illness). Generally, initial therapy by the intravenous route is preferred in a mildly ill patient. After clinical improvement, which occurs usually in about a week and can be expected before radiographic improvement, lower doses (e.g., 8 to 12 million units) can be given intravenously and therapy changed to oral penicillin V, 2 g per day orally, or ampicillin or amoxicillin, 2 g per day (the latter is preferred for absorption). Generally, oral follow-up therapy with this or the other regimens will be required for about 6 to 12 weeks; a stable roentgenographic appearance should be present if complete healing does not occur. Clindamycin, 1.8 to 2.4 g per day (depending on severity) intravenously, is recommended for initial therapy for patients allergic to penicillin. Follow-up oral therapy for these patients is clindamycin, 300 mg orally four times per day. Cefoxitin, which is active against about 90 percent of *B. fragilis* as well as other beta-lactamase-producing anaerobes and the gram-positive organisms, can be given at a dose of 4 to 6 g per day (depending on severity) intravenously in a patient with minor penicillin allergy, as another alternative. Other cephalosporins, such as cefazolin, are likely to be efficacious also, but clinical data are more limited. Tetracycline now has little, if any, role in therapy of lung abscess because of marked resistance among the anaerobes. Chloramphenicol remains active in vitro but its potential for toxicity limits its use.

For seriously ill patients with community-acquired infection, the initial regimen should be either clindamycin, 1.8 to 2.4 g per day intravenously, or penicillin G, 10 to 18 million units per day intravenously, with metronidazole, 2 g per day either intravenously or orally. Follow-up therapy would be either clindamycin, 1.8 to 2.4 g per day orally, or penicillin, V 2 g orally (or ampicillin or amoxicillin 2 g orally), along with metronidazole, 1 to 2 g per day orally (dose of metronidazole depends on severity of illness and patient tolerance). For parenteral agents, penicillin G and metronidazole are less expensive than clindamycin or cefoxitin.

In nosocomial lung abscess, therapy should also be directed against any isolates of *S. aureus* and consideration given to treatment of enterics or *P. aeruginosa* if found. Generally, a penicillinase-resistant penicillin (e.g., nafcillin 9 g per day) or aminoglycosides (gentamicin, tobramycin, or amikacin dosed according to nomograms) may be used in addition to an agent directed against anaerobes. Amikacin should be considered in the setting of resistance to gentamicin. An example of therapy would be (1) clindamycin with an aminoglycoside; (2) penicillin G with nafcillin and an aminoglycoside; or (3) cefoxitin with an aminoglycoside. Obviously, duration of aminoglycoside therapy may be limited by the potential for toxicity. Generally, the role of the antipseudomonal penicillins is limited to treatment of nosocomially acquired lung abscess when their use is directed primarily against aerobic enteric organisms or *P. aeruginosa*; nonetheless, they are active against the majority of anaerobic isolates. The role of the third-generation cephalosporins is not clear, but they have less in vitro activity against the important anaerobes than does cefoxitin. Their use may be considered in nosocomial infection and directed by susceptibility test results, especially in situations in which prolonged aminoglycoside use is to be avoided. The carbapenem drug imipenem does, however, have excellent in vitro activity against virtually all of the important anaerobes as well as the enterics and could be considered for single-agent therapy for nosocomial lung abscess if *P. aeruginosa* is not a major pathogen.

Therapy against the common pathogens such as *S. aureus* in secondary lung abscess would include nafcillin or oxacillin (or an older cephalosporin such as cefazolin in the case of minor penicillin allergy and vancomycin in the case of major penicillin allergy. Combined therapy with cefazolin and an aminoglycoside will generally be required against *K. pneumoniae*, provided that the organism is sensitive in vitro.

Any associated empyema must be drained. Postural drainage should be used. Bronchoscopy may be required to rule out obstruction or tumor. With the exception of surgical drainage of an associated empyema, the role of surgical therapy is now very limited. A small number of cases require surgical extirpation of parenchymal tissue for severe hemoptysis or for smoldering chronic abscesses in bronchiectatic areas after a prolonged trial of antimicrobial therapy. Patients with abscess secondary to obstructing carcinoma may require surgery.

EPIGLOTTITIS (SUPRAGLOTTITIS)

EDWARD B. LEWIN, M.D.

EPIDEMIOLOGY

Inflammation of the supraglottic structures represents one of the true medical emergencies in pediatrics. It is primarily a disease of temperate climates and accounts for 0.5 to 1.0/1,000 pediatric admissions. Supraglottitis is responsible for approximately 5 percent of all pediatric admissions for inflammation of the laryngeal structures. Although the seasonal incidence of supraglottitis is variable, there is generally a winter peak with most cases occurring between October and March. Variation in year-to-year incidence within a particular area is also common.

There is a 3:2 male to female ratio in incidence. In contrast to *Hemophilus influenzae* B meningitis, in which the majority of cases occur in those younger than 2 years of age, supraglottitis typically occurs in the toddler. The mean age of patients with supraglottitis is 3.5 years, but there is considerable distribution around that mean, with 25 percent of cases occurring in children younger than 2 and 20 percent in those older than 4 years of age. By contrast, 57 percent of patients with laryngotracheitis (croup) occur among children younger than 2 years, with the remainder in the older child. Age is therefore a useful but insufficiently discriminatory guide in the differential diagnosis of infectious causes of stridor (Table 1).

Acute supraglottitis in the child is due almost exclusively to *H. influenzae* type B. Rare cases of bacteremic epiglottitis due to *S. pneumoniae* have been reported. The disease in adult compromised hosts may be caused by opportunistic pathogens (e.g., *Candida* species, *Aspergillus*), but even in the adult, *H. influenzae* type B is the most common etiologic agent.

ANATOMY, PATHOLOGY, AND PATHOGENESIS

The epiglottis is a leaf-like cartilaginous structure strategically placed so that the swelling that occurs with inflammation causes rapid encroachment upon the airway. Loosely adherent stratified squamous epithelium covers the anterior and superior one-third of the posterior portion of the epiglottis. A large potential space for the accumulation of edema fluid and inflammatory cells is thereby created. With developing inflammation, the epiglottis curls posteroinferiorly with inspiration, drawing the inflamed structures into the laryngeal outlet, resulting in the typical inspiratory stridor. Other supraglottic structures (e.g., the aryepiglottic folds, valleculae, ventricular bands, and arytenoids) are also involved—hence the term *supraglottitis*. The epiglottic valleculae are pools

TABLE 1 Differential Diagnosis of Acute Obstructions in the Region of the Larynx

Category	*Acute Epiglottitis*	*Bacterial Tracheitis*	*Acute Laryngo-Tracheitis*	*Spasmodic Croup*	*Laryngeal Diphtheria*	*Acute Angioneurotic Edema*	*Foreign Body*
Usual age of occurrence	1 to 8 years	3 weeks to 6 years	3 months to 3 years	3 months to 3 years	All ages	All ages	All ages
Past and family history	Not contributory	Unknown	Family history of croup	Family history of croup; perhaps previous attack	No or inadequate immunization	Allergic history; perhaps previous attack	Occasional history of ingestion
Prodrome	Occasional coryza	URI, brassy cough	Usually coryza	Minimal coryza	Usually pharyngitis	Occasionally cutaneous allergic manifestations	None
Onset (time to full-blown disease)	Rapid; 4–12 hours	5 hours to 3 days	Moderate but variable; 12–48 hours	Sudden; always at night	Slowly for 2–3 day period	Rapid	Usually sudden
Symptoms on presentation							
Fever	Yes; usually 39.5 °C (103 °F)	Yes; usually 38.5 °C–40 °C (101 °F–104 °F)	Yes; variable 37.8 °C–40.5 °C (100 °F–105 °F)	No	Yes; usually 37.8 °C–38.5 °C (100 °F–101 °F)	No	No; unless secondary infection
Hoarseness and barking cough	No	Yes	Yes	Yes	Yes	No	Usually no
Dysphagia	Yes; usually severe	No	No	No	Usually yes	Yes	Frequently yes
Inspiratory stridor	Yes; moderate to severe	Yes	Yes; minimal to severe	Yes; moderate	Yes; minimal to severe	Yes	Variable
Toxic appearance	Yes	Yes	Usually minimal	No	Usually no	No	No
Signs on presentation							
Oral cavity	Pharyngitis and excessive salivation	Normal	Usually minimal pharyngitis	Normal	Membranous pharyngitis	Pale appearance	Normal
Epiglottis	Cherry red and swollen	Normal	Normal	Normal	Usually normal; may contain membrane	Swollen and pale	Normal
Roentgenogram	Swollen epiglottis on lateral film	Subglottic narrowing on PA film	Subglottic narrowing on PA film	Not useful	Not useful	Swollen epiglottis on lateral film	May reveal foreign body
Laboratory							
Leukocyte count	Usually markedly elevated with increased percentage of band forms	Usually markedly elevated with increased percentage of band forms	Mildly elevated with 70% polymorphonuclear cells	Normal	Usually elevated with increased percentage of band forms	Normal; sometimes eosinophilia	Normal unless secondary infection
Bacteriology	Epiglottis and blood cultures yield *H. influenzae*, type B	Tracheal secretions, predominantly *S. aureus*	Only important if secondary infection suspected	Normal flora	Smear and culture from membrane reveals organism	Normal flora	Only important if secondary infection suspected
Clinical course	Rapidly progressive; cardiorespiratory arrest will occur within hours if not treated	Variable speed of progression of obstruction; requires artificial airway and suctioning	Variable speed of progression of obstruction; usually does not require surgical intervention	Symptoms of short duration with treatment; repeat attacks common	Slowly progressive obstruction of the airway	Variable; sometimes leads to rapid asphyxia without therapy	Variable depending upon size and substance of of foreign body

Note: Modified from Cherry JD. Croup. In: Feigin RD, Cherry JD, eds. Textbook of Pediatric Infectious Diseases. Philadelphia: WB Saunders Co, 1981.

where saliva accumulates before deglutition. Inflammation of these structures with consequent dysphagia leads to the drooling so typical in this disease. Inflammation does not extend downward into the vocal cords or subglottic region, and therefore, hoarseness and barking cough are uncommon.

As with *H. influenzae* B meningitis, there may be genetic predisposition to this disease (W-28 and W-17 antigens in the HL-A system, and the NS phenotype in the MNS erythrocytic antigen scheme, are found more commonly in patients with epiglottitis than in controls).

Older infants and children who develop supraglottitis seem to "contain" *H. influenzae* type B better than younger infants who are more prone to develop meningitis. This containment is reflected in a lower serum concentration of *H. influenzae* type B capsular polysaccharide and a more vigorous and sustained antibody response to the invading organism than occurs in their younger infant counterparts who develop meningitis.

CLINICAL MANIFESTATIONS

The typical presentation of supraglottitis is a previously well child in the fourth year of life with a history of less than 24 hours of fever and sore throat that progresses rapidly to difficulty in swallowing (true dysphagia or increased drooling) and is followed by difficulty in breathing (with or without stridor) and a preference for sitting (with or without posturing of the head). It is important to note that as many as one-third of patients on admission may be in shock with cyanosis (with consequent agitation or loss of consciousness) and that the disease may have a history as short as 2 hours in duration from onset to death.

The earliest manifestation is usually the sudden onset of high fever (38.5 °C to 40 °C). Sore throat accompanies fever in 50 percent of the patients.

Complaints related to difficulty in swallowing usually follow the onset of sore throat and fever by a few hours. Excessive drooling as a result of inflammation of the epiglottic valleculae and true dysphagia from involvement of all of the supraglottic structures are prominent at this stage. The voice is often muffled or the patient refuses to speak. (This is in distinction to the hoarse voice heard in laryngotracheitis.) The onset of difficulty in breathing usually occurs within 12 hours of the first clinical manifestations. Stridor eventually appears in more than 50 percent of cases.

During the later stages of the disease, patients often assume a characteristic position. The patient refuses to lie down and demonstrates a preference for the sitting position with the head forward and neck extended.

Cyanosis occurs very late and is not usually clinically evident until the pO_2 is less than 40 mm Hg. Anxiety and restlessness are signs of severe hypoxia and may be precursors of imminent death.

Progression from a moderately ill child to complete obstruction of the airway may occur in minutes. Therefore, rapid assessment and diagnosis, followed by prompt intervention to secure the airway are of the utmost importance to prevent death or hypoxic encephalopathy.

The diagnosis of supraglottitis is a clinical one based upon the history and physical appearance of the child. The picture is usually so characteristic as to dictate the initial course of action: *rapid placement of an artificial airway*. Visualization of the epiglottis in the office or emergency room with a tongue depressor is contraindicated because it may precipitate further swelling of the epiglottis and/or a vago-vagal response in an hypoxic patient, resulting in a fatal cardiac arrhythmia.

The urgency of progressing directly to airway stabilization contraindicates performing other diagnostic procedures (e.g., lateral neck radiography, white blood cell count, blood cultures) before placement of an artificial airway.

MANAGEMENT

Any inpatient service caring for children should have a written protocol to manage patients with suspected supraglottitis. The presence of such a protocol defines the responsibilities of each service in advance and minimizes wasted time and effort.

The first step in the management of patients with suspected supraglottitis is to secure the airway. Nineteen percent of patients with documented supraglottitis will have life-threatening obstruction when first seen, and an additional 17 percent will progress to that point within 6 hours of admission. Eleven percent of all patients with supraglottitis will require emergency airway bypass. This is a hazardous procedure, even in the best of hands, associated with death and/or hypoxic brain damage in 20 percent of patients so treated. Therefore, once the patient is thought to have supraglottitis, he is taken to the operating room immediately, where the obstructed airway is observed directly. If the diagnosis is confirmed, an artificial airway is placed.

Controversy still exists as to whether tracheostomy or nasotracheal intubation is the procedure of choice. The answer depends upon the expertise available at the individual hospital. Where there are capable anesthesiology, otolaryngology, and intensive care personnel, nasotracheal intubation is preferred, since it results in a shorter duration of airway maintenance and hospitalization as well as a diminished rate of immediate and postextubation complications. To aid in reduction of subglottic stenosis secondary to nasotracheal intubation, it is recommended that a nasotracheal tube 0.5 to 1.0 mm smaller than that predicted for the child's age, be utilized (Table 2).

Once the airway is secured, an intravenous line is placed. White blood cell count, differential, blood culture, and an epiglottis culture (swab) are obtained and the patient is begun on antibiotics. Between 15 and 40 percent of strains of *H. influenzae* B produce beta-lactamase and are, therefore, ampicillin-resistant. For this reason, initial therapy with either chloramphenicol or one of the newer cephalosporins (e.g., cefuroxime, cefotaxime, ceftizoxime, or ceftriaxone) should be administered.

TABLE 2 Sizes of Nasotracheal Tubes Recommended for Children with Acute Supraglottitis

Age	*Size in mm*
Birth–6 months	3.0
6 months–2 years	3.5
3 years–5 years	4.0
Older than 5 years	4.5

Note: Cherry JD. Croup. In: Feigin RD, Cherry JD, eds. Textbook of Pediatric Infectious Diseases. Philadelphia: WB Saunders Co, 1981.

Although concurrent meningitis is uncommon, that risk does exist. This, when added to the not-infrequent observation of microabscesses in the epiglottis at postmortem examination, recommends the use of large (meningitic) doses of antibiotics in the treatment of supraglottitis. These dosages are given in Table 3.

If the organism isolated from the blood culture or epiglottis swab is sensitive to ampicillin (beta-lactamase-negative), the original antibiotic can be changed to ampicillin (150 mg per kilogram per day divided every 6 hours). Antibiotic therapy is continued for 7 days.

Management in the Operating Room

Personnel experienced in the delivery of anesthesia to infants and children are the ideal members of the team caring for these patients. An array of appropriate endotracheal tubes (internal diameter, 3.0 to 5.0 mm; laryngoscope blade [Miller 1 to 3]; a rigid bronchoscope; and preparations to perform an emergency tracheostomy with appropriate sized tracheostomy cannulae and tubes) should all be present in the operating room.

The child should be allowed to maintain the position he prefers to maximize air exchange. The parent should be allowed to accompany the child to the entrance of the operating room. While in transit from the emergency room, the anesthesiologist should talk to the patient calmly and in soothing tones, providing reassurance and explaining what is about to happen. The conversation is continued until induction has been successfully accomplished. Movements should be slow and gentle. Induction should be delivered with the child in his position of preference. Halothane and 100 percent oxygen has been particularly successful. It is safer to avoid using muscle relaxants, if possible. Once induction is advanced, a number 20 or 22 teflon intravenous catheter is placed, and diagnostic blood specimens (e.g., for white blood cell count, differential, and blood culture) obtained.

Many anesthesiologists prefer to intubate first with an orotracheal tube and, when secured, replace it with a nasotracheal tube of appropriate size for the patient with supraglottitis (Table 2). Should these attempts fail, a tracheostomy should be performed.

Following insertion, the nasotracheal tube is held in place while tincture of benzoin is applied from ear to ear and over the tube segment outside the nostril. Once dried, strips of half-inch adhesive tape are applied over the benzoin and circumferentially around the tube and secured over the occiput. A nasogastric tube is placed after the airway has been secured.

Before leaving the operating room, the patient is given 0.1 mg per kilogram of intravenous morphine sulfate. This minimizes the agitation and thrashing that may occur during transfer from the operating room to the pediatric intensive care unit.

Management in the Pediatric Intensive Care Unit

All patients with supraglottitis and airway bypass require intensive care unit management. Should a pediatric intensive care unit not be available, the infant or child can be managed in the adult medical ICU, preferably with experienced pediatric nurses working together with medical ICU nursing personnel.

On arriving in the ICU, placement of the tube is evaluated clinically by auscultation and the position of the tube confirmed by chest roentgenogram. If the tube is appropriately placed, it should be marked at the level of the nostril to ensure rapid recognition if inadvertently withdrawn or advanced.

Blood pressure and electrocardiogram should be monitored, particularly in the early hours following intubation. Pulmonary edema associated with the relief of airway obstruction occurs in approximately 7 percent of patients with supraglottitis. This form of pulmonary edema is probably due to increased pulmonary blood volume generated during inspiration against an obstructed laryngeal airway. Exhalation against this obstruction protects the cardiovascular system by decreasing venous return to the thorax. Once the obstruction is bypassed by insertion of an artificial airway, sudden increase in venous return to the central circulation may occur with a consequent increase in pulmonary capillary hydrostatic pressure. To anticipate this problem, 4 to 5 cm of CPAP should be applied as soon as the bypass airway is placed. This is gradually decreased over the next 24 to 36 hours. For 3 to 4 hours after intubation, arterial blood gases should be monitored to detect developing pulmonary edema, which, if present, is treated with assisted ventilation with appropriate levels of PEEP, fluid restriction, and diuretics.

All four extremities should be restrained. Parents or relatives should be encouraged to stay with the child to reduce anxiety. Heavy sedation is important in the

TABLE 3 Recommended Antibiotics in the Treatment of Supraglottitis

Antibiotic	*Dose*	*Interval*
Chloramphenicol	100 mg/kg/day	q6h
Cefuroxime	225 mg/kg/day	q8h
Cefotaxime	200 mg/kg/day	q8h
Ceftizoxime	200 mg/kg/day	q8h
Ceftriaxone	100 mg/kg/day	q12h

management of patients with supraglottitis to reduce agitation and the not-infrequent complication of dislodging of the nasotracheal tube. Sedation also decreases the anxiety produced by having an endotracheal tube in place and the ICU environment; it also minimizes the risks of trauma to the subglottic region that result from motion of the endotracheal tube in the agitated patient. Morphine sulfate, 0.1 to 0.2 mg per kilogram every 2 to 4 hours is preferred for its efficacy and ease of reversibility with naloxone should that be necessary. The major disadvantage in sedation is depression of the agitation that occurs as a result of developing hypoxia (e.g., from a displaced NT tube). Careful attention to this possibility is therefore important.

Adequate humidification to prevent inspissated secretions and CPAP to maintain normal functional residual capacity will help to prevent closure of small airways. One minute prior to endotracheal suctioning, the lungs should be hyperinflated with 100 percent oxygen.

The need for steroids and racemic epinephrine in the initial treatment of this disease are unproved and should not be routinely employed.

Management Following Extubation

The majority of children can be safely extubated 48 hours after intubation. Prior to extubation, the epiglottis is examined at the bedside or in the operating room by fiberoptic or direct laryngoscopy. If the swelling has decreased significantly, the child is taken to the operating room for extubation. Endoscopic examination of the subglottic region is undertaken. If nasotracheal tube is removed, nebulized racemic epinephrine (2%, diluted with sterile saline to a total volume of 3.5 ml) is delivered and the patient begun on a course of dexamethasone 0.5 to 1 mg per kilogram every 6 hours for 24 hours. Should signs of continued subglottic edema persist, racemic epinephrine treatments are reinstituted and administered every 2 hours. Although reintubation is infrequently needed, preparations for this contingency should be made for every patient (e.g., proper size tubes, blades and working blade bulbs at the bedside). Following extubation, the patient is given mist by face mask or tent, transferred to the general pediatric floor, and observed for 24 hours before discharge.

Segmental atelectasis occurs in approximately 25 percent of patients with supraglottitis treated with an artificial airway. This is probably contributed to by poor fluid intake secondary to dysphagia and increase in insensible water loss with high fever and tachypnea in the hours prior to admission, as well as inadequate coughing due to the airway bypass. Vigorous pulmonary toilet is therefore important during this period. The mean duration of hospitalization of patients with supraglottitis treated with a nasotracheal tube bypass is approximately 7 days.

It is generally not necessary to continue oral antibiotic therapy after discharge.

DIFFERENTIAL DIAGNOSIS

Differential diagnosis of acute obstructions in the region of the larynx include bacterial tracheitis, acute laryngotracheitis, spasmodic croup, laryngeal diphtheria, foreign body, and acute angioneurotic edema. The major differential diagnostic features are presented in Table 1.

PREVENTION

Purified *H. influenzae* B polysaccharide vaccine (B-Capsa I) is indicated as routine immunization for all children 24 to 59 months of age. Since 75 percent of patients with supraglottitis are in this age group and because the vaccine is more than 90 percent effective for children of this age, it is now possible to look forward to a significant reduction in the incidence of supraglottitis once widespread immunization is achieved.

COMMON COLD

BARRY M. FARR, M.D., M.Sc.
JACK M. GWALTNEY, Jr., M.D.

The common cold remains the most frequent cause of acute morbidity and of visits to physicians in the United States. Adults average two to four colds per year, and children have six to eight colds per year.

The disease is actually a syndrome of symptoms produced by respiratory infections with any one of more than 100 antigenically distinct viruses (Table 1). A viral etiology has been determined in two of three colds by use of currently available cultural and serologic techniques; the remaining one-third of colds is presumed to be caused by presently unidentified viruses. Colds caused by the various etiologic agents are usually indistinguishable from one another except by viral isolation or serology, but viral culture and serology are both unavailable and unnecessary for routine patient care.

The manifestations of the common cold are so characteristic that the patient's self-diagnosis is usually correct. The key symptoms are nasal discharge, nasal obstruction, sneezing, sore throat, and cough. Similar symptoms due to allergic conditions are usually easily distinguished by their chronic or recurrent pattern and also by relationship to allergen exposure. Fever is usually absent except in

TABLE 1 Etiologies of the Common Cold

Agent	*Number of Antigenic Types*	*Approximate Percentage of Case*
Rhinovirus	89 numbered (plus 20 more awaiting enumeration)	30
Coronavirus	≥3	≥10
Respiratory syncytial virus	1	10–15
Influenza virus	3	
Adenovirus	33	
Parainfluenza virus	3	
Other viruses (enterovirus, varicella, rubeola)		5
Presumed undiscovered viruses		30–40
*Streptococcus pyogenes**		5

* Streptococcal pharyngitis is not always clinically distinct from viral pharyngitis.

the colds of infants or young children. The median duration of symptoms is one week, but colds last for up to two weeks in 25 percent of patients. The severity and duration of cough is often increased in cigarette smokers with a cold.

Physical examination is usually unrevealing except for the occasional presence of visible rhinorrhea or nasal voice. The physicians's most important challenge is to differentiate the uncomplicated cold from the 2 percent of cases with otitis media (mostly children) and the 0.5 percent of cases developing secondary bacterial sinusitis (mostly adults) requiring antimicrobial therapy. A history of change in auditory acuity or earache should be evaluated with pneumatic otoscopy. Pain or tenderness in the maxillary or frontal bones suggests the need for sinus transillumination and/or radiography. Severe sore throat or tonsillar pharyngeal exudate indicates the need for throat culture to exclude streptococcal pharyngitis.

The uncomplicated cold is self-limited and best treated by reassuring the patient and prescribing only those medications needed to relieve the individual patient's symptoms. Combination products containing remedies for all possible symptoms are usually less effective and cause more adverse effects than does specific therapy.

Nasal congestion is best treated with topical vasoconstrictors, such as 0.25% to 0.5% phenylephrine or 1% ephedrine drops or sprays. These nasal drops or sprays must be used regularly every 4 hours for 3 to 4 days. Longer acting compounds, such as oxymetazoline (Afrin) drops or spray, may be used twice a day. Oral administration of decongestants, such as pseudoephedrine (Sudafed), 60 mg by mouth four times a day, offers an alternative that is less effective than topical therapy and may be complicated by increased blood pressure. This may be a significant hazard in patients with prior hypertensive or cardiac disease. Patients should also be warned about the danger of rhinitis medicamentosa following prolonged usage of decongestants. Antihistamines have not been shown to relieve the nasal congestion of colds, which correlates with recent research that did not find elevation of histamine in the nasal secretions of patients with experimentally induced rhinovirus colds. The drying effect of antihistamines on nasal secretions is due to an anticholinergic effect. This benefit must be weighed against antihistamines' other frequent side effect of drowsiness.

Malaise, aches, and low-grade fever are best treated with bed rest and analgesic/antipyretics such as aspirin or acetaminophen. Sore throat is relieved by warm saline gargles and mild analgesics. Cough usually does not require treatment, but moderate to severe coughing may be suppressed with codeine, 15 to 30 mg orally every 4 to 6 hours after the possibility of pneumonia is excluded by history, physical examination, and, if necessary, chest radiography. The patient should be warned that this dosage of codeine may result in constipation which may be counteracted by increasing dietary bulk. Proprietary cough syrups containing dextromethorphan are also effective. The usual adult dose of dextromethorphan is 15 to 30 mg three to four times daily. Smokers should always be advised to stop smoking.

Antibiotics should never be prescribed prophylactically for a patient with an uncomplicated cold as they have no effect on the natural course of the viral infection, they alter the patient's flora to more resistant bacterial species, and they expose the patient to unnecessary risks ranging from mild side effects such as rash and diarrhea to more severe, life-threatening complications such as pseudomembranous colitis and anaphylaxis.

Large-dose therapy with vitamin C has not been shown effective as either prophylaxis or therapy for the common cold. No specific antiviral agent is yet available for prophylaxis or therapy, and vaccines have proved impractical because of the many different viruses involved. Since some cold viruses may be spread by direct hand contact and self-inoculation, handwashing and avoidance of finger-to-nose or finger-to-eye contact is recommended after exposure to a cold sufferer.

INFECTION OF THE MOUTH, SALIVARY GLANDS, AND NECK SPACES

R. BRUCE DONOFF, D.M.D., M.D.

INFECTION OF THE MOUTH

Infection of the oral cavity can be caused by a variety of viral and bacterial agents. The chief site of infection is, of course, the teeth and supporting periodontal structures. The next commonest sites of infection are the mucosal surfaces. The microbiology of oral bacterial infection is complex and reflects the oral flora. Anaerobic bacteria constitute a large part of the normal oral flora. Aerobes include viridans streptococci, group A streptococci, group D streptococci (enterococcus), *Staphylococcus aureus*, diphtheroids, actinomycetes, *Hemophilus influenzae*, and *Bacteroides*. Normal oral flora becomes pathogenic as the result of a number of changes of either a chemical or tissue nature. Selection of the appropriate antimicrobial agent is essential to effective treatment. The main exception to this is found in the immunosuppressed patient. Patients with neutropenia often present in atypical fashion because of their inability to make pus. Gram-negative infections occur in this group, and careful antibiotic selection and observation of clinical response are important. Candidiasis is also more prevalent in this group of patients.

Mucosal Surfaces

Aphthous Stomatitis

Canker sore is probably the commonest lesion of the oral mucosa. It is an ulcerative small lesion that usually heals within 2 weeks. The etiology is unknown, but herpes simplex virus is suspected. The virus has not been isolated from aphthous ulcerations and no anti-HSV antibodies have been demonstrated in these patients. It is seen with increased frequency in higher socioeconomic groups. It may be evoked by stress and anxiety.

The ulcer stage is often preceded by a 2- to 3-day period in which the patient notes some discomfort. Only erythema may be present at this time. A deep ulcerative lesion, which is usually ovoid and has some depth, a yellowish-white necrotic base, and a surrounding zone of erythema, then appears. Lesions rarely exceed 1 cm in diameter. Most commonly, the lesions are found on the buccal, labial, or alveolar mucosa or the ventral surface of the tongue. They uncommonly involve heavily keratinized areas such as the hard palate or attached gingiva. Pain is the primary symptom, and secondary bacterial infection is rare.

The differential diagnosis of ulcerative lesions of the oral mucosa is very extensive. The most important point is that any ulcer which does not show signs of healing within two weeks be considered potentially malignant.

Treatment of canker sores is supportive. Irritating food and drink should be avoided. Topical xylocaine ointment can relieve the pain, and topical steroids like triamcinolone acetonide in Orabase (a mucosal adhesive) is effective. The patient should be instructed to dry the ulcer before applying the medication and to use it three to four times per day.

Herpes Simplex

Herpes simplex virus type I produces a primary and a secondary infection in the mouth. The primary infection is an acute stomatitis, and the secondary form is a chronic, recurrent, localized disease. Primary infection follows the patient's first exposure to the virus. Although commonest among children, it may occur in the adolescent and young adult population. It develops as a classic viral prodrome with oral eruptions in 24 to 48 hours. The mucosa, gingiva, and tongue are involved with vesicles that rupture to form ulcerative lesions. Adenopathy is present and the patient is febrile. The main differential diagnosis is acute necrotizing ulcerative gingivitis, which does not present with a prodrome and is limited to gingival involvement. In healthy patients the disease is self-limited, and unless there is secondary infection, antibiotics are not indicated. Treatment is supportive.

Recurrent herpes simplex type I infections are common. The lesions usually appear on the lips and are referred to as cold sores or herpes labialis. The lesions are recurrent, disappearing and then returning. They are usually quite small (2 to 4 mm). There is no treatment other than keeping the lesions lubricated.

The role of acyclovir in the therapy of infections due to herpes simplex type I is experimental at this point.

Acute Necrotizing Ulcerative Gingivitis

ANUG is a unique bacterial infection that affects the marginal and papillary gingiva. It is referred to as Vincent's disease and trench mouth. It is most often seen in young adults who rarely suffer from typical periodontal disease. The clinical appearance of ANUG is striking. Examination reveals localized or generalized areas of papillary and marginal gingival necrosis. The disease usually begins interproximally (between the teeth) and then spreads laterally. The necrotic areas form a pseudomembrane, and there is necrosis of the interdental papillae, which look crater-like. The etiology is thought to be a localized reduction in tissue resistance, which produces an environment in which fusospirochetes—the principal pathogens—normally present, proliferate. Normal oral flora, including *Fusobacterium fusiforme*, vibrios, streptococci, diplococci, and *Treponema vincentii* are commonly isolated.

The causative organisms are sensitive to penicillin. In the nonallergic patient, a loading dose of 1 g of penicillin V is followed by a 1-week course of 250 mg four times a day. Hydrogen peroxide rinses (a 1:1 dilution of 3% H_2O_2) are helpful to debride the areas. Once systemic symptoms are eliminated, more aggressive local debridement can be performed. In the penicillin-allergic patient, erythromycin in similar dosage is effective. Metronidazole is used extensively in the United Kingdom with excellent results.

Infections of the Teeth and Supporting Structures

Dental Decay

Carious lesions of the teeth, if neglected, involve the pulpal tissue, with subsequent infection developing as abscess formation or cellulitis. Extension of infection through the apex of the tooth results in abscess formation within the alveolar bone. This is painful and usually the patient complains of sensitivity to hot and cold materials. Surgical opening of the tooth is indicated. This is accomplished by opening into the pulp chamber and removing the necrotic pulp. Endodontic treatment along with proper dental restoration can salvage the tooth. Antibiotics should be prescribed. The infection is caused by mixed flora that are usually sensitive to penicillin. Sometimes infection spreads out of the bony environment and results in a tender swelling, usually of the buccal sulcus. Infections spread in this manner in both the mandible and the maxilla. If the swelling is fluctuant, incision and drainage are indicated, with placement of a gauze drain for 24 hours. The offending tooth is usually too painful to operate on under local anesthesia in such situations. Thus, I & D followed by antibiotic treatment usually permits definitive treatment of the tooth with greater patient comfort in a few days. Cellulitis may occur, and it is not unusual to see very toxic and sick patients with such conditions. This is particularly true in patients who neglect dental health. Outpatient antibiotic treatment and the use of warm salt rinses are used to get the infection to localize. The general condition of the patient may warrant hospitalization and the use of parenteral antibiotics.

More than 95 percent of such infections are due to mixed anaerobic oral flora and respond well to penicillin, or erythromycin in the allergic patient. When parenteral antibiotic is needed in the penicilln-allergic patient, clindamycin is very effective. For outpatient treatment of severe infections, the usual dosage of penicillin and erythromycin is a 1-g loading dose, followed by a week of 500 mg four times a day. Clindamycin is used orally in doses of 150 mg three times a day for a week. The possibility of granulomatous colitis must be considered. Parenterally clindamycin is used in doses of 300 mg every 8 hours.

Periodontal Abscess

Infection may track to the apex of a tooth from a periodontal lesion between the tooth and supporting bone. Clinically the patient notes that the offending tooth feels "high," and all other signs and symptoms are identical to those of a periapical abscess due to dental decay. Treatment is directed at establishing drainage of the periodontal pocket and decreasing the bacterial component by the use of antibiotics. The same considerations as discussed above apply.

Pericoronitis

This is a special periodontal infection seen in a younger age group and is due to infection in the area of an impacted wisdom tooth in the mandible. Purulence is observed around the offending tooth, and often the opposing maxillary tooth is traumatizing the area. Treatment is directed at mechanical cleansing of the area by the use of salt rinses, the use of appropriate antibiotics, and, sometimes, removal of the aggravating upper tooth. Such infections usually indicate that the impacted tooth should be removed when the infection is controlled.

INFECTIONS OF THE FACE AND NECK

Infections may spread by three main routes—hematogenous, lymphatic, and direct continuity. The latter is a most important route in oral infections.

Conceptually, it is important to realize that fascial spaces have anatomic connections, thus permitting severe or untreated infections to spread further. A detailed description of the fascial spaces is beyond the scope of this review. For more information the reader is referred to an excellent review of the entire subject (Granite EL. J Oral Surg 1976; 34:34-44). The masticator space contains all the muscles of mastication; thus, infection reaching this space by perforation of the mandible usually causes trismus or inability to open the mouth widely. This space is typically enlarged after removal of impacted wisdom teeth due to inflammation.

Ludwig's angina is a serious infection of odontogenic origin that, by definition, involves the submandibular and sublingual spaces bilaterally. Infection of lower molar teeth may point medially either above or below the insertion of the mylohyoid muscle to affect either of these spaces. Ludwig's angina represents the most severe type of infection of this area. It may cause respiratory embarassment. It is a rapidly progressing gangrenous cellulitis associated with dysphagia, difficulty in breathing, high fever, and a toxic patient. The floor of the mouth and tongue are extremely swollen, but massive edema and induration, rather than pus, are usually found. Early institution of parenteral antibiotics may obviate the need for incision and drainage; however, the patient must be closely observed for respiratory airway obstruction. Fiberoptic intubation is preferred over tracheostomy in this situation. High doses of penicillin (10 million units aqueous penicillin intravenously daily) or cephalosporin derivatives (e.g., ceflorin 6 to 8 g daily) should be employed, but careful observation of response is singularly important.

One last example of fascial spaces is of note. The lateral pharyngeal space is situated between the lateral wall of the pharynx and the fascia overlying the internal pterygoid muscle. There is direct communication between this space and the submandibular space. Infections here are easily confused with infection in the peritonsillar space that lies between the mucous membrane of the lateral wall of the pharynx in the region of the capsule of the tonsil and the fascia covering the superior constrictor muscle. The lateral pharyngeal space may be involved by the spread of a simple pericoronitis. The patient may complain of dysphagia, and a subtle swelling of the soft palate can be noted. This requires a high index of suspicion which can avert serious sequelae such as respiratory embarrassment. The organisms are sensitive to penicillin, but medical treatment should be combined with surgery when indicated.

INFECTIONS OF THE SALIVARY GLANDS

Bacterial infections of the salivary glands are relatively uncommon and may affect both the parotid and submaxillary glands.

Infections of the submaxillary gland are usually due to obstruction by calculi. Typically, the patient complains of swelling with meals, and with decreased salivary flow there is ascending infection by oral flora. On examination, pus may be observed from Wharton's duct and often a stone may be palpated lying in the duct in the floor of the mouth. The gland itself is enlarged and tender. A mandibular occlusal radiograph is helpful in demonstrating the opaque stone. Rarely, a radiolucent stone is encountered. The general condition of the patient is important in deciding upon treatment. If the patient is nontoxic, outpatient treatment may include removal of the stone and oral antibiotics. Penicillin V is the drug of choice in doses of 500 mg four times a day for 1 week. If the patient is toxic and dehydrated admission for supportive care and parenteral therapy is indicated.

The patient with parotitis presents with pain and swelling in the parotid region, usually related to meals. Stones are less common in the parotid duct (Stensen's duct) but debilitation and dehydration are often precipitating factors. Patients with Sjögren's syndrome often present with parotitis. Parotid infections often are caused by *S. aureus* and, therefore, the use of a semisynthetic penicillinase-resistant antibiotic is indicated. If the patient can be treated as an outpatient, dicloxacillin 500 mg four times a day for 1 week is used. If the patient is toxic and requires hydration and supportive care because of debilitation, intravenous oxacillin 6 g per day is indicated. Dilatation of Stensen's duct with lacrimal duct probes is useful to establish drainage. Pus should be cultured. Postoperative parotitis has almost ceased to exist today, but patients with parotitis are often elderly and debilitated. Clinical response should be monitored; defervescence and reduction in leukocytosis mean improvement. It is rare that parotitis or sialoadenitis progress to frank abscess formation requiring incision and drainage.

INTRA-ABDOMINAL INFECTIONS

INFECTIOUS DIARRHEA: A PATIENT IN THE UNITED STATES

CYNTHIA S. WEIKEL, M.D.
RICHARD L. GUERRANT, M.D.

Acute infectious diarrhea is a common problem affecting people of all ages throughout the world. In addition to being a major cause of mortality in crowded, tropical, developing areas, it remains second only to the common cold as a cause of morbidity in the United States. In suburban homes, enteric illnesses affect each person from one to three times each year, with the highest rates among young children and those most closely exposed to young children. In contrast to the summer or rainy season peaks of diarrhea in tropical areas, the predominant season of diarrhea in the United States, as in most developed, temperate areas, is in the winter months, with a lesser peak in the late summer months.

PATHOGENESIS OF INFECTION

Microbial Virulence Factors and Host Defenses

Certain microbial virulence and host-defense factors (Table 1) guide the practitioner's approach to the diagnosis and management of infectious diarrhea. As most enteric infections are acquired either directly or indirectly via the fecal-oral route, the characteristic infectious dose of different microorganisms influences the epidemiologic setting of infection. For example, organisms such as *Shigella* and amebic and giardial cysts are readily transmitted (low infectious dose), which accounts for their frequent spread by close interpersonal contact, as in day care centers or among promiscuous gay males. In contrast, the infectious dose of 10^5 organisms or greater required for *Salmonella, Vibrio*, enterotoxigenic *Escherichia coli*, and others is responsible for the more typical association of these organisms with food or waterborne outbreaks.

Recent advances in our understanding of microbial virulence factors have provided new concepts regarding what constitutes an enteric pathogen. For example, *E. coli* may be a harmless component of the normal flora, enteroadherent (resulting in destruction of the brush border and diarrheal illness), enterotoxin-producing (causing cholera-like diarrhea), or capable of mucosal invasion (resulting in Shigella-like dysentery), all depending on whether specific virulence plasmids are present at a given time in a particular strain. Consequent limitations on the diagnostic usefulness of taxonomic identification of agents without attention to specific virulence traits are obvious. Even among parasitic pathogens such as *Entamoeba histolytica*, recent developments are now clarifying that certain strains appear to be potentially invasive and others are not, possibly related to certain zymodeme (enzyme) markers.

Alteration of several host factors is recognized to predispose to a number of enteric infections. Diminished gastric acidity and, possibly, mucus production may decrease the infectious dose (e.g., of *Salmonella*) required for illness. Hypogammaglobulinemia (especially selective IgA immunodeficiency) is associated with an increased incidence of enteric infections, particularly giardiasis. Disturbance of normal motility of the gut (e.g., as in diabetes mellitus) may predispose to bacterial overgrowth and altered enteric microflora. Antibiotics routinely alter enteric microflora and may establish an ecologic niche for enteric pathogens such as *Clostridium difficile* or *Salmonella*.

Characterization of Diarrheal Illness

It is useful and significant to consider two basic types of acute infectious diarrhea (Table 2). The noninflammatory diarrheas are much commoner than the inflammato-

TABLE 1 Factors Guiding Approach to Diagnosis and Management of Infectious Diarrhea

Host Defenses	*versus*	*Microbial Virulence Factors*
Hygiene		Infectious dose
Gastric acid		Adherence
Mucus		Enterotoxins
Immunity (especially IgA)		Cytotoxins
Motility		Invasiveness
Flora		

TABLE 2 Two Types of Infectious Diarrhea

	Noninflammatory	*Inflammatory*
Mechanism	Enterotoxin or reduced absorptive surface	Mucosal invasion
Characteristic location	Small bowel	Colon
Type of diarrhea	Watery	Dysenteric
Presumptive diagnosis	No fecal WBC	Sheets of fecal PMNs
Examples	*V. cholerae* ETEC, EPEC Rotaviruses Norwalk-like viruses *G. lamblia* *Strongyloides* *Cryptosporidium*	*Salmonella* *Shigella* *C. jejuni* *C. difficile* *Y. enterocolitica* *Vibrio* species *E. histolytica** ? *Aeromonas*

* Although an invasive pathogen, *E. histolytica* may be associated with only pyknotic or absent fecal leukocytes. However, blood in the stool is characteristic.

ry types and arise either from the action of an enterotoxin or from a selective functional impairment that results in net fluid and electrolyte secretion, usually in the upper small bowel. Etiologic agents of noninflammatory watery diarrhea include *Vibrio cholerae*, enterotoxigenic *E. coli* (ETEC), enteropathogenic *E. coli* (EPEC), rotaviruses, Norwalk-like viruses *Giardia lamblia*, and *Cryptosporidium*. With these etiologies, gross blood and pus as well as microscopic evidence of fecal leukocytes are usually absent. In contrast, inflammatory diarrhea usually results from a more distal invasive process, usually in the colon, which causes a dysenteric syndrome with sheets of fecal polymorphonuclear leukocytes on methylene blue examination. Characteristic pathogens that cause inflammatory diarrhea include nontyphi *Salmonella* species, *Shigella, Campylobacter jejuni, Clostridium difficile* (which may also be associated with noninflammatory "antibiotic-associated" diarrhea), and *Yersinia enterocolitica* (certain serotypes). Although amebic dysentery may be characteristically bloody, fecal leukocytes are often pyknotic or absent, perhaps because of the cytocidal effect of this protozoan parasite.

EPIDEMIOLOGY AND DIFFERENTIAL DIAGNOSIS

The list of recognized enteric pathogens has expanded rapidly in the last decade (Table 3). The goal must be to determine the likeliest pathogen on the basis of frequency of occurrence, age of the patient, season of the year, and epidemiologic setting—including travel, sexual history, and food exposures. The differential diagnosis as it relates to a specific epidemiologic setting is summarized in Tables 3 to 6. Particular consideration should be given to the evaluation for potentially treatable pathogens.

Most community-acquired diarrheal illness still remains unexplained. Overall, viruses probably cause most acute, self-limited diarrhea. The major viral causes of enteritis—rotaviruses (especially in children younger than 2 years of age) and Norwalk-like viruses—predominate during winter months, whereas the bacterial and certain parasitic pathogens predominate in the summer and fall months. Although most infectious agents cause diarrhea throughout life, rotaviruses typically cause sporadic and, occasionally, epidemic, illness primarily in children younger than 2 years of age. Diarrhea may last 5 to 8 days and may cause significant dehydration. Although immunity develops in the vast majority of the population, mild illnesses with abdominal cramping and mild diarrhea have been associated with rotaviral infection in close, adult family contacts of infected young children. In contrast, Norwalk-like agents are the leading cause of brief (24 to 48 hours) epidemic gastroenteritis and cause disease primarily in adults.

Travel to a tropical developing area is an important historical point to elicit. Short-lived noninflammatory diarrhea in this setting is most likely due to enterotoxigenic *E. coli*. In contrast, certain parasitic infections—in particular, those due to *Giardia, Cryptosporidium*, and *Stronglyoides stercoralis*—may cause more prolonged noninflammatory diarrhea and/or upper abdominal discomfort. The more serious problem of inflammatory diarrhea in this setting raises a spectrum of possibilities including *C. jejuni, Salmonella, Shigella,* enteroinvasive *E. coli* (EIEC) and *E. histolytica*. In addition, travel within the United States may pose certain risks for diarrheal disease. Both *G. lamblia* and *C. jejuni* infections have been reported among hikers or campers drinking unpurified stream water.

Homosexual men provide an important challenge to the diagnostic skills of the clinician. The potential etiologies for intestinal illness are protean and, more signifi-

TABLE 3 Etiologic Agents of Acute Diarrhea

Bacterial	ETEC EPEC *Campylobacter* (*C. jejuni* and campylobacter-like organisms) *Salmonella* *Shigella* *C. difficile* EIEC *Y. enterocolitica* *Vibrio* species *Aeromonas* *M. avium — M. intracellulare** *Plesiomonas*†
Viral	Rotaviruses Norwalk-like agents Cytomegalovirus* Adenovirus* Coxsackievirus*
Parasitic	*G. lamblia* *Cryptosporidium*‡ *Strongyloides*‡ *E. histolytica*

* Primarily seen in immunodeficient hosts, including AIDS patients and bone marrow transplant recipients.
† Rare cause of diarrhea; the role of antibiotics in therapy is unclear.
‡ Occurs in both immunocompetent and immunodeficient hosts; strikingly severe illnesses may occur in the latter (e.g., 17 liters of stool/day with *Cryptosporidium* or hyperinfection syndrome with *Strongyloides*).

TABLE 4 Intestinal Infections in Homosexual Men

Proctitis	*Neisseria gonorrhoeae* Herpes simplex virus (mostly type 2) *Chlamydia trachomatis* (non-LGV serotypes) *Treponema pallidum*
Proctocolitis*	*Campylobacter* species† *Shigella flexneri* *C. trachomatis* (LGV serotype) E. histolytica C. difficile
Enteritis‡	*G. lamblia*

* Abnormalities in rectal mucosa extend beyond 15 cm on sigmoidoscopic examination.
† Includes *C. jejuni, fetus*, and campylobacter-like organisms.
‡ Normal sigmoidoscopic examination.

cantly, may be multiple in 20 percent or more of patients (Table 4; also see Infections Other Than AIDS Commonly Found in Homosexual Men). Initial evaluation should include rectal Gram stain to evaluate for gonorrhea (gram-negative diplococci are seen in only about 50 percent of culture-positive cases) and anoscopy to identify lesions suitable for darkfield examination and consistent with primary or secondary syphilis. Anorectal herpes simplex viral (HSV) infection is frequently a distinctive syndrome characterized by severe anorectal pain, constitutional symptoms, inguinal lymphadenopathy, and neurologic signs such as difficulty urinating and sacral paresthesias. If these diagnoses cannot be made or the patient has symptoms consistent with enteritis, sigmoidoscopy should be done. This will enable additional specimens for culture to be taken and identify whether the rectal pathology extends beyond 15 cm, which would necessitate further evaluation (e.g., stool cultures and examination for parasites or ova).

Day care centers are an additional epidemiologic setting associated with multiple diarrheal pathogens (Table 5). To date, most outbreaks of diarrhea in day care centers have been associated with *Shigella* or *Giardia* and person-to-person transmission of organisms with a low infectious inoculum (10^1–10^2 bacteria or cysts, respectively). In contrast to shigella infections, which occur in children of all ages, both rotaviral and giardial infections appear to occur primarily in children younger than age 3 who are not toilet trained. Furthermore, outbreaks of diarrhea in day care centers are associated with significant secondary attack rates (10% to 30% in most studies) in the children's families.

Food poisoning is an important, but underestimated, public health problem, with more than 200 reported etiologies. Bacterial contamination of food accounts for more than 90 percent of the total cases in outbreaks where an etiology is determined. However, a specific etiology is identified in only 40 percent of outbreaks. An "outbreak" is defined by the Centers for Disease Control as an incident in which two or more persons experience a similar illness after ingestion of a food epidemiologically implicated as the source of the illness. There are two exceptions: a single case of botulism or chemical poisoning is considered an outbreak.

For convenience in diagnosis, food-poisoning syndromes are best categorized into four groups (Table 6). *Staphylococcus aureus* is the prototypic etiology of short-lived (less than 24 hours) upper gastrointestinal illness due to ingestion of preformed toxin where nausea and vomiting predominate and fever occurs in less than 25 percent of cases. In contrast, ingestion of toxigenic *Clostridium perfringens* results in an illness dominated by noninflammatory diarrhea and abdominal cramps where nausea, vomiting, and fever are uncommon. The commonest recognized cause of food poisoning, *Salmonella*, and other pathogens causing primarily distal ileal and colonic disease, result in inflammatory diarrhea, with polymorphonuclear leukocytes on stool examination with methylene blue.

Recognition of botulism, ciguatera, and certain shellfish poisoning is particularly critical because of the potential for these illnesses to progress to paralysis and respiratory arrest. Shellfish poisoning may be paralytic (associated with ingestion of bivalve mollusks of New England, Alaska, or the West Coast) or neurotoxic and less serious (associated with shellfish from the Florida coastal region). All of the paralytic illnesses may be accompanied by gastrointestinal symptoms including nausea, vomiting, diarrhea, and abdominal cramps. Notably, patients ingesting the neurotoxin(s) of *Clostridium botulinum* will usually develop a symmetrical, descending paralysis with diplopia, ptosis, dysphonia, and, ultimately, respiratory arrest. Distinguishing features of ciguatera poisoning include paresthesias and shooting muscle and dental pains. The features of paralytic shellfish poisoning overlap with those already mentioned, but the implicated food is distinct. In contrast, the nonfatal scombroid fish poisoning results in a histamine-like reaction (flushing, lip swelling, urticaria, dizziness, pruritis) and symptoms of gastroenteritis.

A recent history of antibiotic use should increase the clinician's suspicion of antibiotic-associated diarrhea due to *C. difficile* It is important to note that 25 percent of cases begin up to 6 weeks after antibiotics have been discontinued. Fecal leukocytes are detectable in more than one-half of these patients, and fever and abdominal tenderness or pain may be marked.

Immunocompromised patients are prone to develop diarrheal illness with both common and uncommon pathogens, which, on occasion, leads to serious systemic illness. Table 3 lists pathogens strongly associated with diarrhea in immunodeficient hosts. Important examples of pathogens causing systemic illness following initial gastrointestinal disease include *Campylobacter fetus* subspe-

TABLE 5 Pathogens Associated with Outbreaks of Diarrhea in Day Care Centers

Bacterial	*Shigella* *Campylobacter* *C. difficile*
Protozoal	*G. lamblia* *Cryptosporidium*
Viral	Rotavirus

TABLE 6 Food-Poisoning Syndromes

Pathogen	Source	Incubation Time
Upper gastrointestinal illness (nausea and vomiting predominate)		
*S. aureus**	Meat, poultry, potato and egg salads, cream-filled pastries	1–6 hrs
Bacillus cereus	Rice	1–6 hrs
Heavy metal (Ca, Zn, Cd, Sn)	Acidic or carbonated beverages in rusty or galvanized containers	5 min–2 hrs
Upper small bowel illnesses (noninflammatory diarrhea predominates)		
C. perfringens†	Beef, poultry, ham, lobster	6–24 hrs
B. cereus	Meat, vegetables	6–24 hrs
Distal, ileal, and colonic invasive diseases (inflammatory diarrhea predominates)		
Nontyphoidal *Salmonella*‡ species	Meat, poultry, eggs, fish, salads	6–48 hrs
Shigella species	Waterborne; fish, mixed salads	16–72 hrs
C. jejuni	Poultry, raw milk, waterborne	16–48 hrs
V. parahemolyticus and noncholerae vibrios	Raw or uncooked seafood, waterborne	Usually 24 hrs (range 4–92 hrs)
Y. enterocolitica	Meat, dairy products, waterborne	16–48 hrs
Neurologic disease, usually with gastrointestinal symptoms		
C. botulinium	Usually homemade canned foods; bean or potato salad, meat pies; commercially canned food	6 hrs–8 days; usually 12–36 hrs
Fish poisoning§		
(1) Scombroid	Scombroid fish (tuna including commercially canned; mackeral, bonito, skipjack); dolphin Hawaii/California	1 hr–24 hrs; usually <12 hrs
(2) Ciguatera	Grouper, amberjack, barracuda, red snapper Hawaii/Florida	1 hr–24 hrs; usually <30 min
Shellfish poisoning§ ("red tide")	Bivalve mollusks (mussels, clams, oysters, scallops)	5 min–4 hrs; usually <30 min
Mushroom poisoning	"Wild" mushrooms	Median onset, 2 hrs–12 hrs
(1) Immediate (median onset, 2 hrs): prognosis good; multiple manifestations including gastroenteritis, acute psychosis, parasympathetic hyperactivity and reactions similar to alcohol intoxication or disulfiram use		
(2) Delayed (median onset, 12 hrs): prognosis poor; triphasic illness: phase 1, gastrointestinal illness occasionally with bloody diarrhea; phase 2, occurs 2–3 days later, symptom-free but deterioration of hepatic and renal function; phase 3, hepatorenal failure		

* Commonest cause of food poisoning with an incubation period less than 6 hours.
† Commonest cause of food poisoning with an incubation period of 6 to 24 hours.
‡ The most commonly reported cause of foodborne outbreaks.
§ Fish and shellfish poisoning account for approximately one-half of all food poisonings of chemical etiology.

cies *fetus*, *Y. enterocolitica* (e.g., causing hepatic abscess seen primarily in diabetics and patients with iron overload), *Mycobacterium avium intracellulare* (in particular in AIDS patients), nontyphoidal *Salmonella* species (associated with AIDS and lymphoreticular malignancies), cytomegalovirus, and *S. stercoralis* (syndrome of hyperinfection associated with sepsis due to multiple gram-negative rods; pulmonary infiltrates; and, on occasion, meningitis). In contrast, pasteurized milk products contaminated with *Listeria monocytogenes* may lead to systemic infection without gastrointestinal symptoms. Due to the frequent use of antibiotics in this patient population, antibiotic-associated diarrhea caused by *C. difficile* must be considered in the differential diagnosis. In addition, infections with *G. lamblia* or *Cryptosporidium* may be severe and prolonged in patients with hypogammaglobulinemia. Last, chemotherapeutic agents (e.g., methotrexate, cyclophosphamide, *cis*-platinum, vincristine) must be considered as potential noninfectious etiologies of gastrointestinal disease in the immunodeficient host. Of note, are reports suggesting an association between certain chemotherapeutic agents (i.e., methotrexate) and *C. difficile* disease, although a more significant factor is probably the frequent use of antibiotics in this patient population.

DIAGNOSIS AND MANAGEMENT

As shown in Figure 1, a careful history should be taken for fever, bloody diarrhea, tenesmus, and abdomi-

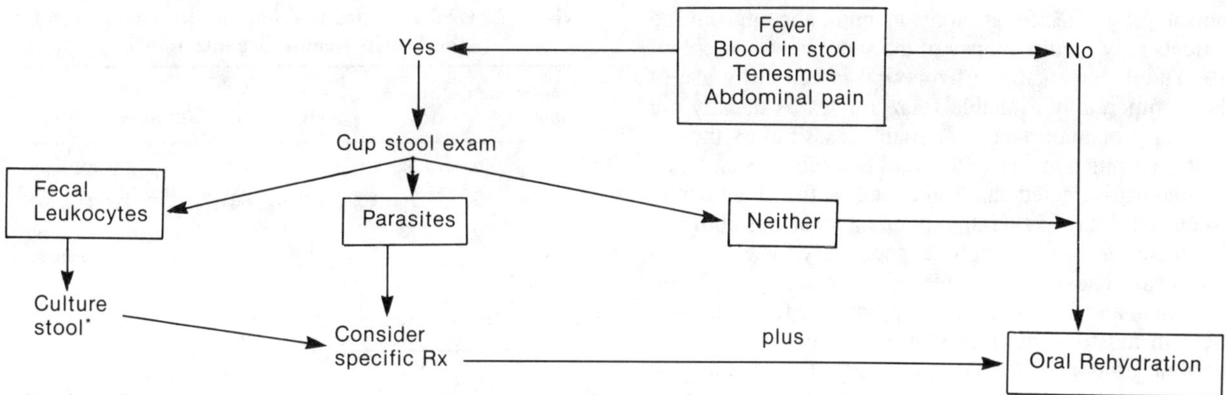

Figure 1 Initial evaluation and management of diarrhea. * Usually for *Salmonella, Shigella,* and *Campylobacter* unless epidemiologic history indicates additional examinations (see text).

nal pain. In addition, a careful epidemiologic history for recent travel, sexual preference, exposure to day care centers, recent foods (e.g., seafood), outbreaks of gastrointestinal illness among others known to the patient, antibiotic use, and conditions associated with immunocompromise must be obtained.

Stool Cultures and Special Examination Procedures

The first decision after obtaining the history and physical examination is whether to get a fecal specimen. Fortunately, several clues can be helpful in selecting those specimens likeliest to yield a useful result. If any epidemiologic or historical features suggestive of an inflammatory diarrhea are elicited, a fecal specimen (obtained in a cup is preferable to a rectal swab) may be useful for both gross and microscopic examination. The presence of blood or leukocytes suggests pathogens associated with an inflammatory process (Table 2) and is important for both therapeutic and epidemiologic reasons. In addition, parasites that may cause acute diarrhea—*G. lamblia, E. histolytica*, or *S. stercoralis*—may be seen in these intial wet-mount preparations. Unfortunately, swab specimens or specimens obtained after any barium radiographic procedures are often falsely negative.

With the burgeoning number of recognized potentially infectious agents that may cause diarrhea, indiscriminate culture and examination of stool specimens for all potential pathogens has become prohibitive. However, if there is a significant history of fever, bloody diarrhea, tenesmus, or abdominal pain or if there are sheets of polymorphonuclear leukocytes on microscopic examination, it is certainly appropriate to culture for *C. jejuni, Salmonella, Shigella*, and, possibly, the recently increasingly appreciated *Aeromonas* species. *Salmonella* and *Shigella* require the standard selective media, whereas *C. jejuni* and *Aeromonas* require special blood agar plates with selective antibiotics.

Special studies for additional agents are dictated by the particular epidemiologic or clinical setting. For example, if unexplained abdominal pain or fever persists, cultures with cold enrichment should be requested for *Y. enterocolitica*. If there is chronic diarrhea beyond 10 days or weight loss, special stains and concentration should be done for *G. lamblia, Cryptosporidium,* and *S. stercoralis* and quantitative cultures of the small bowel for bacterial overgrowth should be considered. Occasionally, small bowel biopsy to identify *Giardia, Cryptosporidium* or pathologic changes consistent with gluten enteropathy, or Whipple's disease may be necessary.

If there is unexplained bloody diarrhea, stool should be examined for *E. histolytica*. If there is seafood or coastal exposure, a special laboratory request for culture for *Vibrio (parahemolyticus, cholerae*, and others) on thiosulfate citrate bile salt sucrose (TCBS) agar should be made. If there has been recent antibiotic use, sigmoidoscopy should be performed to document pseudomembranes (although some patients may have only more proximal colonic involvement), and antibiotics should be discontinued if at all possible. If diarrhea persists or the diagnosis remains unclear, culture for *C. difficile*, or, better yet, direct assay of stool for specifically neutralizable *C. difficile* cytotoxin using culture cells should be obtained.

In the case of suspected food or waterborne outbreaks, the public health department and, possibly, the Centers for Disease Control (in the case of botulism) should be promptly notified, and a food-specific attack rate for the common meal eaten by the affected individuals can be calculated. To be incriminated, a food must have a statistically significantly higher attack rate for those who ate it than those who did not, and almost all of those ill must have eaten the incriminated food. From this information, an incubation period should be estimated and may be diagnostically helpful, as discussed previously.

In the case of diarrhea or rectal symptoms in sexually promiscuous homosexual men, anoscopy and/or sigmoidoscopy may be helpful.

As shown in Table 4, the extent of anatomic involvement is helpful in determining the appropriate pathogens to consider and, thus, the diagnostic tests to be ordered. In the immunocompromised host with diarrheal disease, among other etiologies, one should consider auramine and modified acid-fast stain of stool for detection of *M. avium intracellulare* and *Cryptosporidium*. Furthermore, diagnosis of a specific etiology in immunocompromised patients may require biopsy of the small bowel or colon.

The documentation of rotaviral infection by use of the commercially available rotazyme test is usually not necessary or important in sporadic cases unless the patient is admitted to a hospital ward that requires isolation of rotavirus-infected children or unless this documentation is helpful in excluding other diagnostic possibilities. Likewise, the need to explore specifically for enterotoxins, invasiveness, and cytotoxins, or to serotype *E. coli* is unusual and not required for appropriate fluid management in most cases. Unexplained bloody diarrhea may warrant serotyping of *E. coli* for possible 0157 strains that have increasingly been associated with bloody diarrhea and hemolytic-uremic syndrome in children. Current techniques for identification of Norwalk-like viral agents require either immune electronmicroscopy with acute and convalescent sera or radioimmunoassay, a technique that is not widely available.

TABLE 7 Oral Rehydration Solution Recommended by the World Health Organization

Composition (mmol)		*Ingredients per liter (1.05 quart) of Water*	
Na^+	90	NaCl (salt)	3.5 g (¾ tsp)
Cl^-	80	$NaHCO_3$ (baking soda)	2.5 g (1 tsp)
K^+	20	KCl	1.5 g (1 cup orange juice or 2 bananas)
HCO_3^-	30		
Glucose	110	Sugar	40 g (4 tbsp)

TABLE 8 Treatment of Specific Diarrheal Diseases

Pathogen	*Recommended Therapy**	*Alternative Therapy**
Bacterial		
S. dysenteriae, S. flexneri	Trimethoprim 160 mg + sulfamethoxazole 800 mg PO bid × 3–5 days (1 double-strength tablet bid)	Tetracycline 2.5 g PO once *or* Ampicillin 500 mg PO qid × 3–5 days†
Nontyphoidal *Salmonella*‡ (extraintestinal only)	Trimethoprim 160 mg + sulfamethoxazole 800 mg PO bid × 2 weeks§	Ampicillin 2 g IV q4h × 2 weeks‖ *or* Chloramphenicol 50 mg/kg/day in 4 divided doses PO or IV × 2 weeks
C. jejuni	Erythromycin 250 mg PO qid × 5 days#	Gentamicin 3–5 mg/kg/day in 3 divided doses IV × 7–10 days**
C. difficile	Vancomycin 125–500 mg PO qid × 10 days	Metronidazole 250 mg PO qid ×10 days
Y. enterocolitica (extraintestinal)	Gentamicin 5 mg/kg/day given in 3 divided doses IV × 7–10 days *or* Trimethoprim-sulfamethoxazole	Cefotaxime 12 g/day IV given in divided doses q4h
Enterotoxigenic *E. coli*	Trimethoprim 160 mg + sulfamethoxazole 800 mg PO bid × 3–5 days	Ampicillin 500 mg PO qid × 3–5 days *or* Doxycycline 100 mg PO bid × 3–5 days
Parasitic		
G. lamblia	Quinacrine 100 mg PO tid × 7 days	Metronidazole†† 250 mg PO tid × 7–10 days *or* Furazolidone 100 mg PO qid × 7 days
E. histolytica	Metronidazole 750 mg PO tid × 5–10 days *plus* diloxanide furoate 500 mg PO tid × 10 days *or* Diiodohydroxyquin 650 mg PO tid × 21 days	Tetracycline 250 mg PO qid × 15 days *plus* chloroquine (base) 600 mg, 300 mg, then 150 mg PO tid × 14 days
S. stercoralis	Thiabendazole 25 mg/kg bid × 2 days	NA‡‡

* Dosages are for adults unless otherwise specified.
† Sensitivity testing must be done. Ampicillin-resistant strains are common. Do not use amoxicillin.
‡ Antibiotics for simple salmonella gastroenteritis may prolong carriage of the organism or increase the relapse rate.
§ Drug for IV therapy is not known. Serious gram-negative infections have been treated successfully with TMP/SMZ at dosages of 5–10 mg/kg/day (for the trimethoprim component) given in divided doses q8h.
‖ Sensitivity testing must be done.
Treatment has been shown to eradicate *C. jejuni* from the stool and perhaps to decrease the chance of relapse, but has not been shown to consistently alter the duration of symptoms.
** Reserved for bacteremic disease, which is seen primarily with *C. fetus* subspecies *fetus*.
†† Metronidazole has not been approved in the United States for therapy for giardiasis.
‡‡ NA = Not available.

Therapy

The cornerstone of therapy for all forms of diarrheal illness is fluid and electrolyte replacement. In the vast majority of patients, this is best accomplished by oral rehydration. Table 7 describes the composition and ingredients required per liter of water in the simple oral rehydration solution recommended by the World Health Organization. Furthermore, temporary elimination of milk products from the diet should be recommended. During acute diarrhea, deficiency of lactase in the intestinal epithelial cell brush border may develop and prevent normal absorption of milk products, with a resulting osmotic effect that aggravates the illness. Despite the overall success of oral rehydration, some patients—particularly the very young, the elderly, and those with protracted vomiting or high fever—will require hospitalization and intravenous hydration.

The differentiation of diarrhea as inflammatory—by the fecal leukocyte examination—is critical both to determining the appropriate diagnostic evaluation and to the institution of therapy. In addition to oral fluids, noninflammatory diarrhea may be treated with absorbents such as kaolin plus pectin (Kaopectate), which serve only to change the consistency of the stools, antimotility agents (e.g., diphenoxylate, paregoric) or bismuth subsalicylate (Pepto-Bismol). In general, we discourage the use of antimotility agents because they occasionally increase toxicity and may precipitate toxic megacolon, particularly in patients with inflammatory diarrhea. Similarly, although large doses of bismuth subsalicylate (30 ml or 2 tablespoons orally every 30 minutes for eight doses) have been shown to be beneficial in diarrhea due to enterotoxigenic *E. coli* and, possibly, Norwalk-like viruses, the usefulness of this therapy in diarrhea of other etiologies is unknown.

Antimicrobial agents are indicated in certain bacterial and parasitic enteric infections (Table 8). In patients with high fever, moderate-to-severe abdominal pain and cramping, and/or bloody diarrhea with fecal leukocytes, initial evaluation—including a wet mount to identify the trophozoites of *E. histolytica* and darkfield examination for the darting motility or stool Gram stain (using carbolfuchsin instead of safranin counterstain) for the characteristic "seagull-appearing" gram-negative rods of *C. jejuni*—should be done. If these suggest *E. histolytica* or *C. jejuni* infection, specific theray may be instituted (Table 8). It should be noted that therapy for documented *C. jejuni* infections has not been shown to shorten the course of the illness, but does eradicate the organism from the stool and may decrease the incidence of relapses. If one suspects the diagnosis of shigellosis, therapy with trimethoprim-sulfamethoxazole may be prescribed. Of note, gastroenteritis due to nontyphoidal salmonellae may be associated with fecal leukocytes, and antibacterial therapy has been associated with increasing the risk of symptomatic and bacteriologic relapse and prolonged fecal carriage of *Salmonella* species. If antibiotic-associated *C. difficile* disease is suspected, antibiotics should be discontinued. If the disease persists or worsens, therapy with vancomycin or metronidazole should be considered. *Y. enterocolitica* usually causes a self-limited illness that requires therapy only if systemic complications occur.

The commonest cause of noninflammatory diarrhea among international travelers is enterotoxigenic *E. coli*. Although we do not advocate prophylactic antibiotics to prevent diarrheal disease during international travel, individuals developing noninflammatory diarrhea in this setting or upon returning to the United States may be treated with trimethoprim-sulfamethoxazole, which has been shown in a controlled treatment trial to shorten the duration of illness. The therapy for the common parasitic infections is listed in Table 8.

INFECTIOUS DIARRHEA: A PATIENT OUTSIDE THE UNITED STATES

HERBERT L. DuPONT, M.D.

Approximately 40 percent of persons traveling from a low-risk area, such as the United States, Canada, and northwestern Europe, to an area of high risk for acquiring diarrhea, which includes Latin America, southern and Southeast Asia, and Africa, develop diarrhea. The magnitude of the problem reflects the local rate of endemicity of diarrhea. Food and, to a lesser degree, water are the responsible vehicles of transmission. Bacterial agents cause approximately 80 percent of the illness, which explains the beneficial effect of antimicrobial agents in both the prevention and therapy of travelers' diarrhea.

For the average traveler to a high-risk area, exercising care about where and what one eats and drinks and being prepared to treat the illness should it occur represent the optimal approach. Eating at better restaurants (particularly if a local person can vouch for their safety) and selecting only steaming hot food, citrus fruits, bread, and bottled beverages will reduce the risk. For a select group of travelers, chemoprophylaxis is a useful way to prevent travelers' diarrhea (Fig. 1 and Table 1) Chemoprophylaxis is reasonable for the person on a critically important mis-

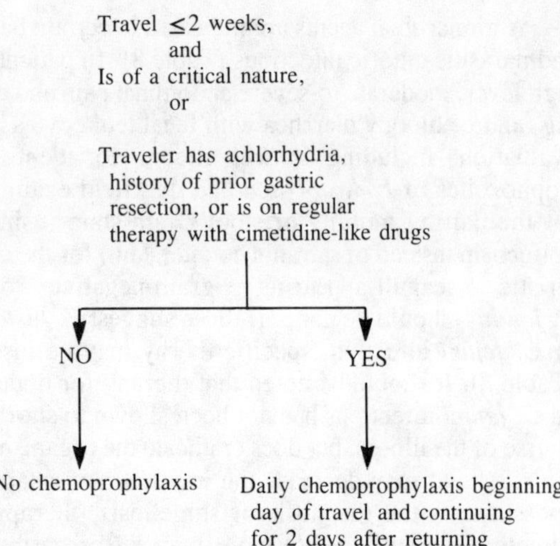

Figure 1 Indications for chemoprophylaxis for selected persons traveling from low- (United States, Canada, northwestern Europe) to high-risk areas (Latin America, southern and southeast Asia, Africa).

TABLE 1 Chemoprophylaxis of Travelers' Diarrhea

	Drugs	*Daily Dosage**
First choice:	trimethoprim-sulfamethoxazole (TMP/SMZ)	1 double-strength tablet (160 mg TMP/800 mg SMZ) once daily
Alternatives:	doxycycline;	100 mg once daily
	bismuth subsalicylate tablets†	2 tablets chewed thoroughly and swallowed 4 × day

* Dosages are for older children and adults.
† Pepto-Bismol.

TABLE 2 Indications for Empiric Therapy of Travelers' Diarrhea

Mild illness (≤3 unformed stools/day) with little or no associated symptomatology	Fluids only
Moderate illness (3–5 unformed stools/day) without fever, dysentery (bloody stools), or disabling associated symptoms	Symptomatic treatment (loperamide or bismuth subsalicylate*)
Severe illness (≥6 unformed stools) or diarrhea with fever, dysentery or disabling associated symptoms	Antimicrobial therapy with or without symptomatic treatment (TMP/SMZ or furazolidone)

* Pepto-Bismol.

TABLE 3 Therapy of Travelers' Diarrhea: Drugs and Dosage for Older Children and Adults

Drugs	*Dosage*
Loperamide	2 capsules initially, followed by 1 capsule after each unformed stool, not to exceed 8 capsules/day
Bismuth subsalicylate (Pepto-Bismol)	30 ml each 30 minutes × 8 doses (one 8-ounce bottle over 3.5 hours)
Trimethoprim-sulfamethoxazole	One double-strength tablet (160 mg TMP/800 mg SMZ) twice a day × 3–5 days
Furazolidone	100 mg four times/day × 5 days

sion or for the person who is either more susceptible to diarrhea or to more serious effects of associated dehydration. This latter group should include patients with achlorhydria, those having had gastric resection, and anyone taking regular antacid therapy (i.e., cimetidine). The shorter the visit, the more reasonable the use of chemoprophylaxis. Stays of less than 1 week are the most appropriate for using this approach, and chemoprophylaxis probably should not be employed if a stay in a high-risk area exceeds 2 weeks. To prevent illness (rather than merely delaying it) the drugs should be started on the day of travel and continued for 1 to 2 days after return to the country of origin. Trimethoprim-sulfamethoxazole (TMP/SMZ) and doxycycline are both effective if used in areas where bacterial enteropathogens are susceptible. Bismuth subsalicylate (Pepto-Bismol) probably is not quite as effective, but it offers some advantages. Problems with the antimicrobial agents include development of rash (5%), sensitivity to sun in persons taking doxycycline, development of resistance of the intestinal flora during drug administration, and more severe but less frequent adverse effects.

In treating the acute diarrhea of travelers to tropical areas, it is reasonable to base drug selection on the affected person's symptoms (Tables 2 and 3). Patients with any form of diarrhea should be encouraged to keep up with fluid and salt losses by drinking liquids, augmented by saltine crackers if necessary. Mild diarrhea with few other symptoms need be treated with no more than fluids. For diarrhea of moderate severity, a drug acting nonspecifically probably represents optimal therapy. Loperamide is probably the most effective drug available of those acting symptomatically. Bismuth subsalicylate (Pepto-Bismol), somewhat less active, reduces the diarrhea by about 50 percent. Antimicrobial agents should be reserved for those with more significant illness. This includes those not improved by symptomatic therapy, as well as any persons with more intense diarrhea (6 or more unformed stools per 24 hours), or if there is fever or dysentery (bloody stools), or if associated symptoms (nausea, abdominal pain, and cramps) are disabling. TMP/SMZ is the optimal drug to treat moderate to severe illness. The major treatable agents that would not respond to the combination drug are *Campylobacter* and *Giardia* (together responsible for about 5% of illness). The response to furazolidone therapy is not as rapid as it is for TMP/SMZ, but the drug has a broader spectrum of activity and includes the two organisms not responsive to TMP/SMZ. Travelers going to tropical areas from industrialized regions probably should go armed with a small supply of the two types of drugs used to treat moderate or severe illness.

TYPHOID FEVER AND ENTERIC FEVER

MYRON M. LEVINE, M.D., D.T.P.H.

Typhoid fever is an acute generalized infection of the reticuloendothelial system, intestinal lymphoid tissues, and gallbladder due to *Salmonella typhi*. A similar disease, paratyphoid fever, follows infection with *S. entertidis* bioserotype paratyphi A and B. These generalized salmonella infections are referred to as enteric fever. Rarely, other serotypes, such as *S. enteritidis* bioserotype typhimurium, can cause enteric fever if they infect compromised hosts, young infants, or the elderly.

Humans are both the only natural host and the reservoir of *S. typhi*, and infection is acquired by ingestion of contaminated food or water. Typhoid and paratyphoid bacilli rapidly pass through the intestinal mucosa and reach the systemic circulation by means of lymphatic drainage and the thoracic duct. As a consequence of this primary bacteremia, the fixed phagocytic cells of the reticuloendothelial system become seeded with *S. typhi* as they ingest the bacilli. Following an incubation period of 9 to 14 days, clinical illness appears, accompanied by the characteristic secondary bacteremia of enteric fever. The clinical picture is typified by fever (which increases in step-wise fashion), malaise, headache, and abdominal pain. In adults, constipation is often present, while in children diarrhea may occur. Typhoid and paratyphoid infections exhibit a spectrum of clinical ilness that includes asymptomatic infection, mild illness with low-grade fever and minimal malaise, or a severe syndrome of very high fever (up to 105 °F to 106 °F), toxemia, and even delirium.

There are many complications that can follow acute enteric fever, but the most important are intestinal perforation and intestinal hemorrhage (which occur in approximately 0.5% of cases) and the chronic biliary carrier state (which occurs in 3% to 5% of cases and is more frequent among females and older patients). In certain areas of the world, such as Indonesia, some patients present with a particularly severe clinical picture of typhoid infection marked by delirium or obtundation.

DIAGNOSIS

Transmission of typhoid or paratyphoid infections within the United States is rare, although occasional outbreaks and sporadic cases still occur. In contrast, enteric fever is a risk for U.S. citizens who travel to less developed areas of the world where these infections are still highly endemic. Microbiology technicians in clinical laboratories comprise another high-risk group since they can acquire the infection while processing cultures. When enteric fever occurs in a very young child in the United States, one should look for a carrier within the household.

If the clinical picture is suspicious, appropriate cultures should be performed. The highest yield of positivity is obtained with a bone marrow culture. This should always be obtained for suspect patients who have had some prior antibiotic therapy; bone marrow cultures in such patients are often positive when blood cultures may be negative. For patients who have not had prior antibiotic therapy, properly performed blood cultures give a high rate of positivity. Three specimens for culture should be obtained, 30 minutes apart, with at least 5 ml of blood per specimen. The blood should be inoculated into a flask containing at least 50 ml of broth to obtain a blood-to-broth ratio of at least 1:10. This dilutes out the factors in blood that may be inhibitory to the salmonellae. Any broth routinely used for blood culture wiil support the growth of *S. typhi*, but medium containing sodium polyanethol sulfonate is preferred.

Since infection of the gallbladder is usual in acute typhoid fever, culture of bilious duodenal fluid is almost as sensitive as a bone marrow culture. This can easily be accomplished by means of a string-capsule device, the Enterotest (Hedeco; Mountain View, Calif). The string device contained within a gelatin capsule is ingested in the morning by a fasting patient and is removed by gentle traction three to four hours later. Fluid for culture is expressed from the bile-stained distal 15 cm using two fingers of a gloved hand. String capsule cultures should be obtained on two consecutive days, even if antibiotics have already been started.

Three stool cultures should also be performed as an adjunct to bone marrow, blood, and bile cultures, although they are positive in only about 50 percent of cases (higher if diarrhea is present).

The Widal test, which measures O and H antibodies to *S. typhi* is not of much practical value. If proper reagents are available and quantitative tube dilutions are performed, elevated titers may be helpful in the nonvaccinated traveler or in children younger than 10 years of age in endemic areas. However, such Widal serologic techniques are not widely available. Healthy adults in endemic areas often have elevated titers, as do recipients of parenteral typhoid vaccine in the United States; in such patients the Widal titers have no value. Aggressive collection of proper culture specimens should preclude the need for a Widal test.

THERAPY

Historically, the therapy of typhoid fever can be divided into three eras: (*1*) prior to 1948, when effective antibiotic therapy did not exist and the case fatality rate was approximately 10 percent; (*2*) the period from 1948 to 1972, during which oral chloramphenicol was shown to be highly efficacious, practical, and economical, particularly in less developed areas of the world; (*3*) from 1973 to the present, when, as a result of some epidemics due to chloramphenicol-resistant strains of *S. typhi* and the advent of trimethoprim-sulfamethoxazole and amoxicillin, alternative drugs appeared to challenge the preeminent role of chloramphenicol as the mainstay of therapy for typhoid fever.

It is helpful to divide the management of acute typhoid fever into three categories: specific antibiotic therapy, general supportive measures, and treatment of the commoner life-endangering complications.

Antimicrobial Agents

Chloramphenicol has been the mainstay of specific therapy of typhoid fever since its first demonstration of efficacy in 1948. Although many other antibiotics of the 1950s and 1960s (such as tetracycline, streptomycin, kanamycin, and colistin) had impressive in vitro activity against *S. typhi*, only chloramphenicol was clinically effective. Chloramphenicol remains the drug of choice in less developed countries because of its practicality, inexpensiveness, and effectiveness when administered orally. Chloramphenicol had reduced typhoid fever from a 3- to 4-week illness with 10 percent case fatality to an illness of 1 week (or less) with a case fatality well below 1 percent. However, a number of observations make chloramphenicol a less-than-ideal drug: (*1*) relapse occurs in approximately 8 to 15 percent of patients; (*2*) it causes irreversible aplastic anemia in approximately 1 in 40,000 to 100,000 recipients; (*3*) occasional patients treated with this drug develop "toxic crises" (Herxheimer-like reactions); (*4*) in recent years the duration of therapy required until an afebrile state occurs has increased; (*5*) the drug is not impressive in preventing development of chronic carriers; and (*6*) epidemics caused by chloramphenicol-resistant strains have occurred (as in Mexico in 1972, in Vietnam in 1973, and in Peru in 1980).

The recommended regimen is 750 mg of chloramphenicol every 6 hours to adults (50 mg per kilogram for children) until the fever subsides (usually 3 to 7 days), followed by 500 mg every 6 hours for adults (50 mg per kilogram for children); the drug is given for a total of 14 days. If the patient is unable to take oral medication, the drug should be given intravenously until the switch to oral medication can be made. Chloramphenicol should not be given intramuscularly because only poor blood levels are achieved. Occasional patients develop a "toxic crisis" following the first doses of drug; it is postulated that this may result from a sudden release of endotoxin secondary to death of the bacteria.

If the *S. typhi* isolate is known to be resistant to chloramphenicol or if epidemiologic data make such infection likely, there are two highly effective alternatives, trimethoprim-sulfamethoxazole and amoxicillin, both of which are administered orally.

Amoxicillin, a congener of ampicillin, shows superior intestinal absorption. Adults are given 1.0 g (children, 100 mg per kilogram) every 6 hours for 14 days. During the 1972 Mexican epidemic caused by chloramphenicol-resistant *S. typhi*, strains began to appear that bore plasmid-mediated resistance to amoxicillin as well. Infections with such strains can be successfully treated with oral trimethoprim-sulfamethoxazole. The dose is 1 tablet of 160 mg trimethoprim and 800 mg sulfamethoxazole twice daily for 14 days. Children should receive 8 mg per kilogram of trimethoprim and 40 mg per kilogram of sulfamethoxazole daily in two divided doses. A large experience with trimethoprim-sulfamethoxazole therapy for typhoid fever caused by chloramphenicol-sensitive strains has shown that it is comparable in efficacy to chloramphenicol in approximately 90 percent of cases. In 8 to 10 percent of infected persons, however, the therapeutic response is retarded, requiring 10 or more days for the body temperature to become normal.

Irrespective of the aforementioned antibiotics selected, the clinical response in typhoid fever is not dramatic. Usually 2 complete days of therapy are required before the fever begins to abate, and a normal temperature is usually not reached for 5 to 7 days.

General Supportive Measures

Because of the high fever, maintenance requirements for water and electrolytes are greatly increased, so the patient should be encouraged to drink fluids liberally. If the patient is too ill to maintain hydration via oral fluids, intravenous fluids must be given; daily maintenance requirements should be increased by 10 percent for each degree of fever above 99 °F (37.2 °C).

Salicylates should not be given to patients with typhoid fever, since they can induce abrupt changes in temperature, hypotension, and even shock. The temperature should be lowered by sponging with tepid water.

Laxatives and enemas should, in general, not be employed because of the danger of precipitating intestinal hemorrhage. If constipation requires relief, oral lactulose should be used; this nonabsorbable disaccharide is a gentle physiologic softener of stool.

COMPLICATIONS

In the preantibiotic era, typhoid fever was a disease marked by a wide array of complications involving virtually every organ system and including intestinal perforation, intestinal hemorrhage, myocarditis, empyema of the gallbladder, encephalopathy, bronchitis, pneumonia, parotitis, osteomyelitis, hepatitis, meningitis, septic arthritis, and orchitis. Since the advent of specific antimicrobial therapy, most of the complications are still encountered with some frequency and are discussed below.

In some areas of the world, such as in Djakarta, Indonesia, an exceptionally virulent form of typhoid fever is seen in a small percentage of patients. These patients with acute typhoid fever present with severe toxemia, delirium, and obtundation and proceed to coma and shock. The case fatality rate in these patients is 55 percent with chloramphenicol alone. However, two days of high-dose dexamethasone drastically reduces the case fatality (to 10%) as the fever and toxemia are reduced. An initial dose of dexamethasone of 3 mg per kilogram should be given intravenously, followed by 1 mg per kilogram every 6 hours for a duration of 48 hours. The use of steroids should be reserved for this rare situation only and otherwise plays no role in the treatment of typhoid fever.

Despite adequate therapy with appropriate antibiotics, 5 to 15 percent of patients manifest relapse. In general, all signs and symptoms are milder in nature than the initial clinical episode, and the treatment is the same as for the initial episode.

Two dreaded complications of typhoid fever are still encountered in approximately 1 percent of cases: intestinal hemorrhage and perforation. When a definitive diagnosis of typhoid fever is made, a unit of blood should be typed and cross-matched as a precaution. Hemorrhage occurs late in the course, often in the second or third week, when the patient is often feeling better. The management of hemorrhage is conservative, utilizing repeated transfusion unless there is evidence of intestinal perforation. In the preantibiotic era, intestinal perforation was almost always fatal. Current consensus favors a combination of medical treatment and surgical intervention. Most surgeons experienced in the treatment of typhoid fever complications favor simple closure of the ulcer. This must be accompanied by additional antibiotics, such as gentamicin, tobramycin, or amikacin (in that order of preference) plus cefoxitin or clindamycin to treat peritoneal contamination by normal enteric flora.

CARRIER STATE

Approximately 3 to 5 percent of persons with acute typhoid fever become chronic biliary carriers. The propensity to carriage increases with age at the time of initial *S. typhi* infection and is greater in females. Most chronic carriers have cholecystitis with stones; occasional carriers lacking gallbladders manifest chronic pathology and infection in the intrahepatic biliary system.

If indicated because of economic or social factors and if the patient is sturdy enough to withstand surgery, cholecystectomy accompanied by 4 weeks of combined intravenous ampicillin and oral amoxicillin therapy can cure the carrier state in approximately 85 percent of instances. When this is not feasible, 3 weeks of high-dose intravenous ampicillin therapy has also shown promising results. Most recently, a moderate success rate has been reported by long-term (at least 4 weeks) amoxicillin therapy (2.0 g three times a day), accompanied by probenecid (0.5 g three times a day).

PREVENTION

In multiple controlled field trials in endemic areas, acetone-killed *S. typhi* parenteral vaccine has been shown to confer 75 to 90 percent protective efficacy against typhoid fever. The protection afforded to persons from nonendemic areas appears to be somewhat less. However, the parenteral vaccine causes fever or adverse local reactions (heat, swelling, erythema) in 15 to 25 percent of recipients. Nevertheless, for persons traveling to highly endemic areas, immunization with two 0.5-ml doses 1 month apart is recommended.

A new, live, oral attenuated *S. typhi* vaccine (strain Ty21a) is becoming available in many countries. Three doses of lyophilized vaccine in enteric-coated capsules was recently shown in field trials in Santiago, Chile, to provide approximately 65 percent protection without causing adverse reactions. This vaccine may become available in the United States in the near future.

INTRA-ABDOMINAL ABSCESS

JOHN G. BARTLETT, M.D.

Intra-abdominal abscesses are localized purulent collections separated from surrounding structures by a fibrous collagen wall.

PATHOGENESIS

Intra-abdominal abscesses are classified as intraperitoneal, retroperitoneal, and visceral. Regardless of location, there are two stages that are quite different in terms of management guidelines. The initial phase is inflammation that may be widespread, such as generalized peritonitis following intestinal perforation, or may be localized, such as a phlegmon, diverticulitis, or appendicitis. The second stage of the infection is the abscess phase. The abscess may occur adjacent to the portal of entry as with periappendiceal abscess, a diverticular abscess, or an abscess at the site of an anastomotic leak; alternatively, there may be extension to distant sites because of failure to localize the infection at the portal of entry. The commonest site with distant spread is the pelvis or lower quadrants, because of gravitational flow, or subphrenic, because of cephalad movement reflecting the negative pressure created by diaphragmatic movements. Intraperitoneal abscesses usually occur in association with disease or operations involving the intestinal lumen, although some cases occur with no apparent explanation. Pelvic abscesses in women often represent complications of pelvic inflammatory disease, childbirth, or gynecologic surgery. Retroperitoneal abscesses usually follow trauma, infection, or malignancy in adjacent organs, especially infected pancreatic pseudocysts, posterior duodenal perforation and intramesenteric abscesses. Visceral abscesses are commonest in the liver, pancreas, fallopian tubes and ovaries, and biliary tract.

DIAGNOSTIC EVALUATION

Abscesses within the abdomen have traditionally presented a formidable diagnostic challenge. The abdominal cavity is the anatomic site that is most difficult to evaluate for the detection of abscesses using physical examination and the usual laboratory tests. Most patients have leukocytosis, and prolonged leukocytosis following laparotomy specifically suggests this diagnosis. Fever is almost invariably present except in occasional elderly patients, patients receiving corticosteroids or antipyretics, or patients with endotoxemia. Patients with a recent laparotomy often have fever, but fever that persists beyond 4 days suggests intra-abdominal sepsis. The physical examination often shows vague findings and may be particularly difficult to evaluate in postoperative patients. The only intra-abdominal abscess that can be frequently detected on physical examination is a pelvic abscess in women. Plain films of the abdomen and contrast studies are often either negative or show only nonspecific findings. The most frequent finding that is regarded as diagnostic is extraluminal gas, but this is seen in only a small portion of cases. Thus, the usual findings are often vague. This accounts for the common recommendation for a laparotomy in patients who had persistent enigmatic fevers in former years. However, the situation has now changed drastically due to the availability of newer scanning techniques.

Radioactive gallium-67 concentrates within purulent collections and shows a sensitivity of up to 80 percent for detecting intra-abdominal abscesses, according to various reports. An advantage is that a whole body image is readily obtained. The problem with this technique is an unacceptably high rate of false-positive tests, lack of specificity (gallium uptake occurs with infections, tumors, and at postoperative sites), and the prolonged time to complete the study (48 to 72 hours). The tracer is excreted in the gut, making interpretation of intra-abdominal collections especially difficult. An alternative is the use of indium-111 labeled white cells, which provides an earlier answer and is generally more specific.

Ultrasonography shows sensitivity exceeding 90 percent according to most studies and has the advantage that it can be performed at the bedside for patients who may be too ill to transport to the radiology suite. The advent of real-time technology permits hundreds of images through multiple scanning planes within 5 minutes. Problems sometimes encountered with ultrasonography are that fluid collections in the gallbladder or bowel may cause occasional false-positive tests; intestinal gas may preclude examination of some areas, and it is difficult to distinguish pus, hematomas, and serous collections.

The most useful test in terms of specificity and sensitivity is computed tomography (CT). Purulent collections show different attenuation values compared with soft tissue, blood, and serous fluid. In addition, the surrounding wall of the abscess may be enhanced with intravenous contrast, and oral contrast material is useful in distinguishing fluid collections within the bowel. My own preference is clearly for CT scan as the most accurate test. Furthermore, I would be reluctant to accept results of the alternative scanning techniques that could not be confirmed with CT scanning. The reason is that false-negative scans, unlike sonography or ^{67}Ga scans, are extremely uncommon. The major causes are very small abscesses or misinterpretation. Nevertheless, the choice of a particular test should be influenced by local expertise, resources, scheduling availability, and the severity of illness. It should also be noted that the scans are often complementary. For example, the gallium scan or ultrasound may be useful for identifying a particular area of interest, so that a subsequent CT scan can be performed with more frequent imaging in areas of suspicion.

Blood cultures should be obtained for any patient with a suspected intra-abdominal abscess, and the recovery of some organisms, particularly *Bacteroides* species, specifically suggests an intra-abdominal focus if there is no alternative explanation. Most of these infections are polymicrobial, but the utility of extensive bacteriologic studies of exudate from abscess contents is controversial. In most instances, the specimen is difficult to obtain except with surgery; when exudate is available, complete bacteriologic studies are arduous to perform, extended periods are usually required to separate and identify individual isolates, and the organisms recovered often simply reflect the technical expertise and resources devoted to the exercise. Most of these infections involve mixtures of aerobic and anaerobic bacteria with rather predictable patterns for specific species. The dominant isolates are coliforms, especially *Escherichia coli*, and anaerobic bacteria, especially *Bacteroides fragilis*.

The published experience with comparative trials of antibiotic regimens provides a suitable guideline for empirically selected regimens in most cases. The greatest use of cultural data is to clarify situations that will modify antibiotic selection, such as the following: (*1*) the recovery of anaerobic bacteria is sometimes important to document in settings where the drug selection has not accounted for these organisms simply to make physicians aware of their presence and importance; (*2*) sensitivity profiles of aerobic gram-negative bacilli may be useful in the drugs selected for this component of mixed infections; (*3*) the pathogenic significance of enterococci is controversial, but the presence of this organism to the exclusion of others or as part of a mixed flora in patients who do not respond may provide necessary information for modifying some of the usual treatment regimens; and (*4*) occasional collections harbor large numbers of fungi, especially *Candida* species, that may require attention. With hepatic abscess it is mandatory to distinguish infections involving *Entamoeba histolytica* from pyogenic abscesses. This distinction may be made on the basis of serologic assays for amebiasis, blood culture results, microbiologic studies of aspirates, or a therapeutic trial with metronidazole.

ANTIBIOTIC SELECTION

Most intra-abdominal abscesses involve multiple bacteria including both coliforms and anaerobes. Most authorities consider both categories of organisms to be important in the pathogenesis of these infections and select antibiotic agents accordingly. Commonly advocated regimens that are considered equally meritorious according to therapeutic trials are the following:

1. An aminoglycoside directed against coliforms
   Gentamicin, 2.0 mg per kilogram, then 1.7 mg per kilogram intravenously every 8 hours; *or*
   Tobramycin, 2.0 mg per kilogram, then 1.7 mg per kilogram intravenously every 8 hours; *or*
   Amikacin, 7.5 mg per kilogram, then 5.0 mg per kilogram intravenously every 8 hours.

2. A second drug directed against anaerobes
   Clindamycin, 600 mg intravenously every 8 hours; *or*
   Cefoxitin, 2 g intravenously every 6 hours; *or*
   Metronidazole, 1 g intravenously, then 500 mg intravenously every 6 hours (the need for a 1 g loading dose is not established); *or*
   Chloramphenicol, 500 mg intravenously every 6 hours.

The following factors may influence the regimen selected:

1. The aminoglycosides are considered equally effective against susceptible coliforms, although sensitivity profiles within an individual institution may influence the choice within the group for patients with hospital-acquired infections. Serum creatinine levels should be monitored regularly during treatment and dose should be adjusted accordingly. My choice is gentamicin for most infections involving coliforms. For *Pseudomonas aeruginosa* infections, tobramycin is preferred. In vitro sensitivity tests obviously influence this choice when these data are available. Peak serum levels are obtained at 30 to 45 minutes after intravenous infusion, with the objective of demonstrating concentrations of 4 to 8 μg per milliliter for tobramycin and gentamicin, and 20 to 40 μg per milliliter for amikacin. Preexisting renal disease should not influence the choice of an aminoglycoside.

2. Cefoxitin may be used as a single agent due to activity against both coliforms and anaerobes. This approach is advocated only in patients who acquire their infection prior to hospitalization and have not received other forms of antibiotic treatment during the preceding 2 weeks.

3. None of the aforementioned regimens have activity against the enterococcus. Many authorities feel this organism is not particularly important in these mixed infections although there are certain exceptions. Treatment directed against enterococci is recommended when this organism is recovered in blood cultures, when it is recovered in exudate in pure culture, and when patients fail to respond with no apparent alternative explanation. Drugs appropriate for enterococci include ampicillin (2 g intravenously every 6 hours) or penicillin G (2 to 4 million units every 4 to 6 hours) when combined with an aminoglycoside.

4. There is considerable controversy concerning the drugs selected for the anaerobic component of the infection, particularly for penicillin-resistant strains, such as the *B. fragilis* group. In vitro sensitivity tests show that virtually all strains of *B. fragilis* are susceptible to chloramphenicol and metronidazole. About 5 to 10 percent of strains are resistant to clindamycin and cefoxitin, although this varies in different institutions. The antipseudomonal penicillins such as ticarcillin and piperacillin also show good activity against about 90 percent of strains. Comparative clinical trials support the use of antipseudomonal penicillins in combination with an aminoglycoside, although the published experience with these drugs is somewhat limited and the minimum inhibitory concentrations are relatively high compared with those of alternative agents. My tack is to not select these agents as preferred regimens, although I do not feel strongly about a change if the patient is doing reasonably well. None of the currently available third-generation cephalosporins offers an advantage with respect to anaerobic bacteria compared with the drugs noted above. A possible exception is moxalactam, which shows in vitro activity against *B. fragilis* comparable with that of cefoxitin, offering the possibility of monodrug therapy is some patients. The problem here is that the risk of a bleeding diathesis dissuades use of moxalactam.

5. Drainage is the most important component of therapy, and no antibiotic regimen can be endorsed with enthusiasm as a substitute. Nevertheless, there are some patients who have had an apparently adequate drainage procedure but have persistent sepsis, which suggests that changes in the antibiotic regimen may make a difference. Factors to consider in such cases are the in vitro sensitivity profiles of gram-negative bacilli, the presence or absence of enterococci, and the detection of other organisms that may have unusual sensitivity profiles. Metronidazole has unparalleled in vitro activity against *B. fragilis* and most other anaerobes. This would be my choice for a patient with persistent sepsis involving anerobes in which the original regimen included the alternative drugs. A similar approach would apply to patients with persistent or recurrent bacteroides bacteremia.

DRAINAGE

Drainage remains the mainstay of treatment for most intra-abdominal abscesses, and the major concern is usually the methods to accomplish this goal.

Abcsesses Not Requiring Drainage

There are two notable exceptions to universal application of the drainage principle. One is tubo-ovarian abscesses, since approximately 70 percent respond to antibiotic treatment without the necessity for surgical intervention. The current guidelines from the Centers for Disease Control include regimens with activity against anaerobes, coliforms, the gonococcus, and *Chlamydia trachomatis*. These regimens are advocated for pelvic inflammatory disease that may involve any of these microbes. However, tubo-ovarian abscesses almost invariably involve anaerobic bacteria with or without coliforms and streptococci. While endorsing the CDC regimens for uncomplicated pelvic inflammatory disease, it is my practice to use the regimens noted above when a tubo-ovarian abscess is present. This decision is obviously influenced by the results of endocervical and rectal cultures for *Neisseria gonorrhoeae*.

The second exception is hepatic abscesses. An established recommendation is to manage amebic abscesses medically and drain pyogenic abscesses surgically. The usual medical regimen for amebic liver abscesses is metronidazole given orally (750 mg three times a day) or intravenously (500 mg intravenously every 6 hours) for 5 to 10 days combined with a luminal amebicide such as diiodohydroxyquin (650 mg three times daily for 20 days) to eliminate cysts from the gastrointestinal tract. Alternatives to metronidazole include emetine given intramuscularly in a dose of 1 mg per kilogram per day to a maximum of 65 mg for 10 days or chloroquine, 250 mg four times a day for 7 days followed by 250 mg twice a day for 3 to 4 weeks. Needle aspiration of these abscesses is not indicated except to help establish the diagnosis, for very large abscesses measuring over 10 cm in diameter, for imminent rupture, or for failure to respond to medical management after 5 days. Open drainage is generally reserved for patients who have failed to respond after 4 to 5 days of medical therapy, primarily for patients with abscesses that are not accessible to needle drainage.

There is recent evidence that pyogenic liver abscesses may be managed medically and in an analogous fashion using antibiotics alone or antibiotics combined with needle aspiration performed at laparotomy or percutaneously with CT, ultrasound, or fluoroscopic guidance. However, despite some enthusiastic reports, it is my current practice to recommend the more traditional method of drainage combined with antibiotics. Drains may be placed surgically using a transperitoneal or extraserosal approach, or by percutaneous insertion using CT or ultrasonic guidance.

On occasions, a patient with a liver abscess receives a trial of metronidazole with or without an aminoglycoside when amebiasis is suspected and shows a good therapeutic response, with serologic assays for *E. histolytica* that subsequently prove negative. In such instances, it seems appropriate to simply continue the antibiotics without the necessity of surgical intervention.

Another exception applies to the patient with multiple, small hepatic abscesses that are simply unrealistic to drain. The mortality of this disease is unacceptably high, but there is little to offer these patients other than an aggressive course of antibiotics based on likely pathogens. With regard to the selection of agents for pyogenic abscesses, any of the regimens cited previously should be appropriate. When using metronidazole combined with an aminoglycoside in such cases, a penicillin is added to provide activity against aerotolerant streptococci.

Surgical Drainage

This is the traditional method of choice for draining intra-abdominal abscesses. The major controversies concern the use of intraoperative peritoneal irrigation, postoperative peritoneal irrigation, the surgical approach, and the method used to close the abdominal wound. All of these are issues that must be dealt with by the operating surgeon, and there are no clear-cut guidelines that will apply to all cases. Antibiotic selection is also controversial, but any of the regimens cited previously appear to be acceptable according to most authorities. With regard to the surgical approach, extraserous drainage is obviously attractive since it is associated with the best prognosis. However, the transperitoneal approach is often preferred since it permits detection of multiple abscesses and associated conditions that account for the abscess when the cause is unclear. At the present time most drainage operations are performed transperitoneally. The extraserous approach is generally reserved for large unilocular abscesses that are likely to be single, such as a subphrenic abscess following left colectomy and splenectomy, a right subphrenic abscess following a Bilroth II resection, a pelvic abscess after a low anterior resection, abscesses contiguous with the abdominal wall, or a pelvic abscess associated with pelvic inflammatory disease. If this approach is correct, there will be rapid resolution of clinical signs of infection following the drainage procedure.

Percutaneous Drainage

An alternative to surgical drainage is percutaneous drainage using ultrasonic or CT guidance. The advantage is avoidance of general anesthesia and postoperative complications. The initial published experience shows an overall success rate of 80 to 85 percent. Nevertheless, this must be recognized as a relatively new procedure that challenges traditional therapeutic modalities and can be recommended only with rather stringent criteria. Factors influencing this recommendation are the following:

1. Technical expertise is required.
2. The procedure is advocated only for only single, well-defined, unilocular abscesses. Contraindications include multiple abscesses, loculations within an abscess, and the presence of poorly defined borders.
3. There must be a safe percutaneous drainage route as indicated by needle placement with CT, ultrasonic, or fluoroscopic guidance. This procedure will also confirm the diagnosis by the detection of purulent material and distinguish other causes of loculated collections such as hematomas, serous collections, or necrotic tumors. The Gram stain and culture are obviously important factors in antibiotic selection.
4. There should be immediate operative capability in the event of a complication. The major complication is hemorrhage; less frequent are septicemia (usually transient), extension of infection, and organ injury due to faulty technique.

There are selected clinical settings in which this technique is particularly attractive. Patients with intra-abdominal abscesses who have a contraindication to surgery constitute one important category. In this instance, percutaneous drainage may be a temporizing procedure for patients who require stabilization prior to the administration of general anesthesia, although percutaneous drainage often represents a definitive procedure. Another setting in which this is particularly attractive is for abscesses following recent abdominal surgery where there is reluctance to reoperate. Patients with abscesses that are easily approached because of large size and easy accessibility are obvious candidates. Failures and complications are commonest with pancreatic abscesses, abscesses within bowel loops, subphrenic abscesses, and abscesses associated with intestinal fistula. Echinococcal cysts and multiple small abscesses represent absolute contraindications.

Technical aspects of the procedure are at the discretion of the person who performs it. General principles are the following:

1. CT scanning is generally viewed as the optimal method to define the anatomy. Drainage may be performed under CT guidance, ultrasound, or fluoroscopy. The catheter may be inserted with the Seldinger technique using a No. 8 to 14 French catheter over a guidewire or the abscess may be drained with a 12- to 16-gauge Argyle catheter inserted by trocar. The latter is generally reserved for large and readily accessible abscesses.
2. Extraserosal drainage and dependent drainage are desirable, but neither is essential.
3. Catheters are managed in a fashion analogous to those placed surgically.
4. Response is monitored by the usual clinical parameters, the amount of drainage, and the size of the abscess as determined by CT scan or ultrasound. Sinograms are generally unnecessary except for suspected enteric fistulae.
5. The expected response is defervescence within 2 to 4 days; drainage usually subsides in 7 to 14 days; and follow-up scans are expected to show resolution of the abscess within 3 weeks. Surgery may be interjected at any time that drainage appears to be inadequate.

BILIARY TRACT INFECTION

CHIN HAK CHUN, M.D.
MARTIN J. RAFF, M.D.

The authors would like to express their appreciation to Mark Malangoni, M.D., Department of Surgery, University of Louisville School of Medicine; and George Drasin, M.D., Department of Radiology, The Jewish Hospital, Louisville, Kentucky, for their helpful comments.

The biliary tract of healthy individuals harbors few, if any, microorganisms. Large volumes of bile flushed through the contracting gallbladder help to clear the biliary tree of bacteria and prevent their multiplication. Interruption of free biliary drainage by mechanical or functional disorders in the gallbladder or cystic and common bile ducts may cause bacterial infection. Cholelithiasis is the most frequent cause of obstruction, and some biliary stones may increase in size or number in the presence of bacteria.

CHOLECYSTITIS

Cholecystitis is, by definition, inflammation of the gallbladder and is most commonly initiated by cholelithiasis. It is estimated that 16 to 20 million people in the United States have gallstones, which are seen in 20 percent of women and 8 percent of men over the age of 40 years. Acute cholecystitis develops in about 25 percent of patients with gallstones.

Pathogenesis

Acute inflammation of the gallbladder wall is a result of obstruction of free biliary drainage by stones in 90 to 95 percent of patients with cholecystitis. In the 5 to 10 percent with "acalculus cholecystitis," the predisposing factors are surgery, trauma, total parenteral nutrition, adenocarcinoma of the gallbladder, periductal adenopathy, torsion of the gallbladder, or parasitic infestation. Inflammation results from lysolecithin chemical injury and other local factors or from ischemia due to increased intramural pressure on the gallbladder wall.

Bacteria are not usually detected during early stages of cholecystitis except in elderly and diabetic patients, although bacterial infection eventually develops in more than 50 percent of patients with cholecystitis. Duodenal bacteria reach the gallbladder via the bile ducts, and lower intestinal flora reaches the biliary tree through the portal circulation or the lymphatics. Bacterial infection may result in gallbladder empyema or gangrene, perforation, peritonitis, cholangitis, septicemia, and pericholecystic, hepatic or, intraperitoneal abscesses. Proliferation of gas-forming bacteria may cause emphysematous cholecystitis, particularly in elderly and diabetic patients. In approximately 80 percent of patients, cholecystitis resolves when stones are spontaneously dislodged from the biliary tree.

Unless precipitating causes are eliminated however, inflammation is likely to recur and to result in chronic cholecystitis.

Clinical Manifestations

More than two-thirds of patients with acute cholecystitis have a history of recurrent epigastric discomfort suggesting cholelithiasis. Acute cholecystitis often begins with upper abdominal discomfort that worsens, localizing to the right hypochodrium. In a smaller number of patients, it begins as acute biliary colic with severe, right upper-quadrant abdominal pain, which may radiate to the interscapular area or shoulder. Eructation and nausea and vomiting are frequent, patients may be minimally icteric, and moderate temperature elevation is often present. Repeated chills, high fever, or jaundice suggest suppurative cholangitis. The right upper-abdominal quadrant is tender to palpation or percussion, and an enlarged tender gallbladder may be palpated. Deep inspiration or cough during palpation of the right subcostal area may induce acute pain (Murphy's sign), even in those whose gallbladders are not palpated.

Laboratory Findings

Leukocytosis in the range of 10,000 to 15,000 cells per cubic millimeter is usual. One-half of patients have an elevated serum bilirubin, 40 percent have a mild increase in serum glutamic oxaloacetic acid transaminase (SGOT); 25 percent have elevated alkaline phosphatase; and 10 percent have small elevations of serum amylase.

Bacteriology

Gallbladder bile is colonized with bacteria in some 40 percent of patients in whom stones are present; they are isolated from about 10 percent of patients with pure pigment stones and from more than 90 percent of patients with bile pigment calcium stones. Bacteria are found in the bile in about 50 percent of patients with acute cholecystitis.

The aerobic bacterium most often isolated is *Escherichia coli*, followed by *Klebsiella*, group D streptococci, *Pseudomonas*, and *Enterobacter* species. *Bacteroides fragilis* is the most frequently isolated anaerobe, followed by *Clostridium perfringens* and anaerobic gram-positive cocci. Infection due to other anaerobic bacteria is rare. A combination of aerobic and anaerobic organisms may be isolated in 30 to 40 percent of patients from whom bacteria are recovered. Microorganisms other than bacteria are rarely found in patients who have not had prior surgical procedures.

Diagnostic Procedures

Plain abdominal roentgenograms are rarely helpful. The presence of radioopaque gallstones, visualized in about 15 percent of patients, does not establish a diagnosis of cholecystitis. Demonstration of gas in the gallbladder wall or lumen however, is virtually diagnostic of emphysematous cholecystitis (usually due to *C. perfringens*).

The oral cholecystogram is of limited diagnostic value in acutely ill patients who are vomiting or jaundiced. Intravenous cholangiography may demonstrate cystic duct obstruction more clearly, but its efficacy is also limited in acutely ill patients, particularly where bilirubin levels are higher than 3.5 mg per 100 milliliters. In addition, the risk of hypersensitivity reactions is appreciable. Provided that either one of these two procedures is used under optimal conditions, one should look for nonvisualization of the gallbladder. Although ultrasonography is noninvasive and accurately measures gallbladder size, it cannot be used to establish the patency of the cystic duct, and the demonstration of cholelithiasis does not aid in differentiating acute from chronic cholecystitis.

The diagnostic procedure of choice is hepatobiliary scanning with one of the ^{99m}Tc-labeled iminodiacetic acid derivatives (e.g., HIDA, PIPIDA), with sensitivity and specificity values of greater than 90 percent (Fig. 1). HIDA or PIPIDA scanning visualizes the functioning hepatobiliary system within the first hour of radionuclide injection. The typical finding in acute cholecystitis is nonvisualization of the gallbladder due to cystic duct obstruction, whereas the liver, hepatic duct, and duodenum are visualized. Ultrasonographic findings consistent with, but not specific for, acute cholecystitis include the presence of stones, a thickened gallbladder wall, a dilated gallbladder lumen, or a pericholecystic collection of fluid. Computerized tomography (CT) is not recommended as an initial diagnostic procedure since it is not as accurate as ultrasonography in detection of stones, does not reveal cystic duct patency, and is significantly more expensive.

Treatment

Patients with acute cholecystitis are best treated in hospital, the majority recovering within 5 to 6 days with supportive treatment including analgesics, intravenous fluids, and nasogastric suction.

Antimicrobial Therapy (Table 1)

Routine antimicrobial therapy does not appear to alter the outcome of acute cholecystitis and does not decrease the frequency of local infectious complications. Most antibiotics fail to reach therapeutic concentrations within an obstructed gallbladder, and bacteria within it cannot be eradicated.

Antimicrobial therapy can be withheld if patients do not appear toxic, or a single antibiotic, such as cefazolin, may be given in a dose of 1 g intravenously every 8 hours for patients who are mildly ill and improving rapidly with supportive therapy. Empiric antimicrobial therapy is recommended for patients prone to bacterial complica-

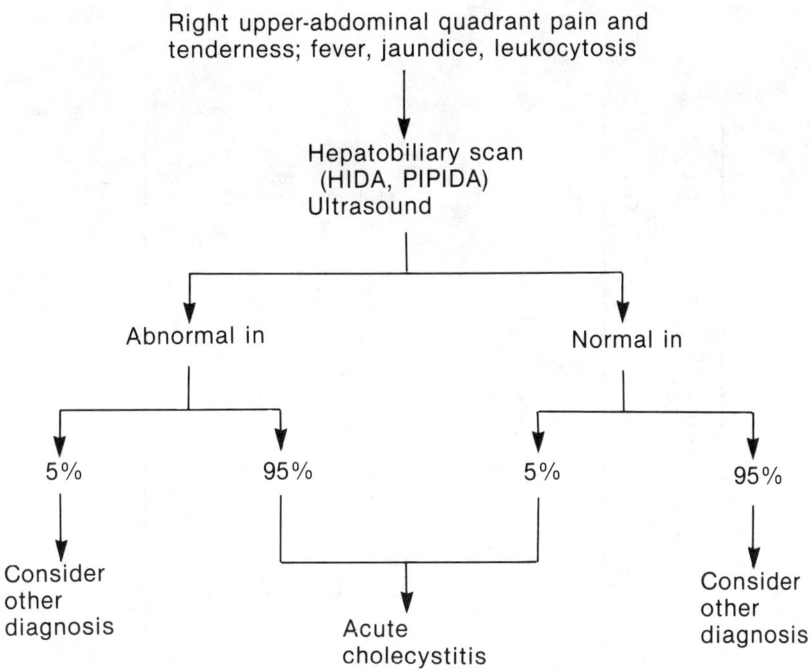

Figure 1 Diagnosis of acute cholecystitis

tions, including (1) those with jaundice and high fever; (2) those older than 60 years; (3) the immunocompromised (including diabetics); and (4) those with emphysematous cholecystitis.

Various combinations of antibiotics might initially be considered appropriate. Patients with exceptionally high fevers, hyperventilation, hypotension, or manifesting other signs and symptoms suggesting a septic state should be treated with a combination of a beta-lactam antibiotic and an aminoglycoside, such as mezlocillin and gentamicin, pending results of cultures of blood and specimens obtained during surgery.

Mezlocillin is currently our choice of expanded-spectrum penicillin derivatives because of low cost, enhanced antibacterial spectrum, reduced toxic potential, and excellent penetration into the bile, occasionally even in the presence of biliary tract obstruction. It is active against most of the commonly isolated strains of gram-negative aerobic bacilli, including many *Klebsiella* strains, the enterococci (which are the third- or fourth-commonest isolates), and many anaerobes, including *B. fragilis*.

Piperacillin has somewhat better antipseudomonad activity in vitro and excellent activity against *B. fragilis*, but is significantly more expensive, and at least one report suggests an unacceptable frequency of drug-induced neutropenia. Once cultures are available it is possible to target therapy more selectively.

In a patient who appears less clinically ill on admission and in whom signs and symptoms of sepsis are lacking, there are those who would withhold the aminoglycoside. We feel, however, that 24 to 48 hours of aminoglycoside therapy will provide a favorable margin of safety without much added cost or risk to the patient, particularly if resistance to beta-lactam antibiotics is common among the Enterobacteriaceae likely to be isolated in your hospital.

Gentamicin is selected primarily on the basis of its low cost, although tobramycin would be an adequate substitute if the risk of nephrotoxicity is considerable in a given patient. If the patient had been in hospital for some time and the nosocomial flora in that facility includes a high number of gentamicin/tobramycin-resistent organisms, amikacin should be used. Clindamycin plus gentamicin is another alternative, although this lacks enterococcal coverage. Cefoxitin or moxalactam may also be employed with or without an aminoglycoside, providing again that enterococci are not a major concern in any given patient. Both of these agents provide coverage against the more common aerobic gram-negative bacilli. Each of the above regimens will provide some coverage against anaerobic bacteria, including many strains of *Bacteroides*.

More specific antimicrobial regimens may be substituted following isolation of pathogens and determination of antibiotic sensitivities. Aqueous penicillin G is the drug of choice for clostridial and anaerobic gram-positive coccal infection, and metronidazole for other obligate anaerobes (particularly *B. fragilis* group). The extended-spectrum penicillins (mezlocillin, piperacillin, or ticarcillin in order of preference), should be used with an

TABLE 1 Antibiotics for Hepatobiliary Infection

Antibiotic (route)	Dosage*	Aerobic Bacteria					Anaerobic Bacteria			
		E. coli	*Klebsiella*	*Enterobacter*	*Pseudomonas*	*Enterococcus*	*B. fragilis*	*Other Bacteroides*	*Clostridium*	*Gram-positive Cocci*
Aminoglycosides (IV, IM)										
Amikacin	5 mg/kg q8h *or* 7.5 mg/kg q12h	4+	4+	4+	4+	Synergy with penicillin	--	--	--	--
Gentamicin	1.5–2 mg/kg q8h	4+	4+	4+	4+	Synergy with penicillin	--	--	--	--
Tobramycin	1.5–2 mg/kg q8h	4+	4+	4+	4+	Synergy with penicillin	--	--	--	--
Penicillins (IV)										
Ampicillin	1–2 g q4h	3+	--	1+	--	4+	--	3+	3+	3+
Piperacillin	2–3 g q4h	3+	3+	4+	3+	4+	3+	3+	4+	4+
Mezlocillin	2–3 g q4h	3+	3+	4+	3+	4+	3+	3+	4+	4+
Cephalosporins (IV, IM)										
Cefazolin	2 g q8h	3+	4+	--	--	--	--	--	2+	3+
Cefoxitin	2 g q4h	3+	4+	1+	--	--	3+	3+	3+	3+
Moxalactam	2–4 g q8h	3+	4+	3+	--	--	3+	3+	3+	3+
Clindamycin (IV)	400–600 mg q6h	--	--	--	--	--	3+	3+	3+	3+
Metronidazole (IV, PO)	500 mg q6h	--	--	--	--	--	4+	4+	3+	2+

Note: 4+, drug of choice; 3+, good activity; 2+, moderate activity; 1+, poor activity; --, not recommended.
* For patients with normal renal function, based on lean body weight.

aminoglycoside (gentamicin or tobramycin, in order of preference) if *Pseudomonas* is isolated. Dosages of antimicrobial agents frequently used in hepatobiliary sepsis are listed in Table 1.

The prophylactic use of antibiotics is recommended in all patients who require surgical intervention for acute cholecystitis. Cefazolin, 1 g intravenously immediately prior to surgery and repeated every 8 hours for 24 hours, should be adequate for this purpose unless resistant organisms are suspected. There do not appear to be any advantages attributable to the use of second- or third-generation cephalosporins. Antibiotics can be discontinued within 24 hours of an uncomplicated cholecystectomy, since the infectious site will have been surgically extirpated, although some surgeons prefer to continue antibiotics for 48 hours.

In patients with perforation, gangrene, or other extensive local infection, the therapeutic antibiotics suggested above should be continued for at least 7 days postoperatively if there has been rapid defervescence and clinical improvement and the patient remains free of overt signs and symptoms of infection. If defervescence and clinical improvement occur less promptly and there is persistence of leukocytosis, continued purulent drainage, or other evidence of incomplete resolution of infection, antibiotic therapy may be prolonged until cure appears evident. Obviously the choice of agents and duration of therapy must be determined on an individual basis by continued close clinical follow-up.

Surgical Therapy

Cholecystectomy is the definitive treatment of acute cholecystitis. Immediate surgery is indicated for emphysematous cholecystitis, perforation with peritonitis, and suspected pericholecystic abscess. The timing of cholecystectomy in patients with seemingly uncomplicated acute cholecystitis is controversial. Some groups favor delaying surgery, allowing 6 to 8 weeks for acute inflammation to resolve. Recent experience from different medical centers, however, supports the concept of early surgery during the acute stages of disease. Cholecystostomy is performed in patients considered too ill for cholecystectomy and should also be considered for patients in whom cholecystectomy may be technically difficult.

CHOLANGITIS

Cholangitis is defined as infection within the bile ducts. Two forms of infective acute cholangitis are recognized: ascending and suppurative.

Incidence

The majority of patients with infective cholangitis have gallstones. Considering however, that cholelithiasis is the most common hepatobiliary pathologic finding in the United States, the incidence of cholangitis is low, accounting for less than 0.2 percent of hospital admissions. Half of these patients are more than 70 years old, and cholangitis is rare in patients under the age of 50 years.

Pathogenesis

Obstruction of biliary flow by stones, stricture, papillitis, tumors, pancreatitis, and parasites increases hydrostatic pressure within the biliary tract. This interferes with function of the sphincter of Oddi and causes reflux of bile. The numbers of bacteria in the duodenum increase in the absence of bile, and they migrate up the common duct, adding to those already multiplying in stagnant bile. Bacteremia frequently occurs at this stage; the increased ductal pressure, edema, congestion, necrosis, and multiplication of bacteria lead to both cholangitis and sepsis. Cholangitis is also a complication of endoscopic retrograde cholangiopancreatography (ERCP).

Ascending cholangitis is usually associated with a partially obstructed biliary system, and purulent material does not accumulate in the biliary tract. Suppurative cholangitis develops in a completely obstructed ductal system and purulent material accumulates in the bile ducts under pressure.

Clinical Manifestations

The onset is usually acute, with high fever, chills, and diffuse, right upper-quadrant abdominal pain. Jaundice is prominent in two-thirds of patients and, because of the high frequency of bacteremia, patients may present in septic shock. Components of Charcot's triad (fever, abdominal pain, and jaundice) may be absent in as many as 15 percent to 30 percent of patients at the time of admission. Occasionally, patients experience only intermittent fever and chills spaced days to weeks apart, and present with fever of unknown origin. Abdominal pain and right upper-quadrant tenderness may be colicky, often radiating to the back or shoulder, and, although the gallbladder may not be palpated, tender hepatomegaly is usually present.

Laboratory Findings

There is usually marked leukocytosis with increased immature forms. The serum bilirubin may be elevated to 4 mg per 100 milliliters initially, increasing as the infection progresses, with serum alkaline phosphatase and SGOT values moderately elevated.

Diagnostic Procedures

Plain abdominal roentgenogram is rarely helpful; the right hemidiaphragm is frequently elevated and right-sided sympathetic pleural effusions may be present, although these are nonspecific. On very rare occasions, gas produced by bacteria will outline the biliary system.

Percutaneous transhepatic cholangiography (PTC) and ERCP will best delineate and often reveal the cause of a dilated biliary system. Samples of bile can be obtained for Gram stain and culture during these procedures, facilitating the selection of appropriate antibiotics. These procedures are invasive however, and may precipitate fulminant sepsis. Ultrasound or CT scanning will demonstrate dilated bile ducts or stones. There is no morbidity associated with these procedures, and they should be utilized before invasive procedures if the clinical presentation is suggestive of cholangitis and exploratory surgery is imminent; their value in patients without dilated bile ducts is limited. Radionuclide hepatobiliary scanning may help to diagnose obstructed common bile ducts if the biliary system and duodenum are not visualized. Oral or intravenous cholecystography is of limited, if any, value in the presence of an elevated bilirubin.

Treatment

Patients with cholangitis are usually severely dehydrated and frequently on the verge of, if not in, septic shock at the time of hospitalization. Intensive resuscitative measures may be necessary to improve the patient's condition prior to surgery; these include plasma volume replacement and correction of electrolyte imbalances. The use of corticosteroids, vasopressors, and other cardiovascular supports may also be required.

Antimicrobial Therapy

Initial antimicrobial regimens should include agents effective against aerobic gram-negative bacilli and anaerobic bacteria. The same antibiotic agents recommended for severe acute cholecystitis, including those effective against anaerobic and aerobic bacteria (Table 1), should be started promptly while awaiting results of blood and bile cultures.

Such combinations may include cephalosporins with anaerobic coverage. Mezlocillin would be our initial choice in combination with gentamicin (other aminoglycosides may be used if risks of nephrotoxicity [tobramycine] or resistant gram-negative bacilli [amikacin] are present). Cefoxitin or moxalactam, in that order of preference, would be excellent alternatives with or without the aminoglycoside, although surgeons may be reluctant to choose the latter compound because of the low incidence of clinically significant bleeding problems that have resulted from interference with platelet aggregation and the hypoprothrombinemia seen in patients with preexisting vitamin K deficiency.

In addition, none of the available cephalosporins should be used in the treatment of enterococcal infection, and these organisms are frequent isolates from the biliary tract. Moxalactam use has been shown to be complicated by an incidence of enterococcal overgrowth of about 3 percent to 5 percent. Clindamycin in combination with gentamicin may be another acceptable alternative.

The total duration of antimicrobial therapy should be determined by the clinical response and adequacy of surgical drainage. Prolonged therapy (two weeks or more) may often be necessary. Patients with obstructive jaundice undergoing PTC or ERCP should receive 1 g of cefazolin prophylactically just prior to surgery if they are not already receiving other antimicrobial therapy. It is unlikely that further doses will be necessary unless the patient manifests signs and symptoms suggestive of active infection, in which case the clinician must make therapeutic, rather than prophylactic, antibiotic choices. Some patients, particularly those with extrahepatic obstruction, may develop sepsis despite prophylaxis, and some investigators feel that all antibiotic use in these patients is therapeutic rather than prophylactic.

Surgical Therapy

Acute cholangitis is a surgical emergency. Prompt operative intervention with common bile duct decompression and T-tube drainage is essential in all patients who do not improve immediately with antimicrobial therapy; patients responding to antibiotics alone invariably require surgery at a later date. The common duct should be explored, operative cholangiography performed, and the gallbladder removed whenever possible.

LIVER ABSCESS

Liver abscesses account for approximately 0.01 percent of hospital admissions. In the United States, 90 percent of liver abscesses are pyogenic, and the remainder, amebic. The liver is protected from invading microorganisms by sinusoidal macrophages and Kupffer's cells. The low incidence of hepatic pyogenic infections may relate to the liver's role as a reticuloendothelial filter for organisms emanating from organs with portal venous drainage.

Pathogenesis

Approximately 70 percent of liver abscesses occur in association with extrahepatic sources of infection, which include the biliary tract (e.g., cholangitis, cholecystitis) in about 30 percent; the portal circulation (e.g., appendicitis, diverticulitis) in about 15 percent; contiguous infection extending directly into the liver in about 15 percent; hematogenous extension from remote sources in about 10 percent; and for the remaining 30 percent, the source is hepatic (e.g., surgery, infarct, trauma, or tumor) in 5 to 10 percent, and unknown in 20 to 25 percent.

Microorganisms appear to invade the hepatic parenchyma through the walls of the biliary tract or, hematogenously, via the hepatic artery or portal vein. There may be extension of infection from adjacent organs directly into contiguous hepatic parenchyma. Trauma leaves devitalized or infarcted liver that may become infected during episodes of transient bacteremia, and abscesses may also develop as a consequence of infected cysts or neoplasms. Abscesses associated with biliary tract infection and bacteremia are usually multiple and diffusely distributed, whereas those emanating from the portal circulation are predominantly single and confined to the right lobe of the liver.

Entamoeba histolytica reaches the liver from the colon primarily via the portal system, although lymphatic migration or direct invasion from contiguous areas is possible. Intrahepatic portal thrombosis and infarction may also predispose to amebic abscesses.

Clinical Manifestations

Early constitutional symptoms include fever, chills, anorexia, and malaise. Symptoms due to the primary infection from which the abscess originated may predominate and dictate the fever pattern. Pain, which may be dull, sharp or pleuritic, is usually in the right upper-abdominal quadrant, epigastrium, right lower chest, or the right shoulder. Tender hepatomegaly, seen in 50 to 75 percent of patients, is the most frequent finding. Pleural friction rubs and right basilar rales may be auscultated, and jaundice is observed in up to 25 percent of patients. Localized swelling over the liver is seen in approximately 10 percent of patients with amebic abscesses, and diarrhea is present in approximately 15 percent. Differentiation of pyogenic from amebic abscesses is not possible on a clinical basis.

Laboratory Findings

Serum levels of bilirubin, SGOT, and alkaline phosphatase are moderately elevated; the latter is occasionally the only abnormal enzyme value. Leukocytosis is common, and blood cultures are positive in 50 percent to 60 percent of patients with pyogenic abscesses.

Diagnostic Procedures

Roentgenograms of the chest or abdomen may show basilar atelectasis, pleural effusion, or elevation of the right hemidiaphragm. Except for those rare occasions when gas is seen within the abscess cavity, plain films can only suggest a peridiaphragmatic inflammatory process. Ultrasonography, CT scan, and ^{99m}Tc sulfur-colloid liver scanning will detect more than 85 percent of hepatic lesions greater than 2 cm in diameter. Ultrasonography and CT, unlike ^{99m}Tc scintiscanning, may distinguish cystic from solid lesions and abscesses from tumors. These two former procedures are also used to guide percutaneous needle aspiration for diagnosis and treatment. One or two of the above procedures is usually sufficient in most cases.

Additional diagnostic modalities include ^{67}Ga or ^{111}In scanning. Both isotopes are concentrated in pyogenic abscesses. In amebic abscesses, ^{67}Ga uptake is increased in the hypervascular abscess rim, with the central area showing decreased uptake.

Percutaneous needle aspirations guided by CT scan or ultrasound help to differentiate pyogenic from amebic abscesses. Malodorous purulent material is more frequently seen in pyogenic lesions. Amebic abscesses usually contain dark brown and sterile fluid in which trophozoites of *E. histolytica* may be found, although amoebae are often found only in the abscess wall. Amoebae can also be grown from the abscess when cultures are available. Serologic tests for amoebae are helpful when abscesses are sterile: positive results in nonendemic areas will suggest an amebic etiology, whereas amebiasis is a less likely diagnosis when serology is negative, although this should not exclude it from consideration.

Microbiology

Pyogenic liver abscesses are frequently polymicrobial. Aerobic gram-negative bacilli, anaerobic gram-negative bacilli, and facultative or microaerophilic streptococci are important pathogens. *E. coli, Klebsiella, B. fragilis* group, and microaerophilic streptococci are frequently isolated. Aerobes and anaerobes are recovered concomitantly in more than 50 percent of patients. Staphylococci are common pathogens in children, frequently causing hematogenous microabscesses. In immunocompromised hosts, alcoholics, and drug abusers, *Candida* species may be isolated as sole pathogens. Sterile abscesses are encountered in less than 10 percent of patients, possibly because obligate anaerobes have been inadequately collected and transported or are difficult to culture. Prior antimicrobial therapy may also make cultures negative, and Gram stains of clinical material at the time of culture may be very helpful.

Treatment

The treatment of pyogenic liver abscesses requires both antimicrobial agents and surgical intervention. Accurate localization and percutaneous aspiration of abscesses has been made possible by ultrasonography and CT scanning.

Antimicrobial Therapy

Antibiotic therapy should be started as soon as a presumptive diagnosis is made, with agents selected to cover both aerobic gram-negative bacilli and anaerobes. If the abscess originated from a discernible primary infection, therapy should be directed against that causative agent. Gentamicin (tobramycin or amikacin may be substituted, as indicated above in section on cholangitis) combined with cefoxitin is recommended as an initial regimen, although moxalactam alone (because of its excellent activity against *B. fragilis*) or a combination of clindamycin or metronidazole with a second-generation cephalosporin can be used alternatively. The dosages and antimicrobial spectra of these antibiotics are listed in Table 1. Metronidazole should be substituted for cefoxitin or clindamycin if pure cultures of obligate anaerobic organisms (particularly *B. fragilis*) are isolated from the abscess or if beta-lactam-resistant obligate anaerobes are likely to be isolated.

The avascular, anaerobic, acidic milieu of the abscess cavity inhibits both antibiotic penetration and leukocyte function and increases binding and degradation of antibiotics. Although there is evidence that clindamycin may enter the leukocyte, neither clindamycin nor the beta-lactam antibiotics are bactericidal against *B. fragilis*, and there have been failures of therapy with these agents despite the presence of organisms against which they appear effective in vitro.

Metronidazole both penetrates into and kills bacteria within the abscess, and has been effective in eradicating obligate anaerobes after clinical failures with other agents. Facultative and microaerophilic streptococci are usually sensitive to penicillins or cephalosporins, but not to metronidazole.

Continuation of aminoglycoside therapy will depend upon the presence of aerobic gram-negative bacilli and their antibiotic susceptibility patterns. Cefoxitin may be continued if the aerobic gram-negative bacilli in polymicrobial abscesses are sensitive, but if clostridia are present, metronidazole or penicillin should be employed. Third-generation cephalosporins do not offer significant advantages unless they obviate the need for aminoglycosides; moxalactam has excellent activity against anaerobes, including *B. fragilis*, and there is in vitro evidence that synergy between cefotaxime and its desacetyl metabolite may produce similar effects.

Antimicrobial therapy should be continued until there is a significant decrease in the size of the abscesses (confirmed by CT scanning or ultrasonography); this may take as long as 2 to 6 weeks.

Metronidazole remains the drug of choice for most patients with amebic abscesses; 750 mg by mouth three times a day for 5 to 7 days is recommended. Other amebicidal drugs equally effective are emetine, dehydroemetine, and chloroquine, but these latter agents produce significant toxic effects, which may severely limit their utility.

Surgical Therapy

Although some patients with small abscesses may recover on antibiotic therapy alone, drainage is often necessary. Percutaneous catheter or needle aspiration, with the aid of ultrasonography or CT, may replace open surgical drainage when the abscesses are accessible. Indications for open surgical drainage include the presence of more than two relatively large abscesses; concomitant drainable intra-abdominal sources of infection (e.g., cholangitis, diverticulitis, appendicitis); abscesses in which the primary source is not obvious, but is suspected to be intra-abdominal (e.g., Crohn's disease, tumor); abscesses with highly viscous purulent contents; and the presence of ascites. Fungal abscesses also require open drainage. Percutaneous drainage is the preferred method for patients with cryptogenic abscesses if there are no more than two cavities and for those patients who are poor surgical risks. The latter method however, while circumventing major surgery, may necessitate prolonged hospitalization.

Amebic abscesses may be successfully treated with antiamebics alone, although initial aspiration may be necessary for diagnostic purposes. Repeated aspiration is indicated only if more than 250 ml of pus was removed at the first aspiration or if pain and constitutional symptoms do not subside.

SPLENIC ABSCESS

Splenic abscesses are uncommon, occurring primarily in patients with infective endocarditis, hemoglobinopathies, or hematologic malignancies or following trauma to the spleen.

Pathogenesis

Splenic infarction appears to be the important antecedent to hematogenous bacterial seeding. Bacteria may also penetrate from infection in contiguous organs, but this is rare.

Diagnostic Procedures

Plain roentgenograms of the chest and abdomen may reveal an elevated left hemidiaphragm, pleural effusion, pulmonary infiltrates or atelectasis; enlarged spleens may displace the stomach or colon, but these findings are nonspecific. Ultrasonography and CT are the preferred diagnostic procedures, but a strong clinical index of suspicion warrants prompt surgical exploration despite the absence of unequivocal radiologic findings, since these lesions are virtually never curable with antibiotics alone.

Bacteriology

Pathogens such as *Staphylococcus aureus* or streptococci, which cause infective endocarditis and bacteremia, are frequently recovered, followed by aerobic gram-negative bacilli, anaerobic bacteria and salmonellae. Patients with hematologic malignancies may develop fungal splenic abscesses.

Clinical Manifestations

Left upper-quadrant abdominal pain and tenderness and fever and chills are the commonest symptoms. Abdominal pain may radiate to the left shoulder. Even when not palpated, the spleen is often tender. Left-sided pleural friction rubs and pleural effusion may occur, and friction rubs may also be auscultated over the spleen.

Treatment

Antimicrobial Therapy

Selection of an initial antimicrobial regimen should be based on the etiology of the primary infection. If this information is not available at the time of diagnosis, antibiotics directed against the most likely pathogen can be started empirically. In those infections occurring secondary to endocarditis, staphylococci and enterococci are frequent pathogens, and a combination of vancomycin, 500 mg intravenously four times a day, and gentamicin, 1.0 to 1.5 mg per kilogram of lean body weight every 8 hours is appropriate, pending identification of the organism.

Surgical Therapy

Splenectomy is mandatory for all patients, since survival in its absence is doubtful at best. Although seldom surgically feasible, uninvolved segments of spleen can be retained to decrease the inherent risk of fulminant sepsis in splenectomized individuals. Splenotomy with drainage is rarely therapeutic.

Infections of the Pancreas

Infections of the normal pancreas are extremely unusual. In children, pancreatitis may occur in association with generalized infections due to mumps or coxsackieviruses A or B, and the same entity occurs rarely in adults. Rising titers of antibody against *Mycoplasma pneumoniae* have also been demonstrated in a few patients with pancreatitis. Bacterial infections of the pancreas are usually complications of preexisting pancreatitis, producing extensive morbidity and high mortality due to pancreatic phlegmon, abscesses, and infected pseudocysts.

Pancreatic abscess occurs in between 1 and 10 percent of patients following episodes of acute pancreatitis; the incidence in patients with chronic pancreatitis is much lower. Pancreatic phlegmon, occurring in up to 18 percent of patients with acute pancreatitis, is a solid mass of indurated pancreatic and adjacent retroperitoneal tissues—as opposed to an abscess that is characterized by collections of pus and necrotic tissue. Secondary infection may occur in 14 to 40 percent of pseudocysts.

Pathogenesis

Pancreatitis is the commonest factor predisposing to pancreatic infection, usually occurring as a result of alcoholism, biliary calculi, surgery, ERCP, and trauma. Bacteria are known to enter the pancreatic duct following reflux of duodenal contents or infected bile. Some bacteria found in the pancreatic juices produce beta-glucuronidase and are capable of deconjugating bile, yielding components of bile acids that are significantly more injurious to pancreatic ducts. Despite these findings, the role of bacteria in the pathogenesis of acute pancreatitis is still not clear.

Acute pancreatitis leads to bacterial infection when bacteria enter and grow on necrotic pancreatic tissue. Reflux of bacterially contaminated or infected bile from duodenal contents, transmural penetration from the adjacent duodenum or colon when either is injured by pancreatitis, and hematogenous seeding are all possible routes for bacterial infection of the pancreas.

Clinical Manifestations

Infectious complications usually develop 1 to 3 weeks after the onset of acute pancreatitis. The commonest clinical course suggestive of pancreatic abscess is an initial therapeutic response of the pancreatitis followed by a recurrence of nausea, vomiting, abdominal pain, tenderness and fever. Some patients may have unremitting fever, leukocytosis, and abdominal tenderness following the initial episode of acute pancreatitis. An abdominal mass is palpated in about 25 to 30 percent, and jaundice may be present in up to 30 percent of patients. Pancreatic pseudocysts develop in 2 to 10 percent of patients with acute pancreatitis, usually about 2 to 3 weeks after the initial attack. Clinical manifestations of infected pseudocysts are similar to those of pancreatic abscesses.

Laboratory Findings

Elevated serum amylase levels occur in 20 to 70 percent of patients with pancreatic abscesses; serum levels of bilirubin, alkaline phosphatase, and SGOT are usually minimally elevated; leukocytosis is common. There are no laboratory tests diagnostic of pancreatic abscess or infected pseudocyst.

Diagnostic Procedures

Plain roentgenogram of the abdomen reveals a paralytic ileus in 70 to 80 percent and small bowel obstruction, rarely, in patients with pancreatic abscesses. Gas in the abscess (soap-bubble sign) may be seen in less than 20 percent of cases. Barium studies of the upper gastrointestinal tract will invariably demonstrate an extrinsic mass displacing the stomach or widening of the duodenal loop.

Ultrasonography and CT scanning are the preferred procedures, revealing the abscess in 80 to 90 percent of patients. It may be difficult to differentiate abscesses from pseudocysts. Gallium-67 or indium-111 scans would be nonspecific in view of the diffusely inflamed pancreas unless a focal area of intense accumulation is seen. Percutaneous needle aspiration guided by ultrasound or CT scan can be diagnostic if purulent material is obtained.

Bacteriology

The bacteria recovered from pancreatic abscesses frequently include *E. coli, Enterobacter, Klebsiella* and *Pseudomonas* species, and enterococci. Anaerobic organisms are isolated from less than 20 percent of reported cases, but the considerable number of sterile abscesses suggests a greater role for these organisms. Recovery of *Candida* species and other yeast-like fungi appears to have increased recently, although the numbers are not significant. The etiologic agents of phlegmons or infected pseudocysts are presumed to be similar to those causing pancreatic abscesses.

Treatment

Pancreatic abscess is invariably fatal if not treated surgically, and early intervention is of paramount importance.

Supportive Therapy

Conventional therapy for acute pancreatitis, including nasogastric suction, intravenous fluids, and correction of electrolyte imbalances should be continued. Total parenteral nutrition should be started in most patients, although the infectious risks associated with this must be kept clearly in mind.

Antimicrobial Therapy

Antimicrobial therapy does not reduce the severity of acute hemorrhagic pancreatitis or lower the incidence of pancreatic abscess, and routine use of antibiotics is not recommended for acute pancreatitis. Once infectious complications are diagnosed, a combination of gentamicin and mezlocillin should be started (other broad-spectrum penicillins such as ticarcillin or piperacillin may be substituted as indicated above).

The regimen containing mezlocillin is adequate against aerobic enteric bacilli, including most strains of *Klebsiella* and enterococci. As an alternative, clindamycin may provide better activity against anaerobic organisms (piperacillin also has good activity against *B. fragilis*), but will be inadequate for gram-negative bacillary or enterococcal infections. A more specific antimicrobial regimen should be substituted when the results of blood and abscess cultures are available (the dosages and antimicrobial activity of antibiotics mentioned above are listed in Table 1).

Recovery of *Candida* species from pancreatic infection in a nonsurgical patient warrants antifungal therapy with amphotericin B and flucytosine. If *Candida* species are isolated from the superficial wound or drainage tubes, cultures should be performed on blood and pancreatic tissue to document the presence of deep-seated infection before antifungal treatment is started.

Surgical Therapy

Adequate surgical debridement with external drainage should be performed whenever possible. All pancreatic, peripancreatic, and retroperitoneal abscesses must be located and drained despite the fact that this may be technically quite difficult because of the extensive inflammation, secondary adhesions, and peripancreatic tissue necrosis. Pancreatic abscesses may extend to the mediastinum or burrow down the retroperitoneal space to the scrotum or femoral triangle. The role of percutaneous catheter drainage in treating pancreatic abscess is quite limited. Surgical treatment for an infected pseudocyst is external drainage, which may incapacitate patients for months. Percutaneous catheter drainage is technically simple, the duration of drainage may be shortened significantly, and it should be considered for uncomplicated infected pseudocysts.

Pancreatic phlegmon usually responds to medical therapy alone. An initial therapeutic response to antibiotics followed by relapse within 3 weeks or an absence of prompt improvement accompanied by clincial manifestations of sepsis indicates underlying complications that should precipitate rapid surgical intervention.

VIRAL HEPATITIS

DAVID J. GOCKE, M.D.

DIFFERENTIAL DIAGNOSIS

When faced with a patient with jaundice and/or hepatic enzyme abnormalities, one needs first to decide whether the patient has one of the classic forms of viral hepatitis or is suffering from liver injury due to some other cause. Hepatic injury of an acute nature (i.e., evolving over days rather than weeks or months) can be caused by nonviral as well as viral agents. Chief among the nonviral causes is acute alcoholic hepatitis, which is common and usually accompanied by evidence of intoxication or binge drinking. Chemically induced hepatic injury is also fairly frequent and should be revealed by a careful medication and environmental history. Other nonviral etiologies such as biliary obstruction or metastatic carcinoma may occasionally present rather acutely, but the diagnosis is usually suggested by other accompanying features.

Among viral causes of acute hepatic injury, one must consider in the differential diagnosis the occasional case of severe infectious mononucleosis due to the Epstein-Barr virus, which may cause enzyme elevations and, rarely, jaundice. Almost invariably such patients have florid disease with fever, lymphadenopathy, and splenomegaly, which makes the diagnosis obvious. A mononucleosis-like illness with a negative mononucleosis test is due to cytomegalovirus infection and can also be associated with hepatic injury. This may be more confusing because the serologic test is negative, but again, the hepatic manifestations are usually minor compared with the systemic features. Other viruses (and, for that matter, other infectious agents) cause liver injury so rarely as to be negligible in the scope of this discussion.

Having considered the above possible causes of acute hepatic injury and concluded that one of the hepatitis viruses is the most likely etiology, the next step is to differentiate one type of viral hepatitis from another. This is not just an academic exercise because knowledge of the particular hepatitis virus responsible for the illness has important epidemiologic and therapeutic implications in management of the patient. Clinical and epidemiologic features of the illness may suggest that one or another of the hepatitis viruses is responsible. Some of these features are summarized in Table 1. However, there is considerable variation and overlap with regard to these features and, in the individual case, one must depend on serology to make a specific diagnosis.

In the past 15 years, the discovery of specific viral antigens and antibodies associated with the type A and type B hepatitis viruses and development of reliable, widely available tests for these markers now permits specific differentiation of these two infections. In addition, clinical application of these tests has led, by a process of exclusion, to the recognition of so-called non-A, non-B (NANB) hepatitis, a serious form of hepatitis previously unappreciated. Even more recently, the discovery of the Delta hepatitis agent has revealed another new and important facet of viral hepatitis. Figure 1 illustrates the process involved in the serologic differentiation of acute viral hepatitis. The results of these sensitive, specific, and reliable assays for antibody to the hepatitis A virus (anti-HAV) and to the hepatitis B markers (HBsAg, anti-HBs and anti-HBc) are usually available within 48 to 72 hours. As with most infectious diseases, the finding of viral antigen in the patient's serum usually indicates acute infection with the agent. Thus, the finding of a positive test

TABLE 1 Clinical and Epidemiologic Features in Viral Hepatitis

Type	*Source*	*Risk Factors or Settings*	*Significance*
Hepatitis A	Ingestion of contaminated food or water	Shellfish Day-care centers Institutions for retarded Prisons Male homosexuality Foreign travel	Often anicteric Usually self-limited Rarely fatal (<1%) No carrier state No chronic infection Requires public health intervention
Hepatitis B	Parenteral inoculation of contaminated blood or blood products; sexual contact	Transfusion of blood or blood products Drug abuse Male homosexuality Sexual contact Health care professions Institutions for retarded Prisons	Often icteric High morbidity May be fulminant (1%–2%) 6%–10% become carriers and/or develop chronic hepatitis Hepatoma
Non-A, Non-B hepatitis	As for hepatitis B	As for hepatitis B	May be icteric May be fulminant 20%–60% become carriers and/or develop chronic hepatitis
Delta hepatitis	As for hepatitis B (Delta infection requires "help" from HBV, always occurs in patient concomitantly infected with HBV)	Transfusion of blood or blood products Drug abuse	Requires coinfection with HBV Increases severity of liver damage →fulminant hepatitis→death (10%–20%) →progressive chronic active hepatitis

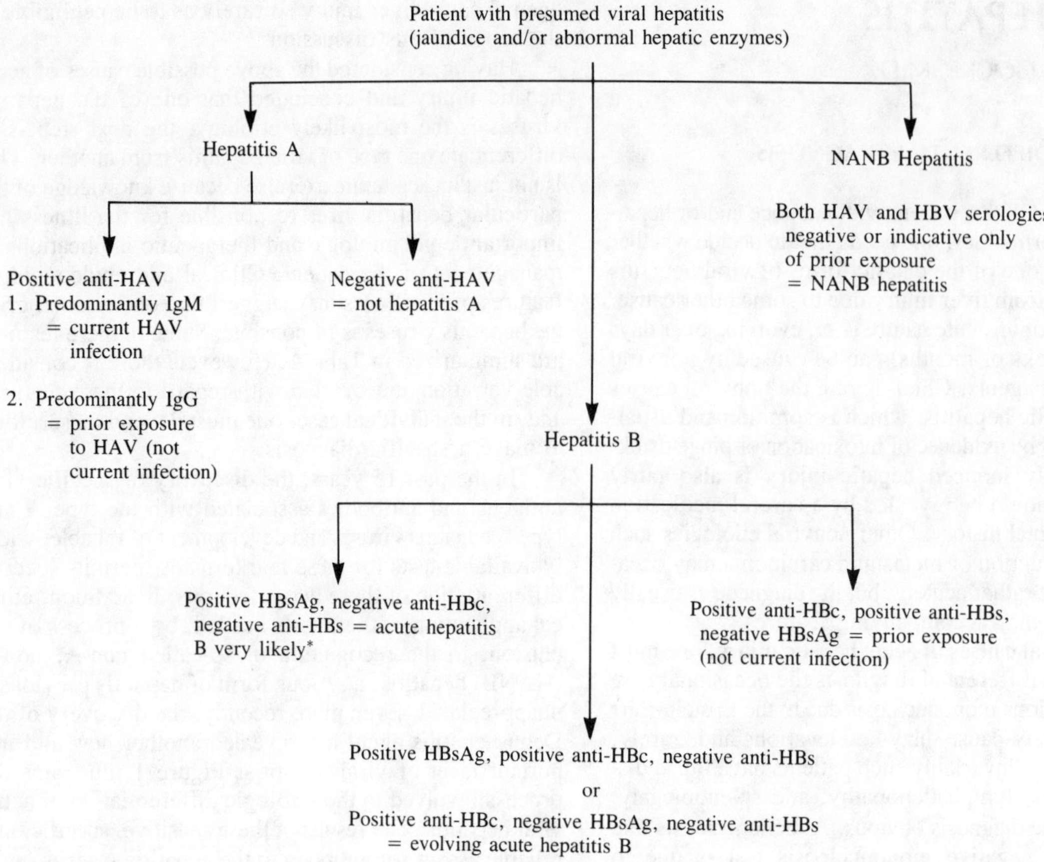

Patient with presumed viral hepatitis
(jaundice and/or abnormal hepatic enzymes)
Hepatitis A
NANB Hepatitis
Both HAV and HBV serologies negative or indicative only of prior exposure = NANB hepatitis
Positive anti-HAV
1. Predominantly IgM = current HAV infection
2. Predominantly IgG = prior exposure to HAV (not current infection)
Negative anti-HAV = not hepatitis A
Hepatitis B
Positive HBsAg, negative anti-HBc, negative anti-HBs = acute hepatitis B very likely*
Positive anti-HBc, positive anti-HBs, negative HBsAg = prior exposure (not current infection)
Positive HBsAg, positive anti-HBc, negative anti-HBs
or
Positive anti-HBc, negative HBsAg, negative anti-HBs
= evolving acute hepatitis B
* Occasionally (5%–10%) patients presenting with apparent acute hepatitis B are actually having an acute exacerbation of an underlying chronic hepatitis B (see text).

Figure 1 Schema for serologic differentiation of acute viral hepatitis

for HBsAg in the serum of a patient with acute hepatic injury very likely signifies acute hepatitis B infection. One caveat to this is the occasional HBsAg-positive patient with what appears to be an acute process who is actually having an acute exacerbation of an underlying, previously unrecognized chronic form of hepatitis B. This exception may not become apparent without long-term follow-up of the patient and/or liver biopsy, but does not alter management for the acute episode. The presence of antibody to the infectious agent may represent either recent infection or prior exposure to the agent that is unrelated to the current illness. Differentiation of IgM and IgG components of the antibody response helps to distinguish recent from remote exposure. Thus, a positive test for anti-HAV predominantly of the IgM type is strongly suggestive of current HAV infection, whereas an IgG or mixed IgG/IgM response probably represents only prior exposure. Of the tests for hepatitis B virus (HBV) markers, detection of a positive anti-HBc in the presence of a negative anti-HBs is often useful in differentiating hepatitis B in the acute phase because the anti-HBc response appears earlier during the acute illness than the anti-HBs response, which may not be seen until the patient has recovered. When both the anti-HBc and anti-HBs are positive, this finding is compatible with either remote exposure to HBV unrelated to the current illness or with the late convalescent phase of an acute HBV infection. Thus, these tests always need to be interpreted in terms of the point in the patient's course when the blood was tested. Of course, documentation of recent seroconversion from negative to positive for any of the antibody tests is also strong evidence of recent infection. Finally, the tests for hepatitis Be antigen (HBeAg) and antibody (anti-HBe) are usually reserved for evaluation of patients with chronic forms of hepatitis B (see below).

The significance of making a specific diagnosis of hepatitis A is that one can be assured the patient will almost always recover without serious sequelae. Chronic forms of hepatitis and the carrier state are essentially unheard of with this disease, and fulminant hepatitis is rare. However, this diagnosis should be prompt epidemiologic investigation for the source of infection and institution of appropriate control measures (as discussed below). A diagnosis of hepatitis B, on the other hand, has more serious implications. The patient is more likely to be hospitalized or incapacitated for an extended time and has a significant chance of developing a major complication of HBV infection (fulminant disease, chronic hepatitis, the carrier state, hepatoma). These problems demand careful follow-up and proper management. Also, identification of contacts and immunization procedures need to be considered, as outlined below.

If a diagnosis of neither hepatitis A or B can be established after applying the above criteria, then one has arrived at a diagnosis of NANB hepatitis by exclusion. Obviously, this is not a specific way to make a diagnosis, but lacking tests for specific markers of the NANB agents, it is the best we can do at present. Occasionally, a case may be misdiagnosed in this manner, but this exclusion process is probably accurate at least 90 percent of the time. Clearly, NANB hepatitis is a real entity. At least two types of NANB agents have been demonstrated by epidemiologic and transmission studies, but these are not usually differentiated in the clinical setting at present. The major significance of establishing a diagnosis of NANB hepatitis is that it alerts the physician to the development of chronic disease, which occurs with disturbing frequency (20% to 60% of patients in various studies) and which requires appropriate follow-up and management.

Delta hepatitis is a newly discovered form of hepatitis caused by a defective or incomplete RNA virus that cannot produce infection by itself. This agent has an absolute requirement for coinfection with HBV, which provides essential help for replication of the Delta agent. Delta infection always occurs in a person who is concomitantly infected with HBV, either chronically or acutely. Delta "superinfection" may make an acute hepatitis much more severe (leading to fulminant hepatitis) or may exacerbate chronic hepatitis B (leading to early cirrhosis and hepatic insufficiency). Tests for Delta antigen and antibody are not yet widely available, but may appear in the next year or two.

MANAGEMENT

General Recommendations

When first seen, the course of the patient with presumed viral hepatitis is still unpredictable. Many recover uneventfully. Others develop serious, life-threatening complications that cannot be predicted at the outset. There is no specific antiviral therapy at present, but good management involves much more than benign neglect.

Early Recognition of Impending Hepatic Insufficiency. The syndrome of fulminant hepatitis leading to hepatic insufficiency, coma, and death is the least common but most dreaded complicaton of viral hepatitis. It occurs in less than 1 percent of patients with hepatitis A, in 1 to 2 percent of patients with hepatitis B or NANB hepatitis, and in 10 to 20 percent of hepatitis B patients superinfected with the Delta agent. Once coma occurs, the survival rate is only 30 to 40 percent in experienced key to successful management is early recognition—before coma supervenes. The best predictor of impending hepatic insufficiency is the prothrombin time, which should be ordered along the bilirubin, hepatic enzymes, and viral markers as a part of the initial evaluation. The level of bilirubin, hepatic enzymes, and blood ammonia are not reliable guides, but if the prothrombin time is increased, especially if more than 20 seconds, the possibility that the patient will progress to full-blown hepatic insufficiency and coma is great. Deterioration can occur in a few hours, so close observation is required. The aim should be to start anticholemic measures (consult standard texts for details) before coma develops, rather than after.

When to Hospitalize the Patient with Hepatitis. There are only two indications for hospitalization of a patient with acute viral hepatitis. One is an elevated prothrombin time, as discussed above. The other is the patient with severe nausea and vomiting who is unable to maintain fluid balance or who is so weak and incapacitated as to be unable to care for himself at home. Most patients with acute hepatitis can and should be cared for at home in order to avoid unnecessary exposure of hospital staff and utilization of expensive hospital beds.

Isolation? All forms of viral hepatitis are capable of person-to-person transmission and certainly represent a hazard. In the hospital setting, both stool and needle/syringe precautions should be employed until the type and stage of hepatitis is defined (usually within 72 hours) and then modified along the following lines. Type A hepatitis is essentially never viremic in the acute phase (so serum precautions are not needed), and virus disappears from the stool very early in the acute phase (so even stool precautions are not needed in the convalescent phase). Types B and NANB require only needle/syringe precautions (not stool), but it is especially important that specimens sent to the laboratory and contaminated waste material be double-bagged and flagged to protect hospital personnel. A private room in the hospital is usually not necessary, unless the patient is a perambulatory child, has a bleeding diathesis, or is incontinent of stool or urine.

In the home setting, knowledge of the type and stage of hepatitis is also a guide. For hepatitis A, the patient should practice careful hand washing and good personal hygiene and avoid preparation of food for other family members. Decontamination of clothing, linen, and dishes can be satisfactorily achieved with conventional washing machines and dishwashers. Bear in mind that by the time the patient presents to a physician and a diagnosis is established, the virus has usually disappeared from the stool. Once the bilirubin and enzymes begin to decline in hepatitis A, isolation is no longer necessary. With hepatitis B and NANB, however, viremia may persist for weeks, months, or years, even though the bilirubin and enzymes are improving. Such patients may transmit disease. With hepatitis B, as long as the patient's blood contains HBsAg, he must be regarded as potentially infectious. In HBV infection, the presence of HBeAg in the serum is known to be associated with a high degree of infectivity, whereas patients with anti-HBe are much less infective, but this is only relative. For NANB hepatitis, since there is no antigenic marker to follow, one can be guided only by persistent enzyme elevations. The primary hazards for transmission of both type B and NANB disease in the home setting are close personal contact (usually sexual) and the sharing of toothbrushes, razors, and other articles that may be blood contaminated. Thus, it is the spouse or sexual partner who is at greatest risk of acquiring the infection and should be evaluated for evidence of infecton and immunized if not already infected. Other members of the household are at much lower risk, except in special situations (a home dialysis patient, communal intravenous drug abuse, open wounds). Recommendations on immunization for hepatitis B are given below.

Diet. During the acute anorectic phase of viral hepatitis, the primary concern should be maintenance of caloric intake and fluid and electrolyte balance, orally, if possible, or with intravenous supplements, if necessary. Otherwise, the patient need only be instructed to eat and drink what appeals to him. As nausea subsides and the appetite returns, most patients resume an adequate intake. The old idea of urging high-carbohydrate, high-calorie diets on an anorectic patient is counterproductive and has never been shown to hasten hepatic recovery. As noted above, if impending hepatic coma is suspected, protein restriction (20 g per day) or elimination (a no-protein diet) may be indicated.

Alcohol and Other Drugs. Alcohol is a direct hepatic toxin and acts in an additive fashion with viral hepatic injury. Alcohol should be strictly prohibited, not only in the acute phase but until the enzymes have returned to normal. Also, remember that the half-life of medications metabolized in the liver may be prolonged. Sedatives and tranquilizers should especially be avoided.

Activity. There is no evidence that strict bed rest speeds recovery in the average patient. However, most patients with hepatitis do not feel like doing much. Thus, limited activity around the home is advisable, but confinement to bed is unnecessary. The patient should be cautioned to resume normal activity only gradually and as tolerated. In some cases, the patient may not recover his usual stamina and well-being for 3 to 6 months.

Steroids. Corticosteroids are not indicated in the management of acute hepatitis of any type. Although steroids make the patient feel better transiently, they do not alter the ultimate course of the disease, may prolong full recovery, and are often associated with serious rebound hepatitis when discontinued.

Problems To Look For. Early recognition and treatment of impending hepatic insufficiency has been discussed above. As the acute phase passes and improvement begins, the next question is whether the patient will develop persistent infection, either in the form of an asymptomatic carrier state or some form of chronic hepatitis. As noted previously, this is rare with hepatitis A, but 6 to 10 percent of patients with hepatitis B and 20 to 60 percent with NANB develop some form of persistent infection. Thus, periodic follow-up (every 2 to 4 weeks) is indicated until it can be documented that the hepatic enzymes have returned to normal and stay normal and, in the case of hepatitis B, that HBs antigenemia has cleared. In some cases, this requires several months, during which time the comments made above about potential infectivity, alcohol prohibition, and activity still apply. An error commonly made in patients whose enzymes are still abnormal after 2 to 3 months is the unwarranted institution of steroid therapy. After 6 months, however, if the enzymes are still abnormal, liver biopsy is indicated. The management of chronic forms of hepatitis is beyond the scope of this discussion. Suffice it to say here that this is a difficult and controversial area that should be handled by an experienced hepatologist.

Specific Recommendations on Immunization

Guidelines for hepatitis immunization are given in Table 2.

Hepatitis. There is no hepatitis A vaccine available at present (although a candidate vaccine is currently in clinical trials and may be available in 1 to 2 years). Pools of normal human serum globulin (NSG) contain significant antibody to HAV and will prevent or ameliorate HAV infection if given within 2 weeks of exposure. Postexposure prophylaxis for close contacts of patients with hepatitis A and for individuals exposed in common-source outbreaks of hepatitis A is clearly indicated. The definition of "close contact" should be limited to members of the same household, not to entire schools, offices, neighborhoods, or social contacts. Preexposure prophylaxis of hepatitis A is indicated for travelers to areas of the world highly endemic for hepatitis A (basically, all the underdeveloped countries). The recommended dose of NSG is 0.04 ml per kilogram. In the event of continuing exposure, as with prolonged travel in endemic areas, this dose should be repeated every 3 to 4 months.

Hepatitis B. A safe, highly effective hepatitis B vaccine is now widely available. It is clearly indicated in persons at high risk of developing hepatitis B, i.e., those with exposure to contaminated blood and blood products. This includes susceptible health care workers (including surgeons, dentists, pathologists, and clinical laboratory workers), male homosexuals, and household contacts of hepatitis B patients. Regarding household contacts, if the patient is a chronic hepatitis B carrier (so that exposure may be prolonged), both active immunization with the hepatitis B vaccine and passive immunization with hepatitis B immune globulin (HBIG) are indicated for the susceptible contacts. This combination of passive/active immunization confers immediate protection from the HBIG pending later development of active immunity from the vaccine. This is especially important for sexual contacts of the infected carrier. This passive/active immunization against hepatitis B is also now the recommended approach for neonates born to HBsAg-positive mothers. To determine the susceptibility of contacts, and to rule out ongoing HBV infection, these individuals should be tested for anti-HBc, HBsAg, and hepatic enzyme levels. The presence of HBsAg and/or abnormal enzymes indi-

TABLE 2 Summary of Hepatitis Immunization Recommendations

	Vaccine		*Immune Globulin*	
	Setting	*Dose*	*Setting*	*Dose*
Hepatitis A	(Vaccine not currently available)		Postexposure: household contacts common-source outbreaks	0.04 ml IG/kg IM
			Preexposure: travel to endemic area	0.04 ml IG/kg IM every 4–6 months
Hepatitis B	Postexposure: sexual contact* neonatal* Preexposure: risk of blood contact	3 doses† 20 μg each IM at 0, 1, and 6 months	Postexposure: needle stick sexual contact* neonatal*	0.06 ml HBIG/kg IM
			Preexposure: not indicated (use vaccine)	
Non-A, Non-B hepatitis	(Vaccine not currently available)		Postexposure: ? needle stick ? neonatal	0.04 ml IG/kg IM (controversial!)
			Preexposure: not indicated	

Note: Abbreviations, IG=normal serum globulin; HBIG=hepatitis B immune globulin
* Use combined active/passive immunization with both HB vaccine and HBIG
† Dose in children <12 years old = 10 μg each injection

cates current infection, whereas the presence of anti-HBc with negative HBsAg and normal enzymes indicates immunity. However, in any postexposure situation, early protection is important and administration of vaccine and HBIG to an individual already infected is not dangerous, so immunization should not be excessively delayed while waiting for test results. The hepatitis B vaccine must be given in three intramuscular injections (20 μg each) at 0, 1, and 6 months for optimal response. Children younger than 12 years require only half doses (10 μg each), and immunocompromised hosts (i.e., dialysis patients) require larger doses (40 μg each). Finally, the usual dose of HBIG is 0.06 ml per kilogram.

For prophylaxis in the case of limited or one-time exposures—as in medical personnel with contaminated needle sticks, after limited sexual contact, or where the patient has promptly reverted to HBsAg-negative—adequate protection may be achieved with HBIG alone in the doses noted. In such cases, a second dose of HBIG should be given 1 month later.

Non-A, Non-B Hepatitis. There is no vaccine or hyperimmune globulin for NANB hepatitis. Whether normal serum globulin (IG) preparations contain enough antibody against NANB agents to be helpful is a controversial issue. However, since ordinary IG is inexpensive and harmless, many authorities would administer IG in high-risk situations, such as for contaminated needle sticks or the infant born of a mother with NANB hepatitis.

INFECTION CAUSED BY INTESTINAL HELMINTHS

RAMÓN H. BERMÚDEZ, M.D.

The majority of human infections caused by worms are associated with the gastrointestinal tract or liver. These multicellular organisms may parasitize the lumen of the gut, the biliary tract, or the portal venous system, but in some circumstances, tissue invasion may occur as well. Intestinal helminthic infections may be asymptomatic; disease manifestations may, however, be localized to the gastrointestinal tract or there may be more systemic clinical features. Because of their worldwide prevalence, intestinal helminthic infections cause considerable morbidity and mortality. For the purpose of this discussion, worm infections are divided according to their human anatomic habitat and to their general taxonomic features (Table 1).

EPIDEMIOLOGY

Intestinal helminths cause common infections in many parts of the world. Although their prevalence has

TABLE 1 Major Intestinal Helminths in Humans

Final Habitat in Humans	*Type and Species*	
Small intestine	Nematodes	*Ascaris lumbricoides*
		Ancylostoma duodenale
		Necator americanus
		Strongyloides stercoralis
	Cestodes	*Taenia saginata*
		Taenia solium
		Diphyllobothrium latum
		Hymenolepsis nana
	Trematodes	*Fasciolopsis buski*
Large intestine	Nematodes	*Trichuris trichiura*
		Enterobius vermicularis
Liver	Nematodes	*Toxocara canis*
		Toxocara cati
	Trematodes	*Clonorchis sinensis*
		Fasciola hepatica
		Opisthorchis viverrini
	Cestodes	*Echinococcus granulosis*
Portal venous system	Trematodes	*Schistosoma mansoni*
		Schistosoma japonicum

decreased in the developed countries, they still constitute a reason for concern, particularly in the immunocompromised host. Worm infections in general are characterized by a complex host-parasite relationship. Intestinal worms vary in size from 1 cm to several meters, and their life cycle may require more than one host. Parasitic worms do not multiply within humans; an increase in worm load within a specific individual must, therefore, be the result of further exposure to the infective stage. This general rule applies to all worm infections discussed except strongyloidiasis and echinococcosis; in these infections, massive parasite loads may develop in humans because of special worm characteristics.

Most infected individuals harbor a low worm burden and only a small proportion acquire serious infections. Although there is no satisfactory explanation for this peculiar epidemiologic pattern of worm infections, it is of major clinical and therapeutic significance; pathologic changes and disease due to helminths have been shown to correlate with intensity of worm loads, and low helminth burden has been shown to result in little or no clinically significant disease. These epidemiologic features, which have only recently been fully appreciated, are now being used as the basis for planning strategies for control of worm infections in general.

CLINICAL PRESENTATIONS AND DIFFERENTIAL DIAGNOSES

Worm infections of the gastrointestinal tract and liver may result in local, distant, or systemic clinical manifestations. Such a protean nature poses a major problem in making an etiologic diagnosis. Symptomatic patients with any of the several intestinal helminths may complain of abdominal pain or diarrhea, whereas organomegaly, ascites, or jaundice are the common features of hepatic disease. Furthermore, distant or systemic manifestations or both may occur in some intestinal worm infections such as epilepsy in cystiscercosis or vitamin B_{12} deficiency in diphyllobothriasis. In spite of these common clinical presentations, recognizing certain clinical associations, obtaining careful geographic history, and performing the correct diagnostic procedures should be of considerable help in diagnosing a specific worm infection.

Most intestinal helminthiases are diagnosed by examination of stools for parasite eggs, larvae, or segments. It is essential that a close coordination between patient, physician, and laboratory personnel be established to obtain appropriate samples and perform the necessary examinations. This is particularly important because the routine stool examination procedures may be grossly inadequate. For example, testing fecal material for *Enterobious vermicularis* eggs is commonly unrewarding; the infection is diagnosed by obtaining samples from the perianal region. It may also be necessary to use special procedures to examine stools for *S. stercoralis* larvae or for cestode segments. Additional diagnostic procedures, such as duodenal aspiration or serology, may be helpful in achieving the correct diagnosis, and others, such as hepatic or intestinal biopsy, are rarely if ever needed.

Peripheral blood eosinophilia may be a useful clinical sign suggesting worm infections. Eosinophilia is defined as total cell count in peripheral blood of more than 350 per cubic millimeter. These or higher levels of eosinophilia have consistently been reported in indviduals with tissue-migrating worm infections. In contrast, worms that parasitize the gut lumen (for example, *Ascaris lumbricoides* and hookworms) are associated with eosinophilia only during their migratory phase in the lungs. Furthermore, in some intestinal worm infections, such as strongyloidiasis and visceral larva migrans, tissue invasion is a common feature; in these situations, peripheral blood, as well as tissue eosinophilia, is marked. Eosinophilia also occurs in association with worm infections of hepatic parenchyma and not the biliary tract. In *Fasciola hepatica* infection, eosinophilia may be noted during larval penetration of the hepatic capsule and migration into the parenchyma, but it decreases when the parasites reach their final habitat in the bile canaliculi.

THERAPY

Treatment of intestinal helminthic infections should take into consideration several important principles. Because most worm infections are asymptomatic and because worms do not multiply within the human host, chemotherapy may not be needed in lightly infected individuals with no clinical disease and no opportunity for reinfection. Chemotherapy, if effective, will markedly reduce worm burden; this also may be associated with recovery from clinical features of disease. Exceptions are particularly relevant in some intestinal worm infections; hookworm anemia necessitates additional iron therapy and diphyllobothriasis-associated pernicious anemia is corrected only by vitamin B_{12} administration. Furthermore, removal of worms may not necessarily result in control

TABLE 2 Diagnosis and Treatment of Infections Due to Intestinal Nematodes (round worms)

					Drug of Choice		*Alternative Regimen*	
Infecting Organism	*Diagnostic Stage*	*Specimen*	*Diagnostic Test (Routine)*	*Diagnostic Test (Specialized)*	*Generic (Trade) Name*	*Usual Dose and Route*	*Generic (Trade) Name*	*Usual Dose and Route*
Ascaris lumbricoides (ascariasis)	Egg Larvae Adult worm	Stool Sputum Stool	O & P Examine visually	Direct wet smear Serology	Mebendazole (Vermox)	100 mg PO bid × 3 days	Pyrantel pamoate (Antiminth) Piperazine citrate (Antepar) Levimazole (Ketrex)	11 mg/kg single dose PO (maximum 1 g) 75 mg/kg/day × 2 4 mg/kg PO
Ancylostoma duodenale (ancylostomiasis)	Egg Larvae	Stool Stool	O & P O & P	Baerman Harada-Mori Petri dish	Mebendazole (Vermox)	100 mg PO bid × 3 days	Bephemium hydroxy-naphthoate Pyrantel pamoate	5 g (2.5 g of base) PO bid × 3 days 10 mg/kg/day PO × 3
Necator americanus (hookworm infection)	Egg Larvae	Stool Stool	O & P O & P	Baerman Harada-Mori Petri dish	Mebendazole (Vermox)	100 mg PO bid × 3 days *or* 1.0 g single dose PO	Pyrantel pamoate Thiabendazole (Mintezol)	11 mg/kg single dose PO × 3 days 25 mg/kg PO bid × 2 days (maximum 3 g/day)
Strongyloides stercoralis (strongyloidiasis)	Egg Larvae	Duodenal material Stool	O & P	Enterotest Duodenal aspirate or drainage Serology	Thiabendazole (Mintezol)	25 mg/kg PO bid × 2 days	Pyrantel pamoate	11 mg/kg single dose PO; repeat every 6 weeks × 2
Trichuris trichiura (whipworm infection)	Egg Adult worm	Stool Stool	O & P O & P		Mebendazole (Vermox)	100 mg PO tid × 3 days Repeat 2 courses if necessary	Hexylresorcinol	500 ml of 0.2% solution Retention enema (30 min)
Enterobius vermicularis (pinworm infection)	Egg Adult worm	Anal impression Smear Stool/tape	Scotch tape Smear Smear		Pyrantel pamoate (Antiminth, Combatrin)	11 mg/kg single dose PO Repeat q6 weeks × 2	Mebendazole (Vermox) Pyrivinium pamoate (Povan, Vamquin)	100 mg single dose PO 5 mg/kg single dose PO (maximum 350 mg, repeat after 2 weeks)
Cutaneous *Larva migrans* (creeping eruption)	Larvae	Skin	Biopsy	Serology	Thiabendazole (Mintezol)	25 mg/kg PO bid × 5 days; repeat in 2days if active lesions persist	Thiabendazole (Mintezol)	Topical application
Visceral *Larva migrans* (toxocariasis, *Toxocara* species) *Capillaria heptica*	Larvae	Tissue	Biopsy	Serology	Thiabendazole (Mintezol)	25 mg/kg PO bid until symptoms subside or toxicity precludes further treatment (7–28 days)	Diethylcarbamazine (DEC, Hetrazan)	5 mg/kg/day PO for 3 weeks

TABLE 3 Diagnosis and Treatment of Infections Due to Cestodes

Infecting Organism	Diagnostic Stage	Specimen	Diagnostic Test (Routine)	Diagnostic Test (Specialized)	Drug of Choice: Generic (Trade) Name	Drug of Choice: Usual Dose and Route	Alternative Regimen: Generic (Trade) Name	Alternative Regimen: Usual Dose and Route
Diphyllobotrium latum (fish tapeworm)	Gravid proglottid	Stool	Visual ID	None	Niclosamide (Niclocide, Cestocide, Yomesan)	1.0 g (2 tablets) PO, chewed, then 1 hr later 1.0 g (2 tablets) more = 2 g	Paromomycin	1.0 g PO q15min × 4 doses
	Egg	Stool	O & P				Praziquantel	10 mg/kg PO single dose
Taenia saginata (beef tapeworm)	Gravid proglottid	Stool	India ink injection		Niclosamide (Niclocide, Cestocide, Yomesan)	1.0 g (2 tablets) PO, chewed, then 1 hr later 1.0 g (2 tablets) more = 2 g	Paromomycin	1.0 g PO q15min × 4 doses
	Egg	Stool	O & P	Scotch tape swab			Praziquantel	10 mg/kg PO single dose
Dipylidium caninum (dog tapeworm)	Gravid proglottid	Stool	Visual ID	None	Niclosamide (Niclocide, Cestocide, Yomesan)	1.0 g (2 tablets) PO chewed, then 1 hr later 1.0 g (2 tablets) more = 2 g	Paromoycin	1.0 g PO q15min × 4 doses
	Egg packet	Stool	O & P					
Hymenollepsis nana (dwarf tapeworm)	Egg	Stool	O & P	None	Niclosamide (Niclocide, Cestocide, Yomesan)	2 g daily = 5 days	Paromomycin	45 mg/kg/day PO single dose × 7
							Praziquantel	25 mg/kg PO × 7 days
Taenia solium (pork tapeworm)	Gravid proglottid	Stool	India ink injection		Niclosamide (Niclocide, Cestocide, Yomesan)	1.0 g (1 tablets) PO chewed, then 1 hr later 1.0 g (2 tablets) more = 2 g	Paromomycin	1.0 g PO q15min × 4 doses
	Egg	Stool	O & P				Praziquantel	10 mg/kg PO single dose
							Mebendazole (Vermox)	100 mg PO bid × 3 days
Cysticercosis	Larvae	Subcutaneous nodules; brain cysts	Biopsy	Serology	Praziquantel (Biltricide)	20 mg/kg PO tid × 10 days	Surgical resection	
					Prednisone	10 mg PO tid start 1 day before, through 3 days		
Echinococcus granulosus and *multilocularis*	Hydatid Sand	Hydatid Fluid	Sedimentation or centrifugation of fluid	Squash prep Serology	Mebendazole (Vermox)	40 mg/kg/day PO × 3 mo up to 14 g; in multilocular cysts: Rx may be continued for 3 years with decreased symptoms, but larvae still viable	Complete surgical excision of unilocular cyst	

TABLE 4 Diagnosis and Treatment of Infections Due to Trematodes (Flukes)

					Drug of Choice		Alternative Regimen	
Infecting Organism	*Diagnostic Stage*	*Specimen*	*Diagnostic Test (Routine)*	*Diagnostic Test (Specialized)*	*Generic (Trade) Name*	*Usual Dose and Route*	*Generic (Trade) Name*	*Usual Dose and Route*
Clonorchis sinensis (liver fluke)	Egg	Stool Duodenal material	O & P Wet preparation	None Entero test	Praziquantel (Biltricide)	25 mg/kg PO tid × 1 day	None	
Heterophyes heterophyes (intestinal fluke)	Egg	Stool	O & P	None	Praziquantel (Biltricide)	25 mg/kg PO tid × 1 day	Tetrachloroethylene	0.12 ml/kg PO (maximum, 5 ml)
Metagonimus yokogawai (intestinal fluke)	Egg	Stool	O & P	None	Praziquantel (Biltricide)	25 mg/kg PO tid × 1 day	Tetrachloroethylene	0.12 ml/kg PO (maximum, 5 ml)
Opisthorchis viverrini (liver fluke)	Egg	Stool Duodenal material	O & P Wet preparation	None Entero test	Praziquantel (Biltricide)	25 mg/kg PO tid × 1 day	None	
Fasciola hepatica (sheep liver fluke)	Egg	Stool	O & P	Serology	Praziquantel (Biltricide)	25 mg/kg PO tid × 1 day	Bithionol (Actamer, Bitin)	50 mg/kg PO every other day × 15 doses
Paragonimus westermani (lung fluke)	Egg	Stool	O & P Sputum concentrate	Serology	Praziquantel (Biltricide)	25 mg/kg PO tid × 1 day	Bithionol (Actamer, Bitin)	50 mg/kg PO every other day × 15 doses
Schistosoma haematobium (genitourinary bilharziasis)	Egg	Urine Collection between 10 AM & 2 PM at 24 °C	Urine sedimentation concentrate	Membrane filtration Hatching test Serology	Metrifonate (Bilarcil)	10 mg/kg PO q2–4 weeks (maximum 3 doses)	Praziquantel (Biltricide) Niridazole (Ambilhar) Lucanthone (Miracil D)	20 mg/kg PO tid in 1 day (not <4 hrs or >6 hrs between doses 25 mg/kg PO daily × 7 days 20 mg/kg PO × 8–20 days
Fasciola buski	Egg	Stool	O & P	None	Praziquantel (Biltricide)	25 mg/kg PO tid × 1 day	Tetrachloroethylene (NEMA worm capsule, veterinary)	0.12 ml/kg PO (maximum, 5 ml single dose)
Schistosoma mansoni (intestinal bilharziasis)	Egg	Stool	O & P	Tissue from sigmoidoscopy Hatching test Serology	Oxamniquine (Vansil)	15 mg/kg once (western hemisphere) 15 mg/kg PO bid × 2 days (Africa-Middle East	Praziquantel (Biltricide)	20 mg/kg PO tid in 1 day (not <4 hrs or >6 hrs between doses)
Schistosoma japonicum (oriental schistosomiasis)	Egg	Stool	O & P	Tissue from sigmoidoscopy Hatching test Serology	Praziquantel (Biltricide)	20 mg/kg PO tid in one day	Niridazole (Ambilhar)	25 mg/kg PO daily × 10 days (maximum 1.5 g)

of clinical disease; this is especially the case with the chronic permanent pathologic sequelae seen in disease with *Schistosoma mansoni* or *japonica*. Management of some worm infections should therefore be designed after careful evaluation; chemotherapy still plays a central role, but other modalities, either medical or surgical, may be needed.

The objectives in treating an individual patient with a specific worm infection are different from those in effect when chemotherapy is used to control these infections in endemic areas. Although eradication of infection is a feasible goal when treating an individual patient, significant reduction of intensity of infection in selected populations may be the strategy for control in endemic areas, particularly in those areas with limited resources.

The following section deals with chemotherapy of the various intestine-related worm infections. A deliberate attempt was made to select only one effective chemotherapeutic agent. Alternative therapy has been included in the tables presented. Most of these agents have been introduced over the last decade or so. They are administered orally, mainly in single doses or short courses, and have proven efficacy and safety. There are no absolute or relative contraindications to the use of any of the chemotherapeutic agents recommended. Their adverse effects are relatively minor and do not usually require interruption of therapy.

Intestinal Round Worms (Nematodes)

The drug of choice for treatment of ascariasis, hookworm infection and trichuriasis is mebendazole. For these three infections, mebendazole is administered orally, 100 mg twice daily for 3 days. Similar doses are used in children more than 2 years of age. In ascariasis, patients thought to have intestinal or biliary obstruction should receive piperazine citrate because of its relaxing effect on worm musculature. Piperazine citrate is given orally, 75 mg per kilogram per day for 2 days.

Strongyloidiasis in immunocompetent hosts of all ages can easily be treated with oral thiabendazole, 25 mg per kilogram twice daily for 2 days. For the hyperinfection syndrome seen in immunocompromised individuals, strongyloidiasis treatment is much more complex. Thiabendazole should be administered in similar doses, but for 10 days. The serious sequelae of the hyperinfection syndrome are usually due to bacterial infections and associated compromise of cardiopulmonary function. Appropriate antibiotics, medical management, and reduction of immunosuppressive therapy are essential elements in the treatment of this syndrome (Table 2 illustrates the diagnosis and treatment of these infections).

Intestinal Tapeworms (cestodes)

Individuals with any of the four common tapeworm infections (*Taenia saginata, Taenia solium, Diphyllobothrium latum* and *Hymenolepsis nana*) are treated with niclosamide. It is administered orally in a single 2-g dose that must be chewed thoroughly. The niclosamide dose for children is 0.5 g for those weighing 11 to 34 kg and 1 g for those above 34 kg. When niclosamide is given to children, the tablets should be crushed to a fine powder and mixed with a small amount of water. In *H. nana* infection, the same dose of niclosamide is recommended for a course of 5 days.

Recently, mebendazole and praziquantel have been shown to be effective against *T. solium* and may be used as alternative drugs (Table 3 presents the diagnosis and management of cestode infections).

Intestinal Flukes (Trematodes)

Praziquantel is currently the drug of choice for treatment of *Fasciolopsis buski* infection. It is administered orally, 25 mg per kilogram three doses a day. This results in elimination of most parasites. Similar doses are used in children. Praziquantel has become the drug of choice for most of the infections due to intestinal trematodes.

Liver Flukes (Trematodes)

Praziquantel is also the drug of choice for treatment of *Clonorchis sinensis, F. hepatica*, and *Opsthorches viverrini* infections. It is used in the same dosage as described for intestinal flukes.

Liver Cestodes

Echinococcus granulosis cysts in the liver are the most common clinical feature of this infection. In many cases cysts are found on routine abdominal roentgenographic examination. Calcified, small, or asymptomatic cysts are better left alone. A trial of mebendazole may be given. Large, or symptomatic cysts, on the other hand, necessitate surgical intervention; cysts contents must be killed by hypertonic saline before their removal either by marsupialization or partial hepatectomy.

Blood Flukes

Oxamniquine is the current drug of choice for treatment of schistosomiasis mansoni. It is administered as a single oral dose of 20 mg per kilogram. The same dose is used for children.

For individuals infected with *S. mansoni* in Africa, a higher dose of 60 mg per kilogram may be required. For *S. japonicum* infection, praziquantel is the currently recommended drug. It is given orally, 20 mg per kilogram three times a day in one day. Praziquantel is also effective against other human schistosomes (*S. mansoni* and *S. haematobia*, see Table 4 for details).

Chemotherapy for schistosomiasis mansoni or japonica may, in addition to eliminating worms, also result in regression of disease (hepatosplenomegaly) or arrest its development. This is particularly true if chemotherapy is given to infected children. Once the chronic fibro-obstructive sequelae have developed, chemotherapy results in little clinical improvement. These patients need medical management of complications such as esophageal varices, hematemesis, and ascites.

CENTRAL NERVOUS SYSTEM INFECTIONS

MENINGITIS IN CHILDREN

GARY D. OVERTURF, M.D.

ETIOLOGY AND DIAGNOSIS

Bacterial meningitis is predominantly a childhood disease with approximately three-fourths of all cases occurring in children younger than 5 years of age. *Hemophilus influenzae* is responsible for at least 67 percent of cases of bacterial meningitis in children from 2 months to 10 years of age, followed in incidence by *Neisseria meningitidis* (20%) and *Streptococcus pneumoniae* (10% to 15%). Thus, these three pathogens account for more than 97 percent of all cases of bacterial meningitis in children, with attack rates of approximately 3.0, 1.2, and 0.8 cases per 100,000 children per annum for hemophilus, meningococcal, and pneumococcal meningitis, respectively.

The etiology of bacterial meningitis not acquired in the community is more variable and may be divided broadly into two groups: (1) those episodes associated with predisposing causes such as neurologic trauma and (2) immunodeficiency states (sickle cell anemia, agammaglobulinemia, or specific complement deficiencies) or chronic ear and sinus disease. Of those children who undergo shunt insertions, *Staphylococcus epidermidis* and *Staphylococcus aureus* are responsible for 50 percent and 25 percent respectively, whereas enterococci, alpha streptococci, meningococci, pneumococci, *Hemophilus* species, *Bacillus subtilis*, enteric organisms, and diphtheroid species are the causes of the remainder of cases. Clustering of these infections within 2 months of surgery and similar rates of infection for ventriculoatrial and ventriculoperitoneal shunts suggest that the infecting organisms are probably introduced during the perioperative period. Children with deficiencies of complement function, splenic function, and agammaglobulinemia have a much increased incidence of infections due to all the usual meningeal pathogens, particularly pneumococci. Patients with sickle cell disease, particularly those younger than 5 years of age, have an incidence of pneumococcal meningitis that is several hundredfold that of the general population, with rates of five to six infections per 100 patient years. A few patients with deficiency of some of the terminal components of complement have been described with recurrent episodes of infections due to species of *Neisseria*.

Evaluation of febrile children must be performed with an appreciation for the possibility of bacterial meningitis. Specific meningeal symptoms (i.e., Brudzinski's and Kernig's signs) are not reliably present, particularly in children younger than 12 to 18 months of age. Therefore, the admonition to perform a lumbar puncture at the least suspicion is mandatory. Although the typical CSF from a child with bacterial meningitis will be characterized by more than 1,000 neutrophils per milliliter in association with a low glucose level and high protein concentration, one-third of children at initial lumbar puncture will have a CSF cell count less than 1,000 per milliliter, one-third will have a normal glucose concentration, and one-fifth will have a normal protein concentration.

The initiation of correct antibiotic therapy in an individual patient hinges on the accurate identification of the causative organism. Although antibiotic therapy as traditionally recommended is an empiric exercise, the specific choice should consider epidemiologic factors coupled with a meticulous microscopic survey of the Gram stained CSF sediment. Positive CSF Gram stains under optimal examination, can be expected in approximately 85 percent, 80 percent, and 60 percent of children with hemophilus, pneumococcal, and meningococcal infections, respectively. Latex particle agglutination (LPA) and coagglutination (with staphylococcal protein A) are very accurate in the early diagnosis of hemophilus infections, but have much higher failure rates in pneumococcal and meningococcal disease. LPA and coagglutination are essentially as accurate as standard microbiologic tests (culture) in hemophilus disease and can detect as little as 0.2 ng of antigen per milliliter. LPA appears to be more sensitive and is therefore preferable to coagglutination. Measurements of serum CRP and CSF concentrations of lactic acid may also be useful nonspecific indicators of bacterial infections. Levels of lactic acid of 35 or more mg per deciliter have generally been a sensitive indicator of the presence of bacterial meningitis. Similarly, elevated serum levels of CRP may be useful in indicating the presence of bacterial infection.

Approximately one-half of children with bacterial meningitis will have received partially effective antibiotics before evaluation. Such partially effective drugs include penicillins, cephalosporins, TMP/SMZ, and sulfonamides. Most characteristics of the spinal fluid in partially treated patients are similar to those of children who are untreated except for the Gram stain and culture. Cases due to *Hemophilus* are likely to still have positive cultures and Gram stains, but the frequency of negative CSF cultures and Gram stains increases for pneumococcal and meningococcal infections. The nonspecific tests listed above may be helpful in deciding whether a bacterial infection is present, but a decision to initiate therapy must be based upon the clinical presentation and spinal fluid findings. A repeated lumbar puncture after an interval of 8 to 12 hours may reveal a change from polymorphonuclear leukocyte predominance to mononuclear predominance, thus strongly suggesting a viral etiology for the meningitis.

THERAPY

Supportive Therapy

Associated fever, vomiting, poor oral intake, and general physiologic stress may contribute to fluid and electrolyte disturbances in children with bacterial meningitis. Severe dehydration (hypovolemia) is unusual in bacterial meningitis, but should be treated with aggressive fluid replacement if it occurs. More frequently, hypotension is associated with septic shock, and therapy directed solely to simple hypovolemia alone will not correct the hypotension.

A number of investigators have confirmed the presence of a nearly universal syndrome of inappropriate secretion of antidiuretic hormone (SIADH) in children with bacterial meningitis. A significantly elevated arginine vasopressin concentration in the CSF of children with bacterial meningitis may be yet another operative factor in the production of cerebral edema, since this agent produces a significant alteration of the brain's ability to regulate water permeability. Therefore, fluid administration is restricted to 1,000 to 1,200 ml per square meter (or approximately two-thirds to three-fourths maintenance) in most children for at least 24 to 48 hours or until signs of intracranial pressure have resolved and serum sodium concentrations are normal and stable.

Convulsive disorders are common among children with bacterial meningitis and primarily occur during the first 12 to 48 hours of illness, presumptively as a result of cerebral cortical irritation. Seizures occur in up to 33 percent of children during the acute disease. The usual initial control of seizures is accomplished with diazepam (0.25 mg per kilogram intravenously infused over 1 to 5 minutes). Should this fail to control seizures, or if they recur, phenobarbital, 10 mg per kilogram intravenously, should be used, followed by maintenance doses (5 mg per kilogram per day) to maintain serum concentrations at 10 to 20 μg per milliliter. If seizures are limited to only the first 48 to 72 hours and are easily controlled, subsequent administration of anticonvulsant medications will usually not be necessary.

Measures to reduce increased intracranial pressure (ICP) in bacterial meningitis have been limited to osmotic agents and controlled ventilation. The dose of mannitol is 0.5 to 2.0 g per kilogram intravenously given as a single bolus over 10 to 15 minutes; it may be repeated two or three times at 2- to 4-hour intervals, but is usually used only once to assist stabilization of a patient thought to be suffering uncal herniation. Rebound in increased intracranial pressure may occur at 2 to 12 hours following a dose, and repeated administration is often complicated by hypovolemia and electrolyte depletion. The goal of controlled ventilation is to induce a mild respiratory alkalosis. The patient must be intubated and if necessary, respiratory effort must be controlled with pancuronium (0.04 to 0.1 mg per kilogram). Blood gases should be monitored, such that a PCO_2 of 25 to 27 Torr is achieved with a PO_2 of 85 to 95 Torr.

Monitoring of ICP via an intraventricular catheter has been utilized infrequently in children with bacterial meningitis. Although the advantage of monitoring ICP via an intraventricular catheter is to provide specific information regarding the response to various therapeutic manipulations and a modality to remove excess CSF, the presence of infection is thought by most authorities to be a relative contraindication to the placement of intraventricular catheters, since placement of the catheter must traverse an infected space (subarachnoid) to a potentially noninfected space (ventricle). It is possible that the subarachnoid screw or bolt may be an adequate substitute for patients with bacterial meningitis who require monitoring.

Corticosteroids are neither advantageous nor detrimental to patients less than 16 years of age, although death was significantly more likely among steroid-treated patients more than 16 years of age in double-blinded prospective studies. Therefore, their routine use cannot be advocated. Disseminated intravascular coagulation (DIC) occurs frequently in meningococcal meningitis and correlates with the presence of shock. DIC may also occur in hemophilus or pneumococcal disease. Heparin therapy does not appear to enhance survival. Improvement in the associated hypotension contributes the major factor in abolishing DIC and reducing mortality.

Specific Therapy

Although CSF Gram stained smears or antigen tests are utilized for the diagnosis of bacterial meningitis, their accuracy is limited by the experience and diligence of the microbiology laboratory. Therefore, children should be treated routinely with drugs active against the three commonest meningeal pathogens: *H. influenzae*, *S. pneumoniae*, and *N. meningitidis*. Bacterial meningitis in children younger than 10 years of age may be treated effectively with combinations of chloramphenicol and ampicillin (Table 1). If the initial Gram stain or antigen tests positively confirm pneumococcal or meningococcal infection, it is reasonable to dispense with the use of chloramphenicol. Conversely, if these tests confirm hemophilus infection, combined therapy should be employed initially until the antibiotic susceptibility of the

TABLE 1 Choice of Antibiotics by Etiologic Agent and Usual Duration of Therapy for Bacterial Meningitis

Bacteria	*Antibiotics*	*Alternative(s)**	*Duration (days) of Treatment*
Gram-negative			
H. influenzae	Chloramphenicol *or* ampicillin	Cefotaxime *or* ceftizoxime *or* ceftriaxone, *or* cefuroxime, *or* moxalactam	10–14†
N. meningitidis	Penicillin G *or* ampicillin	Chloramphenicol *or* listed cephalosporins	10
Enteric gram-negative	Ampicillin plus an aminoglycoside *or* cefotaxime, ceftriaxone, *or* moxalactam		21–28†
Bacteroides species	Chloramphenicol *or* metronidazole		10–14†
Gram-positive			
Enterococci	Ampicillin plus gentamicin	Vancomycin plus gentamicin	14–21†
Other streptococci (including pneumococci)	Penicillin G *or* ampicillin	Cefotaxime *or* ceftriaxone	10–14†
Staphylococci	Nafcillin *or* methicillin, *or* oxacillin	Vancomycin	10–14†
L. monocytogenes	Ampicillin	Chloramphenicol	14

* Alternatives may be indicated if etiology is unconfirmed (i.e., purulent unknown).
† Depending on response.

organism is determined; thereafter, therapy should be continued with the single, least toxic effective agent. Chloramphenicol remains the appropriate agent in all penicillin-allergic patients.

The use of two drugs at the beginning of therapy is justified because of a 10 to 40 percent resistance to ampicillin, and rarely, resistance to chloramphenicol or to both antibiotics. In addition, in the United States, up to 10 percent of isolates of *S. pneumoniae* are relatively resistant to penicillin (MIC, 0.1 to 1.0 μg per milliliter). Although in the past, isolated cases of failures of penicillin G in cases of meningitis due to pneumococci with similar susceptibility patterns have been reported, there is no evidence that the currently observed in vitro "resistance" patterns of pneumococci have been correlated with a generally more frequent failure of penicillin therapy. If beta-lactamase-producing as well as chloramphenicol-resistant *H. influenzae* or penicillin-resistant pneumococci become more widespread, current recommendations for antibiotic therapy will require reevaluation.

Several newer cephalosporin compounds have activity against *H. influenzae, S. pneumoniae,* and *N. meningitidis* and may serve as alternatives in meningitis of undetermined etiology or cases caused by ampicillin- and chloramphenicol-resistant isolates of *H. influenzae*. Moxalactam can only be used for hemophilus and meningococcal infections since it has inadequate activity against pneumococci. Cefotaxime, ceftizoxime, ceftriaxone, ceftazidime, and cefuroxime are alternatives for any of the three major meningeal pathogens.

Less common bacterial causes of meningitis are treated with antimicrobial agents appropriate for each organism. In particular, gram-negative bacillary infections may be more effectively treated with one of the newer cephalosporins—moxalactam, cefotaxime, or ceftizoxime—and aminoglycosides may supplement these agents or be used when the results of susceptibility studies indicate resistance to the newer agents.

All antimicrobial agents are best administered intravenously. Penicillins and cephalosporins are usually administered intravenously, although occasional doses of intramuscular antibiotics are acceptable when intravenous access is impossible (Table 2). Chloramphenicol can be administered orally as the base or the palmitate ester. CSF and serum concentrations following oral use are equivalent to those following intravenous administration. However, oral use is generally confined to that period after the initial 5 days of therapy or when intravenous access is impossible.

There is no evidence that specific CSF criteria better define the duration of antibiotic therapy than clinical response alone or that their use results in fewer relapses following therapy. However, repeated lumbar punctures at 24 to 36 hours of treatment and subsequently at the end of therapy may assist the physician in documenting CSF sterilization (early) and provide a posttreatment CSF baseline (late) for defining problems that may arise during convalescence. Experience suggests that antibiotic therapy for 10 days is sufficient in most cases (Table 2).

Computerized tomography (CT) may be indicated for evaluation of seizures, hemiparesis or other focal neurologic signs, prolonged fever, or a significant alteration in mental status. One may expect to find subdural collections (in 25%), cerebral swelling (10%), ependymitis (15%), contrast-enhancing basal meninges (5%), focal cortical necrosis (10%), ischemic infarct (20%), and ventricular widening (65%). CT scan should be utilized only to evaluate symptomatic problems as they arise during the course of treatment.

The prevailing approach to subdural effusions is (1) daily transillumination and/or neurologic examination, (2) daily measurement of frontal occipital circumference, and

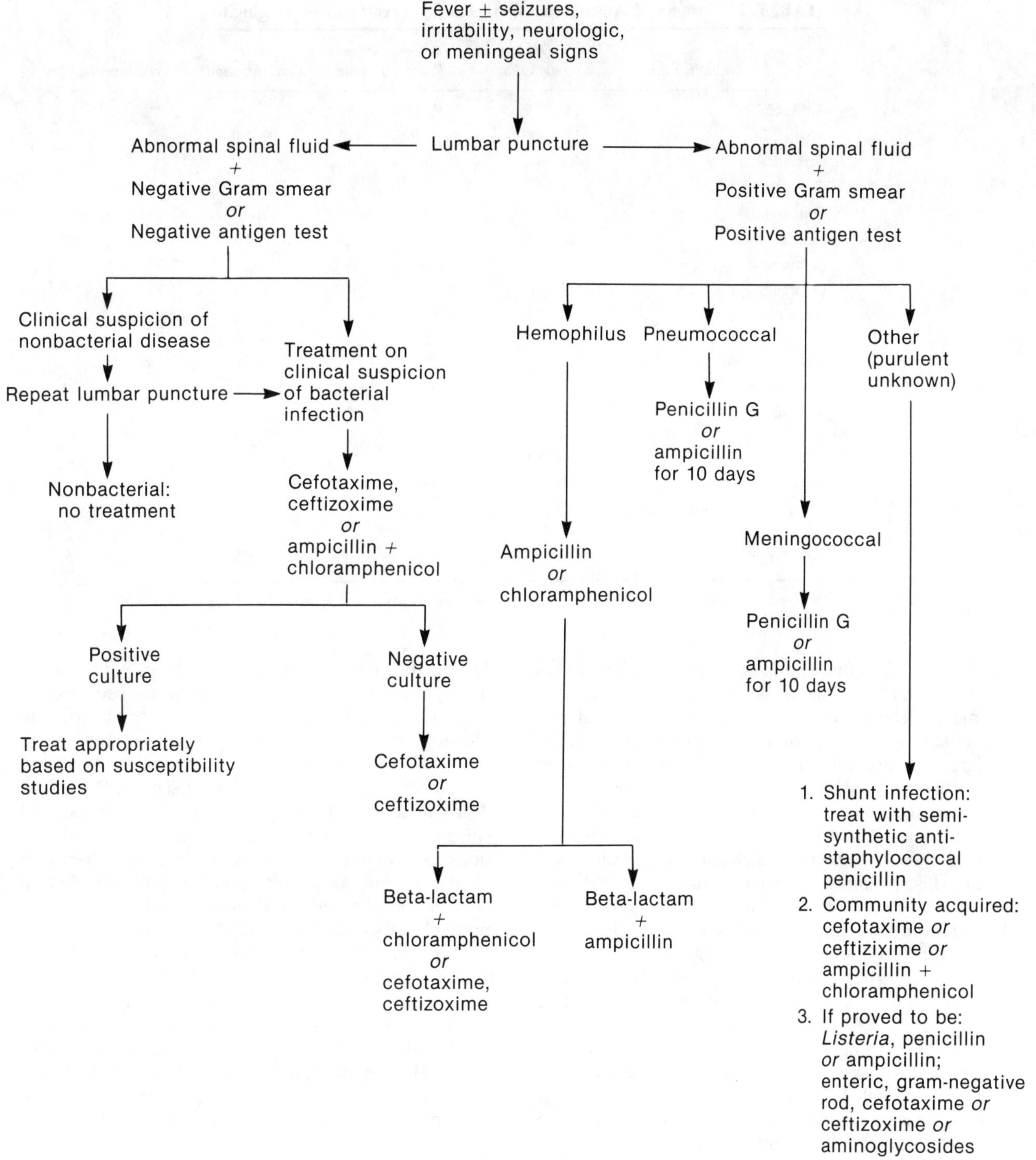

Figure 1 Evaluation and management of bacterial meningitis

TABLE 2 Dosages of Antimicrobial Agents for Treatment of Meningitis

Antibiotic	*Dosage (mg/kg/day)*	*Route*	*Interval (hours)*	*CSF Concentration**
Amikacin	15–22.5	IV, IM	8	
Ampicillin	150–400	IV, IM	4–6	0–2.0
Carbenicillin	400–600	IV	4	0–4.0
Cefotaxime	200	IV	6	2–8
Ceftizoxime	200	IV	6–8	2–8
Ceftriaxone	100	IV	12	5–10
Cefuroxime	200	IV	6	1–5
Chloramphenicol	75–100	IV, PO	6	5–10
Gentamicin	6 (children), 7.5 (infants)	IV, IM	8	0–1.0
Methicillin, naficillin, oxacillin	200	IV	4–6	NA†
Moxalactam	200	IV	6–8	5–15
Metronidazole	7.5	IV	6	10–50
Penicillin G	155 (200,000 units)	IV	4	0–2.0
Ticarcillin	400	IV	4	NA
Trimethoprim-sulfamethoxazole	12 TMP/ 60 SMZ	IV	6	
Vancomycin	20–40	IV	6–8	0–1.5

* Expected range of CSF concentration in bacterial meningitis during administration of the dosages listed (μg/ml).
† Not applicable.

(3) CT scan to evaluate an abnormality of either. Initial subdural paracentesis should be performed to exclude empyema. Repeated paracentesis should be considered only for relief of specific neurologically correlated symptoms or large midline shift on CT scan. Surgical procedures are rarely required, even in massive effusions.

Persistent and recurring fevers are the most frequent complications. Persistent fever often remains unexplained. In some cases, it is due to localized infections such as septic arthritis, pneumonia, sinusitis, mastoiditis, subdural empyema, or, very rarely, brain abscess or pericarditis. Recurrent fever may be due to thrombophlebitis or drug fever, particularly with beta-lactam antibiotics after 7 days of therapy. Sterile collections of subdural fluid may also explain persistent or recurrent fever, usually appearing during the second week of illness.

Antibiotic prophylaxis is recommended for certain household contacts of meningococcal or haemophilus disease. A household contact is conventionally defined as a person with a contact of 4 hours duration daily for 5 to 7 days per week. For meningococcal infection, rifampin is recommended for all household contacts as follows: adults, 600 mg every 24 hours in four doses; children (12 months of age or older), 20 mg per kilogram every 24 hours in four doses. Although still controversial, the American Academy of Pediatrics recommends antibiotic prophylaxis for contacts of hemophilus disease in households where other children younger than 4 years of age reside: adults 600 mg every 24 hours in four doses; children 20 mg per kilogram every 24 hours in four doses. In the case of hemophilus infection, it has been recommended to treat the index case with rifampin prior to discharge from care. Among the current major impediments to rifampin prophylaxis is the lack of a pediatric formulation. Patients should be warned of the limitations of prophylaxis, and febrile episodes among contacts of patients with meningococcal or hemophilus disease should be promptly investigated. Outbreaks of disease in schools and day care centers should be reported to a central public health agency, and, usually, decisions regarding prophylaxis should be formulated by such authorities.

Mortality rates from meningitis are low (1% to 10%) in otherwise healthy children. However, permanent sequelae are frequent: pneumococcal meningitis is associated with the highest incidence of neurologic injury (30% to 60%), whereas meningococcal disease is the most benign. Hemophilus infections are associated with a sequelae rate of 20 to 30 percent. Such sequelae may include mental retardation, spasticity, epilepsy, blindness, deafness, or specific learning defects. It may be impossible to judge the degree of permanent impairment at the time of hospital discharge and children should be carefully observed for a minimum of 12 months with at least some specific evaluation of neurologic functioning, hearing, vision, and sequential standardized evaluation of development (Gesell testing or Denver Developmental Test). Figure 1 provides a summary of the techniques used to evaluate and manage bacterial meningitis.

BACTERIAL MENINGITIS IN ADULTS

RICHARD B. ROBERTS, M.D.
JOHN A. ROMANKIEWICZ, Pharm.D.

Bacterial meningitis is a serious, life-threatening infection. It is a medical emergency that necessitates early recognition and institution of appropriate supportive and antimicrobial therapy. The reported annual incidence in the United States is 2.9 cases per 100,000 population, although this figure reflects gross underreporting, and the true incidence is probably closer to 10 cases per 10,000. *Hemophilus influenzae, Neisseria meningitidis,* and *Streptococcus pneumoniae* are responsible for the majority of these infections, although defects in nonimmunologic and immunologic host defenses predispose patients to meningitis due to other bacterial pathogens.

The clinical presentations of bacterial meningitis are quite similar regardless of the causative organism. Clinicians must rely on age of the patient, the epidemiologic and clinical setting, and, most important, the isolation and identification of the causative agent in order to direct appropriate antimicrobial therapy. Deficiencies, however, exist in our current therapeutic approach to patients with bacterial meningitis, including both host and drug factors. Examples of the former include the immunocompromised host and inadequate host-defense mechanisms of the central nervous system. Factors that limit the usefulness of antimicrobial agents include penetration into the cerebrospinal fluid (CSF) following systemic therapy, development of resistance by many bacteria, necessity for bactericidal (not bacteriostatic) antibiotics, and the low therapeutic index of aminoglycosides. The development of the new beta-lactam antibiotics, however, provides agents that possess a wide spectrum of gram-negative activity, are bactericidal, and achieve adequate concentrations in spinal fluid following parenteral therapy.

PREDISPOSING FACTORS AND MICROBIOLOGY

Patient Age

Hemophilus influenzae, N. meningitidis, and *S. pneumoniae* account for more than 80 percent of bacterial meningitis in children and adults; the former two are commonest in young children and the latter, in adults. As shown in Table 1, the relative frequency of bacteria associated with meningitis depends in part on the patient's age and underlying condition. Thus, *S. pneumoniae* accounts for one-third to one-half of adult cases, followed in decreasing order of frequency *N. meningitidis* (10% to 30%), staphylococci (5% to 15%), and *Listeria monocytogenes* (5%). Gram-negative bacilli and *H. influenzae*, the commonest pathogens in neonates and children respectively, account for only 1 percent each in the adult population.

Impaired Host Defenses

The bacteria associated with meningitis in patients with impaired immunologic host-defense mechanisms are shown in Table 2. The encapsulated bacteria *H. influenzae, N. meningitidis*, and *S. pneumoniae* are most frequently associated with B-cell deficiencies such as are seen in thymoma with agammaglobulinemia, Bruton-type agammaglobulinemia, and multiple myeloma. Other impaired immunologic host-defense mechanisms that result in a predisposition for meningitis due to encapsulated bacteria are sickle cell disease, functional asplenia, and splenectomy. In addition, deficiencies in the latter components of the complement cascade impair the direct serum bactericidal activity against the pathogenic *Neisseriae* including *N. meningitidis. L. monocytogenes* and *Mycobacterium tuberculosis*, two intracellular pathogens that require an intact cell-mediated immune system for control and eradication, are frequent bacterial pathogens in T-cell deficiencies, such as in patients with underlying lymphoma, Hodgkin's disease, or in those receiving immunosuppressive therapy.

Anatomical Defects

Patients who have anatomical defects with direct communication to the subarachnoid space are also at high risk for developing bacterial meningitis. These defects may be congenitally acquired, as occurs with spina bifida and meningomyelocele, or as a result of accidental or surgical trauma. As shown in Table 3, the pathogens responsible for meningitis in these patients are normal flora of the skin (i.e., *Staphylococcus aureus* and *Staphylococcus epidermidis* or gram-negative bacilli) or of the upper respiratory tract (i.e., encapsulated bacteria). In the latter case, patients may have spinal fluid leakage resulting in CSF rhinorrhea and multiple episodes of encapsulated bacterial meningitis.

PATHOGENESIS AND ROUTES OF INFECTION

A description of the anatomy of the meninges and the formation of CSF is beyond the scope of this discussion. The following factors bear directly on the susceptibility and response to infection. The inadequate host defense mechanisms of the central nervous system are reflected in the CSF and most likely play a role in the pathogenesis of bacterial meningitis. Reduced immunoglobulin and complement levels have been noted in normal and infected CSF, accounting for the impaired phagocytic activity necessary in host defense against encapsulated bacteria. A diminished polymorphonuclear leukocyte (PMN) response, as reflected in the low ratio of PMNs to bacteria in infected CSF, also contributes to impaired phagocytosis.

Bacteria gain access to the meninges either by direct

TABLE 1 Bacterial Causes (%) of Meningitis in Different Age Groups

Neonate (*under 2 months*)	*Children* (*2 months to 15 years*)	*Adults* (*over 15 years*)
Gram-negative bacilli (55%–60%) (*E. coli, Klebsiella* species)	*H. influenzae* (35%–45%)	*S. pneumoniae* (30%–50%)
	N. meningitidis (30%–40%)	*N. meningitidis* (10%–30%)
Group B streptococci (10%–25%)	*S. pneumoniae* (10%–20%)	*S. aureus, S. epidermidis* (5%–15%)
L. monocytogenes (2%–10%)	*S. aureus, S. epidermidis*	*L. monocytogenes* (5%)
S. aureus, S. epidermidis (5%)	Gram-negative bacilli	*H. influenzae* (1%)
S. pneumoniae		Gram-negative bacilli (1%)
N. meningitidis		Group B streptococci
H. influenzae		
Group A streptococci		

Note: Incidence is in decreasing order of frequency.

extension from a contiguous site of infection or via the blood that can carry bacteria to the brain from remote sites of infection. Direct extension may result from infected structures of the upper respiratory tract such as in otitis media, mastoiditis, or sinusitis. Anatomical defects permitting communication of the subarachnoid space with either the nasopharynx or skin also predispose patients to bacterial meningitis. As noted above, such defects may be congenital (i.e., associated with meningomyelocele or spina bifida) or from accidental and surgical trauma.

The bloodstream is the usual route by which bacteria reach the meninges. The initial infected site for bacteremia is often the respiratory tract. It is assumed that bacteria that colonize and infect the respiratory tract may have a predilection for the central nervous system (tissue tropism), although data to support this hypothesis are lacking.

DIAGNOSIS

Clinical Evaluation

Patients with bacterial meningitis present with symptoms and signs related to their systemic illness, the initial focus of infection, and the central nervous system. The relative frequency of symptoms and neurologic signs in bacterial meningitis are listed in Table 4. The duration of systemic symptoms such as fever, chills, headache, and vomiting is often short, i.e., 24 to 48 hours. Changes in mentation—from lethargy, confusion, and disorientation to coma—may progress rapidly and help to distinguish bacterial from viral meningitis; this progression is usually not seen in viral meningitis. Alteration of mental status implies some process other than pure meningitis, e.g., increased intracranial pressure, cortical vein thrombosis, or encephalitis. Evidence of meningeal irritation, either by stiffness of the neck or positive neurologic signs, is observed in the majority of patients. These signs and symptoms may be absent in neonates and the elderly. The clinical diagnosis of bacterial meningitis may be difficult in patients with already altered mental status.

Upper respiratory tract infections, such as pharyngitis, otitis media, and sinusitis, may occur in more than 50 percent of patients presenting with bacterial meningitis. On physical examination, patients are usually febrile, with evidence of meningeal irritation. Except for changes in mental status (e.g., impaired alertness, confusion, convulsions), the neurologic examination may be unrevealing. Increased intracranial pressure should be suspected in the presence of papilledema. A careful physical examination for extra-central nervous system sites of infection, including parameningeal structures, should always be performed.

In addition to a detailed clinical history and physical examination in patients suspected of having bacterial meningitis, important information may be obtained from a careful evaluation of the clinical and epidemiologic set-

TABLE 2 Bacterial Meningitis Associated With Impaired Host-Defense Mechanisms

B-cell deficiency
S. pneumoniae
H. influenzae
N. meningitidis
T-cell deficiency
L. monocytogenes
M. tuberculosis

TABLE 3 Bacterial Meningitis Associated With Anatomical Defects

Congenital defects
S. aureus
S. epidermidis
Gram-negative bacilli
Acquired defects
Communication with nasopharynx
S. pneumoniae
H. influenzae
N. meningitidis
Communication with skin
S. aureus
S. epidermidis
Gram-negative bacilli

TABLE 4 Frequency (%) of Symptoms and Signs of Bacterial Meningitis

Symptoms	*Neurologic Signs*
Fever (45%–85%)	Nuchal rigidity (11%–50%)
Chills (3%–38%)	Kernig's and Brudzinski's signs (81%)
Headache (25%–47%)	Coma (30%)
Vomiting (25%–70%)	Neurologic abnormalities (25%)
Confusion (37%–56%)	
Seizures (40%)	
Photophobia (0%–4%)	

ting. Information regarding age, season of the year, family illness, medications, underlying illnesses, and recent travel may be helpful in indicating specific exposures or specific complications of underlying illnesses.

Laboratory Evaluation

Examination of the CSF is the single most important laboratory test in patients with bacterial meningitis. Obtaining CSF requires an invasive procedure (lumbar puncture) that can be associated with certain complications (iatrogenic meningitis, paraspinal hematoma). A careful lumbar puncture should be performed, especially in patients with evidence of increased intracranial pressure and thrombocytopenia. If the procedure has to be delayed to evaluate or treat these parameters, empiric antimicrobial therapy should be instituted. The CSF should be handled expeditiously and appropriate studies be performed immediately. Red blood cells and PMNs lyse when CSF is left standing, and fastidious encapsulated bacteria cannot be isolated unless directly inoculated on appropriate laboratory media. Laboratory studies that should be performed on all CSF specimens include the following: (*1*) appearance of CSF and opening pressure, (*2*) presence of red and white blood cells, (*3*) protein and glucose determinations with simultaneous blood glucose (the CSF should be at least two-thirds the blood glucose), (*4*) Gram stain (positive in 70% to 80% of patients) and acid-fast stain, and (*5*) appropriate cultures. As a guideline, the laboratory results of these CSF parameters for different causes of meningitis are shown in Table 5.

Other tests, if indicated, include serologic evidence for neurosyphilis, viral isolation and serology, India ink stain, antigen detection, cultures for fungi, and cytology for malignant cells. The laboratory tests that are currently available to demonstrate the etiology of bacterial meningitis are listed in Table 6. In addition to demonstrating bacteria by stain, Quellung reaction, and culture, specific bacterial antigens may be detected by use of counterimmunoelectrophoresis or latex-agglutination techniques. Nonspecific tests reported by some to be helpful, but which are not readily available, include limulus lysate gelation for endotoxin and lactic acid, lactate dehydrogenase (LDH) isoenzymes, and C-reactive protein determinations. We do not use these latter tests routinely.

Antimicrobial therapy administered prior to the first CSF examination will result in alterations of total leukocyte and differential counts in addition to negative Gram stains and cultures. Because of these findings, patients who have received antibiotics prior to diagnosis usually receive a full 14-day course of antimicrobial therapy. In patients with early viral (aseptic) meningitis, the total and differential counts may be consistent with bacterial meningitis. Repeat CSF examination within 6 to 12 hours may demonstrate a differential count with increased numbers of mononuclear cells, and antimicrobial therapy can be withheld in such patients.

Other laboratory tests that should be performed in patients with suspected meningitis include cultures of blood and other clinically indicated specimens and x-ray studies of the chest, mastoids, and sinuses to identify an initial source of infection.

Complications

The early- and late-onset complications that may be observed in patients with bacterial meningitis are listed in Table 7. An appreciation of these complications is critical in the management and follow-up of these patients. Many of the early complications seen during the initial hospitalization are related to the severity of the systemic illness and include upper gastrointestinal hemorrhage, vasculitis with digital gangrene, herpes labialis, shock,

TABLE 5 Cerebrospinal Fluid Profile in Meningitis

	Leukocytes			
	Total No. (cells/mm³)	*Morphology*	*Protein (μl = <45 mg%)*	*Sugar (μl = >⅔ of serum glucose)*
Bacterial	>200	PMN	Increased	Decreased
Viral	<200	Mononuclear	Normal	Normal
Fungal	<200	Mononuclear	Increased	Decreased
Carcinomatous	<200	Malignant cells	Increased	Decreased

TABLE 6 Diagnostic Laboratory Tests of Cerebrospinal Fluid in Bacterial Meningitis

Demonstration of bacteria
- Gram-stain, acid-fast bacilli (AFB) stain
- Quellung reaction
- Culture

Detection of specific bacterial antigens
- Counterimmunoelectrophoresis (CIE)
- Latex agglutination

acute respiratory distress syndrome (ARDS), disseminated intravascular coagulation (DIC), and inappropriate antidiuretic hormone (ADH) secretion with hyponatremia.

Early-onset neurologic complications include generalized seizures, cerebellar or temporal lobe herniation secondary to increased intracranial pressure, transient focal signs secondary to superficial cortical vein thrombosis, and sterile subdural effusions. The latter is more commonly recognized in neonates prior to closure of the fontanelle and may be the cause of persistent fever or seizure activity. Diagnostic aspiration is recommended both to relieve pressure and to ensure sterility of the effusion.

Late-onset complications are predominantly neurologic and include perceptual learning defects, mental retardation, seizure disorders, deafness, motor deficits, and hydrocephalus. The latter complication most commonly follows basilar granulomatous meningitis due to tuberculosis or the systemic mycoses.

THERAPEUTIC CONSIDERATIONS

General Supportive Measures

All patients with bacterial meningitis should be hospitalized and isolated for respiratory pathogens for the first 48 hours until the etiologic agent is identified. Intensive care is mandatory, and the following emergency measures should be instituted: (*1*) if needed, establishment of a patent airway to prevent aspiration and maintain adequate ventilation, especially in comatose patients; (*2*) maintenance of intravenous access for adequate hydration and various therapeutic drugs; (*3*) monitoring vital signs and maintenance of systolic blood pressure above 90 mm Hg. Caution must be exercised in the administration of intravenous fluids so that congestive heart failure and pulmonary edema are not precipitated by overhydration. Overhydration may also increase the likelihood of cerebral edema, resulting in cranial nerve palsy or respiratory arrest from herniation of the temporal lobe and cerebellum, respectively. Administration of mannitol (1 to 2 g per kilogram as a 15% to 20% solution given over 30 to 60 minutes intravenously) and subsequent diuresis may decrease intracranial pressure due to cerebral edema.

Anticonvulsants should be used to control seizures, but should not be given prophylactically because they may interfere with the monitoring of mental status. Although there is some controversy involved, steroids are generally contraindicated in patients with bacterial meningitis except when acute hydrocephalus due to basilar meningitis is strongly suspected.

Disseminated intravascular coagulation (DIC) may complicate any cause of bacterial meningitis, but is most commonly seen in patients with meningococcal or pneumococcal (with asplenia) meningitis. DIC may be suspected clinically when petechiae and bleeding at needle puncture sites are observed. Measures of coagulation should be obtained immediately and depleted clotting factors replaced. The beneficial role of heparin has not been substantiated, although it is recommended by most hematologists. Full-dose intravenous heparin is initiated by pump: 5,000 units initially, followed by 1,000 units every hour. Response to heparin therapy is determined by the normalization of depleted clotting factors and reduction of fibrinogen levels. The platelet count and prothrombin time are unreliable because the former may also be reduced because of bone marrow suppression from infection and the latter, elevated because of heparin therapy. It has been reported that because DIC in these patients is endotoxin-mediated, efforts to remove endotoxin by plasmaphoresis or to neutralize it by immunotherapy has met with some clinical success. At present, we have not routinely used these methods.

Antimicrobial Therapy

The properties of an ideal antimicrobial agent for bacterial meningitis include: (*1*) bactericidal activity, (*2*) high therapeutic to toxic ratio, and (*3*) sufficient CSF penetration to achieve levels at least several times the minimum bactericidal concentration (MBC) against the infecting bacteria.

TABLE 7 Complications of Bacterial Meningitis

Early-onset
- Gastrointestinal hemorrhage—stress ulcer
- Vasculitis with distal digital gangrene
- Herpes labialis
- Congestive heart failure
- Shock
- Acute respiratory distress syndrome
- Disseminated intravascular coagulation
- Inappropriate antidiuretic hormone (ADH) secretion with hyponatremia
- Neurologic
  - Generalized seizures
  - Cerebellar or temporal lobe herniation
  - Transient focal signs due to cortical vein thrombosis
  - Subdural effusions

Late-onset (neurologic)
- Perceptual learning deficits
- Mental retardation
- Seizure disorder
- Deafness
- Motor deficit
- Hydrocephalus

CSF Penetration

The determinants of CSF penetration of an antimicrobial agent include the degree of inflammation of the meninges and the physical properties of the drug, including protein binding, ionization, lipid solubility, and carrier transport. Nearly all large molecules are excluded from the CSF; any bound portion of a drug would also be excluded because only free drug crosses the choroid plexus. Drugs that are salts are highly ionized and, therefore, lipid insoluble. The ability of a drug to pass through the choroidal cells is a function of its lipid solubility at body pH. Drug concentration is also dependent on its elimination or removal from the CSF. The recognized mechanisms of drug removal include bulk (mass) flow of CSF, diffusion of lipid soluble substances, and an active transport system, especially for ionized drugs, through the arachnoid villi. Inflammation of the meninges increases capillary permeability and, thereby, enhances drug entry and inhibits active transport out of the CSF, thus increasing the CSF concentration.

The penetration of various antimicrobial agents into the CSF in the presence and absence of inflamed meninges is outlined in Table 8. Data concerning the CSF penetration of various agents are often from single case reports and determined by different methods. Recent studies with animal models have been useful, although the extrapolation of these data to humans is always questionable. In general, CSF penetration increases with inflammation of the meninges, although conflicting results have been reported correlating CSF penetration with increased leukocytes or protein in the CSF. The range of drug concentrations in the CSF of patients with meningitis is shown in Table 9.

Bactericidal Activity

Ideally, an antibiotic should be bactericidal against the infecting bacteria. Chloramphenicol is bactericidal against the encapsulated bacteria *H. influenzae, N. meningitidis*, and *S. pneumoniae* and is effective in bacterial meningitis caused by these bacteria. However, chloramphenicol is bacteriostatic against the aerobic gram-negative bacilli (MIC, 2 to 6 μg per milliliter; MBC, more than 60 μg per milliliter) and is not generally effective as a single agent in gram-negative bacillary (GNB) meningitis. Emergence of resistance to chloramphenicol has also been documented during therapy. Furthermore, experimental in vitro studies have shown that the combination of chloramphenicol and gentamicin is antagonistic, suggesting that a ''static-cidal'' drug combination may not be optimal for the treatment of bacterial meningitis. Similar antagonistic results were previously observed in patients with pneumococcal meningitis who received penicillin and tetracycline.

Drug Toxicity

The aminoglycosides have a low therapeutic index and their dose-related ototoxicity and nephrotoxicity preclude achieving CSF levels many times the MBC of gram-negative bacilli following parenteral administration.

Route of Administration

To achieve adequate CSF concentrations, antimicrobial agents must be given by the intravenous route. Because of the unidirectional flow of CSF, adequate ventricular drug levels cannot be obtained following intrathecal administration by the lumbar route. For drugs that do not adequately enter the CSF after intravenous administration (i.e., aminoglycosides), intraventricular injection may be required. This has been especially true in GNB meningitis because ventriculitis occurs in 70 percent of patients. Unfortunately, intraventricular administration of the aminoglycosides has been associated with local tissue injury and panencephalopathy following repeated injections. Antibiotics can also be delivered into the ventricles by an Ommaya or Rickham reservoir;

TABLE 8 Penetration of Antibiotics into Cerebrospinal Fluid

Good With or Without Inflammation	*Good With Inflammation*	*Unreliable Even With Inflammation*	*No Passage*
Sulfisoxazole	Penicillins	Cephalothin and other	Polymyxin B
Sulfadiazine	Penicillin G	first-generation	Colistin
Trimethoprim-sulfamethoxazole	Ampicillin	cephalosporins	Bacitracin
Chloramphenicol	Carbenicillin	Cefamandole	
Metronidazole	Ticarcillin	Cefoxitin	
Isoniazid	Methicillin	Tetracycline	
Ethionamide	Oxacillin	Clindamycin	
Cycloserine	Nafcillin	Erythromycin	
Flucytosine	Vancomycin	Aminoglycosides	
	New beta-lactams	Gentamicin	
	Cefotaxime	Tobramycin	
	Moxalactam	Amikacin	
	Cefoperazone	Netilmicin	
	Ceftizoxime	Amphotericin B	
	Rifampin		
	Ethambutol		

TABLE 9 Range of Drug Concentrations in Patients With Bacterial Meningitis

Drug	*Range of CSF Concentration (µg/ml)*	*Percentage of Serum Concentration*
Penicillin	1.0–10	--
Ampicillin	3.0–28	11–65
Methicillin	1.3–2.8	8–23
Nafcillin	2.7–9.8	14–30
Chloramphenicol	10–20	40–50
Gentamicin	0.2–3.0	10–30
Cephalothin	0.5–3.0	4–10
New beta-lactams (cefotaxime, moxalactam, cefoperazone, ceftizoxime)	5.0–30	15–45
Trimethoprim-	0.2–2.35	52–233
sulfamethoxazole	5.0–35	35–90
Metronidazole	12–27	100

however, this requires an invasive neurosurgical procedure that is sometimes associated with complications. Intrathecal antibiotics are given (at dosages listed in Table 10) in 3 to 5 ml of nonpreservative 5% dextrose in water or normal saline. Cefotaxime, because of its activity against GNB and excellent penetration into CSF following intravenous administration, is now the preferred agent in meningitis caused by susceptible GNB.

Suspected Pathogen and Susceptibility

In addition to the pharmacologic properties and toxicity of the antimicrobial agent, the suspected pathogen and its susceptibility must be considered in the choice of an antimicrobial agent. As described above, the pathogen may be suspected on the basis of the patient's age and underlying condition and the clinical setting and epidemiologic factors, but is confirmed only by isolation from the CSF or blood. Over the past several years, emergence of resistance of many of the pathogens responsible for bacterial meningitis has been noted, including ampicillin-resistant *H. influenzae*, multiply resistant *S. pneumoniae*, and ampicillin-resistant *Escherichia coli*.

The antimicrobial agents commonly used for treatment of bacterial meningitis and their unique properties include the following:

Penicillin G penetrates inflamed meninges and achieves CSF concentrations well above the MBC of susceptible organisms. It is the drug of choice for pneumococcal and meningococcal meningitis.

Ampicillin penetrates inflamed meninges slightly better than does penicillin G and is bactericidal against not only pneumococci and meningococci but also group B streptococci and *L. monocytogenes*. Emergence of resistance of *H. influenzae* and *E. coli* has limited its usefulness in infections due to these pathogens.

Chloramphenicol is bactericidal and effective as alternate therapy in *H. influenzae*, meningococcal, and pneumococcal meningitis. Less than 1 percent of *H. influenzae* isolates and multiply resistant pneumococci have been resistant to chloramphenicol. Chloramphenicol is bacteriostatic against enteric gram-negative bacteria.

Aminoglycosides do not achieve adequate CSF concentrations, are less active at the lowered pH of inflamed tissues and fluids, and have a low therapeutic index, limiting their usefulness in GNB meningitis. Their only role at the present time is in multiple resistant nosocomial GNB meningitis in which intraventricular administration may be necessary to achieve bacteriologic cure.

New beta-lactams (cefotaxime, moxalactam, cefoperazone, ceftizoxime) achieve excellent CSF levels 50 to 1,000 times the MBC of most susceptible bacteria. Because of their extended half-lives, high serum levels, and possible CSF accumulation, a steady state is reached in the CSF that persists between doses. These agents are active against ampicillin-sensitive and -resistant *H. influenzae*, meningococci, penicillin-sensitive pneumococci, and most Enterobacteriaceae, including *E. coli* and *Klebsiella* species. *Pseudomonas* strains are variable in their sensitivity, and *Acinetobacter* species and *L. monocytogenes* are resistant to the new beta-lactams. It is not recommended that one of these be used as a single agent for empiric therapy. Cefotaxime is our first choice among these agents; it has been used to successfully treat GNB meningitis. Cefoperazone is not approved for this use and reported data are based only on in vitro studies. Moxalactam is not used to treat pneumococcal meningitis.

The CSF penetration of the first- (cephalothin, cefazolin) and second- (cefamandole, cefoxitin) generation cephalosporins is unreliable, and these agents should not be used in bacterial meningitis. Pneumococcal and *H. influenzae* meningitis have developed in patients receiving cephalothin and cefamandole, respectively.

Wide-spectrum penicillins (azlocillin, mezlocillin, piperacillin) have been used to treat meningitis in only a limited number of patients. Although there is evidence that they penetrate inflamed meninges, none is approved for use in the treatment of meningitis.

Initial Therapy

The agents chosen for initial therapy of bacterial meningitis prior to the isolation of the pathogen should be based on the patient's age and the clinical setting and include either ampicillin (12 g per day) or penicillin G (24 million units per day). Alternative choices are either chloramphenicol (4 g per day) or cefotaxime (12 g per day). Drug therapy specifically directed against the causative organism should be instituted when identification and antimicrobial sensitivity are known. The primary and alternative antimicrobial regimens are listed in Table 10.

Duration of Therapy and Monitoring

The duration of parenteral antimicrobial therapy of uncomplicated bacterial meningitis is 2 weeks. Daily

TABLE 10 Antibiotic Therapy for Bacterial Meningitis in Adults

	Preferred Therapy		*Alternative Therapy*		
Organism	*Antibiotic*	*Dosage/24 hours*	*Antibiotic*	*Dosage/24 hours*	*Adjunctive Therapy*
Gram-positive					
Pneumococcus	Penicillin G	24 million units IV	Chloramphenicol *or* New beta-lactam *except* moxalactam	4 g IV 12 g IV	
Multiply resistant	Vancomycin	2 g IV			Vancomycin 2–5 mg (IT)‡
Group A and B *Streptococcus*	Penicillin G	24 million units IV			
S. faecalis	Ampicillin	12 g IV	Vancomycin	2 g IV	
S. aureus	Nafcillin	12 g IV	Vancomycin	2 g IV	
Methicillin resistant *S. aureus*	Vancomycin	2 g IV			Vancomycin 2–5 mg IT
L. monocytogenes	Ampicillin	12 g IV	Trimethoprim-sulfamethoxazole	12 ampules IV	Gentamicin 3–5 mg/kg IV
Gram-negative					
H. influenzae	Ampicillin	12 g IV	New beta-lactams*	12 g IV	
Ampicillin resistant *H. influenzae*	Chloramphenicol	4 g IV	New beta-lactams*	12 g IV	
Meningococcus	Penicillin G	24 million units IV	Chloramphenicol New beta-lactams*	4 g IV 12 g IV	
Aerobic gram-negative bacilli					
Enterobacteriaceae	New beta-lactams*	12 g IV			
Pseudomonas	New beta-lactams* *or* Carbenicillin *plus* Aminoglycoside†	12 g IV 30–40 g IV IV			Aminoglycoside† (2–5 mg) intraventricularly

* Preferred beta-lactam is cefotaxime 2 g q4h IV; others, on the basis of in vitro sensitivity, are moxalactam, or ceftizoxime 3 g q6h.
† Choice of aminoglycoside based on in vitro sensitivity: gentamicin and tobramycin 4–6 mg/kg IV and amikacin 15 mg/kg IV.
‡ IT = intrathecal

monitoring for the complications outlined in Table 7 should be performed. Repeat lumbar punctures should be performed only in the case of suspected complications or emergent resistance.

PROPHYLAXIS

Antimicrobial Prophylaxis

The risk that close contacts of patients with meningococcal meningitis will develop clinical disease is 500 to 600 times that of noncontacts in endemic disease situations and 15,000 times that of noncontacts in epidemic disease. Recent studies suggest that close contacts younger than the age of 4 years of patients with *H. influenzae* have an increased risk of 200 to 400 times normal. Close contacts include immediate family members, children in day care centers, and hospital personnel who have had intimate contact (i.e., mouth-to-mouth resuscitation) with the patient's respiratory secretions. Since most secondary cases in susceptible close contacts occur within 48 to 72 hours, antimicrobial prophylaxis should be given to contacts immediately upon recognition of the index case. For meningococcal prophylaxis, oral rifampin (600 mg twice daily) for 2 days is recommended. Sulfisoxazole (500 mg twice daily) for 2 days or minocycline (150 mg twice daily) for 4 days may be given if the isolate is known to be sensitive to sulfadiazine in the former case or if patients are allergic to rifampin. If the organism is resistant to sulfisoxazole, minocycline may be used; minocycline, however, has been associated with a high incidence of vestibular reactions. For *H. influenzae* prophylaxis, oral rifampin, 20 mg per kilogram per day for 4 days, is recommended for close contacts under 4 years of age.

Immunoprophylaxis

At the present time a tetravalent meningococcal polysaccharide vaccine (groups A, C, Y, W-135) and a 23-valent pneumococcal polysaccharide vaccine (Danish types 1, 2, 3, 4, 5, 8, 9N, 12F, 14, 17, 19F, 20, 22F, 23F, 6B, 10A, 11A, 7F, 15B, 18C, 19A, 9V, 33F) are available for clinical use. Indications for meningococcal immunoprophylaxis include routine prophylaxis in military training installations, outbreaks in civilian closed-population groups, individuals traveling to foreign countries where disease is epidemic, and as an adjunct to antibiotic prophylaxis for family and day care center contacts. Such prophylaxis is effective because 30 percent to 40 percent of secondary disease occurs more than 5 days after exposure to the index case. The frequency and severity of pneumococcal meningitis is increased in patients with splenic dysfunction and asplenia, (i.e., children with sickle cell disease), and indications for pneumococcal immunoprophylaxis include these patients as well. Unfortunately, the bacterial polysaccharide vaccines are not regularly immunogenic in children under 2 years of age, and other forms of prophylaxis are necessary for that age group.

A type B *H. influenzae* vaccine has recently been approved for the following high risk patients: (1) all children at 24 months of age; (2) children at 18 months of age, particularly those with underlying conditions, (e.g., sickle cell disease, primary antibody deficiency) or attendees of day care facilities under 5 years of age. These latter children may require revaccination within 18 months to ensure adequate protection.

ASEPTIC MENINGITIS

JACK MENDELSON, M.D.

Aseptic meningitis and atypical pneumonia are analagous conditions, for they both refer to infectious processes where the "usual" bacteria (in meningitis these include *Streptococcus pneumoniae, Neisseria meningitidis,* and *Hemophilus influenzae*) are not cultured from fluids from the infected site in a patient not on antibiotic therapy. The diagnosis and management of aseptic meningitis presents one of the more difficult problems in infectious diseases, because, on the one hand, cases caused by viruses generally have no available specific therapy, and on the other, failure to adequately treat a partially treated bacterial meningitis may have devastating consequences.

Patients who have received only a day or two of oral antibiotics usually do not present a great problem, since bacterial meningitis is not often masked in this situation. Thus, cultures are usually positive, and patients should be treated with appropriate antibiotics. However, patients who received small amounts of antibiotics before admission should not automatically be treated, but, rather, should be observed only if they are not toxic and if the cerebrospinal fluid findings are compatible with an aseptic process; however, should the condition deteriorate or changes occur in the CSF that suggest a bacterial etiology, therapy should be instituted even if the cultures remain negative.

At times it is difficult to be certain that one is actually dealing with meningitis; the classic nuchal rigidity may not be dramatic, and headache may be the most prominent complaint. A rapid onset of symptoms usually suggests a viral etiology, whereas a prolonged history and gradual onset support other etiologies such as tuberculosis, brain abscess, or cryptococcal disease. Once a diagnosis of possible meningitis is entertained, then one must be certain that it is safe to perform a lumbar puncture (LP) based on normal funduscopic examination and absence of signs and symptoms of greatly increased intracranial pressure. Examination of CSF is one of the most critical facets in the work-up of the patient.

Meningitis is an inflammation of the meninges, and the symptoms usually include headache, stiff neck, and fever. Once cerebral function becomes impaired—as manifested by progression to coma, impairment of sensorium, or onset of focal neurologic symptoms—the patient must be subjected to other procedures such as CT scan, electroencephalogram, brain scan, and possible brain biopsy if herpes simplex encephalitis is considered.

No strict guidelines can be given regarding the CSF findings in aseptic meningitis. Naturally, no bacteria are noted on Gram stain of the fluid, and routine bacteriologic cultures are negative. The number of leukocytes found can vary tremendously from as few as 10 to 20 to thousands per cubic millimeter. The demonstration of neutrophils does not necessarily suggest a bacterial etiology since these cells are found at an early stage in viral meningitis. Elevated levels of CSF protein are almost inevitable, but the degree of elevation generally does not suggest any particular group of pathogens. In viral meningitis the CSF glucose levels are usually not depressed, as is often the situation with bacterial meningitis, but, here again, there are exceptions: mumps and lymphocytic choriomeningitic (LCM) infections may present with low CSF glucose levels.

Let us imagine, then, a patient who presents with headache, fever, stiff neck, and modest pleocytosis with 200 white blood cells per cubic millimeter, 75 percent of which are neutrophils. If one is faced with this problem early in the course of the patient's disease, then most often one is dealing with a viral process, particularly if the patient is not very toxic and has received no previous antibiotics. Antibiotics may be withheld, but the patient must be kept under close observation. If the patient deteriorates clinically, a repeat LP should be performed for analysis, and the decision to treat with antibiotics will depend on changes in the CSF, such as an increase in numbers of neutrophils, a lowering of the CSF glucose levels, and an elevation in the protein level. Assuming that the Gram stain is still negative for microorganisms, latex agglutination assays for pneumococcal, meningococcal, or haemophilus antigens may be performed; the latex tests are more sensitive and rapid than counterimmunoelectrophoresis (CIE), where false-negative results are frequent. Once antibiotic therapy has been instituted, the patient should receive a full course of antimicrobial treatment, even if the latex test is negative. Other ancillary tests (other than microbiologic cultures) may be necessary in order to solve this difficult clinical problem. Acute and convalescent serum determinations are not helpful in clarifying the situation early on. CIE or latex agglutination tests (as noted above) may be helpful in the diagno-

TABLE 1 Epidemiology, Diagnosis, and Treatment of Aseptic Meningitis

Etiology of Disease	*Epidemiologic and Clinical Clues*	*CSF Characteristics*	*Ancillary Tests*	*Treatment*
Enterovirus (polio, rare)	1. Mainly children, young adults; rare >40 yrs 2. Late summer, early autumn	1. PMNs, then lymphocytes (20-2,000/mm³) 2. Glucose normal 3. Protein ↑ (rarely >100 mg%)	1. Viral culture 2. Serology only if virus isolated	----
Mumps	1. 90% of disease occurs in children <14 yrs 2. January to May 3. Parotitis and/or orchitis usually present	1. PMNs, then lymphocytes (20-2,000/mm³) 2. Glucose normal (low in up to 30%) 3. Protein ↑ (rarely >70 mg%)	1. Viral culture 2. Serology	----
Herpes simplex (type 1 or 2)	1. Usually adults 2. May progress to encephalitis 3. No seasonal variation 4. May occur in association with genital herpes	1. PMNs, then lymphocytes 2. Glucose normal 3. Protein ↑ 4. May see RBCs	1. Viral isolation from CSF rare 2. Serology	ARA-A?
Varicella-zoster	1. Varicella rash 2. Shingles	1. As for enteroviruses	1. Viral isolation from vesicle on skin 2. Serology	----
Lymphocytic choriomeningitis	1. Mainly young adults 2. Laboratory workers handling mice, hamsters, etc. 3. Fall, winter and spring 4. Occasional associated arthritis, parotitis, orchitis	1. Lymphocytes (may be >2,000/mm³) 2. Glucose may be ↓ (25%) 3. Protein ↑ (average, 100 mg%)	1. Viral isolation from CSF 2. Serology	----
Partially treated meningitis	1. History: antibiotic use 2. Rash (meningococcal) 3. Childhood (*H. influenza*) 4. Otitis, sinusitis mastoiditis (*S. pneumoniae*)	1. Gram stain (+) in 60% 2. PMNs >1,200/mm³ 3. Glucose <30 mg% 4. Protein >150 mg%	1. Culture (may be negative) 2. CIE* not very sensitive (pneumococcus, *H. influenzae*) 3. Latex agglutination (sensitive and rapid) 4. Lactic acid >35 mg% 5. Limulus lysate test (for gram-negative organisms) 6. CSF amino acid levels	1. *S. pneumoniae*: penicillin G, 2 million units IV q2h × 10–14 days 2. *N. meningitides*: as above, but treat for at least 5 days after patient becomes afebrile 3. *H. influenzae*: ampicillin 300 mg/kg/day IV q4h plus chloramphenicol 100 mg/kg/day IV q6h until sensitivities available (alternate regimens include cotrimoxazole, moxalactam)
M. tuberculosis	1. Subacute or chronic 2. Evidence of miliary TB 3. In U.S. mainly in adults, elderly 4. Cranial nerve palsies	1. Acid-fast stain often negative (75%) 2. PMNs, then mononuclears (100–500/mm³) 3. Glucose ↓ (25 mg% = mean) 4. Protein ↑ (30 mg% = mean)	1. Culture-positive approx. 60% (send large volumes of CSF for culture)	1. INH† 300 mg daily 2. Rifampin 600 mg daily 3. Ethambutol 15 mg/kg/day; Treat for 18–24 months

* CIE = counter immunoelectrophoresis (latex agglutination preferred)
† INH = isoniazid

TABLE 1 Epidemiology, Diagnosis, and Treatment of Aseptic Meningitis (Continued)

Etiology of Disease	*Epidemiologic and Clinical Clues*	*CSF Characteristics*	*Ancillary Tests*	*Treatment*
Spinal epidural abscess	1. Back pain, leg pain 2. May be postoperative (back surgery) 3. Evidence of vertebral osteomyelitis 4. Mostly males 5. Deficits in motor, sensory, or sphincter function	As those found in aseptic meningitis syndrome	Myelography (not CT scan)	1. Immediate surgery, and cloxacillin 2 g IV q4h for 4 weeks at least 2. (*S. aureus* is pathogen in 90% of cases)
Brain abscess	1. Presence of bronchiectasis, lung abscess 2. Poor dental hygiene 3. Congenital heart disease 4. Seizures 5. Focal neurologic findings 6. Usually males	LP may be dangerous and is not advised because of the possibility of herniation	1. CT scan 2. Brain Scan 3. Aspiration or excision	1. Surgery (usually aspiration or excision) 2. Based on bacteriologic results: Penicillin G 2 million units IV q2h for 6–8 weeks *or* Chloramphenicol 1 g IV q4h for 6–8 weeks *or* Metronidazole 15 mg/kg infused IV over 1 hour followed by 7.5 mg/kg infused over 1 hour IV q6h for 6–8 weeks
Secondary syphilis	1. Rare (2% of cases) 2. May be male homosexual 3. Rash (including palms and soles) 4. Mucous membrane lesions 5. Lymphadenopathy 6. Usually subacute	1. Lymphocytes 2. Glucose normal 3. Protein ↑	1. VDRL 2. FTA-abs‡ 3. CSF darkfield	Benzathine penicillin G 2.4 million units IM once
Leptospirosis	1. Usually young adult male 2. Summer and early fall 3. Indirect contact with infected animal's urine via water, soil 4. Occupational exposure (veterinarians, farmers) 5. History of camping, swimming 6. Uveitis in 2% 7. Headache very intense	1. PMNs, then mononuclears 2. Protein normal to 300 mg% 3. Glucose normal	1. Agglutination tests (≥1:100) 2. Isolation of organism from blood, CSF, or urine using Fletcher's medium, EMJH, and Tween 80 albumin medium 3. Hamster inoculation	Treat within first 4 days: Penicillin G 1 million units IV q6h for 1 week
Lyme disease (*Borrelia* species)	1. Most cases in U.S. Northeast (but not all) 2. Classic rash, erythema chronicum migrans	1. Lymphocytes (25–450/mm^3) 2. Glucose normal	1. IFA test§	Early manifestations: tetracycline 500 mg PO QID for 10 days

‡ FTA-abs = fluorescent treponemal antibody absorption test
§ IFA = indirect fluorescent antibody

TABLE 1 Epidemiology, Diagnosis, and Treatment of Aseptic Meningitis (Continued)

Etiology of Disease	*Epidemiologic and Clinical Clues*	*CSF Characteristics*	*Ancillary Tests*	*Treatment*
	3. Arthritis 4. Cardiac arrythmias 5. Summer or early fall 6. Tick bite (recalled by only 20%)	3. Protein normal		
Cryptococcus neoformans	1. Half of patients may be on steroids, and/or have lymphoreticular malignancies 2. Indolent onset 3. Symptoms may wax and wane 4. Minimal nuchal rigidity 5. 20% have cranial nerve palsies	1. Mainly lymphocytes (40–400/mm³) 2. Glucose ↓ in 50% 3. Protein ↑	1. Culture 2. India ink stain 3. Latex agglutination test on CSF	1. Amphotericin B 0.3 mg/kg/day IV for 6 weeks *and* 2. Flucytosine 37.5 mg/kg PO q6h for 6 weeks
Coccidioidomycosis	1. Occurs in 7 southwestern U.S. states or after travel to area 2. May occur more often in Immunosuppressed patients Pregnant females Filipinos Hispanics Blacks 3. Usually within 6 months after primary pulmonary infection 4. Signs of meningeal irritation usually absent 5. Cranial nerve palsies	1. Mainly lymphocytes (<500/mm³) 2. Glucose ↓ 3. Protein ↑ 4. May see eosinophils	1. Culture 2. CSF, CF[ll] titres ↑ in 95% 3. Blood CF tests	1. Intrathecal amphotericin B beginning with 0.025 mg and increasing to 0.5 mg if tolerated; administer thrice weekly for 3 months, then twice weekly for 2 months tapering to once every 1–6 weeks; treat until CSF has been normal for 1 year *and* 2. Amphotericin B IV to a total of 1 g (for other system involvement, which is common with meningitis) *or* 3. Miconazole therapy still experimental

[ll] CF = complement fixation

sis of a partially treated pneumococcal, meningococcal, or hemophilus meningitis. A positive limulus lysate test on CSF may indicate a gram-negative meningitis and has its greatest usefulness in two clinical situations. The first is in the neonatal period and the second is in the post-craniotomy patient. A positive CSF VDRL test would suggest syphilis. Recently, a CSF latex agglutination test for cryptococcal meningitis has proved to be an extremely useful diagnostic procedure. Myelography (not CT scan) may aid in the diagnosis of an epidural abscess, whereas CT or a brain scan are of great value in the demonstration of an early brain abscess (see chapter *Localized Infection of the Central Nervous System*).

Epidemiologic and clinical clues are extremely important areas of information in solving the problem of the etiology of an aseptic meningitis and must be sought early on in the work-up of the patient. Enteroviruses and mumps infect mainly children, and herpes simplex and LCM are more often infections of adults. Laboratory workers acquire LCM infections, whereas veterinarians and farmers develop leptospirosis. Enteroviral meningitis, Lyme disease, and leptospirosis occur mainly in summer and late autumn; mumps occurs from January to May. Varicella, herpes simplex, tuberculosis, brain abscess, syphilis, and cryptococcosis know no season.

The methods of diagnosis of the latter conditions noted above vary tremendously. Enteroviral, mumps, and LCM infections are diagnosed by the isolation of the virus from spinal fluid. Leptospires may be isolated from the spinal fluid during the first 10 days of the disease and from the urine later on by the use of special media (e.g., Fletcher's) that are not readily available in most laboratories. A darkfield examination of the spinal fluid may reveal the spirochetes. Finally, serologic testing, e.g., slide agglutination, is a useful screening procedure for leptospirosis. For Lyme disease, it is much more difficult to visualize organisms directly in the CSF. Antibody titer tests are more widely used, but the presence of the characteristic rash is most useful in confirming the diagnosis (see chapter *Lyme Disease*).

Various other historical, epidemiologic, and clinical clues may be helpful. Recent travel to the northeastern United States may suggest Lyme disease, particularly if a rash is present, whereas coccidioidomycosis enters the differential if someone has been to one of the seven southwestern states, especially if the patient is immunosuppressed, pregnant, Hispanic, black, or Filipino. Of utmost importance, as noted above, is the history of recent antibiotic administration; without such information it may be impossible to exclude a bacteriologic etiology and necessitate antibiotic therapy. Leg and back pain, particularly in a male who has had recent back surgery, suggests a spinal epidural abscess, and focal neurologic findings (also more frequent in males) may be a manifestation of brain abscess.

Immunosuppressed patients are more predisposed to cryptococcal and tuberculous meningitis. These patients generally have a history of more chronic onset of disease. In the case of cryptococcal meningitis the patients, besides possibly being immunosuppressed, may have evidence of cryptococcal disease elsewhere and should have an India ink or latex agglutination test performed on the spinal fluid. The latex test is very sensitive and is widely used. If one suspects tuberculosis, particularly if the patient is immunosuppressed or has a history of tuberculosis or evidence of pulmonary tuberculosis, acid-fast stains of spinal fluid should be done. These are rarely rewarding, and even cultures may be negative. Once the decision to treat has been made on the basis of the above considerations, antituberculous therapy should be continued even if cultures remain negative (see chapter *Tuberculosis*).

In the table that follows, many of the aspects relating to the diagnosis and management of aseptic meningitis have been discussed above, and many others are included below. As well, specific therapy is outlined when indicated. The clinician faced with the difficult problem of aseptic meningitis will be better able to approach it in a more rewarding manner using all the clinical information that is available.

LOCALIZED INFECTION OF THE CENTRAL NERVOUS SYSTEM

KENNETH L. TYLER, M.D.

Localized infections of the central nervous system (CNS) produce a wide variety of clinical signs and symptoms. Diagnosis of these infections often requires the use and interpretation of specialized diagnostic techniques including computerized tomography (CT scan) and cerebral angiography. Successful therapy depends on a combination of prompt and aggressive medical management and the use of appropriate neurosurgical intervention. Because of the unique features of each type of infection, they are each discussed separately in terms of etiology, pathogenesis, clinical features, laboratory and diagnostic studies, and treatment.

Other CNS infections including bacterial meningitis, aseptic meningitis, and viral encephalitis are discussed in separate chapters as are specific infections such as tuberculosis, syphilis, and certain parasitic diseases.

Dr. Tyler is supported by a physician-scientist award from the National Institute of Allergy and Infectious Diseases, by a fellowship grant from the Muscular Dystrophy Association, and by a grant from the William P. Anderson Foundation.

CEREBRAL SUBDURAL EMPYEMA

Subdural empyema (SDE) can be defined as a collection of pus in the preformed space between the cranial dural and arachnoid membranes. Spinal subdural empyema is a rare form of localized infection of the spinal cord and is discussed separately.

Etiology

Infection of the paranasal sinuses is now the most frequent antecedent to SDE (70% of cases). In most cases, the frontal sinuses are involved, but SDE may follow maxillary sinusitis, and sphenoidal sinusitis may precede SDE in the area of the sella turcica (perihypophyseal abscess). SDE usually follows acute rather than chronic sinusitis. In the preantibiotic era, otitic infections were a common antecedent to SDE, but they now account for less than 30 percent of cases; in these cases, SDE often follows an acute exacerbation of chronic otitis. Unusual antecedents of SDE include secondary infection of a subdural hematoma, cranial osteomyelitis, extension through a dural fistula of an epidural abscess, septic thrombophlebitis of the cerebral veins or sinuses, and metastatic spread from a distant primary site of infection. Chronic septic labyrinthitis or petrous apicitis are rare cases of SDE in the posterior fossa. In children, subdural empyema may develop during the course of acute meningitis.

Pathogenesis

Otogenic infections can spread to the subdural space by direct erosion through the adjacent bone of the tegmen tympani and the underlying dura. Infection usually spreads along the tentorium to the falx, and may extend into the posterior fossa or laterally over the temporal lobe. Patients with sinusitis may develop septic thrombophlebitis of the mucosal veins, with subsequent spread of infection to the dural veins and venous sinuses, resulting in SDE. SDE may also result from direct extension of infection from the sinuses to the subdural space. In these cases, there is often pathologic evidence of osteomyelitis of the adjacent bone. When associated paranasal sinusitis is present, infection of the subdural space often originates near the frontal pole of the skull and then extends posteriorly.

Clinical Features

The clinical features of SDE are due to *(1)* signs and symptoms of any antecedent local infection (e.g., sinusitis or otitis), *(2)* signs and symptoms of increased intracranial pressure, and *(3)* signs and symptoms of focal neurological dysfunction. Local pain referred to the region of an infected ear or sinus is quite common. Typically, there is also pain and tenderness over the brow or between the eyes that is exacerbated by percussion of the involved sinus. Orbital swelling and mild proptosis frequently occur and presumably reflect infection involving the orbital veins. Scalp swelling or cellulitis, if present, should suggest the possibility of an associated extradural abscess or of cranial osteomyelitis.

General signs and symptoms include the almost invariable presence of fever, severe headache, and nuchal rigidity. Nausea and vomiting accompany the headache in one-half to two-thirds of cases. Patients generally appear to be severely ill. A change in the level of consciousness occurs with progression of the illness. Early on, patients often seem to be sleepy, confused, or inattentive. With further disease progression, they become somnolent, stuporous, and ultimately comatose. Patients with increased intracranial pressure may develop bradycardia, systolic hypertension, and Cheyne-Stokes breathing. Papilloedema is uncommon, and when it appears, there is usually coexisting sinus thrombosis.

Within a few days of the onset of illness, a wide variety of focal signs and symptoms appear. Contralateral hemiparesis or hemiplegia is the commonest focal symptom and eventually develops in almost all patients. Weakness is typically maximal in the face and arm (faciobrachial paresis). The deep tendon reflexes may either be increased or diminished, but the ipsilateral plantar response is usually extensor. Bilaterally upgoing toes should suggest the possibility of transtentorial herniation with compression of the brain stem.

Many patients develop a paresis or palsy of conjugate gaze toward the side opposite the lesion. In more obvious cases, this may result in a resting deviation of the eyes toward the side of the lesion.

Close to 50 percent of patients with SDE will develop seizures. Commonly, focal motor or Jacksonian seizures will antedate more generalized convulsions. Status epilepticus can occur.

Aphasia occurs in many patients with SDE, involving the dominant (typically left) hemisphere. These patients often make naming errors (anomic aphasia), although the full syndrome of either Broca's or, less commonly, Wernicke's aphasia may be seen.

Laboratory and Diagnostic Studies

Computed cranial tomography (CT scanning) has become the cornerstone of diagnosis of SDE. The CT scan is abnormal in virtually all cases. Typically, there is a crescent-shaped region of decreased attenuation between the inner table of the skull and the cerebral cortex. Midline structures are displaced away from the side of the SDE, and there is typically compression of the ipsilateral lateral ventricle. Contrast injection often produces irregular enhancement of the peripheral margin of the SDE. In cases of intrafalcial empyema, there is a lucent area running sagittally between the cerebral hemispheres.

In doubtful cases, cerebral angiography may prove valuable. The angiogram typically shows a displacement of vessels away from the inner skull table, suggesting the presence of an extra-axial avascular mass. Particular attention should be paid to the position of the meningeal arteries and the dural sinuses. Displacement of these structures away from the inner skull table suggests extradural, rather than subdural, location of a mass. In the rare cases of intrafalcial empyema, the proximal branches of the anterior cerebral artery are displaced contralaterally and the distal branches ipsilaterally. This results in distinctive S-shaped configuration of the anterior cerebral artery.

Routine radiographic studies are often of value in identifying the presence of sinusitis, mastoiditis, or cranial osteomyelitis. The CT scan may also provide evidence suggesting sinusitis or mastoiditis.

The EEG (electroencephalogram) is rarely of significant diagnostic value. The EEG may show decreased voltage and slow waves on the side of the SDE.

Lumbar puncture (LP) should be avoided in cases of suspected SDE. The LP rarely adds important diagnostic information and can result in cerebral herniation in patients with increased intracranial pressure. When CSF has been obtained in cases of SDE, the findings are quite variable. The CSF pressure is increased in about 70 percent of cases. Pleocytosis is seen in almost all patients, but the cell count varies from 15 to 1,000 cells. In patients with cell counts greater than 1,000, the possibility of rupture of the SDE into the subarachnoid space should be considered. In infants this number of cells suggests that SDE may have resulted as a complication of acute meningitis. The cells may be either predominantly polymorphonuclear leukocytes (PMNs) (60% of cases) or predominantly lymphocytes (40%). The protein is typically elevated, but rarely more than 200 mg per deciliter. The glucose is normal. Organisms are not seen and CSF cultures are negative unless there is an associated meningitis.

Pathology

A detailed discussion of the pathology of SDE is beyond the scope of this chapter. On gross examination, the subdural exudate usually covers a large part of one cerebral hemisphere. The empyema does not ''wall off,'' and there is no evidence of a limiting membrane surrounding the exudate. Underneath the SDE, the brain is almost always depressed, and there is often evidence of an underlying purulent subarachnoid exudate and thrombosis and/or thrombophlebitis of the subarachnoid veins. Microscopic studies show evidence of infiltration of the dura with inflammatory cells, typically PMNs. The inner surface of the dura is lined with a PMN exudate. The outer layer of the cerebral cortex and subcortical white matter often show evidence of necrosis.

Infecting Agents

The commonest organisms isolated from SDE are aerobic and anaerobic streptococci and *Staphylococcus aureus*. Gram-negative organisms (*Escherichia coli, Proteus* species, *Klebsiella* species, *Pseudomonas* species) may be found in cases that follow otitis or mastoiditis but are rare following paranasal sinusitis. Anaerobic bacteria are often present and may be overlooked unless special culture techniques are utilized.

Therapy

SDE is a fulminating and often life-threatening intracranial infection. Definitive therapy must be initiated without delay. Once the diagnosis is confirmed, operative drainage should be performed urgently. Drainage can be done through burr holes or following craniectomy. In most cases, a surgical approach directed toward the lateral frontal region results in the best drainage of the SDE. Obviously, the surgical approach should be modified according to the best available information on the location of the SDE. Local instillation of penicillin or other antibacterial agents may be helpful and is favored by some neurosurgeons. Surgical therapy should be combined with high doses of parenteral antibiotics in all cases. The combination of (doses are for adults with normal renal function) nafcillin, 2 g intravenously every 4 hours, or oxacillin, 2 g intravenously every 4 hours (these are therapeutically equivalent), and chloramphenicol, 1.5 g intravenously every 6 hours, usually provides satisfactory initial coverage until culture results are available. If the patient is penicillin allergic, vancomycin, 500 mg intravenously every 6 hours may be used in place of oxacillin or nafcillin.

Anticonvulsants are administered for treatment of seizures, and osmotic agents are used, when necessary, to control increased intracranial pressure.

CEREBRAL EPIDURAL ABSCESS

Etiology and Pathogenesis

Epidural abscess (EA) is the rarest of the localized intracranial suppurative infections. Pus collects between the external layer of the dura and the inner table of the skull. EA is typically associated with an overlying focal cranial osteomyelitis. Infection often spreads across the dura through the emissary veins and produces a subdural empyema as well. EA may follow localized infections of the middle ear or paranasal sinuses. EA may also follow either accidental or surgical penetration of the cranial bones. Implanted foreign bodies (dural grafts, tantalum implants, ventricular shunts, Crutchfield tongs) that penetrate the calvarium may become infected and result in the development of EA. Rare causes of EA include spread of septic dural sinus thrombosis (e.g., infectious cavernous sinus thrombosis), spread of a subdural empyema through a dural fistula, and metastatic spread of infection from a distant site.

Clinical Features

The clinical features of EA do not differ significantly from those described for subdural empyema, and distinction between these two conditions on purely clinical grounds may be difficult. Typically, signs and symptoms of a local infection, such as sinusitis or mastoiditis, are followed by severe generalized headache and high fever. With large abscesses there may be progressive alteration in mental status and focal neurologic signs. In these cases, contralateral hemiparesis is particularly common. Smaller abscesses may produce an isolated contralateral monoparesis. Focal motor convulsions occur with frequency and may generalize. An epidural empyema situated near the petrous pyramid may produce ipsilateral facial pain and sensory loss combined with diplopia due to an ipsilateral lateral rectus palsy (Gradenigo's syndrome).

Laboratory and Diagnostic Studies

The CT scan has become the primary diagnostic study for the diagnosis of EA. The typical picture is one of an extracerebral zone of low density. Evidence of sinusitis or osteomyelitis may be seen. Contrast enhancement of the outer margin of the EA is commonly found. Mass effect—including a contralateral shift of midline structures and compression of the ipsilateral lateral ventricle—is usually seen. It may be impossible to differentiate SDE and EA on CT scan.

The typical angiographic features of an epidural mass lesion were discussed in the section on SDE.

Conventional radiographic or polytomographic studies may help suggest the diagnosis of EA by demonstrating the presence of mastoid or paranasal sinus infection or by showing evidence of cranial osteomyelitis.

Lumbar puncture rarely adds valuable diagnostic information and may result in the development of herniation. When CSF has been examined, it typically shows a mild to moderate pleocytosis in which PMNs or lymphocytes may predominate. The protein is almost invariably elevated. The CSF pressure may be normal or elevated. The CSF glucose levels are normal and organisms are not seen or cultured.

Pathology

Extradural empyemas are often small and circumscribed, although large lesions are occasionally seen. Pus is found between the outer surface of the dura and the inner table of the skull. The dura itself often shows evidence of inflammation. In autopsy studies, an associated subdural empyema is found in up to 80 percent of cases, and an associated brain abscess in 15 to 20 percent.

Infecting Agents

The major infecting agents are similar to those responsible for subdural empyema.

Treatment

Optimal treatment of EA requires the combination of surgical debridement and drainage with parenteral antibiotic therapy. Infected bone should be removed, and the abscess should be drained as completely as possible. Antibiotic therapy is similar to that for SDE and should be modified as indicated by operative cultures.

BRAIN ABSCESS

Etiology

Brain abscesses usually arise from direct extension of infection from contiguous sites (e.g., middle ear, paranasal sinuses), from metastatic spread of distant infections, or from either accidental or surgically induced cranial trauma. Even after careful consideration of each of these possibilities, about 15 to 25 percent of intracranial abscesses are idiopathic in nature.

The two major sources of direct spread of infection are the middle ear/mastoid region and the paranasal sinuses. Otogenic abscesses result when infection in the middle ear erodes through the tegmen tympani or tegmen mastoideum. Spread via the lateral or other sinuses may provide an additional route. Chronic otitis, rather than acute disease, is usually the antecedent infection. Frequently, there is a history of an acute exacerbation of chronic otitis immediately preceding the first symptoms of the brain abscess. In adults otogenic abscesses most commonly occur in the temporal lobe, followed by the cerebellum. In children, a higher percentage of otogenic abscesses are cerebellar. As a corollary to this rule, an otogenic source should always be suspected when an abscess is found in the temporal lobe or cerebellum. The abscesses following infection of the frontal or ethmoid sinuses are commonly located in the frontal lobes. Sphenoidal sinusitis may result in frontal lobe, temporal lobe, or even intrasellar abscesses.

Hematogenous dissemination of infection accounts for about 25 percent of all brain abscesses. In about 20 percent of these cases, multiple abscesses are present. The most frequent site of primary infection is the lung. A wide variety of pulmonary infections including lung abscesses, pneumonia, empyema, and bronchiectasis may predispose to brain abscess development. There is also a higher-than-expected incidence of brain abscesses in patients with cystic fibrosis and pulmonary arteriovenous fistulas (e.g., Osler-Weber-Rendu syndrome). Pulmonary alveolar proteinosis predisposes patients to nocardial brain abscesses. Certain cardiac diseases also predispose to the development of brain abscess. Patients with cyanotic congenital heart disease and a right-to-left shunt are at particular risk. Bacterial endocarditis only rarely results in the production of macroabscesses (more than 1 cm diameter) in the brain, although microabscesses (less than 1 cm) are quite common. A variety of other primary infections including peritonsillar abscess, odontogenic abscess, abdominal infections, and infected intrauterine devices account for occasional cases of metastatic brain abscess. Heroin addicts and other intravenous drug abusers also appear to be at higher risk for developing brain abscesses.

Traumatic brain abscesses may be delayed for years or even decades after the acute trauma. Retained bone or metallic fragments seem to increase the risk.

Clinical Features

The signs and symptoms of brain abscess are produced by the primary infection, if one is present, by the focal effects of the brain abscess on the CNS, and by increased intracranial pressure.

General symptoms include fever, chills, and malaise. Fever is more commonly present in acute cases and much less frequent in chronic ones. In most instances the fever appears to be due to the primary infection (e.g., otitis or sinusitis), rather then to the brain abscess. Since fever is only present in about 40 percent of patients and is often low-grade, its absence does not exclude the diagnosis. Signs of increased intracranial pressure can include headache, nausea and vomiting, and alteration in mental status.

Headache may be either generalized or focal and is present in 50 to 70 percent of cases. Its absence does not exclude the diagnosis of brain abscess. Papilloedema has been reported in 25 to 50 percent of patients, but it may be a late finding. Paralysis of one or both VIth cranial nerves may result from increased intracranial pressure. Alterations in mental status—ranging from lethargy to stupor or even coma—are found in 50 to 70 percent of patients. Nuchal rigidity occurs in 20 to 50 percent of patients. Seizures may be focal or generalized and occur in about one-third of cases.

A wide variety of focal neurologic signs can occur and may provide a clue to localization. Hemiparesis occurs in about 50 percent of patients, and abnormalities of the visual fields in 5 to 20 percent. Frontal lobe abscesses may produce deterioration in memory function and attention. Temporal lobe abscesses may result in aphasia, hemiparesis, and superior quadrantopsia. Abscesses in the cerebellum often produce suboccipital headache, which radiates to the neck and interscapular area. Signs of cerebellar dysfunction may be subtle and can include incoordination, ataxia, hypotonia, conjugate gaze palsies, and nystagmus.

Laboratory and Diagnostic Studies

The peripheral white blood cell count is above 10,000 per cubic millimeter in about 50 percent of patients, but exceeds 20,000 in only 10 percent. The ESR is increased in about 75 percent of patients and may be a helpful clue in differentiating brain abscess from other mass lesions.

Of the neurodiagnostic tests, the CT scan is unequivocally the most important aid in diagnosis. It permits accurate localization of the abscess, evaluation of its size, and delineation of associated edema and mass effect. The CT scan identifies virtually 100 percent of cases of brain abscesses. The abscess appears as a mass lesion, often with a central lucent zone and a surrounding area of edema. Contrast enhancement is seen as a rim of increased density around the abscess periphery. The development of this pattern of ring enhancement has been attributed to the vascularity of the abscess capsule. Early in its natural history, an abscess appears as a zone of hypodensity without a clear capsule (cerebritis). After 3 to 6 weeks, ring enhancement is seen on CT scan, and after this point, the abscess becomes well demarcated. It is important to remember that ring-enhancing lesions are also produced by primary and metastatic tumors and, occasionally, by hematomas and hemorrhagic infarcts. The visualization on CT scan of septae inside the lesion and of ependymal or meningeal enhancement favors the diagnosis of an abscess.

Angiography is rarely used today to identify or localize brain abscesses. The usual finding is one of an avascular mass, although an area of increased vascularity corresponding to the abscess capsule may be seen. Angiography is reasonably sensitive in localizing abscesses in the temporal lobe, but frontal and parietal abscesses may be missed. The angiogram does not usually allow a precise etiologic diagnosis to be made, but simply identifies the presence of a mass lesion.

The EEG is no longer a primary diagnostic tool in cases of suspected brain abscess. It is abnormal in 75 to 90 percent of cases of supratentorial brain abscesses. The findings may include focal high amplitude slow (delta) waves, epileptiform discharges, or asymmetric fast activity.

Lumbar puncture should be avoided in cases of suspected brain abscess. The LP rarely adds useful diagnostic information, and it may result in abrupt neurologic deterioration or death. This type of deterioration occurs in up to one-third of patients within 24 to 48 hours of an LP. Reported CSF results generally include increased intracranial pressure, a pleocytosis (more than 10 cells per cubic millimeter) in 70 percent, and an elevated protein in two-thirds of cases. Cell counts of about 10,000 should raise the possibility that ventricular extension has occurred. Cell counts tend to be higher before the abscess is encapsulated and in abscesses located near the ventricles or subarachnoid space. The glucose levels are normal and cultures are negative unless there is an associated meningitis.

Infecting Agents

The bacteriology of brain abscesses is extremely variable. The most frequently isolated organisms are *S. aureus*, aerobic and anaerobic streptococci, *Streptococcus pneumoniae, Bacteroides* species, and gram-negative bacteria. Reports of isolation of a large number of other organisms have appeared. *Listeria monocytogenes* is an important pathogen in immunosuppressed patients. *Clostridia* species and *S. aureus* are often found in post-traumatic abscesses. Multiple pathogens are found in 20 to 30 percent of cases. The reported incidence of anaerobic organisms varies widely and probably depends on the techniques used to culture specimens.

Therapy

The optimal approach to the treatment of brain abscesses is combined medical and neurosurgical therapy. The choice of optimal antibiotic therapy depends on the causative organisms. Every attempt should be made to obtain an aspirate of the abscess material for aerobic, anaerobic, and special cultures. Frequently, a sterotactic aspiration under CT guidance is possible.

Prior to identification of the causative organism(s),

empiric antibiotic therapy of abscesses associated with paranasal sinusitis should include intravenous penicillin G, 2 million units every 2 hours, plus chloramphenicol, 1.5 g every 6 hours. Nafcillin or oxacillin, 2 g every 4 hours intravenously, should be substituted for penicillin in abscesses of metastatic or traumatic etiology.

Therapy should be continued for a minimum of 4 weeks or until follow-up CT scans demonstrate resolution of the abscess. Several new agents including moxalactam, TMP/SMZ, and metronidazole may prove to be valuable adjuncts to therapy in specific situations.

There remains controversy over the optimal form of surgical therapy for brain abscess. Some neurosurgeons favor repeated aspirations of the abscess, whereas others feel that total excision is the treatment of choice. In general, definitive therapy involves total excision, although careful consideration of both options should be made for each case in consultation with the neurosurgical staff.

In addition to antibiotic therapy, the use of prophylactic anticonvulsants is warranted in most cases due to the high incidence of seizures. Either diphenylhydantoin (300 mg per day after an initial loading dose of 1 g in divided doses) or carbamazepine (200 mg twice a day increasing in 200-mg increments every 2 days to 200 mg four times per day) are suitable anticonvulsants. Doses should be adjusted to maintain therapeutic blood levels. (Diphenylhydantoin, 10 to 20 μg per deciliter; carbamazepine, 8 to 12 μg per deciliter). Osmotic agents may be required to control increased intracranial pressure. Steroids should be avoided whenever possible as they may inhibit antibiotic penetration into the abscess cavity.

Medical therapy alone is generally not advisable in the treatment of brain abscess. It should be considered only in cases of small abscesses (less than 2.5 cm diameter) with poorly developed or absent capsules.

THROMBOPHLEBITIS OF THE INTRACRANIAL VEINS AND SINUSES

Etiology and Pathogenesis

The etiology of dural sinus or cerebral vein infections varies according to the sinus or vein involved. Infective thrombosis most commonly involves the lateral, cavernous, and petrous sinsues. The superior sagittal sinus (SSS) and straight sinus are more commonly the site of noninfective thrombotic processes.

Lateral Sinus Etiology

The lateral sinus includes the transverse and sigmoid sinuses and terminates at the level of the jugular bulb. In many individuals one of the paired lateral sinuses, typically the right, is dominant. The lateral sinus lies in close relation to the middle ear and mastoid bone. Infection that spreads to the sinus commonly begins as mastoiditis or otitis media. A more unusual cause of lateral sinus infection is retrograde spread, via the jugular vein, of infections in the neck or pharynx (e.g., pharyngitis, adenitis, cellulitis, boils).

Clinical Features

Patients with suppurative lateral sinus thrombosis have fever and chills. Septicemia occurs in about 50 percent of cases. Septic emboli to the lungs, joints, or skin can occur. Local signs include retroauricular pain and pain on tilting or rotation of the neck. A firm cord (the jugular vein) may be felt along the anterior border of the sternocleidomastoid muscle. Involvement of the emissary veins results in swelling, erythema, and venous enlargement behind the ear, over the inion, and in the upper neck. If infection involves the dominant sinus signs of increased intracranial pressure including headache, nausea and vomiting occur. Papilloedema is present in 50 percent of cases. The presence of papilloedema or other signs of increased intracranial pressure should suggest the possibility that the contralateral sinus is hypoplastic or that infection has spread to the torcular or superior sagittal sinus. Unilateral papilloedema is usually indicative of spread of infection to the ipsilateral cavernous sinus.

Cranial nerve involvement commonly occurs. Involvement of the Vth and VIth nerves (Gradenigo's syndrome) results from petrous apicitis or disease in the inferior petrosal sinus. Sixth cranial nerve involvement can also result from increased intracranial pressure. The clinical findings in Gradeningo's syndrome include facial pain and hypesthesia and diplopia due to lateral rectus muscle palsy. Spread of infection to the jugular bulb can result in paralysis of the IXth, Xth, and XIth cranial nerves (Vernet's syndrome). Symptoms include hoarseness and dysphagia. There is usually a diminished gag reflex, poor palatal movement on one side, and decreased sensation in the peritonsillar area. Weakness of the ipsilateral sternocleidomastoid muscle and trapezius can occur. Ipsilateral tongue weakness may result from involvement of the XIIth nerve in the hypoglossal canal.

Focal CNS symptoms are uncommon with lateral sinus infection and usually indicate dissemination of infection. Involvement of the inferior anastomotic vein of Labbé can result in contralateral hemiparesis, aphasia, visual field abnormalities, and focal or generalized seizures.

Cavernous Sinus Etiology

Infection of the cavernous sinus (CS) generally occurs via one of three routes. Localized infections in the orbit, paranasal sinuses, or upper half of the face can spread to the CS from the ophthalmic veins. Infections near the teeth, tonsils, or jaw can produce sphenoid sinus infection with subsequent spread to the CS. Finally, ear infections or lateral sinus infections can spread to the CS by way of the petrosal sinuses. Although most cases of CS infection begin unilaterally, they quickly become bilateral because of the interconnection of the two CSs through the circular sinus.

Clinical Features

The onset of CS infection is abrupt, and most patients are acutely ill with high fever. Local signs and symptoms include eye pain, photophobia, proptosis, corneal clouding, orbital swelling and edema, and chemosis of the eyelid and conjunctiva. Cyanosis of the upper face, including the eyelids and the root of the nose, may be seen.

Cranial nerve palsies are invariably found and produce progressive external ophthalmoplegia. The VIth cranial nerve is usually involved initially, with subsequent involvement of the IIIrd and IVth nerves. The first division, and less commonly the second division, of the Vth (trigeminal) nerve can be involved producing facial pain, paresthesias or hypesthesia, and a diminished corneal reflex. Papilloedema results from impaired venous return. Disease of the optic nerve may result in decreased visual acuity and the appearance of scotomas. The pupils may be increased or decreased in size and are commonly sluggish or unreactive.

Superior Sagittal Sinus Etiology

As indicated earlier, septic thrombosis of the superior sagittal sinus (SSS) is far less common than noninfectious thrombosis. Infection of the SSS may result from nasal infections or infections of the paranasal sinuses. Infection may also spread directly through a contaminated compound skull fracture, or from a subdural empyema, epidural abscess, or meningitis. Metastatic infection from a distant primary site and retrograde spread of infection from tributary dural venous sinuses are often causes of SSS infection.

Clinical Features

Patients generally present with headache, fever, and signs of increased intracranial pressure. Edema of the forehead and scalp may result from involvement of emissary veins.

Focal CNS symptoms include paresis of one or both legs, cortical sensory loss, and unilateral seizures. Focal motor seizures or Jacksonian seizures are particularly common. When hemiparesis is present, the face is often relatively spared, and the weakness is more pronounced in the legs than in the arms. Many of the focal CNS signs and symptoms reflect thrombosis of cortical veins with subsequent hemorrhagic cortical infarction rather than SSS involvement per se.

Diagnosis of Intracranial Thrombophlebitis

The diagnosis usually depends on a high index of clinical suspicion. The CT scan is often helpful in excluding other causes of intracranial suppuration (e.g., brain abscess). The finding on CT scan of single or multiple hemorrhagic cortical infarctions, especially in the parasagittal area, may suggest cortical vein thrombosis. In some cases a high density serpiginous cord—representing a thrombosed cortical vein—can be seen on nonenhanced scans. This sign is virtually pathognomonic of cerebral vein thrombosis. With SSS occlusion, there may be contrast enhancement of the outer margin of the sinus and a hypodense center (''empty delta'' sign).

The most informative test is cerebral angiography. The venous sinuses and cortical veins are well visualized in the late or delayed phases of a cerebral angiogram. Signs of venous sinus occlusion include absent filling, filling defects, dilation or tortuousity of veins, slow venous filling, and reversal of the direction of venous flow. The major venous sinuses are extremely well visualized by digital subtraction angiograhy. In centers where this test is available, it often replaces conventional angiography as the diagnostic procedure of choice.

Lumbar puncture should only be performed if there are no signs of increased intracranial pressure. The spinal fluid usually shows a mild to moderate lymphocytic pleocytosis and a normal or slightly elevated protein. The presence of xanthochromia or frank hemorrhage is indicative of cortical vein thrombosis. The glucose is normal and cultures are sterile unless there is an associated meningitis. Manometric studies are not reliable. The Queckenstedt and Toby-Ayer tests of spinal fluid manometrics are only rarely performed but may be valuable in specific situations.

Therapy

Appropriate therapy consists of antibiotics and, in many cases, neurosurgical intervention. Empiric antibiotic therapy is directed toward adequate coverage of aerobic and anaerobic streptococci, *S. aureus*, and *S. pneumoniae*, and assorted anaerobes. Gram-negative organisms may be important in certain situations, especially with otogenic infections. Fungal infection (mucormycosis) is a special problem in diabetics. Empiric therapy should consist of nafcillin or oxacillin, 2 g intravenously every 4 hours, plus chloramphenicol, 1.5 g intravenously every 6 hours. Nafcillin and oxacillin are therapeutically equivalent.

Surgery should be performed if there is evidence of localized infection (e.g., osteomyelitis, mastoiditis, sinusitis). The roles of thrombectomy or of ligation of infected sinuses or of the jugular vein have not been established, and these procedures should not be routinely performed. The use of anticoagulants is also controversial. These agents should not be used if there is evidence of cortical vein thrombosis or hemorrhagic infarction. Anticoagulants may be of value for patients who develop progressive sinus thrombosis or episodes of septic embolization. Intracranial hypertension may require the use of osmotic agents or ventricular shunting procedures. Anticonvulsants are not used prophylactically, but are required in patients who develop focal or generalized seizures, especially in the setting of cortical vein thrombosis.

INTRACEREBRAL MYCOTIC ANEURYSMS

Etiology and Pathogenesis

Mycotic aneurysms are a rare complication of bacterial endocarditis and occur in less than 5 percent of cases. They constitute about 5 percent of all intracranial aneurysms. In acute bacterial endocarditis (e.g., due to *S. aureus*), mycotic aneurysms tend to develop early in the course of infection, whereas in subacute endocarditis (e.g., due to viridans streptococci), they characteristically appear late. Dissemination of infection to a site of arterial damage may produce a mycotic aneurysm even when bacterial endocarditis is not present.

The pathogenesis of these aneurysms remains unclear. In most cases, septic embolization to the vasa vasorum appears to be the inciting factor. In other cases septic intraluminal arterial emboli appear to produce an endarteritis that subsequently spreads outward through the vessel wall. Spread of infection from contiguous areas to adjacent arteries may be a third mechanism of pathogenesis.

Mycotic aneurysms are solitary in 80 percent of cases and multiple in 20 percent. They tend to involve vessels near their branching points. The distal portion of the middle cerebral artery is probably the most commonly involved site.

Clinical Features

In many cases, mycotic aneurysms, like congenital berry aneurysms, appear to be asymptomatic unless they leak or rupture. Some patients develop severe, unremitting, localized headache. When this symptom develops in a patient with known bacterial endocarditis, aneurysm should be strongly suspected. Many patients will have evidence of cerebral embolization in the period immediately preceding the development of a mycotic aneurysm. Patients with endocarditis who develop focal CNS findings should have a CT scan, followed in most cases by a lumbar puncture. An aseptic CSF pattern (lymphocytic pleocytosis, normal or elevated protein levels, normal glucose level) is usually indicative of embolism, brain abscess, or mycotic aneurysm. The first two possibilities can usually be excluded on the basis of the history and the results of the CT scan. A hemorrhagic spinal fluid (more than 200 red blood cells per cubic millimeter in all tubes after a nontraumatic LP) should always suggest mycotic aneurysm.

Diagnostic Studies

Patients who develop severe and persistent focal headache in the setting of endocarditis should undergo cerebral angiography. Patients with endocarditis and hemorrhagic spinal fluid or evidence of intracerebral hemorrhage by CT should also undergo angiography. Angiography remains the definitive diagnostic test for identification of mycotic aneurysms. However, small aneurysms may be missed. Improved techniques for digital subtraction angiography will make this test increasingly valuable in the future. Due to the incidence of multiple aneurysms (about 20%), injection of both carotid arteries is advisable. Mycotic aneurysms of the posterior circulation are rare. A vertebral injection is probably not routinely required and should be used only when indicated by the clinical situation or when visualization of the carotid circulation does not reveal an aneurysm. Subtraction and magnification views are essential. Patients with an intracerebral hematoma who have a negative angiogram during the acute stage should have the test repeated after the mass effect of the hematoma has resolved. The small size of aneurysms makes CT of limited value in direct diagnosis. The CT scan may be helpful in excluding other diagnoses (e.g., abscess, infarct) or in indirectly suggesting mycotic aneurysm by demonstrating intracerebral or subarachnoid blood.

The mortality of patients with endocarditis and a ruptured mycotic aneurysm exceeds 80 percent. The goal must be to identify patients with unruptured aneurysms and treat them aggressively. Controversy exists about the appropriate role of antibiotic therapy alone in the treatment of mycotic aneurysms. Antibiotic therapy alone results in resolution of almost 50 percent of recognized peripheral mycotic aneurysms. The mortality rate in patients treated with medical therapy is about 15 percent, although mild to moderate neurologic deficits are seen in 25 to 50 percent of survivors. Patients treated medically should have follow-up angiography on a weekly or biweekly basis. If there is an increase in aneurysm size, any evidence of bleeding, or no decrease in aneurysm size over 4 to 6 weeks, then surgery should be performed. The choice of antibiotics depends on isolation of the etiologic agent from the bloodstream or other sites (e.g., embolic material). Regimens for staphylococci and streptococci are listed below.

Streptococcal Endocarditis and Mycotic Aneurysm

Aqueous penicillin G, 2 million units intravenously every 2 hours, plus streptomycin, 0.5 g intramuscularly every 12 hours. These doses should be modified once organism sensitivities are available. Toxicity may require alteration of the streptomycin dose or dosing interval. Therapy should be continued for a minimum of 4 to 6 weeks. If the aneurysm is decreasing in size but has not resolved, therapy should be continued and a decision about surgical therapy made.

Staphylococcal Endocarditis and Mycotic Aneurysm

Nafcillin or oxacillin, 2 g intravenously every 4 hours (for penicillin allergic patients: vancomycin, 500 mg intravenously every 6 hours). Nafcillin and oxacillin are therapeutically equivalent. Duration of therapy is as noted above.

LOCALIZED INFECTIONS OF THE SPINAL CORD

Localized infections of the spinal cord can be classified according to their anatomic location as epidural, subdural, or intraspinal. Epidural abscesses are considerably more frequent than are either subdural or intraspinal infections. Localized infections of the spinal cord are medical and neurosurgical emergencies that require rapid institution of appropriate therapy. Therapeutic delay often results in tragic sequelae for the patient, including permanent paraplegia or quadriplegia and even death.

Pathogenesis

The possible routes of initiation of localized infections of the spinal cord include *(1)* direct extension from contiguous infection (e.g., vertebral osteomyelitis, perinephric or retroperitoneal abscess); *(2)* hematogenous spread from a distant site of infection; *(3)* introduction of infected material (e.g., following knife or gunshot injury, lumbar puncture, operation. In rare cases (''primary''), none of the factors noted above can be identified. Metastatic infection probably accounts for 50 percent of cases of epidural and intraspinal abscess and an even higher percentage of cases of spinal subdural empyema. The primary infection can be in the skin (furunculosis, carbuncles, cellulitis), the lungs (pneumonia, empyema, bronchiectasis), the heart (endocarditis), the genitourinary system (prostatic abscess, purulent cystitis), or the oropharynx (retropharyngeal or tonsillary abscess, dental abscess). Septic abortion may be a site of primary infection in pregnant women.

Clinical Features

Distinction between epidural and subdural infections can rarely be made clinically. These infections appear to occur with increased frequency in immunosuppressed patients, diabetics, and intravenous drug abusers. The initial symptom is usually severe, localized pain, typically in the back. In cases of epidural empyema, pain is increased by percussion or local pressure. Patients with subdural empyema or intraspinal abscess frequently do not have percussion tenderness. With both epi- or subdural infection, patients typically hold the spine rigid and try to avoid any undue motion. At this stage, patients are usually acutely ill. Fever is almost invariably present, and there may be chills or rigors. Headache and meningeal signs are also commonly present. Most patients have radicular pains involving the chest or, less commonly, the arms or legs. Symptoms are followed quickly (in 24 to 48 hours) by signs of an acute transverse spinal cord lesion. Patients develop flaccid paraplegia (or quadriplegia), loss of reflexes, a sensory level, and sphincter disturbances. Babinski's sign is present bilaterally. Flaccidity may subsequently evolve into spasticity with hyperactive reflexes once the period of ''spinal shock'' is over.

Some patients, especially those whose infection is caused by fungi or mycobacteria (see below), follow a slower (''chronic'') course, which can mimic other extradural compressive lesions such as tumors.

Most cases of intraspinal abscesses present with a clinical picture similar to that of epidural or subdural lesions. Constitutional symptoms such as fever, malaise, rigors are followed by back pain with or without meningeal symptoms. Within hours to days, there is paraplegia (flaccid, arreflexic), anesthesia with a sensory level, and disorder of bowel and bladder function. Specific signs pointing to an intramedullary lesion (e.g., dissociated sensory loss, sacral sparing) are frequently obscured by the rapid progression of the illness.

Pathology

A complete discussion of pathology is beyond the scope of this chapter. Most epidural and subdural infections are located posterior (dorsal) to the spinal cord. Infections are more common in the thoracic region, although cervical, and less commonly, lumbar, sacral, or cauda equina lesions occur. In most cases of epidural abscess, the infection extends for several (e.g., three to six) cord segments. Subdural empyema may be present at multiple levels. Intraspinal abscesses are typically located centrally in the cord or in the region of the posterior horns. They are most common in the cervical region and may extend into the brainstem. Abscesses are usually single, but multiple abscesses are not rare. The abscess size is quite variable, from microscopic to the entire length of the cord. Most lesions extend for at least five segments. These abscesses rarely encapsulate.

Infecting Agents

The commonest cause of acute localized spinal infections are bacteria. Cases of chronic epidural abscess are frequently due to mycobacteria, actinomyces, and fungi (blastomycosis, cryptococcosis, aspergillosis, nocardiosis) and, occasionally, result from other agents (e.g., *Echinococcus*). Of the bacterial agents, *S. aureus* is clearly the most frequently encountered and is responsible for one-half to two-thirds of all cases of localized spinal infection. *Staphylococcus* should be particularly suspected in patients with a history of antecedent trauma or skin infection. Streptococci and pneumococci may be encountered in patients with primary pulmonary infections. In intravenous drug abusers and patients with antecedent genitourinary infections, gram-negative organisms

(*Escherichia coli, Pseudomonas Aeruginosa, Serratia marcescens, Enterobacter cloacae, Proteus* species) are commonly found.

Laboratory Tests

Patients with acute localized spinal infections will almost invariably have a leukocytosis and an elevated erythrocyte sedimentation rate. Radiographs of the spine are often normal, but may show evidence of localized osteomyelitis with bony destruction and disk-space narrowing. Blood cultures are positive in up to 50 percent of cases. Myelography remains the definitive diagnostic procedure and should be performed immediately in all systemically ill patients who develop severe back pain, radicular symptoms, or signs of spinal cord compression. Ideally, metrizamide myelography should be combined with CT scan of the spine for the best delineation of the lesion. Cervical puncture should be performed for introduction of dye to diminish the risk of entering the abscess if it is located in the lumbar area. In almost all cases of epidural infection or subdural infection, myelography will demonstrate either a complete (80%) or partial (20%) block to the flow of dye. An attempt should be made to define the upper and lower extent of the lesion. CT scan, even without the addition of dye into the subarachnoid space, will often demonstrate an epidural abscess. Patients with intraspinal abscess will commonly have swelling of the spinal cord seen by myelography or CT. In some cases the swelling is severe enough to result in either partial or complete CSF block.

Lumbar puncture is best deferred until the time of myelography. The CSF in patients with acute epidural or subdural infection usually has a polymorphonuclear pleocytosis (50 to 500 cells), an elevated level of protein, and a normal level of glucose. In patients with epidural abscess, the CSF culture is positive in approximately 20 percent. If the CSF pleocytosis is excessive and the glucose is depressed, a concomitant spinal meningitis is usually present. Patients with chronic infections may only have an elevated CSF protein. In cases of suspected epidural abscess, the LP needle should be advanced slowly and aspirated frequently. If frank pus is withdrawn, the procedure should be terminated to avoid introducing infection into the subdural or subarachnoid space.

Therapy

Once a localized spinal infection has been diagnosed and localized, a bilateral exploratory laminectomy should be performed immediately. In cases of intraspinal abscess puncture or incision of the cord and aspiration to evacuate pus should be done. In patients with epidural infection, care should be taken to avoid opening the spinal dura. Aspiration of pus should probably be followed by local antibiotic irrigation (e.g.,bacitracin, 50,000 units per 50 milliliters of normal saline). Drains should be placed between the epidural space and the skin surface. Material obtained at operation should be sent for aerobic and anaerobic bacterial culture and for fungal and mycobacterial culture in all chronic cases. Pathologic material should be examined microscopically for bacteria, mycobacteria, fungi, and for the presence of granulomas. Gram stain, Ziehl-Neelson stain, and other appropriate stains should be performed immediately on some of the available material.

Definitive antibiotic therapy should be based on cultures obtained at operation. Initial antibiotic therapy should be instituted as soon as the diagnosis is suspected. Because of the high frequency of *S. aureus* infections, a semisynthetic penicillin in high doses should be used, e.g., nafcillin sodium, 2 g every 4 hours, intravenously, or (therapeutically equivalent) oxacillin sodium, 2 g every 4 hours, intravenously (alternate therapy if patient is penicillin-allergic: vancomycin hydrochloride, 500 mg every 6 hours intravenously).

In drug addicts or patients with preexisting genitourinary disease, an aminoglycoside should be added, e.g., tobramycin sulfate or gentamicin sulfate, 1.5 mg per kilogram every 8 hours intravenously (4.5 mg per kilogram per day). Serum levels should be monitored. Subsequent doses adjustments should be made on the basis of drug levels. Dose reduction is invariably required in patients with renal insufficiency. Infection caused by tuberculosis should be treated with triple therapy (isoniazid, ethambutol, rifampin, or streptomycin). Amphotericin B or miconazole with or without fluorouracil should be used for fungal infections.

VIRAL ENCEPHALITIS

MARTIN S. HIRSCH, M.D.
DAVID D. HO, M.D.

This chapter was supported by the Mashud A. Mezerhane B. Fund.

Encephalitis, defined as inflammation of the brain, is not a rare disease. Approximately 1,400 to 4,300 cases are reported annually in the United States to the Centers for Disease Control, although the actual numbers are certainly much higher. Patients with encephalitis frequently also have meningeal inflammation, perhaps making meningoencephalitis a more appropriate term.

Meningoencephalitis has diverse causes. Despite the wide variety of agents that can cause encephalitis in the United States, 50 to 75 percent of all cases remain etiologically undefined. Although viruses cause the majority of the remainder, nonviral diseases can also present with an encephalitic picture (Table 1). Since the morbidity and mortality of certain forms of encephalitis are high (5% to 10% overall fatality rates, but 70% to 80% with herpes simplex and eastern equine encephalitis), early recognition is important. Because antiviral agents can reduce the mortality from herpes simplex encephalitis, accurate diagnosis and prompt therapy have become imperative. A systematic diagnostic approach is necessary when patients present with altered mental status, fever, and headache. Analysis of cerebrospinal fluid and attempts to evaluate focal abnormalities by physical examination, electroencephalography (EEG), computed tomography (CT), or technetium brain scans are indicated. If focal abnormalities are found, brain biopsy is required to confirm the diagnosis.

This chapter will concentrate on acute meningoencephalitides caused by herpes simplex virus and arboviruses and will present guidelines for the diagnosis and management of patients with these disorders.

HERPES SIMPLEX VIRUS, TYPE I (HSV-I)

Herpes simplex virus accounts for 10 percent of all reported cases of encephalitis, and estimates of its frequency in the United States range from several hundred to several thousand cases a year. Individuals of all ages are susceptible, though neonates are usually infected by HSV-II and others by HSV-I. Beyond the newborn period, herpes simplex encephalitis may result from either primary infection (30%) or reactivation (70%). HSV-I has a predilection for involvement of the temporal lobe, possibly related to retrograde spread by olfactory or trigeminal pathways.

Previously healthy individuals of both sexes are most often affected. Presentation may be abrupt or insidious, following a nonspecific prodrome. Fever, headache, nuchal rigidity, and obtundation are the common presenting features. Personality change occurs in 85 percent of patients, dysphasia in 76 percent, seizures in 67 percent, autonomic dysfunction in 60 percent, and ataxia in 40 percent. Focal findings (hemiparesis, cranial nerve deficits, localized seizures) are present in 85 percent of patients.

TABLE 1 Important Nonviral Causes of Encephalitis

Mycobacterium tuberculosis
Mycoplasma pneumoniae
Rickettsia rickettsii
Lyme disease
Leptospira interrogans
Treponema pallidum
Coccidiodes immitis
Naegleria species
Toxoplasma gondii, Cryptococcus neoformans, Listeria monocytogenes in immunosuppressed patients
Atypical presentation of bacterial meningitis, brain abscess, parameningeal infection, infective endocarditis*
Collagen vascular disease

* In addition, it is important to recognize that many conditions may mimic encephalitis. These include metabolic and toxic encephalopathies, carcinomas, lymphomas, and cerebrovascular accidents.

Cerebrospinal fluid (CSF) formulas can range from normal (3%) to markedly abnormal, with neutrophils early and lymphocytes later in illness. Erythrocytes may be present, protein levels are usually elevated, and glucose levels are usually normal. Cultures of CSF for HSV are negative in more than 95 percent of patients.

Among neurodiagnostic tests, the EEG is the most sensitive early in herpes encephalitis. The characteristic pattern is one of periodic temporal spike and slow waves and is found in the majority of cases. Focal findings on technetium scan (enhanced localized radionuclide uptake) or CT scan (edema, mass effect, low-density lesion with contrast enhancement, hemorrhage) are seen in approximately 50 percent of patients. None of these neurodiagnostic findings, however, is specific for herpes encephalitis.

Brain biopsy is the only reliable way to confirm the diagnosis. The yield from an open biopsy is extremely high and morbidity is low (2%). If one relies on clinical impressions alone, the diagnosis of herpes encephalitis is incorrect approximately 50 percent of the time. Biopsy can not only confirm this impression, it can also provide alternative, treatable diagnoses. Proper ways to process biopsy specimens are discussed below (Clinical Guidelines).

Randomized, double-blinded, placebo-controlled, multicenter studies have demonstrated efficacy for vidarabine (adenine arabinoside) in reducing mortality from herpes simplex encephalitis. Age and state of consciousness at onset are important variables influencing outcome. More recent controlled trials in the United States and in Sweden showed that intravenous acyclovir was more effective than vidarabine in improving survival. Thus, at present, acyclovir (30 mg per kilogram per day in three divided doses) is the treatment of choice for herpes encephalitis. Individuals who are younger than 30 years of age fare better than those who are older, and patients who are merely lethargic respond to treatment better than those who are comatose.

ARBOVIRUSES

Although no longer an official taxonomic term, arbovirus refers to a group of more than 250 enveloped RNA viruses transmitted by arthropods. Nearly all cases of arbovirus encephalitis in the United States are due to St. Louis encephalitis (SLE), eastern equine encephalitis (EEE), western equine encephalitis (WEE), and California encephalitis (CE). Together these arboviruses account for about 10 percent of all cases of reported encephalitis, but this figure can be as high as 50 percent during an epidemic year.

St. Louis encephalitis is the commonest arboviral disease in the United States. The largest epidemic of SLE occurred in 1975, with nearly 2,000 cases reported from the East Coast to Arizona; the case fatality rate was 10 percent. In urban areas of the Midwest, SLE virus is transmitted by *Culex* mosquitoes, which breed in stagnant sewage water. In the West, the disease occurs primarily in irrigated rural areas, whereas in Florida, the mosquito vector and disease are prevalent in both urban and rural areas. Asymptomatic or mild infections are common, particularly in children. Severe disease is more likely to involve the aged. In addition to typical encephalitic findings, dysuria, pyuria, and inappropriate ADH secretion may occur. There are no unique CSF or EEG findings. As with all of the arboviruses causing encephalitis in the United States, viral isolation from CSF or blood is uncommon, although the agent can be isolated from affected brain tissue by inoculation of appropriate cell cultures or suckling mice. Serology, however, is the mainstay of arboviral diagnosis, and a variety of techniques are used to assay for both serum and CSF antibodies. No effective antiviral treatment is yet available for SLE or any of the other arbovirus encephalitides.

Eastern equine encephalitis occurs sporadically near freshwater marshes of the Atlantic and Gulf coasts. Although cases are generally limited in number, mortality rates often exceed 50 percent. Birds are the main reservoir, and the virus is transmitted by a mosquito that does not ordinarily bite humans. Disease in neither horse nor man plays a role in the subsequent spread of virus. Disease is most frequent in those younger than 10 or older than 55 years. Often, EEE has an abrupt onset and a fulminant course, with progressive loss of consciousness and seizures. Cranial nerve abnormalities and periorbital edema are occasionally seen. The CSF often contains fewer than 1,000 leukocytes per cubic millimeter, with a preponderance of neutrophils. Survivors are often left with significant neurologic sequelae, including mental retardation, seizure disorders, or emotional lability.

Western equine encephalitis occurs sporadically in irrigated rural areas in the western two-thirds of the United States. As in EEE and SLE, birds are the major reservoir for infection. Highest attack rates are in infants younger than 1 year or those older than 55 years. Mild and inapparent infections are frequent, and case fatality rates are low (2% to 3%). However, children under 2 years may develop mental retardation, seizures, or spasticity after recovery.

California encephalitis has a wide geographic distribution, but is particularly common in the upper Mississippi Valley. Among 10 subtypes of CE virus, the LaCrosse strain is the most prevalent and virulent. The vector is a forest-dwelling mosquito, and the reservoirs are small rodents such as squirrels; this explains the predilection of the vector for woodland campers. Disease occurs primarily among children in the 5- to 9-year-old age group, with adults usually having mild or asymptomatic infections. Fatalities are rare, but persisting personality problems or recurrent seizures are seen in up to 15 percent of affected children.

OTHER VIRUSES

Central nervous system manifestations can complicate many other viral infections. Varicella encephalitis can present as acute cerebellar ataxia with nystagmus and dysarthria. This syndrome is associated with an excellent prognosis. However, varicella encephalitis can also begin with seizures and focal neurologic deficits, with a mortality rate as high as 35 percent. Herpes zoster encephalitis is rare and largely seen in elderly immunosuppressed patients; it is usually self-limited and has a low mortality.

Encephalitis due to Epstein-Barr virus can be diffuse or localized to the temporal lobe or cerebellum. When seen in the setting of heterophile antibody–positive infectious mononucleosis, the diagnosis can be readily made. However, encephalitis may be the only manifestation of EBV infection, requiring determination of specific antibodies to viral capsid or early antigens.

Cytomegaloviral encephalitis is exceedingly uncommon in previously healthy individuals, but may occur in the setting of immunodeficiency. Disorientation, obtundation, paresthesias, and psychotic behavior occur. A syndrome of subacute encephalitis once thought to be secondary to CMV has been observed in patients with acquired immunodeficiency syndrome (AIDS). This disorder is characterized by apathy, depression, and progressive dementia. Recent studies suggest that the encephalopathy of AIDS is actually a consequence of brain infection by human T lymphotropic virus type III (HTLV-III).

Enteroviral encephalitis occurs primarily in children during summer months. Although enteroviruses cause 30 to 50 percent of all cases of viral meningitis, they account for only 2 percent of encephalitis cases. Outcomes are generally benign, except in newborns where fulminant encephalitis may occur, and in children with agammaglobulinemia, who sometimes develop chronic encephalitis.

Rabies virus encephalitis following animal bites is discussed elsewhere in this text. Lymphocytic choriomeningitis is a rare cause of encephalitis and is suggested by very high CSF lymphocyte counts and/or high protein values in the setting of recent exposure to rodents such as mice or hamsters.

Parainfectious encephalitides may follow viral infections or vaccinations and are thought to result from immunopathologic mechanisms. Most cases of measles encephalitis are thought to be parainfectious. Varicella, mumps, rubella, or influenza virus infections, as well as ill-defined upper respiratory infections, may be followed in 4 to 14 days by encephalitis clinically indistinguishable from that caused by direct viral involvement. Permanent neurological sequelae are infrequent except in the setting of measles.

CLINICAL GUIDELINES

Alteration in brain function distinguishes viral meningoencephalitis from viral aseptic meningitis (see Table 2). Once this differentiation is made, the physician must consider epidemiologic features for clues concerning season, geography, prodromal illness, and insect or animal exposure. A summer case of encephalitis occurring near freshwater marshes of Massachusetts results in a different list of diagnostic possibilities than a winter case in

TABLE 2 Management of Viral Encephalitis

Is encephalitis present?	Check for brain dysfunction
Are there epidemiologic clues?	Review information such as season, geography, animal or insect exposure, prodromal illness
Are there cerebrospinal fluid or serum abnormalities?	Check CSF cell and differential counts, protein, glucose, and obtain cultures or antigen tests for bacteria, fungi, mycobacteria Obtain CSF and peripheral viral cultures and appropriate studies on serum (heterophil and viral antibodies)
Are there focal neurologic abnormalities?	Review physical examination and consider EEG, CT scan, technetium scan
Should the site of focal abnormality be biopsied?	Culture biopsy material for viruses and examine by histology and immunofluorescence
Should treatment be started?	Begin acyclovir (10 mg/kg q8h) IV Continue for 10 days if brain biopsy herpes cultures are positive; discontinue on day 5 if herpes studies are negative

Nebraska. In addition, nonviral, often treatable illnesses that may mimic viral encephalitis must always be considered (Table 1). Searching for such clues may occasionally lead to a laboratory test, such as a mono spot test or heterophile antibody determination, that provides the diagnosis.

Clinical features alone cannot usually establish an etiologic diagnosis. However, hints of temporal lobe involvement (focal seizures, speech difficulties, olfactory hallucinations) should suggest the diagnosis of herpes simplex encephalitis. The temporal sequence of the disease may also be helfpul. Encephalitis following a viral exanthem by 1 to 2 weeks is more likely to be parainfectious, whereas a rapid progressive clinical course without prodrome suggests herpes or eastern equine encephalitis.

Examination of CSF is important and can usually be performed following early lumbar puncture. If there is concern about elevated intracranial pressure and possible herniation, a cisternal puncture can be performed. If the CSF shows a neutrophilic response, bacterial processes are likely, although early viral infections of the central nervous system can demonstrate a similar picture. A normal CSF formula suggests a toxic or metabolic encephalopathy, but does not rule out an early viral encephalitis. If the clinical suspicion is high, a repeat lumbar puncture may be necessary. A lymphocytic pleocytosis in the CSF is most frequently found in viral encephalitis, although fungal and mycobacterial processes must be excluded. Appropriate cultures, stains, and antigen testing must be performed on individual specimens. Attempts should be made to determine whether the process is generalized or localized in the central nervous system. Electroencephalography, CT scanning, and radionuclide scanning can all provide useful information. Anatomic definition is also helpful in directing the approach of neurosurgeons in subsequent brain biopsies. The need for a biopsy should be evaluated for each case. However, if a frontotemporal lesion is defined, we favor open biopsy of the involved area.

The brain biopsy specimen should be immediately cultured for virus and processed for histopathology. Immunofluorescence for herpesvirus antigens can provide confirmatory data, often within hours of biopsy. However, culture of the biopsy material remains the sine qua non for diagnosis. In herpes encephalitis, viral cultures are often positive within 24 to 48 hours, and the great majority are positive by day 5. Compared with viral isolation, histopathologic changes, e.g., intranuclear inclusions, lack sensitivity (56%), but are reasonably specific (86%). Immunofluorescence is quite sensitive (70%) and specific (91%). Electron microscopy for herpesvirus particles is insensitive (45%), but highly specific (98%).

Serology may be useful in making a retrospective diagnosis of herpes encephalitis. Measurement of specific HSV-I antibodies in CSF and comparison of serum to CSF antibody levels are not sufficiently sensitive (50%) during the first 10 days of illness to influence management decisions. Measurement of early antibody to arboviruses may be more useful. If the physician's index of suspicion for arboviral encephalitis is high, several state and federal laboratories can detect small amounts of serum or CSF antibodies to these viruses early in the course of disease.

Because the level of consciousness is a critical prognostic factor in the outcome of herpes encephalitis, therapeutic decisions must be made prior to definitive diagnosis, which follows biopsy. Therapy with acyclovir, 30 mg per kilogram per day infused intravenously in three divided doses, should be instituted immediately after biopsy. If cultures of herpes virus are positive, treatment is continued for 10 days. If all assays are negative by the fifth day, acyclovir should be discontinued.

Treatment for other forms of viral encephalitis remains supportive. Attention must be directed toward reducing cerebral edema, if present, by agents such as dexamethasone or mannitol. Seizures are managed with intravenous anticonvulsive agents. Respiratory support may be required, and care is needed to prevent or treat secondary bacterial infections.

Approaches to diagnosis and treatment of viral meningoencephalitis are still in their infancy. Nevertehlss, important advances have been made over the past decade. With the development of sensitive antigen- and nucleic acid–detection techniques, as well as advances in antiviral therapy, even more significant strides should occur in the relatively near future.

URINARY TRACT INFECTIONS AND SEXUALLY TRANSMITTED DISEASES

BACTERIURIA AND PYELONEPHRITIS

DENIS A. EVANS, M.D.

The evaluation and treatment of a patient with urinary tract infection depends on the type and anatomic location of the infectious process, the setting in which it occurs, the particular pathogen involved, and the severity of the associated symptoms. For convenience of discussion, urinary tract infections can reasonably be considered according to the presumed anatomic location, with this usually being judged from the patient's symptoms only. For example, bacteriuria associated with fever, flank pain, nausea, and severe constitutional symptoms will be presumed to represent kidney infection and called pyelonephritis, whereas bacteriuria accompanied by frequency and dysuria but without fever or severe constitutional symptoms will be thought of as cystitis. It must be emphasized that these distinctions are based more on a theoretical construct than on empiric verification of the anatomic involvement. The wide category of asymptomatic bacteriuria that is not easily classified under this anatomic system also must be carefully considered.

DIAGNOSIS OF BACTERIURIA

Because it is difficult to obtain urine specimens completely free from bacteria from the skin and genitals—especially in women—and because most bacteriologic techniques are designed to maximize the recovery of any organisms which may be present in a specimen, the separation of urine specimens containing bacteria from the urinary tract from those specimens contaminated during voiding was difficult until the use of semiquantitative cultural techniques became widespread. Such techniques rely on the observation that urinary tract infections are usually accompanied by high numbers of bacteria in the urine, typically, 10^7 or 10^8 per milliliter, whereas contaminating bacteria are present in much lower numbers, usually 10^3 or fewer. With good collection techniques, relatively few specimens should contain 10^4 or 10^5 organisms. Bacteriuria may be defined as the presence of sufficient bacteria in the urine so that one is reasonably certain that they represent bacteria from the urinary tract and not merely contaminants. In usual clinical practice, a criterion of greater than or equal to 10^5 organisms per milliliter is usually used. Recent studies have suggested that a lower criterion of 10^4 or even 10^2 gram-negative bacilli per milliliter may be appropriate in young symptomatic women especially if pyuria is present (see chapter *Acute Dysuria in Women and Initial Management of Urethritis in Men*). Although they are often difficult to obtain, especially when treating symptomatic patients, repeat urine specimens prior to therapy will often greatly clarify the meaning of intermediate numbers of organisms or atypical organisms. A second specimen that contains no organisms or organisms of a different species suggests that the first specimen was contaminated. The repeated isolation of the same organism as in the original specimen, even if in a lesser quantity than typical, is more suggestive of infection.

Bacteriuria may be caused by any of a large number of different organisms. Most organisms will be enteric gram-negative bacilli. For infections occurring in the community, *Escherichia coli* is by far the commonest pathogen, usually accounting for three-quarters or more of the urinary tract infections seen. *Proteus mirabilis* and *Klebsiella* are also frequently seen in community-acquired infections, but other species of gram-negative rods are uncommon. Coagulase-negative staphylococci and enterococci can also cause urinary tract infection. Isolation of these gram-positive cocci can lead to difficulties in interpretation since they are also very frequent contaminants of voided urine specimens. Repeat urine cultures are especially useful in distinguishing contamination from bacteriuria for these organisms.

The spectrum of organisms accounting for urinary tract infections seen in hospitals is usually quite different from that seen in the community. This spectrum of pathogens will vary from institution to institution, reflecting the organisms that are responsible for hospital-acquired infections in each one. Organisms such as *Enterobacter*, *Serratia*, indole-positive *Proteus*, and *Pseudomonas aeruginosa*, which are very uncommon causes of infection in the community, are seen much more frequently in hospitals. In general, the organisms seen in hospitals will exhibit much more resistance to antimicrobial agents than those seen in the community.

ASYMPTOMATIC BACTERIURIA

In our current state of knowledge, the best treatment of asymptomatic bacteriuria (defined as two consecutive cultures with more than 10^5 CFU of a single species per milliliter) varies according to the setting in which it is found. Bacteriuria is very common in the general population of adult women. About 3 percent to 5 percent of women will be bacteriuric at any given time. The proportion with bacteriuria increases strongly with increasing age. Most of these women have few or no symptoms attributable to the condition. Bacteriuria is distinctly uncommon among adult men until the age of about 70 years. Bacteriuria is found in about 1 percent of newborns. Newborn boys appear to have higher risk of bacteriuria than do newborn girls. Bacteriuria is found in about 1 percent to 2 percent of school-aged girls and is very uncommon among school-aged boys.

Treatment of asymptomatic bacteriuria is advisable in several situations. Among pregnant women, bacteriuria has been demonstrated to predispose to symptomatic pyelonephritis during the pregnancy or soon after delivery, and treatment has been shown to be of benefit. The possible link of bacteriuria to low birth weight also argues for treatment in pregnancy. The screening of all pregnant women at the first prenatal visit and the treatment of those found to be positive, even if asymptomatic, is strongly recommended. Those women found to be bacteriuric and treated should be checked for recurrence of bacteriuria for the remainder of the pregnancy, and any recurrence should be treated.

Boys with bacteriuria appear to be at substantial risk of underlying anatomic abnormalities of the urinary tract, so radiographic evaluation, including intravenous pyelograms and voiding cystourethrograms, is to be undertaken as is cystoscopy. Careful follow-up and treatment of recurrent infection is appropriate, especially among those found to have anatomic abnormalities. For girls, vigorous evaluation, including intravenous pyelography and voiding cystourethrography, is appropriate for those with bacteriuria apparent at an early age, i.e., in the neonatal or preschool period. Again, follow-up to detect recurrent infection and treatment of any infections detected is needed, especially for children found to have urologic abnormalities. There are insufficient data to permit a consensus regarding the extent of evaluation needed for bacteriuria among school-aged girls. Some argue that radiographic and urologic evaluation as outlined above for preschool girls is appropriate, and others restrict such evaluations to those with recurrent infections. Delaying evaluation of the urinary tract until it is demonstrated whether the infection will recur is to me the most reasonable approach, provided that the initial episode is treated and the follow-up necessary to detect and treat recurrent infection is undertaken.

Men with bacteriuria should be carefully evaluated. If the bacteriuria appears clearly related to a recent episode of urinary tract instrumentation—most commonly catheterization—treatment of the episode with a short course of an appropriate antimicrobial agent and follow-up for clearance of the infection and of all urinalysis abnormalities is appropriate. For those men who do not have a clear history of recent instrumentation in whom the infection recurs after treatment or for whom the follow-up urinalysis shows a residual abnormality such as persistent hematuria or pyuria, further evaluation, usually including intravenous pyelography, voiding cystourethrography, and cystoscopy is appropriate.

The largest group with asymptomatic bacteriuria, by far, is women. Some studies have raised the possibility of adverse effects, including increased mortality associated with bacteriuria, in this group. To date, however, this evidence is not sufficiently strong to warrant the large-scale screening and treatment effort that would be necessary to effectively deal with the condition in the general population. Since bacteriuria tends to recur frequently after apparently successful antimicrobial treatment, most of the effort involved in effective treatment would be for the detection and therapy of recurrences. For women with bacteriuria, on the basis of our current knowledge, treatment is best reserved for symptomatic episodes, with the exception that, in the setting of frequent recurrent symptomatic infections, the treatment of asymptomatic episodes of bacteriuria is often necessary because such asymptomatic episodes may quickly become symptomatic.

Bacteriuria is substantially more frequent among hospitalized men and women and among both men and women residents of long-term-care institutions such as nursing homes than it is in the general population. The acquisition of bacteriuria in hospitals, and probably in long-term-care institutions, is strongly related to urinary tract instrumentation, especially the use of indwelling urinary catheters.

Recent information suggests that among patients in general hospitals who have indwelling urinary catheters placed, those who acquire bacteriuria have substantially increased risk of death during the hospitalization compared with those who remain free of bacteriuria. The cause of the increased risk has not been demonstrated, but is thought to be undetected spread of infection. It has not yet been determined if treatment is effective in eradicating bacteriuria in this group is or if such treatment prevents mortality. Further, it is not clear whether similar risks apply to noncatheterized patients with bacteriuria in the hospital. Although definitive advice concerning therapy of bacteriuria among catheterized patients awaits studies addressing these issues, several suggestions may be offered now. (Catheter-related infections are discussed in more detail in the chapter, *Catheter-Associated Urinary Tract Infection.*) All reasonable steps should be taken to reduce the acquisition of bacteriuria by catheterized patients. The most important single step is to reduce the number and duration of indwelling urinary catheterizations to those essential for good medical care. Of particular importance is reducing the duration of catheterization by discontinuing catheters promptly when the need for them has passed. For those undergoing catheterization, the use of sterile, closed drainage systems and careful attention to avoiding breaks in the integrity of the system, such as disconnecting the catheter from the bag, are of great importance in reducing risk of infection. Sealed-junction catheters with a plastic band sealing the catheter to the drainage bag should be used whenever possible. Careful attention to cleansing of the periurethral area and aseptic technique should be emphasized at the time of catheter insertion. All medical care personnel should be trained to avoid inadvertent carriage of organisms from one patient to another, mainly through careful handwashing. Other steps to reduce infection have not been uniformly successful. Irrigation of the bladder with antiseptic solutions has not been shown to be useful in the general hospital setting, but is probably worth considering for those patients who will have the catheter disconnected periodically. Although movement of organisms along the interface between the catheter and urethral mucosa is probably a major route of acquiring bacteriuria, the use of antiseptic ointment at the urethral meatus has not been shown to be useful. The addition of antiseptic solutions to drainage bags may be useful in certain settings, particularly in units with numerous patients having long-term catheters and bacteriuria with resistant organisms, but drainage-bag antiseptics are probably of little use in the usual general hospital setting.

The proper management of those who have acquired bacteriuria despite these preventive measures is less clear. For most patients in general hospitals, the duration of catheterization is short (an average of about 3 days). For such patients who acquire bacteriuria and remain asymptomatic, the most prudent course seems to be to watch the patient carefully for a few days until the catheter is removed and then treat with a short (5 to 7 days) course of an antibiotic to clear the bacteriuria. Those patients who develop symptoms while being monitored should be promptly treated according to the severity of the signs and symptoms (see below). It is considerably more difficult to outline a satisfactory approach to treatment of infections among persons with long-term indwelling urinary catheters. At the present time, there is not sufficient evidence to support uniform and wide-spread use of antimicrobial agents among patients with urinary catheters in place for prolonged periods. These patients should be treated if there is any clear evidence of harm from the infection, including the presence of symptoms referable to the urinary tract or fever or leukocytosis without other obvious cause. In addition, treatment may be prudent for those with impaired renal function, if this treatment can be accomplished with the use of agents with low risk of nephrotoxicity. In general, courses of antibiotic therapy for catheterized persons with urinary tract infection should be very brief, usually a few days. Patients who continue to be catheterized will very likely reacquire bacteriuria and the cycle of careful observation and short-term treatment when indicated repeated over and over.

CYSTITIS AND THE URETHRAL SYNDROME

A variety of overlapping terms are used to refer to symptoms of burning and pain on urination, urgency, and frequency—usually not accompanied by constitutional symptoms. This group of symptoms is far commoner among women than among men. Because it is accompanied by bacteriuria, only about one-half or slightly more of the time, the terms *urethral syndrome* or *frequency-dysuria syndrome* are sometimes used to refer to the symptom complex regardless of etiology. Alternatively and confusingly, these terms are sometimes used to refer only to this complex of symptoms occurring in the absence of bacteriuria. When accompanied by bacteriuria, these symptoms are often referred to as cystitis, implying only bladder involvement in contrast to the more serious systemic symptoms associated with pyelonephritis. Therapy of dysuria in women is considered more fully in the chapter, *Acute Dysuria in Women and Initial Management of Urethritis in Men*.

One has considerable latitude in the choice of an antimicrobial agent for treatment of initial symptomatic urinary tract infection in a community setting. Many agents and schedules of therapy have been shown to produce bacteriologic clearance of infection within a short period. The strong tendency for infection to recur after apparently successful initial treatment is a major difficulty in the therapy of urinary tract infections, but no agent or schedule of therapy suitable for routine use for initial symptomatic infections has been convincingly shown to be superior to any other in lessening recurrences. An agent suitable for routine therapy of symptomatic infection should have several properties: it should be effective against the range of pathogens usually responsible for these infections; it should be effective after oral administration; there should be a low risk of adverse effects; and the cost of the agent should not be excessive.

Fortunately, a large number of commonly used antimicrobial agents satisfy these criteria, and there are not strong grounds for choosing among them. The commonest approach is to give the antimicrobial orally for 5 to 10 days. Over the past several years, a number of single-dose regimens for treating urinary tract infections in women have also been evaluated. In general, the results of single-dose therapy appear equivalent to those achieved with longer terms of treatment. From limited data, however, it appears that the single-dose schedules may be less effective in pregnant women, so it seems prudent to use 7 to 10 days of treatment for these patients.

A great many specific antimicrobial treatment regimens have proved useful in treatment of symptomatic urinary tract infections. Among them are ampicillin, 250 mg four times a day for 7 days; sulfisoxazole, 500 mg, four times a day for 7 days; or trimethoprim-sulfamethoxazole, 160 mg and 800 mg (one double-strength tablet), twice a day for 7 days. Useful single-dose regimens include amoxicillin, 2.0 g; trimethorpim-sulfamethoxazole, 160 and 800 mg; or sulfisoxazole, 1.0 g. There are not strong grounds for favoring one of these over another.

Plans of treatment must take into account the usual situation that the results of the urine culture will be unknown at the initial visit, but the patient will require symptomatic relief at this point. A reasonable procedure is to obtain a brief history and examination sufficient to rule out the presence of systemic signs and symptoms suggesting pyelonehritis or, on the other hand, symptoms such as vaginal discharge suggesting alternative sources of urethral symptoms. A urinalysis and urine culture should also be performed. If symptoms are quite bothersome, it is reasonable to prescribe either a 5- to 7-day course of treatment or a single-dose regimen. The patient can be asked to telephone in 24 to 48 hours to find the results of the urine culture. If the culture shows bacteriuria and a several-day regimen has been initiated, treatment is completed. It is probably prudent to reculture those women found to have bacteriuria 1 to 2 weeks after completion of therapy to detect the few individuals who will have a relapse of infection (see below) since such relapses may indicate a higher risk of anatomic abnormality within the urinary tract. If the initial culture is negative and the symptoms have abated, the course of antibiotic may be terminated, and further follow-up will depend on any symptomatic recurrences. If the initial culture is negative and symptoms perist, then further evaluation for other causes of the symptoms including pelvic examination and repeat urine culture is warranted (see chapter, *Acute Dysuria in Women and Initial Management of Urethritis in Men*).

FREQUENTLY RECURRING SYMPTOMATIC URINARY TRACT INFECTIONS

Frequently recurring symptomatic urinary tract infections can greatly interfere with patients' lives, while providing a difficult therapeutic challenge. Recurrences are usually divided into two groups: relapses—recurrences of infection with the same organism—suggesting a persistent focus of incompletely treated infection; and reinfections—recurrences of infection with a different organism—implying a new infection ascending via the urethra from the pool of colonic flora. Relapses tend to occur soon after the completion of therapy, are thought to indicate a stronger risk of an anatomic abnormality of the urinary tract, and are much less common than reinfections. A practical problem is that techniques usually available in the clinical microbiology laboratory are not adequate at times to detect differences in organisms causing recurrences, leading to some reinfections being misclassified as relapses.

The approach to treating recurring infections should emphasize obtaining adequate information, especially urine cultures, and an orderly approach to assessing several questions about each recurrence: *(1)* Is this recurrence of symptoms due in fact, to a urinary infection, or is it due to some other process? Practically, this question is usually answered by deterining whether or not bacteriuria is present. *(2)* Do the cultural data and timing suggest a relapse or a reinfection? *(3)* Is the infection responding promptly to treatment, that is, is a urine culture obtained soon after beginning therapy, negative? *(4)* How quickly is termination of treatment followed by recurrence of bacteriuria, that is, is a culture a few weeks after completion of a course of therapy negative? Answering these questions demands a considerable amount of effort, especially in obtaining cultures, but the answers are extremely useful in guiding therapy.

There is no clear consensus concerning the criteria for radiographic or urologic evaluation of adult women with recurrent urinary tract infections. The proportion of women found to have anatomic abnormalities of the urinary tract by such evaluations is small. Further, most of the abnormalities that are found are not suitable for surgical correction. An intravenous pyelogram and serum creatinine level seem appropriate for women with three or more documented recurrences of infection or for women with clear evidence of relapses rather than reinfections. If an initial radiographic evaluation for recurrent infections is normal, repeat of the study is rarely useful. Follow-up determinations of serum creatinine to assess renal functions are appropriate for those with frequently recurring infections. Intravenous pyelography and further urologic evaluation should also be undertaken for women in whom pyuria or hematuria persists after the bacteriologic resolution of infection.

A number of other tests have been used to attempt to identify women at higher risk of possible sequelae of recurrent urinary tract infection. Most of these procedures attempt to distinguish upper urinary tract infection or pyelonephritis from lower tract infection or cystitis. Available tests include bladder washout procedures, examination of the urine for the excretion of kidney-specific enzymes, and a number of tests for antibody to the infecting organisms in the urine or serum, the most recent of which is the test for antibody-coated bacteria in the urine. Unfortunately, none of these tests currently has a sufficiently secure interpretation to be reliably useful in the care of individual patients in clinical practice.

As long as symptomatic recurrences are relatively widely spaced—no more than one every 6 or 12 months—and the culture results suggest reinfection rather than relapses, repeated short courses (7 to 10 days) of antimicrobials probably represent the best management. If cultures suggest relapses with the same organism, therapy is usually given for a longer time, 6 to 12 weeks, in the hope of eradicating a focus of infection.

If symptomatic recurrences are closely spaced and significantly interfere with the quality of life, longer term therapy should be considered. Such therapy is usually given for a period of 6 to 9 weeks at first and then discontinued to see if symptomatic infection quickly recurs. If it does, therapy is given for a longer time—for approximately 3 months—again discontinued to see if infection recurs and if it does, given for periods of about 6 months at a time, discontinuing after each prolonged course of treatment to see if the patient will remain symptom free without antimicrobial treatment. The dose of antimicrobial used should be low, just sufficient to maintain a sterile urine. For many agents, about one-quarter of the usual daily dose for acute urinary tract infection administered once a day will suffice.

The suitability of antimicrobial agents for long-term therapy of recurring urinary tract infections may be assessed using the criteria noted previously for agents useful in short-course therapy of initial urinary infections: efficacy against the range of pathogens anticipated, suitability for oral administration, low risk of adverse reactions, and acceptable cost. Since resistant oragnisms are a greater problem in recurring urinary tract infections, the breadth of the antimicrobial spectrum of an agent is of more concern than for therapy of initial infections, and an attention should be given to an additional criterion, that of being unlikely to give rise to resistant organisms during prolonged therapy.

This final criterion is difficult to satisfy, but is reason to give special consideration to the group of antimicrobial agents usually designated as urinary tract antiseptics. These agents provide useful antimicrobial activity only in the urine, the major route of excretion. The concentrations present in the blood and extracellular space are below those needed to inhibit susceptible organisms. Although the subject has not been extensively investigated, it appears that urinary tract antiseptics are less likely to alter the colonic flora through the emergence of resistant organisms than are agents that achieve effective antibacterial activity in most body fluids. This consideration is important since most recurrences of urinary tract infections are reinfections with new organisms arising from the colonic pool of gram-negative flora. One might anticipate that long-term therapy with urinary tract antiseptics would be less likely to lead to reinfections with resistant organisms, but this issue has not been well studied.

Frequently used urinary tract antiseptics include nitrofurantoin, methenamine mandelate, methenamine hippurate, and nalidixic acid. Nitrofurantoin is effective against many of the frequently encountered pathogens causing urinary tract infections, although *Pseudomonas aeruginosa*, many isolates of *Enterobacter*, and many strains of *Proteus* are resistant. Although a dose of 100 mg four ties per day is commonly emloyed, excellent results can be obtained with 50 mg four times per day with less risk of gastrointestinal side effects. Emergence of resistant organisms during treatment has been infrequent. Adverse effects have been commoner than with some other agents. Gastrointestinal upset, which is dose related and which can usually be eliminated by reducing the dose of the drug and taking it with meals, has been the most frequent, but hypersensitivity reactions, peripheral neuropathy, and pulmonary reactions have been seen uncommonly. Therapy with nitrofurantoin should not be attempted in the presence of renal impairment since adverse effects appear to be increased (presumably reflecting increased serum concentrations of the drug) while urinary excretion of the agent is usually insufficient to clear the urinary tract infection. Methenamine mandelate and methenamine hippurate are each a combination of two unrelated agents, methenamine and an organic acid, in a single salt. Both drugs are active only under quite acidic conditions. Two methods of increasing the acidity of the urine are commonly tried: an acidifying agent such as ascorbic acid may be given, but the effect on urinary pH is usually very small. The usual initial dose of methenamine madelate and methenamine hippurate is 500 mg four times per day. The dose of the methenamine-organic acid salt may be increased, relying on the organic acid component of the salt to lower pH, but this approach may be limited by side effects including dysuria and gastric distress. It is often necessary to use a dose of 1 g four times a day. Much higher daily doses, up to 12 g per day, have been used by some clinicians, but dysuria and gastric distress occur frequently with these doses and experience with such high doses is extremely limited. Resistance to methenamine mandelate or methenamine hippurate appears to be uncommon but is difficult to measure; the usual laboratory methods cannot be used since the agents are effective only under acidic conditions. Nalidixic acid has a wide spectrum of antimicrobial activity, but the rapid development of resistance has been observed both in vitro and in vivo and limits the usefulness of the drug for treating recurrent urinary tract infections.

PYELONEPHRITIS

The usual basis for the diagnosis of pyelonephritis is the coincidence of laboratory evidence for urinary tract infection with abdominal signs or symptoms or severe constitutional symptoms. These signs and symptoms may include flank pain, nausea, vomiting, abdominal tenderness and such constitutional symptoms as fever and malaise, or, in severe cases, intense toxicity and prostration. As noted earlier, the correspondence between this complex of symptoms and actual anatomic localization of infection to the kidney is not certain. Nevertheless, both the severity of the associated symptoms and the possibility of renal involvement are reasonable grounds for treating this type of urinary tract infection with special care.

In deciding on the best treatment for a particular patient, it is necessary to take into account both the setting in which the infection occurs and the associated signs and symptoms. With regard to setting, the most relevant distinction is probably between infections occurring in a hospital or long-term-care facility and those arising in the community. Resistant gram-negative bacilli are much more likely to be the responsible pathogens among hospitalized patients or, on the basis of incomplete data, among patients in long-term-care settings. In assessing the patient with pyelonephritis, it is always prudent to consider the possibility of gram-negative rod bacteremia. Again, the hospital setting is relevant because such bacteremias are an important cause of mortality and morbidity among hospital patients and because one-half or more of the gram-negative bacteremias occurring in U.S. hospitals arise from urinary tract infection. The signs and symptoms associated with the infection provide important clues to the possibility of bacteremia and suggest the types of supportive care that will be most important while awaiting a response to antimicrobial agents. Chills, especially with rigors, prostration, confusion or somnolence, tachycardia, hypotension, and coolness or pallor of the extremities are among the signs suggesting the possibility of bacteremia. (A more complete discussion of the assessment and therapy of patients with gram-negative bacteremia may be found in the chapter *Gram-Negative Bacteremia*.)

Pyelonephritis occurring in the community can often be treated without admission to the hospital, especially if the associated constitutional symptoms are mild or moderate, the nausea and vomiting are not so prominent as to preclude the effective use of oral antimicrobials, and the patient is likely to understand and comply with the prescribed regimen. Hospitalization is usually advisable if these conditions cannot be met.

It is always advisable to obtain the necessary specimens for bacteriologic evaluation prior to beginning antibiotic therapy. A properly obtained urine specimen is necessary for both culture and urinalysis. If there are any signs and symptoms suggesting bacteremia, two or more blood cultures obtained from separate sites by venipuncture are advisable. Very often, one must choose an antibiotic and initiate treatment before the results of the culture and antibiotic susceptibility testing are available. In the temporary absence of such data, presumptive choice of an antimicrobial agent for treating pyelonephritis again depends on the setting in which the illness occurs and the signs and symptoms of infection. For patients who are hospitalized and for patients in whom there is a substantial possibility of bacteremia, it is advisable to take little chance of resistance to the presumptive regimen, since this would leave a potentially life-threatening infection untreated for a period of time, and one will accept some increased risk of adverse effects such as nephrotoxicity, if necessary, to assume adequate treament. A knowledge of the antimicrobial susceptibility patterns occurring in the individual hospital in which one practices is extremely useful in making this choice. In general, an aminoglycoside antibiotic such as gentamicin, amikacin, or tobramycin is a reasonable presumptive choice for seriously ill hospitalized patients pending the results of antibiotic susceptibility testing since enteric gram-negative bacilli are the usual pathogens in pyelonephritis, and resistance to these agents is uncommon among such organisms. If the susceptibility results of a particular hospital show that resistance to the antibiotic of interest is uncommon in that institution, third-generation cephem antibiotics such as cefoperazone, cefotaxime, moxalactam, ceftizoxime, ceftriaxone, or ceftazidime are also worth considering. Clinical experience with these agents is more limited, but the risk of nephrotoxicity or ototoxicity appears to be less than with aminoglycoside agents. It is entirely reasonable to change from the agent chosen presumptively to an agent with lower potential for toxicity or cost once antimicrobial susceptibility results are available that demonstrate susceptibility of the pathogen to the agent with lower risk of toxicity. For seriously ill patients, parenteral administration of the antibiotic is advisable until substantial improvement is clear. In addition, most agents suitable for presumptive therapy of serious gram-negative bacillary infection in the temporary absence of susceptibility test results are not effective after oral administration. After clear improvement has occurred and if bacteremia was not found, the course of antimicrobial therapy can be continued with an orally administered agent if such an agent can be identified with the results of susceptibility tests. There is insufficient information to provide definitive guidance regarding duration of therapy in pyelonephritis, but, for seriously ill patients, a total duration of approximately 2 weeks seems reasonable.

For less seriously ill patients with pyelonephritis, especially those who have community-acquired infection and do not have other major medical problems, a somewhat different approach can be taken. As with the seriously ill, hospitalized patient, obtaining adequate specimens for bacteriologic evaluation prior to initiating antibiotic therapy is extremely important, and it is usually necessary to choose initial antimicrobial therapy before the cultural and susceptibility data from these specimens are available. Since community-acquired infections are much less likely to be due to resistant organisms, however, and since the consequences of possibly ineffective therapy for 2 days while awaiting antimicrobial susceptibility results are less threatening, it is reasonable to initiate therapy with an agent having low risk of toxicity and the convenience of oral administration at the sacrifice of some increase in the possibility of resistance to this initial agent. Agents such as ampicillin, 500 mg four times a day, or trimethoprim-sulfamethoxazole, one double-strength tablet twice a day, are appropriate choices. Duration of therapy, again, is not a settled matter, but a 10-day to two-week course appears reasonable based on current knowledge.

ACUTE DYSURIA IN WOMEN AND URETHRITIS IN MEN

WALTER E. STAMM, M.D.

ACUTE DYSURIA IN WOMEN

Acute dysuria occurs commonly in adult women and usually reflects the presence of lower genitourinary tract infection: cystitis (generally due to *Escherichia coli* or *Staphylococcus saprophyticus*), vaginitis (due to *Candida albicans, Trichomonas vaginalis*, or bacterial vaginosis), or urethritis (due to *Chlamydia trachomatis, Neisseria gonorrhoeae* or herpes simplex virus). The relative proportion of cases due to each of these agents depends upon the age and sexual activity of a given patient population. Symptoms produced by these various infections overlap to such a degree that accurate diagnosis depends on the physical examination and simple laboratory tests. Of particular importance are the vaginal speculum examination, microscopic examination of vaginal secretions, and urinalysis. Recent studies clarifying the etiology of acute dysuria in women have demonstrated that, in acutely symptomatic women with *E. coli* infections and with pyuria, bacterial counts in midstream urine may often be in the range of 10^2 to 10^4 CFU/ml. Determination of a specific etiologic diagnosis is a necessity for optimal treatment.

Initially, women with dysuria should be evaluated to determine if their symptoms are attributable to vaginitis, urinary infection, or urethritis (Fig. 1). Women with vaginitis often characterize dysuria as external (that is, occurring as the urine contacts the inflamed labial tissue). Additional symptoms of vaginal discharge, pruritis, and vaginal odor suggest the presence of vaginitis, which can be readily confirmed by pelvic examination. Complaints of suprapubic pain, hematuria, and urgency are infrequent with vaginitis and should direct the evaluation to other etiologies.

The absence of symptoms and signs of vaginitis necessitates an assessment of the dysuric patient for urinary tract infection and urethritis. The presence of pyuria in a midstream urine specimen is a sensitive indicator of probable infection, but does not discriminate between the site or type of infection. Fever, flank pain, and costovertebral angle tenderness strongly suggest the presence of pyelonephritis. On the basis of clinical presentation alone, distinction between cystitis and urethritis can often be difficult. A history of previous urinary tract infections and complaints of either gross hematuria or suprapubic pain suggest cystitis. Infection with *N. gonorrhoeae* or *C. trachomatis* should be suspected in young, sexually active women who have had a recent change in sex partners or a history of previous sexually transmitted disease (Fig. 1).

The presence of one or more bacteria per oil immersion field on microscopic analysis of a gram-stained, uncentrifuged urine specimen correlates with more than 10^5 organisms per milliliter in a urine culture and is helpful in the diagnosis of urinary infection when positive. To confirm the result of Gram stain, or in the absence of this finding, quantitative culture of a midstream urine specimen remains the preferred means to evaluate patients for urinary infection. The presence of lower quantitative counts (10^2 to 10^4 per milliliter of urine) of coliforms (*E. coli, Klebsiella*, etc.) in cultures of urine from dysuric women—particularly if the patient has concomitant pyuria—usually indicates acute urinary infection with these organisms.

Women with dysuria and pyuria in whom urinary infection is not confirmed by Gram stain (or culture if Gram stain is negative) or women whose illness suggests the presence of chlamydial or gonococcal infection should have a pelvic examination (Fig. 1). Findings consistent with mucopurulent cervicitis should be carefully sought in these women, and cultures for *N. gonorrhoeae* and *C. trachomatis* should be performed. If chlamydial cultures are not available, the presence of a negative urine culture, pyuria, and a negative clinical and microbiologic evaluation for gonorrhea in a sexually active woman with suggests infection with *C. trachomatis*. Examination of the patient's sexual partner may be useful in establishing a diagnosis as well.

Treatment of dysuric women should be directed against the specific etiologic agent identified. Urinary infections due to coliforms and *S. saprophyticus* are treated effectively by several antimicrobial agents including trimethoprim-sulfamethoxazole (TMP/SMZ), sulfonamides, trimethoprim, amoxicillin, and nitrofurantoin. In a number of studies, single-dose therapy has been equal in efficacy to conventional 7- to 10-day courses of therapy for acute lower urinary tract infections. Because of the increased compliance, decreased adverse effects, and diminution in cost afforded by single-dose treatment, this mode of therapy is preferred for uncomplicated lower tract infections. Based on current data, single-dose TMP/SMZ (4 single-strength tablets given orally) appears to be the best treatment regimen. Alternative single-dose regimens include 3.0 g amoxicillin, 2 g of sulfamethoxzole, or 400 mg of trimethoprim. Patients with recurrent or persistent infection following single-dose therapy should receive 7 days of therapy as well as careful posttherapy evaluation to ensure eradication of infection.

Management of chlamydial, gonococcal, and other sexually transmitted infections should include evaluation and therapy of the sexual partner(s). For specific details regarding treatment of these infections the reader is referred to the appropriate chapters in this volume. Women with acute dysuria without pyuria should be treated with pyridium (one tablet four times daily) to relieve symptoms and asked to return for reevaluation if symptoms persist. In most instances, symptoms will resolve spontaneously, and no further therapy is necessary.

INITIAL MANAGEMENT OF URETHRITIS IN MEN

Urethritis is the most frequent sexually transmitted disease (STD) syndrome seen in men. Customarily, cli-

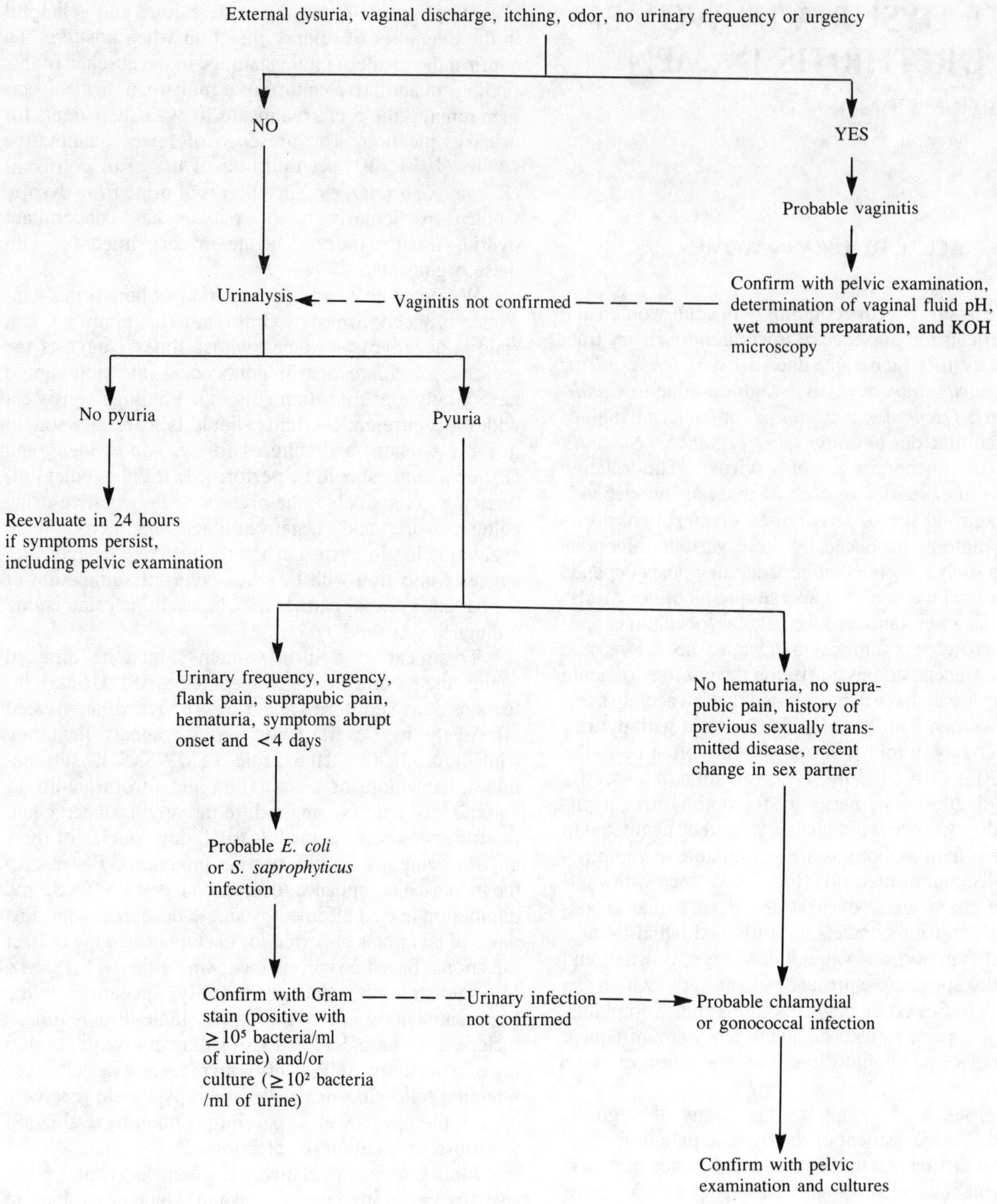

Figure 1 Evaluation of women with acute dysuria

nicians categorize urethritis into gonococcal and nongonococcal etiologies. The relative frequency of nongonococcal urethritis (NGU) and gonococcal urethritis in a given clinic depends upon the racial and socioeconomic characteristics of the population served. *C. trachomatis* causes approximately 40 percent of cases of NGU, and *Ureaplasma urealyticum* may cause an additional 10 to 20 percent of cases. The remaining cases probably result from sexually transmitted pathogens, but their precise etiology remains unclear. Occasionally, urethritis results from infection with *T. vaginalis* or herpes simplex virus. Most patients with urethritis due to genital herpes infection will have obvious herpetic penile lesions, and many with urethritis due to *T. vaginalis* will have sex partners with vaginitis.

The diagnostic approach to men with urethritis be-

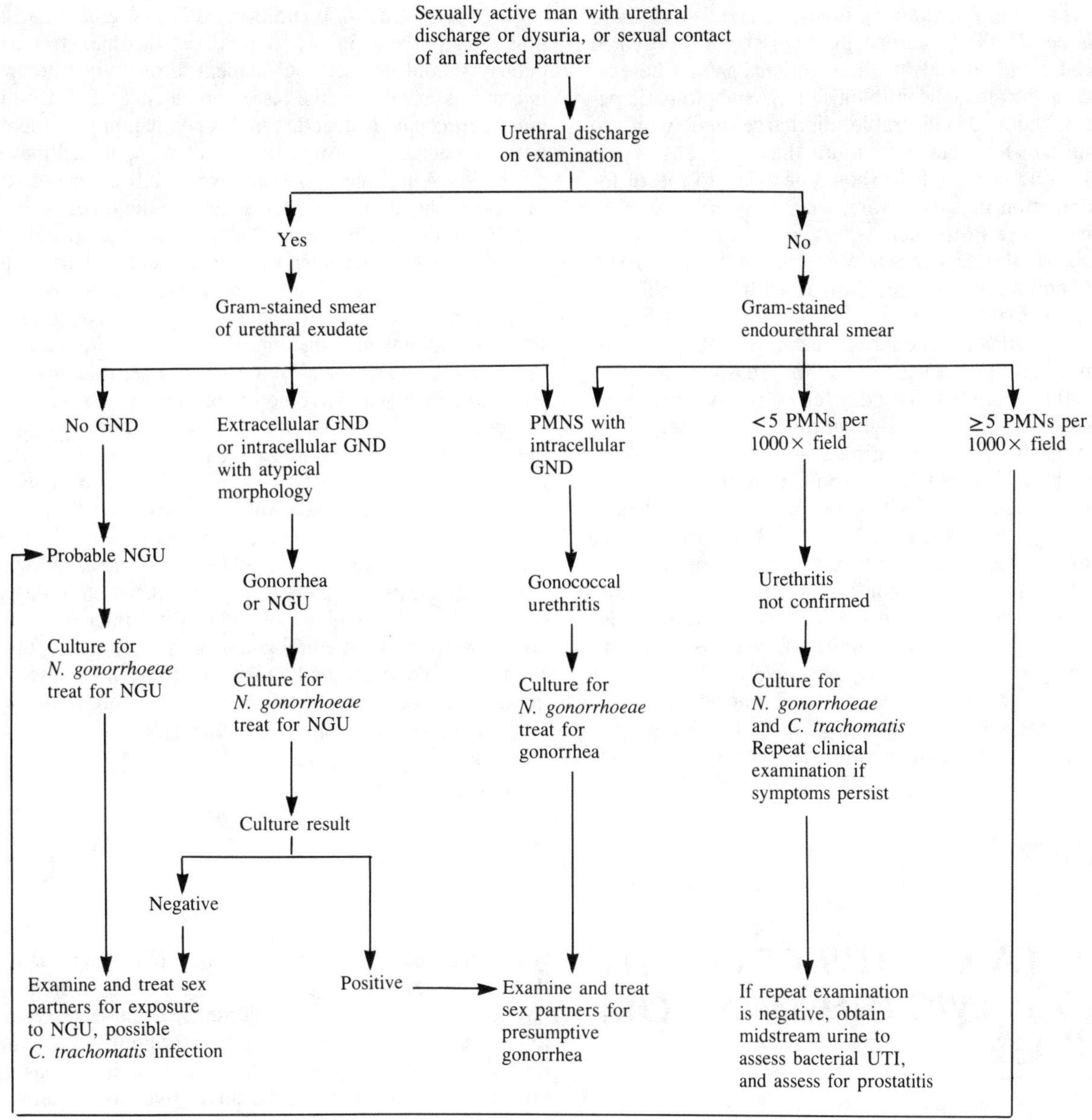

Figure 2 Management of a male with possible urethritis

gins by distinguishing those patients who have urethral discharge on examination from those who do not (Fig. 2). Patients with a demonstrable discharge should be treated for NGU or gonococcal urethritis based upon the results of Gram stain of urethral secretions. Either a positive Gram stain showing intracellular gram-negative diplococci (98% sensitive and specific as compared with culture) or a positive culture confirms the diagnosis of gonococcal urethritis. Men with a urethral discharge on examination—but negative smears and cultures for *N. gonorrhoeae*—have, by definition, NGU. The Gram stain in patients with NGU usually shows five or more polymorphonuclear leukocytes (PMNs) per 1,000× field. It is generally unnecessary to make a specific etiologic diagnosis (i.e., perform chlamydial or ureaplasmal cultures) in men with NGU.

Patients without a demonstrable urethral discharge upon examination but with urethral symptoms or a history of an infected partner should also have urethral Gram stains done. Patients whose smears show PMNs with intracellular gram-negative diplococci should be treated for gonorrhea. In patients whose smears are not diagnostic of gonococcal urethritis, the number of PMNs per 1,000× microscopic field should be determined. Patients with fewer than five PMNs per 1,000× microscopic field, no history of recent contact with a known infected partner, and no symptoms should be advised that their examination results are normal and that they should return for reexamination only if symptoms arise or persist. Patients with fewer than five PMNs per 1,000× microscopic field but with history of contact with an infected partner should be epidemiologically treated in an appropriate manner.

Patients having symptoms of urethritis and five or more PMNs per 1,000× microscopic field should be treated for NGU, and contacts of these patients should be examined and treated epidemiologically. Asymptomatic patients without demonstrable discharge and with no exposure history but with more than five PMNs per 1,000× microscopic field should be asked to return for reexamination in 7 days—or sooner if symptoms arise. If five or more PMNs per 1,000× microscopic field are still present, if discharge is now present, or if the *C. trachomatis* culture is positive, the patient and his contacts should be treated for NGU.

Men with NGU should be treated with tetracycline, 500 mg orally four times per day for 7 days, or doxycycline, 100 mg orally twice a day for 7 days. Alternatively, erythromycin, 500 mg orally four times per day for 7 days can be used. The latter regimen should also be used in men with NGU who fail to respond to tetracycline therapy. Heterosexual men with gonococcal urethritis should be treated with amoxicillin, 3.0 g plus 1.0 g probenecid, as a single oral dose, followed by tetracycline, 500 mg orally four times per day for 7 days to treat the concomitant chlamydial infection present in 25 percent of patients. Alternatively, 4.8 million units of aqueous procaine penicillin G (APPG) intramuscularly plus 1.0 g probenecid, or 250 mg of ceftriaxone intramuscularly followed by tetracycline, 500 mg orally four times per day for 7 days can be used. In homosexual men with gonococcal urethritis, 4.8 million units of APPG intramuscularly, plus 1.0 g probenecid or 250 mg of ceftriaxone intramuscularly should be used; subsequent tetracycline therapy is unnecessary due to the lesser prevalence of concomitant *C. trachomatis* infection in this population. In patients with suspected or proven infection with penicillinase-producing gonococci, spectinomycin, 2.0 g, or cefoxitin, 2.0 g, should be used instead of amoxicillin or APPG.

It should be emphasized that clinical features alone do not reliably distinguish between gonococcal and nongonococcal urethritis. For this reason, a microscopic examination of the urethral smear and appropriate cultures must be undertaken to distinguish the two disorders. Further, heterosexual men seen in high-risk settings, such as an STD clinic, who have no history or signs of urethral symptoms and no history of contact with an infected partner should also have a urethral Gram stain and cultures or antigen detection tests for *Chlamydia* and *N. gonorrhoeae*. Some of these men will have asymptomatic gonorrhea or NGU, as evidenced by persistent urethral leukocytosis and/or a positive *C. trachomatis* culture. Since homosexual men are at less risk than heterosexual men of developing NGU or chlamydial infection, and since asymptomatic urethral gonorrhea is rare in this population, routine screening by urethral smear or chlamydial culture is not necessary for asymptomatic homosexual men who have no known infected partners.

VULVOVAGINITIS, CERVICITIS, AND PELVIC INFLAMMATORY DISEASE

GARY E. GARBER, M.D.
ANTHONY W. CHOW, M.D.

GENERAL CONSIDERATIONS

Lower genitourinary symptoms are common complaints among adult women in primary care settings as well as in specialty clinics for sexually transmitted diseases. Among such women, vaginal symptoms are more than five times as common as urinary symptoms. Genital and urinary infections may often coexist, and their clinical distinction is not always clearcut. Furthermore, symptoms or signs of an abnormal vaginal discharge may be caused by a diverse variety of conditions or their combination (Table 1). Lack of uniformity in the clinical definition of these conditions, and of a consistent approach to laboratory confirmation also contributes to the diagnostic uncertainties and refractory response to therapy in many instances. Not surprisingly, considerable difficulty is also encountered clinically in differentiating true inflammatory conditions of the female genital tract from physiologic, functional, or psychosomatic causes of symptoms. For these reasons, a systematic approach to the diagnosis and management of urogenital infections is essential. Special emphasis should be given to the following considerations: (*1*) the history and physical examination should focus primarily on the epidemiology and anatomic localization of the likely sites of infection or inflammation; (*2*) specific etiologic diagnosis will require additional office or laboratory tests since the clinical diagnosis is imprecise and often misleading; (*3*) concomitant infection with multiple pathogens at different sites are common; (*4*) the presence of potentially serious but asymptomatic infection (e.g., cervicitis) should be excluded; (*5*) an important therapeutic goal should include prevention of upper genital tract infection and its sequelae in addition to eradication of lower genital symptoms and epidemiologic control of major sexually transmitted infections. A critical initial step in the evaluation of all lower genital symptoms, therefore, should be directed to detection and effective treatment of cervicitis or coexisting salpingitis.

An algorithm approach to the management of adult women with lower genital complaints is summarized in Figure 1.

TABLE 1 Conditions Associated with Vaginal Discharge

Infectious	*Noninfectious*
Vulvovaginitis Bacterial vaginosis Candidiasis Trichomoniasis	Excessive mucorrhea and physiologic discharge Atrophic vaginitis
Cervicitis Chlamydial infection Gonorrhea Genital herpes	Desquamative inflammatory vaginitis Foreign body, trauma, irradiation, hypersensitivity, or chemical irritation
Salpingitis	
Other sexually transmitted diseases	Endometriosis, neoplasms cysts, or polyps
Toxic shock syndrome	Others
Miscellaneous vulvovaginal pyogenic infections	

SYSTEMATIC APPROACH TO DIAGNOSIS

History

Historical features are relatively nonspecific, but are useful for defining the epidemiology and natural history of specific infections. Inflammation of the cervix and vagina often produce similar symptoms, such as external dysuria, introital dyspareunia, and increased amount or altered quality of vaginal discharge. Patients with cervicitis often complain of intermenstrual or postcoital spotting. Abdominal pain or systemic complaints are uncommon with vulvovaginitis or uncomplicated cervicitis and should prompt a diligent search for accompanying pelvic inflammatory disease. Presence of fever may suggest acute salpingitis or primary genital herpes. Fever and multisystem involvement beginning during a menstrual period should raise the possibility of toxic shock syndrome.

The color and amount of discharge as perceived by the patient has little value in differential diagnosis. Although trichomoniasis and candidiasis can cause marked vaginal irritation, their clinical presentation can vary greatly from individual to individual. Vaginal odor may be the only symptom in bacterial vaginosis, a condition often associated with little vaginal irritation. The complaint of vaginal discharge does not in itself indicate a pathologic process. Physiologic discharge (mucorrhea) may be heavy enough to stain underwear, but it is not usually associated with external dysuria, vulvar irritation, or odor. The amount of discharge may vary with the phase of the menstrual cycle, and may be increased by oral contraceptive use or pregnancy. Because the onset of physiologic discharge often coincides with the onset of sexual activity, women who feel anxious or guilty about their sexual activity may attach inordinate importance to small changes in normal vaginal discharge.

A complete and detailed sexual history is particularly important, since exposure to a new sexual partner increases the likelihood of sexually transmitted disease. The sexual history should include the number of recent new partners, patterns of sexual behavior, previous sexually transmitted diseases, and partner's sexual history. This line of questioning is often disconcerting for both the physician and patient. The patient is far more likely to freely discuss intimate sexual details if the impression projected is that of a routine but necessary and confidential procedure. This skill is acquired only with practice.

General Physical Examination

Particular attention should be directed to the skin, palms, soles, eyes, mouth, pharynx, anorectum, pubic hair, lymph nodes, and joints. Examination of the abdomen should include careful listening for diminished bowel sounds and evidence of peritoneal, suprapubic, or perihepatic inflammation. The pubic region should be inspected for lice and other pediculosis. The inguinal and femoral regions should be palpated for adenopathy. An anorectal examination by proctoscopy and digital palpation should be routinely performed.

The Pelvic Examination

The labia and the perineum should be examined for erythema, excoriation, and discrete lesions. Diffuse perineal erythema or edema may accompany trichomoniasis, candidiasis, or early toxic shock syndrome. Examination of extravaginal surfaces may reveal lesions of genital herpes, syphilis, chancroid, condylomata accuminata, molluscum contagiosum, or scabies. Vulvovaginal pyogenic infections such as abscesses involving Bartholin's and Skene's glands, infected labial inclusion cysts, furunculosis, and suppurative hidradenitis are readily apparent.

Next, the urethral meatus is examined and gently stripped with a finger placed inside the introitus. If urethral discharge is expressed, such material should be examined microscopically and cultured. A vaginal speculum, moistened with warm water and without lubricant, is then gently inserted. In the presence of severe genital herpes, or occasionally trichomoniasis, insertion of the speculum may be impossible due to intense discomfort. In such cases, a preliminary etiologic diagnosis is sometimes made from material recovered on a cotton swab gently inserted into the vagina.

After insertion of the speculum, the cervix is first examined, since cervicitis is a serious condition and is often asymptomatic. The cervix should be wiped clean and cotton-tipped swabs of endocervical secretions obtained through the cervical os. Mucoid material is normally observed at the cervical os and is present in increased amounts in women taking oral contraceptives. Normal cervical discharge is usually clear or white and is nonhomogeneous and viscous. Purulent or mucopurulent

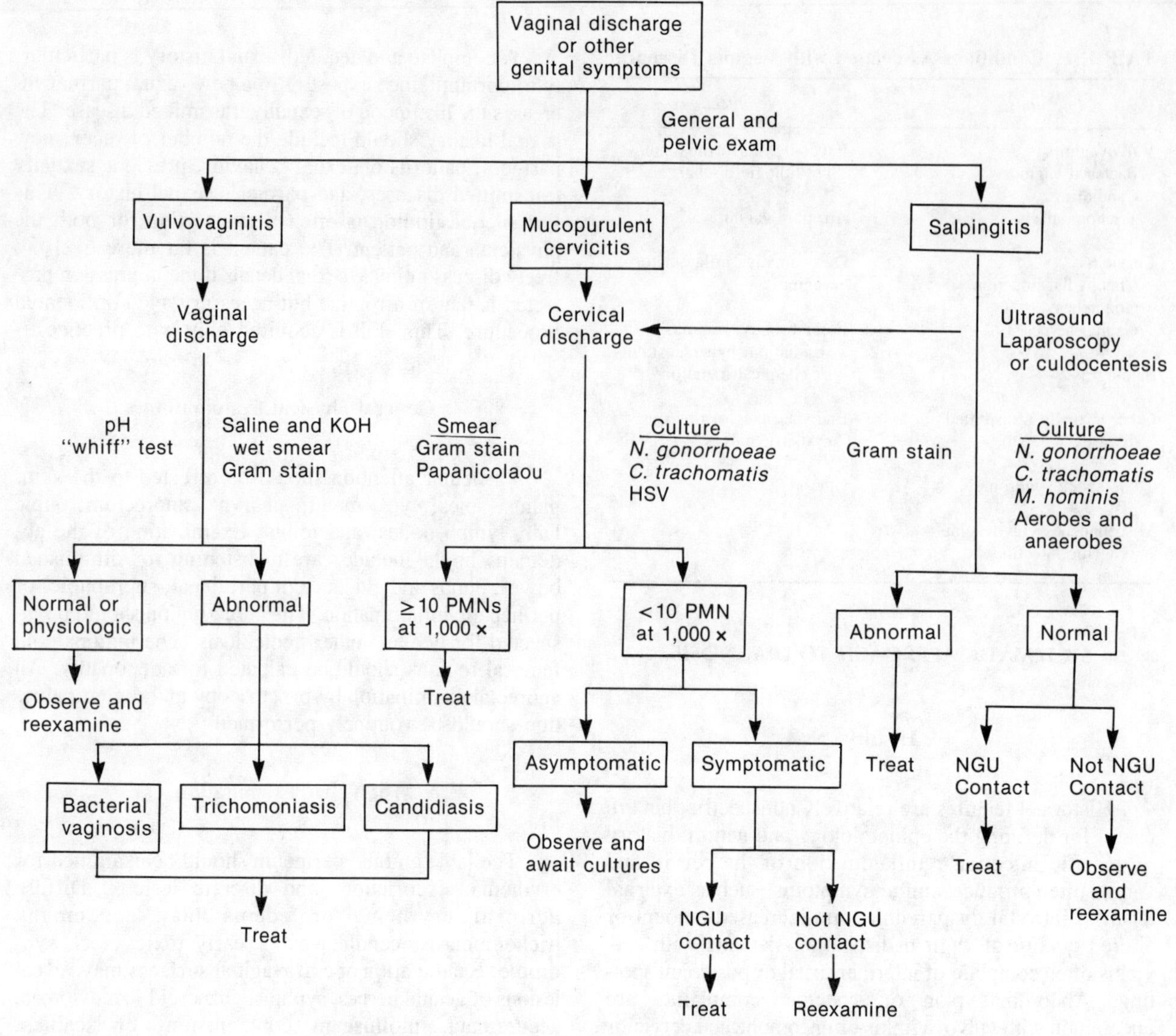

Figure 1 Approach to genital symptoms in premenopausal women.

cervical discharge is associated with infective cervicitis and is readily recognized by the appearance of yellow or green exudate on the white cotton-tipped swab. The cervix should also be observed for erosions, friability, or easy bleeding. Mucopurulent cervicitis is most commonly caused by *Chlamydia trachomatis, Neisseria gonorrhoeae*, or both, and must be differentiated from cervicitis caused by herpes simplex virus (HSV), from vaginitis, and from simple cervical ectopy without inflammation. Cervical ectopy represents the presence of columnar endocervical epithelium in an exposed portion of the ectocervix and appears redder than the surrounding stratified vaginal epithelium. Ectopy, when not associated with visible or microscopic endocervical mucopus or with colposcopic epithelial abnormalities, is a normal finding and requires no therapy. Its prevalence is increased at the onset of menarche, by oral contraceptive use, and by pregnancy, but gradually declines through later adolescence. Hypertrophic cervicitis manifests as intensely red, congested areas that appear to project from the surface of the cervix. It can be distinguished from ectopy in that it is usually asymmetrical and irregular around the cervical os, is rather friable and bleeds easily, and is usually accompanied by a mucopurulent cervical discharge. Presence of hypertrophic cervicitis is highly suggestive of chlamydial cervicitis, but it is an uncommon clinical finding. Cervical secretions should be collected for Gram stain and for culture (or other testing, depending on availability) of *N. gonorrhoeae, C. trachomatis*, and HSV. A Papanicolaou smear may identify trichomonads or cytologic findings characteristic of HSV infection.

After establishing the presence or absence of cervicitis, efforts should then be directed to establishing the presence or absence of vaginal infection. Not infrequently, cervicitis coexists with vaginal infection, particularly with bacterial vaginosis or trichomonal vaginitis. The amount, consistency, color, odor, and location of the discharge within the vagina should be noted. The character of vaginal discharge is relatively nonspecific. A yellow or green discharge is suggestive of trichomoniasis, but this occurs in less than one-fifth of infected women. Similarly, a frothy discharge is seen in only one-tenth of women with trichomoniasis, is nonspecific, and is equally suggestive of bacterial vaginosis. The amount of discharge in vulvovaginal candidiasis is highly variable, and one does not always see the classic curdy discharge. The vaginal wall should also be inspected for erythema, edema, and ulceration. Vaginal ulcers tend to occur in the right vaginal fornix, are chronic, and are associated with the use of tampons in some patients. A sample of discharge should be removed with a swab from the vaginal wall, avoiding contamination with cervical mucus. The vaginal pH should be determined directly by rolling the swab containing the specimen onto pH indicator paper. An additional specimen should be removed with a swab and mixed first with a drop of saline, then with a drop of 10 percent potassium hydroxide (KOH) on a microscope slide. The odor released after mixing the specimen with KOH is noted, and separate cover slips are placed on the saline and KOH wet mounts for microscopic examination to detect the presence and quantity of normal epithelial cells, clue cells, polymorphonuclear leukocytes (PMNs), motile trichomonads, or fungal elements.

Finally, the bimanual examination is performed to determine adnexal or cervical motion tenderness, and to exclude the presence of palpable adnexal or cul-de-sac masses. Adnexal tenderness is uncommon with local vaginal infections and suggest salpingitis; palpation of an abnormal adnexal or cul-de-sac mass may indicate tuboovarian abscess, ectopic pregnancy, or malignancy and requires prompt gynecologic or surgical consultation.

In most patients, the constellation of symptoms and signs together with the microscopic findings in vaginal secretions will allow a preliminary etiologic diagnosis of vulvovaginitis, and further studies are unnecessary (Table 2). However, it is prudent to request that the patient remain undressed in the examination room in case microscopic examination of the wet smear is unrevealing and further microbiologic studies are indicated. Patients generally do not mind waiting for 2 to 3 minutes for the results of the wet mount before the examination is continued. Depending on the clinical findings, these further studies may include culture for *Candida albicans* and *Trichomonas vaginalis* or Gram stain of vaginal fluid to differentiate between normal flora and the flora characteristic of bacterial vaginosis. In women with prominent vaginal complaints but no abnormal findings, each of these additional microbiologic tests may be indicated to differentiate vaginal infection from functional complaints and other causes of vaginal symptoms.

Routine Office and Laboratory Investigations

A number of bedside and office evaluations of clinical specimens are invaluable in the etiologic diagnosis of

TABLE 2 Diagnostic Features of Vaginitis in Premenopausal Adults

	Normal or Physiologic Discharge	*Bacterial Vaginosis*	*Candidal Vulvovaginitis*	*Trichomonal Vaginitis*
Etiology	Uninfected; *Lactobacillus* predominant	*G. vaginalis* and various anaerobic bacteria	*C. albicans* and other yeasts	*T. vaginalis*
Predominant symptoms	None	Malodorous discharge	Vulvar itching and/or irritation; increased discharge	Profuse discharge, often malodorous
Vulvitis	None	Rare	Usual	Occasional
Inflammation of vaginal epithelium	None	None	Erythema	Erythema; occasional petechiae
Discharge				
Amount	Variable, but usually scant	Moderate	Scant to moderate	Profuse
Color	Clear or white	White or grey	White	Yellow
Consistency	Nonhomogeneous, flocular	Homogeneous, low viscosity, uniformly coating vaginal walls; occasionally frothy	Clumped, adherent plaques	Homogeneous, low viscosity; often frothy
Usual vaginal pH	<4.5	≥ 4.5	<4.5	≥ 5.0
Amine odor with 10% KOH ("whiff test")	None	Positive	None	Often positive
Microscopy (saline or KOH wet smears, Gram stain)	Normal epithelial cells; lactobacilli predominate	Clue cells; few PMNs; lactobacilli outnumbered by profuse mixed flora nearly always including *G. vaginalis* plus anaerobes	PMNs, epithelial cells; yeast or pseudohyphae in up to 80%	PMNs, motile trichomonads in 80–90%

Note: Modified with permission from Holmes KK: Lower genital tract infections in women: cystitis/urethritis, vulvovaginitis, and cervicitis. In: *Sexually Transmitted Diseases*. Holmes KK, Mordh P-A, Sparling PF, Wiesner PJ (eds), New York: McGraw-Hill, 1984:583.

vulvovaginitis and cervicitis. These include vaginal pH, KOH "whiff" test, and microscopic examination of wet smears and Gram stains of vaginal and cervical specimens. Cervical and vaginal cultures should be obtained only for specific and selected pathogens, and should be interpreted with caution.

Vaginal pH. The pH of vaginal discharge can be estimated at the bedside by use of pH indicators such as nitrazine paper, when the pH is between 4.5 and 7.0. A vaginal pH of 4.5 or less is most consistent with physiologic discharge or with vulvovaginal candidiasis. Vaginal pH greater than 4.5 is seen in patients with trichomoniasis or bacterial vaginosis.

KOH Whiff Test. Vaginal secretions from patients with bacterial vaginosis, when added to several drops of 10% KOH on a microscope slide will elicit a pungent fishy, amine-like odor. A positive whiff test can be expected in more than 90 percent of women with bacterial vaginosis and an undefined proportion of patients with trichomoniasis, but is absent in women with vulvovaginal candidiasis or physiologic discharge.

Microscopic Examination of Vaginal Specimens. The wet mount of vaginal discharge is the single most useful technique in making an initial etiologic diagnosis of vulvovaginitis (Table 2). The following specific information is sought: (*1*) the nature of the vaginal epithelial cells and the presence of clue cells; (*2*) the presence and number of PMNs; (*3*) the presence of specific and readily identifiable pathogens such as motile trichomonads, budding yeasts, or pseudohyphae. Normal vaginal epithelial cells are flat and clean looking. The edges are sharply defined, and the nuclei, easily visible. Clue cells, which strongly suggest bacterial vaginosis, are squamous epithelial cells covered with coccobacilli, giving them a granular appearance with indistinct cell edges and nucleus. Presence of large numbers of PMNs may be either cervical or vaginal in origin. The number of PMNs is usually normal in bacterial vaginosis (i.e., one would not see an intense inflammatory response) and may be normal or increased in candidal vulvovaginitis or trichomoniasis. The presence of excessive PMNs should prompt further search for an inflammatory genital focus, but the absence of excessive PMNs does not rule out notable infection. The composition and normality of the bacterial vaginal flora is effectively assessed by Gram stain of vaginal fluid. Normal vaginal secretions contain predominantly gram-positive rods resembling lactobacilli, with or without gram-variable coccobacilli resembling *Gardnerella vaginalis*. In bacterial vaginosis, vaginal fluid contains few or no lactobacilli with a predominance of *G. vaginalis* plus other organisms resembling anaerobic gram-negative *Bacteroides* species gram-positive cocci, or curved rods.

Microscopic Examination of Cervical Specimens. The Gram stain of endocervical secretions examined at 1,000× is the most useful and practical tool for the etiologic diagnosis of symptomatic or asymptomatic cervicitis. Visualization of yellow, mucopurulent endocervical secretions on a white swab or presence of 10 or more PMNs per 1,000× field are positively correlated with cervical *C. trachomatis* infection. Neither *N. gonorrhoeae* nor HSV infection is significantly associated with endocervical PMN leukocyte concentration or presence of macroscopic mucopus. On the other hand, demonstration of intracellular gram-negative diplococci in the Gram stain of endocervical secretions has a sensitivity of 60 percent and specificity close to 100 percent for the diagnosis of gonococcal infection. This compares favorably to isolation of *N. gonorrhoeae* from a single endocervical culture, which has a sensitivity of 80 to 90 percent. Giemsa-stained smears of endocervical scrapings are of less value for the diagnosis of chlamydial cervicitis since chlamydial inclusions can be identified in only a minority of infected women. Multinucleated giant cells and Cowdry type A intranuclear inclusions suggest HSV cervicitis; but in the presence of extensive tissue necrosis, the cellular architecture is distorted, and the typical cytologic findings are seen in less than one-third of infected patients. Similarly, the typical cytologic findings of HSV infection in Papanicolaou smears are reliable indicators of disease only when observed, but the sensitivity of this technique has been questioned.

Cultures. Prevalence is sufficient to recommend that endocervical, urethral, and anorectal cultures be obtained routinely for confirmation of gonorrhea and for detection of beta-lactamase production by *N. gonorrhoeae* isolates. Although endocervical cultures for *C. trachomatis* and HSV are desirable, they are not readily available in many centers. Routine aerobic and anaerobic vaginal cultures are not recommended, and results should be interpreted with great caution since the vagina is normally colonized by a wide variety of microorganisms. As an example, isolation of *G. vaginalis* from the vagina, even in high concentration, is not specific for the diagnosis of bacterial vaginosis.

Special Diagnostic Procedures

Fluorescent antibody staining of cervical scraping will correctly identify *C. trachomatis* in two-thirds of infected women. Isolation of *C. trachomatis* requires cultural techniques that are extremely labor-intensive and may not be available. The presence of ectocervical lesions suggestive of HSV infection should warrant laboratory confirmation by viral isolation and differentiation of HSV-1 and HSV-2 serotypes by use of type-specific monoclonal antibodies. Cytologic and immunofluorescent antigen detection techniques for genital herpes are 50 percent and 70 percent, respectively, as sensitive as viral isolation. Cultures for *Ureaplasma urealyticum* and *Mycoplasma hominis* from cervical and urethral secretions may be helpful in instances of postpartum fever or recurrent pregnancy loss.

A variety of selective media are available for isolation of *T. vaginalis* from vaginal secretions, and culture is the most sensitive method for diagnosis of vaginal trichomoniasis. Vaginal cultures for yeast and *T. vaginalis* are particularly useful when symptoms or signs are suggestive of one or the other, but neither can be demonstrated by direct microscopy of wet smears. Gas-liquid chromatography of vaginal fluid from women with bacterial vaginosis may show a characteristic pattern of organic acid metabolites: the concentration of lactate, the major metabolite of lactobacilli, is reduced, while succinate, acetate, propionate, butyrate and other organic acids produced by the abnormal flora are increased. Toxin-producing *Staphylococcus aureus* may be isolated in high concentration from vaginal cultures of women with symptoms and signs suggestive of toxic shock syndrome (TSS). Toxic shock syndrome toxin-1, the major staphylococcal exotoxin implicated in TSS, can be detected in vaginal washings of some patients by solid-phase enzyme-linked immunosorbent assay during the acute illness; serum antitoxin antibodies in such patients are typically low in titer.

Colposcopy is increasingly used to evaluate women with abnormal cytologic smears consistent with cervical intraepithelial neoplasia. Colposcopy also has great potential utility in high-risk populations (e.g., in clinics treating sexually transmitted diseases), for screening of flat condylomata of the cervix or vagina and for cervicitis. Laparoscopy is invaluble for the visual diagnosis of salpingitis, and both laparoscopy and culdocentesis are helpful for microbiologic sampling and specific etiologic diagnosis of salpingitis and other pelvic conditions (Table 3). Ultrasonography is particularly useful for detection and localization of tuboovarian abscess.

MANAGEMENT OF SPECIFIC SYNDROMES

Vulvovaginitis

Vulvovaginitis may be the most frequent cause of genital symptoms in women. The cardinal manifestations are increased yellow or green discharge; vulvar itching, irritation or burning; external dysuria; introital dyspareunia; and malodor that is often increased following sexual intercourse. Treatment should be based on specific etiologic diagnosis that can usually be made at the time of initial clinical evaluation (Table 2). The commonest cause of all vaginal discharge is bacterial vaginosis, which is also known as nonspecific vaginitis, followed in frequency by vulvovaginal candidiasis and trichomoniasis. Multiple and concomitant vaginal infections are not infrequent, especially trichomoniasis coexisting with *G. vaginalis*-associated bacterial vaginosis. Cervicitis may also present as vaginal discharge and must first be ruled out. Other causes of abnormal vaginal discharge, such as atrophic vaginitis, desquamative inflammatory vaginitis, and vaginal fistula or ulcers, are rare. In a patient with persistent vaginitis for which a specific pathogen cannot be identified, examination of the sexual partner may often provide the answer.

TABLE 3 Differential Diagnosis of Pelvic Infection Based on Gross Characteristics of Culdocentesis Fluid

Bloody	*Cloudy*	*Purulent*
Ruptured ectopic pregnancy	Acute salpingitis	Ruptured tubo-ovarian abscess
Ruptured corpus luteum cyst	Pelvic peritonitis	Ruptured appendix
Uterine perforation	Twisted adnexal cyst	Ruptured diverticular abscess
Gastrointestinal bleeding	Peritonitis due to other causes	---
Ruptured spleen or liver	---	---
Retrograde menstruation	---	---

Note: Modified with permission from Chow AW: Female genital infections. In: *Infectious Diseases - Diagnosis and Management*. Yoshikawa TT, Chow AW, Guze LB (eds), New York: John Wiley and Sons, 1980:159.

Common pitfalls that lead to misdiagnosis and treatment failure in the management of vulvovaginitis include: (*1*) diagnosis based exclusively on macroscopic appearance of discharge, with failure to perform a wet smear; (*2*) "telephone" diagnosis and treatment; (*3*) broad-spectrum, "shotgun" remedies; (*4*) failure to use appropriate antimicrobial agents; and (*5*) failure to treat the sexual partner. Recommended therapeutic regimens for the most frequent causes of vulvovaginitis and cervicitis are summarized in Table 4. Adjunctive measures, such as warm tub baths to ease pain and reduce edema, careful attention to personal hygiene, and abstinence from sexual intercourse, are also important. Patients whose symptoms respond promptly to specific therapy should be seen about 1 week after completion of therapy for repeat clinical and microscopic evaluation. Women with physiologic discharge should be given a careful explanation of the conditiion. Persistence of worrisome symptoms in a woman in whom thorough and repeated evaluation has failed to reveal genital pathology may indicate psychosexual problems; such patients may well benefit from counselling provided by a trained therapist.

Bacterial Vaginosis or Nonspecific Vaginitis

Current evidence indicates that *G. vaginalis* (formerly known as *Hemophilus vaginalis* or *Corynebacterium vaginale*) in conjunction with high vaginal concentrations of anaerobic bacteria (particularly *Bacteroides* species, *Peptococcus* species, *Peptostreptococcus* species, and motile curved rods known as *Morbiluncus* species is the primary cause of this condition. It is characterized clinically by symptoms of slightly increased, malodorous, watery vaginal discharge, with little pain or itching. The malodor may increase postcoitally (possibly due to release of amines by semen, which is alkaline). Examination often reveals a nonviscous, homogeneous, grey-white, uniformly adherent vaginal discharge, without gross inflammation of the vaginal mucosa. Bacterial vaginosis should be suspected in the presence of three of four of the following findings: (*1*) characteristic vaginal discharge; (*2*) vaginal pH above 4.5; (*3*) positive whiff test; (*4*) presence of clue cells. Symptoms alone are not reliable for diagnosis since many patients are asymptomatic. The diagnosis is readily confirmed by the characteristic

TABLE 4 Recommended Regimens for Treatment of Vulvovaginitis, Cervicitis, and Acute Salpingitis

Infection	*Choice*	*Alternate*
Vulvovaginitis		
Bacterial vaginosis	Metronidazole (500 mg PO BID) for 7 days	Ampicillin (500 mg PO QID) for 7 days
Candidiasis	Miconazole or clotrimazole vaginal cream (100 mg HS) for 7 days	Nystatin vaginal cream (100,000 units BID) for 7–14 days *or* Boric acid capsules (600 mg intravaginally HS) for 14 days
Trichomoniasis (sexual partner treated)	Metronidazole or tinadazole (2 g PO) single dose	Clotrimazole vaginal cream (100 mg HS) for 7 days
(sexual partner not treated)	Metronidazole or tinadazole (250 mg PO TID) for 7–10 days	Clotrimazole vaginal cream (100 mg HS) for 7 days
Cervicitis		
Chlamydial or mucopurulent	Tetracycline (500 mg PO QID) for 7 days	Doxycycline or minocycline (100 mg PO BID) for 7 days *or* Erythromycin (500 mg PO QID) for 7 days
Gonococcal		
PPNG not suspected	Ampicillin (3.5 g PO), amoxicillin (3 g PO), or APPG (4.8 μ IM), each with probenecid (1 g PO) and followed by tetracycline (500 mg PO QID) for 7 days	Tetracycline (500 mg PO QID) for 5 days
PPNG suspected	Spectinomycin (2 g IM) or cefoxitin (2 g IM) plus probenecid (1 g PO), each followed by tetracycline (500 mg PO QID) for 7 days	Trimethoprim/sulfamethoxazole 80-mg/400-mg tablets (9 tablets PO OD) for 3 days
Genital Herpes		
Primary or first episode	Acyclovir (5 mg/kg IV q8h or 200 mg PO q4–6h) for 5–7 days	Acyclovir cream topically to external genital lesions, 6 times daily for 7–14 days
Recurrent episodes	Routine therapy in immunocompetent hosts not recommended	
Salpingitis		
Inpatient	Cefoxitin (2 g IV q6h) plus doxycycline (100 mg IV q12h) for 10–14 days	Metronidazole (500 mg IV q6h) plus doxycycline (100 mg IV q12h) for 10–14 days *or* Clindamycin (600 mg IV q6h) plus tobramycin (1.5 mg/kg IV q8h) for 10–14 days
Outpatient	Cefoxitin (2 g IM) plus probenecid (1 g PO), followed by doxycycline (100 mg PO BID) for 10–14 days	Ampicillin (3.5 g PO), amoxicillin (3 g PO) or APPG (4.8 μ IM), each with probenecid (1 g PO) and followed by doxycycline (100 mg PO BID) for 10–14 days *or* Trimethoprim/sulfamethoxazole 80-mg/400-mg tablets (2 tablets PO BID) plus clindamycin (300 mg PO TID) for 10–14 days

changes in vaginal flora observed on Gram stain and by demonstration of a high ratio of succinate to lactate (greater than 0.4) or presence of specific amines (putrescine and cadaverine) in vaginal washings of affected patients. The latter two techniques may be useful if confirmation of diagnosis by the four findings above is difficult. The presence or absence of clue cells per se is not helpful since both false-positive (due to adherence by lactobacilli to desquamated vaginal epithelial cells) and false-negative (possibly due to presence of local IgA, which blocks bacterial attachment to vaginal cell surfaces) findings can occur. Culture of vaginal fluid is also not useful since isolation of *G. vaginalis*, even in high concentration, is not specific for bacterial vaginosis.

The recommended therapy of bacterial vaginosis is metronidazole, which appears to eradicate or suppress *G. vaginalis* and obligate anaerobes while promoting recolonization with lactobacilli (Table 4). Single-dose therapy, as used in the treatment of trichomoniasis, is associated with a high failure rate and is not recommended. Treatment with ampicillin is associated with success rates ranging from 33 to 100 percent. Erythromycin and doxycline are ineffective, as are local measures such as triple-sulfa vaginal cream, or providone-iodine vaginal tablets. Interestingly, treatment of the male sexual partner with metronidazole does not appear to prevent recurrence of bacterial vaginosis among women who had been treated with metronidazole.

Candidal Vulvovaginitis

This entity accounts for approximately one-third of all cases of vaginitis in office practice. Candidal vulvovaginitis is commoner during menstruation and in pregnancy and is associated with diabetes mellitus, immunosuppression, and use of broad-spectrum antibiotics, corticosteroids, or oral contraceptives. As high as 10 to 27 percent of male sexual partners of infected women may be found to have balanoposthitis. Clinically, candidal vulvovaginitis is characterized by symptoms of vulvar itching, burning, or other irritation, often associated with external dysuria and with scant, nonmalodorous discharge. Examination usually reveals reddened, inflamed vaginal mucosa with a thick, white, "cottage cheese" discharge. The vaginal pH is less than 4.5. Mixed infection with bacterial vaginosis or trichomoniasis is relatively uncommon. The diagnosis is confirmed by the presence of fungal elements either in saline or KOH smears or Gram stain of vaginal secretions. The KOH smear is considered the most sensitive noncultural method of diagnosis. Two drops of 10 percent KOH are mixed with the discharge on a glass slide under a cover slip and heated until boiling. This destroys the PMNs and epithelial cells and leaves intact the candidal budding and pseudohyphal forms. Cultures should be obtained if the clinical presentation is suggestive of vulvovaginal candidiasis but the wet smear is negative. Although *C. albicans* is the commonest isolate, other *Candida* species (e.g., *Candida glabrata* have also been implicated.

The recommended treatment for candidal vulvovaginitis is local application of antifungal imidazoles such as miconazole or clotrimazole nightly for 7 days (Table 4). Three-day therapy with double strength clotrimazole has also been shown to be effective. Intravaginal nystatin cream can also be used, but requires twice daily applications for 2 weeks. More recently, the use of 600 mg boric acid powder in gelatin capsules, inserted intravaginally each evening for 14 days, has been found to be equally effective to nystatin, but has the advantage of lower cost. Oral therapy with ketoconazole does not provide added advantage in cure rate or prevention of recurrence and is not recommended except for patients with chronic mucocutaneous candidiasis. The presence of *Candida* species per se in any asymptomatic woman does not require treatment. The need for treatment of the male sexual partner has not been determined.

Trichomonal Vaginitis

Symptoms associated with *T. vaginalis* vaginitis are highly variable and appear to correlate with the severity of the inflammatory response in a given host. *T. vaginalis* may also be associated wth asymptomatic infection, which almost invariably leads to symptomatic disease eventually. In patients with minimal or no inflammatory response despite the presence of trichomonads, excessive vaginal discharge may be the only symptom. In more severe cases, the infection is characterized by a profuse, watery, foul-smelling vaginal discharge associated with burning, dysuria, and intermenstrual spotting. Examination shows a foamy, bubbly discharge adherent to an erythematous or often edematous vaginal mucosa with multiple petechiae. The vaginal pH is usually greater than 5.0. Numerous PMNs are seen in the wet smear. Diagnosis is confirmed by the presence of motile trichomonads in the saline preparation of vaginal discharge. In patients with minimal symptoms, the wet smear may not be sufficiently sensitive, and culture for *T. vaginalis* on selective medium (such as Diamond's medium) is highly recommended.

Systemic treatment with oral nitroimidazoles, such as metronidazole or tinidazole, are the only regimens consistently effective for *T. vaginalis* vaginitis (Table 4). Simultaneous treatment of the male sexual partner is important for prevention of relapse or reinfection and is particularly important if the 2-g single-dose regimen is used. The presence of *T. vaginalis*, even in the absence of vaginal symptoms, should be treated since these women almost invariably develop symptomatic disease eventually. The commonest causes of recurrent *T. vaginalis* infection, or apparent treatment failure, are due to reinfection or patient noncompliance with therapy. Persistent infection despite good compliance and avoidance of reinfection should suggest the possibility of infection due to metronidazole-resistant *T. vaginalis*. Such patients may require 7- to 14-day retreatment regimens consisting of oral metronidazole, 2 to 3 g daily by mouth, together with a vaginal metronidazole tablet, 500 mg, inserted nightly each day until vaginal symptoms have completely subsided. Metronidazole remains the drug of choice for symptomatic trichomonal vaginitis during pregnancy; the dosage is the same as for a nonpregnant individual. Clotrimazole can be administered intravaginally as a topical trichomonicide, but it is clearly less effective than metronidazole.

Cervicitis

Infection of the cervix by sexually transmitted pathogens may lead to several potential complications, including endometritis and salpingitis leading to ectopic pregnancy or infertility; premature rupture of membranes, chorioamnionitis, and puerperal infection during pregnancy; and initiation or promotion of cervical neoplasia. Cervicitis can be difficult to diagnose because many women are asymptomatic, and infection is often discovered only after a sexual partner presents wih urethritis. Alternatively, cervical infection may be misdiagnosed as vaginitis if a thorough pelvic examination is not performed. The typical finding of cervicitis is an inflamed cervix, with a mucopurulent exudate emanating from the os. The principal infectious causes are *C. trachomatis, N. gonorrhoeae*, and HSV. Although cervical infection with any of these pathogens is more likely to present with a mucopurulent endocervical discharge, only HSV is associated with characteristic ectocervical ulcerations, and only *C. trachomatis* is associated wtih the presence of mucopus or with 10 or more PMNs per high-power field in cervical mucus. *C. trachomatis* frequently coexists with *N. gonorrhoeae* in cervicitis; treatment for both gonococcal and nongonococcal cervicitis should, therefore, also be effective against *C. trachomatis*.

Mucopurulent or Chlamydial Cervicitis

Chlamydial infection should always be suspected in women with mucopurulent cervicitis whether or not gonorrhea is also found. Similar to the case of gonococcal urethritis in men, women with gonococcal infection treated with 4.8 million units of procaine penicillin G plus probenecid were associated with a significantly higher rate of posttreatment cervicitis and pelvic inflammatory disease as compared with similar women treated with agents effective against both *N. gonorrhoeae* and *C. trachomatis*. Tetracycline, 500 mg four times daily for 7 days, is currently the most effective regimen for mucopurulent cervicitis and eradication of *C. trachomatis* from the cervix (Table 4). Doxycycline or minocycline are useful alternative agents. Erythromycin is recommended in women allergic to tetracycline or during pregnancy. If coexisting gonococcal infection is found, additional therapy for gonorrhea should be provided in areas where tetracycline is no longer highly effective against *N. gonorrhoeae*.

Gonococcal Cervicitis

Whenever endocervical gonorrhea is suspected, the urethra as well as paraurethral glands should also be carefully examined. Cultures should be obtained from multiple sites including the anorectum and the oropharynx. A confirmatory test for *C. trachomatis* is also desirable in women with cervicitis, even if gonococcal infection is found, since more than 40 percent of women with gonorrhea have coexisting chlamydial infection. Initial empiric therapy, therefore, should also be effective against *C. trachomatis* (Table 4). Single-dose ampicillin or amoxicillin plus probenecid followed by 7 days of tetracycline is the regimen of choice for infections in which penicillinase-producing *N. gonorrhoeae* (PPNG) is not suspected. The combined regimen of ampicillin or amoxicillin followed by tetracycline will also eradicate pharyngeal gonococcal infection, for which ampicillin, amoxicillin and spectinomycin are not highly effective. Patients allergic to penicillin or in whom PPNG or pregnancy is suspected may be treated with spectinomycin, ceftriaxone, or cefoxitin plus probenecid. Trimethoprim-sulfamethoxazole appears to be a useful alternative to ampicillin-tetracycline combination for dual endocervical infection with *N. gonorrhoeae* and *C. trachomatis*.

Herpes Simplex Cervicitis and Genital Infection

The first episode of genital herpes is frequently accompanied by systemic as well as local manifestations. Concomitant cervicitis occurs in the majority of cases (80% to 90%), in contrast to recurrent episodes (10% to 20%). Several anatomic sites besides the cervix may be involved including the urethra, vulva, pharynx, and extragenital cutaneous regions. Primary HSV genital infection tends to be more severe in women, and complications occur more frequently than in men. The most prominent local symptoms include pain, dysuria, tender inguinal adenopathy, and neurologic complications such as sacral anesthesia, urinary retention, and constipation. The cervix may show diffuse friability with necrotic and ulcerative lesions of both the exocervix and endocervix. The presence of HSV is confirmed either by culture or direct immunofluorescent staining of scrapings from active lesions. Recurrent genital herpes is less severe and of shorter duration than primary or first episodes of infection. There is, however, considerable variability in the intensity and duration of symptoms and in the frequency of recurrence. Recurrent viral shedding from the cervix can also occur in the absence of symptoms or external genital lesions. This is of clinical importance particularly in late pregnancy because of concern of intrapartum transmission of HSV infection to the neonate. Pregnant women with a history of recurrent genital herpes should be closely monitored virologically or cytologically near term, usually starting between 32 and 36 weeks of gestation. Women with active external genital lesions or cervical viral shedding at the time of labor should be delivered by cesarean section. Women with two sequential negative viral cultures or cytologic studies performed 3 to 4 days apart and absent genital lesions at the time of labor may be delivered vaginally.

Acyclovir is effective in reducing some of the manifestations of primary genital HSV infection and in shortening the duration of viral shedding (Table 4). Oral acyclovir is also effective in suppressing recurrent episodes among patients receiving continuous therapy and may be indicated in selected patients with severe underlying disease and immunosuppression. Topical acyclovir is useful for the treatment of external genital lesions in women during primary or first episodes of HSV infection. It is not approved for intravaginal use since the polyethylene glycol base is irritating and may cause vaginal erythema. Routine use of topical acyclovir in recurrent genital herpes is not recommended since it has no established role either in prophylaxis of recurrence or in prevention of acquisition of new infection.

Acute Salpingitis

Acute salpingitis, or pelvic inflammatory disease (PID), is believed to result from ascending infection, by contiguous spread of sexually transmitted pathogens and/or indigenous vaginal microflora, from the endocervix and endometrium. Major risk factors for salpingitis include an intrauterine device, previous gonococcal infection, previous episodes of PID, lower socioeconomic status, nulliparity, and number of sexual partners. Use of oral contraceptives appears to have a protective influence. The microbiology of acute PID is complex. Cultures obtained directly from inflamed fallopian tubes either at laparoscopy or laparotomy clearly indicate a polymicrobial etiology, including *N. gonorrhoeae, C. trachomatis, Mycoplasma hominis*, and mixed aerobes and anaerobes (Table 5). Clinically, acute PID associated with endocervical gonorrhea tends to occur more frequently during the first 10 days of the menstrual cycle, and affected patients are more severely ill than those with nongonococcal PID. On the other hand, patients with nongonococcal PID are more likely to have a history of previous PID, a less optimal response to conventional antimicrobial therapy, and are more likely to develop late sequelae such as recurrent PID, adnexal abscess, and infertility.

The clinical diagnosis of acute PID by history and physical findings alone is often inaccurate. The classic manifestations include fever, chills, malaise, and bilateral lower abdominal pain that is often aggravated by movement of the iliopsoas muscles. Pelvic examination reveals a mucopurulent cervical discharge, and exquisite tenderness on movement of the cervix. The adnexal regions are tender and thickened, and an adnexal or cul-de-sac mass may be palpable if infection is recurrent or chronic. Visual confirmation of tubal inflammation by colposcopy or laparoscopy can be very helpful and should be undertaken, particularly if the clinical diagnosis of acute PID is in doubt, or when the clinical presentation is atypical. Analyses of specimens obtained by culdocentesis for presence of PMNs and microorganisms by Gram stain and culture are helpful, but not very reliable for the diagnosis of chlamydial salpingitis. Cervical secretions should be routinely examined for PMNs as well as both *N. gonorrhoeae* and *C. trachomatis*. Since appropriate collection and microbiologic testing of specimens from the fallopian tubes are neither practical nor desirable in all cases of PID, treatment is often empiric, based on selection of antimicrobial agents active against the major recognized pathogens (Table 4). Any IUD should be removed, and all sexual partners within 2 months prior to the patient's illness should be examined and empirically treated with a regimen effective against both *C. trachomatis* and *N. gonorrhoeae* before and irrespective of cultural results. Hospitalization should be considered for acutely ill patients, particularly if pelvic peritonitis is present, if the diagnosis of acute PID is in doubt and other surgical emergencies are possible, if an adnexal or cul-de-sac mass is palpable, or if the patient is pregnant.

It should be noted that none of the currently recommended regimens for acute salpingitis outlined in Table 4 are considered optimal therapy, and their relative efficacy remains to be established by controlled clinical trials. The cefoxitin-doxycycline regimen is theoretically most attractive, since cefoxitin has excellent activity against the anaerobes most frequently isolated in PID, as well as aerobic and microaerophilic streptococci, coliforms and gonococci, whereas doxycycline is effective against *C. trachomatis* and *M. hominis*. The metronidazole-doxycycline combination is attractive since excellent tissue concentrations can be achieved by oral administration of these agents. However, this regimen may not be reliably effective against Enterobacteriaceae or against *N. gonorrhoeae* in areas where moderate tetracycline resistance is encountered. The clindamycin-aminoglycoside regimen is the least attractive since it does not provide optimal coverage for either *C. trachomatis* or *N. gonorrhoeae*. The combination of trimethoprim-sulfamethoxazole plus clindamycin for outpatient treatment of acute PID appears promising and deserves critical evaluation. Approximately 5 to 15 percent of women fail to respond to initial antimicrobial therapy, 20 percent have at least one recurrence, and 15 percent are left infertile. It is clear that a comprehensive assessment of any therapeutic regimen for PID must include evaluation for late sequelae such as recurrence, infertility, and ectopic

TABLE 5 Recommended Regimens for Treatment of Vulvovaginal and Tubo-ovarian Abscess

Infection	*Choice*	*Alternate*
Vulvovaginal abscess		
Inpatient	Cefoxitin (1.5 g IV q8h) for 5–7 days	Metronidazole (500 mg IV q6h) or clindamycin (600 mg IV q8h) plus gentamicin or tobramycin (1.5 mg/kg IV q8h) for 5–7 days
Outpatient	Ampicillin (500 mg PO QID) plus metronidazole (500 mg QID) for 7–10 days	Trimethoprim/sulfamethoxazole 80-mg/400-mg (1 tablet PO BID) plus clindamycin (300 mg PO TID) for 7–10 days
Tubo-ovarian abscess		
Inpatient	Clindamycin (600 mg IV q8h) plus tobramycin (1.5 mg/kg IV q8h) for 10–14 days	Metronidazole (500 mg IV q6h) or cefoxitin (1.5 g IV q8h) or ticarcillin (3 g IV q4h), each plus gentamicin or tobramycin (1.5 mg/kg IV q8h) for 10–14 days *or* Cefotaxime (1.5 g IV q6h) ± gentamicin or tobramycin (depending on severity) (1.5 mg/kg IV q8h) for 10–14 days
Outpatient	Ampicillin (500 mg PO QID) plus metronidazole (500 mg PO QID) for 6–8 weeks	Trimethoprim/sulfamethoxazole 80-mg/400-mg (2 tablets PO BID) plus clindamycin (300 mg PO TID) for 6–8 weeks

Note: Regimens are applicable after exclusion of endocervical or paraurethral *N. gonorrhoeae* or *C. trachomatis* infection.

pregnancy, as well as the immediate response to acute symptoms.

Vulvovaginal and Tubo-ovarian Abscess

Pyogenic Vulvovaginal Infections

These include abscesses of Bartholin's and Skene's glands, infected labial inclusion cysts, labial abscesses, furunculosis, and hidradenitis. Mixed infection due to both aerobic and anaerobic vaginal bacteria is the general rule, and coliforms, *B. fragilis, B. bivius*, and anaerobic cocci are commonly involved. Coexisting *N. gonorrhoeae* should be excluded. Surgical drainage is the primary therapeutic modality, and antimicrobials are of secondary importance. In the absence of specific cultural and antibiotic susceptibility data, initial selection of drugs should include those effective against both aerobic and anaerobic bacteria of vaginal origin (Table 5). Subsequent modification of antimicrobial therapy should be guided by the clinical response and by microbiologic data based on specimens obtained by direct needle aspiration of lesions (avoiding contamination by normal vaginal flora).

Tubo-ovarian Abscess

Tubo-ovarian abscess (TOA) occurring in the absence of obstetric and postoperative infections, is generally a consequence of acute or chronic PID. Unilateral presentation of TOA is not uncommon and is not uniquely associated with IUD usage. Tubo-ovarian abscesses are often polymicrobial, caused by mixed aerobes and anaerobes including *Escherichia coli, B. fragilis, B. bivius, Peptococcus* species, *Peptostreptococcus* species, and aerobic streptococci. The recommended antimicrobial regimens for initial empiric treatment of TOA are outlined in Table 5. The optimal duration of treatment has not been clearly established. The general recommendation is that antibiotics should be continued by oral administration for 6 to 8 weeks, until the adnexal mass is no longer palpable. Medical therapy with antimicrobial agents alone is successful in 40 to 70 percent of cases. Surgical intervention is indicated if rupture is suspected or imminent or if suboptimal clinical response is observed after 72 hours of initial antimicrobial therapy. Conservative initial management of TOA, particularly in young, nulliparous patients, is indicated in the majority of cases. Serial ultrasonography is particularly useful in assessing the therapeutic response and resolution of mass effect during follow-up.

PROSTATITIS, EPIDIDYMITIS, AND BALANOPOSTHITIS

GERALD W. CHODAK, M.D.

PROSTATITIS

Current treatment of inflammatory diseases of the prostate still results in dissatisfied patients and frustrated physicians. Despite significant progress, there is a persistent difficulty in explaining why some patients respond so well to a short course of therapy and others have persistent or recurrent symptoms, even when prolonged therapy is employed. Nevertheless, a systematic approach to evaluation will enable the physician to localize the source of infection and determine whether it is likely to respond to antibiotic therapy.

Diagnostic Evaluation and Culture Techniques

In addition to the routine history and physical examination, information about the prostate can be obtained from microscopy and culture of the prostatic fluid. In order to localize the bacteria to the prostate, samples are taken from different parts of the voided urine as well as from fluid expressed by prostatic massage. At the time of evaluation, the patient should have a relatively full bladder. The urine is divided into the first 10 ml of voided urine (urethral sample) and the midstream urine (bladder sample). A digital examination is then performed, and fluid from the prostate is expressed into the urethra and collected (EPS). Another urine sample is then collected (VB3), which also contains prostatic fluid. The laboratory should be informed of the physician's interest in finding low densities of organisms. Evaluation of this test is difficult, but if pyuria is present, low counts of bacteria can be considered significant if no other diagnostic finding points to a differential diagnosis. The pathogens are usually the same as those causing urinary tract infections and include *Escherichia coli, Klebsiella, Enterobacter, Proteus*, and *Pseudomonas* species.

Microscopic Evaluation of Prostatic Fluid

Two criteria used to diagnose an inflammatory process in the prostate are the presence of leukocytes and lipid-laden macrophages (oval fat bodies) in the expressed prostatic fluid. The fluid must be compared with the first 10 ml of voided urine, which contains urethral contents. Normal prostatic fluid contains fewer than 10 WBC per high-power field, and more than 15 or 20 WBC per high-power field are considered abnormal. Oval fat bodies are not typically found in the urethra, so that an increase in these cells in the prostatic fluid is also evidence for an inflammatory response.

Interpretation of Cultural Results

A bacterial infection in the prostate may not produce a count of more than 100,000 CFU per millilter. Therefore, the diagnosis is made by comparing the prostatic cultures with those of the urethra and bladder. A prostatic infection is present when the urine from the bladder (VB2) contains fewer than 10,000 CFU/ml and the prostatic cultures (EPS and VB3) contain 10 times as many bacteria as does the urethral culture (VB1). In order to diagnose bacterial prostatitis when the bladder urine contains significant bacteria, the patient must first be treated for a few days with nitrofurantoin, which sterilizes the urine while not greatly affecting the prostate. Reculture at that time will permit the same comparison between the urethral sample and the VB3 and EPS cultures.

ACUTE BACTERIAL PROSTATITIS

Diagnosis

Patients with acute prostatitis present with fever, chills, and irritative voiding symptoms that include dysuria, frequency, and pain. Examination of the prostate reveals a tender prostate, and prostate massage is not recommended because of the possibility of producing a bacteremia. One underlying cause of this disorder is acute or chronic urinary retention which is assessed by palpating an enlarged bladder. If significant residual urine is suspected following voiding, then the bladder is catheterized and an indwelling catheter is left in place when more than 100 ml is present.

Treatment

Hospitalization is usually advised for patients with high fever (greater than 101 °F) and significant pain. Bed rest, hydration and analgesics provide symptomatic relief. Antibiotic therapy is instituted with gentamicin (3 mg per kilogram intravenously in three divided doses) and ampicillin (2 g intravenously every 6 hours) until the cultures and sensitivities are available. When the fever has defervesced, the antibiotic can usually be changed to trimethoprim (160 mg) and sulfasoxazole (800 mg) orally twice a day. The usual course of therapy is 2 weeks.

CHRONIC BACTERIAL PROSTATITIS

Diagnosis

Most men with chronic prostatitis complain of chronic irritative symptoms and pain in the pelvic area or in the penis following ejaculation. Patients may have recurrent urinary infections with the same organism and/or positive EPS or VB3 cultures.

Treatment

Optimal therapy requires obtaining high levels of antibiotic in prostatic secretions rather than in prostatic tissue. The most effective treatment is trimethoprim (160 mg) and sulfamethoxazole (800 mg) orally taken in combination twice a day. Patients treated with short courses of therapy are more likely to have recurrences than those taking a longer course. The best approach is to initiate therapy for 12 weeks. Patients who develop recurrent symptoms after therapy is discontinued may improve following administration of low-dose daily therapy consisting of 80 mg of trimethoprim and 400 mg of sulfamethoxazole for another 1 to 3 months. An alternative therapy is carbenicillin indanyl sodium (382 mg, two tablets orally four times per day) for 4 weeks, which may be as effective, although it has a substantially higher cost. In some cases, patients fail to obtain prolonged relief of their symptoms, and these may warrant surgical intervention, which involves either transurethral prostatectomy or total prostatovesiculectomy. Although the transrethral procedure has far fewer adverse effects, the patient should be informed that his symptoms may not be totally cured because some residual tissue will still remain. Urologists are generally reluctant to recommend surgery to treat this disorder.

NONBACTERIAL PROSTATITIS

Patients complain of the same symptoms found in bacterial prostatitis, and the prostatic fluid also contains more than 15 to 20 WBC per high-power field; however, the urine, EPS, and VB3 cultures are negative. There is no conclusive evidence that *Chlamydia* is a primary cause of this problem, and, yet, a trial of tetracycline, 500 mg orally every 6 hours for 10 to 14 days may be warranted. If little or no response occurs, no additional antibiotics are warranted. Patients with negative cultures should not be placed on long-term antibiotic therapy. The optimal treatment is based on symptoms. Patients often feel better by taking hot sitz baths two or three times per day. Prostatic massage has no proven value in the management of this illness. Patients should be encouraged to maintain their normal sexual activity and physical exercise and should be informed that the problem is not serious but the symptoms are likely to persist for a variable period of time. Many patients notice that alcohol and caffeine worsen their symptoms, so that reducing these items from their diet may improve their symptoms.

ACUTE EPIDIDYMITIS

Acute epididymitis is a disorder characterized by an abrupt onset of pain and swelling in the tail of the epididymis and may be followed by diffuse swelling of the entire epididymis, ipsilateral testicle, and hemiscrotum (epididymo-orchitis). The causes may be either sexual or nonsexual and nonsexual causes are more likely to have

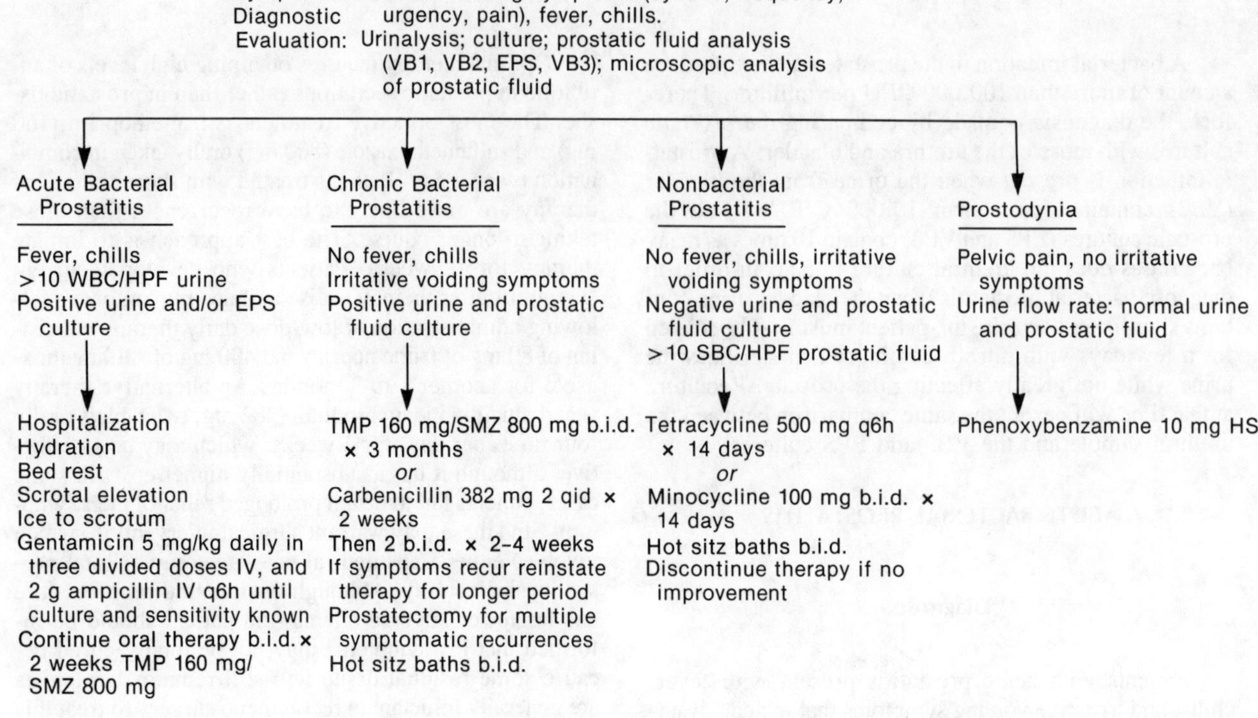

Figure 1 Diagnosis and treatment of prostatitis.

an anatomic basis. Patients over 40 years of age who develop epididymitis usually have an associated urinary tract infection, which is due to some obstructive process such as a urethral stricture or benign prostatic hypertrophy.

Diagnosis

The initial diagnosis is made based on clinical findings, which include swelling and marked tenderness along the epididymis. As the disease progresses, epididymo-orchitis may develop as the testicle also becomes swollen and tender.

The cause of epididymitis in patients who have a history of sexual exposure may be determined by performing a Gram stain of a urethral smear obtained prior to voiding. If intracellular gram-negative diplococci are identified, then *Neisseria gonorrhoeae* is the cause. If no organisms are identified, then a culture must be performed to rule out gonococcal infection. In the absence of neisseriae, *Chlamydia trachomatis* is usually the responsible organism in this group.

For patients who develop epididymitis secondary to a urinary tract anomaly, a urine culture and sensitivity will identify the causative organism.

An important cause of epididymitis in the older population is urinary obstruction associated with an inability to empty the bladder. When the history or physical examination suggests a significant residual urine, a catheter is passed and left in place if more than 100 ml remains in the bladder following voiding.

Treatment

The optimal treatment of acute epididymitis depends on the underlying cause. Febrile patients with epididymitis secondary to bacteriuria are treated initially with ampicillin, 1 g intravenously every 6 hours, and tobramycin, 3.0 mg per kilogram intravenously in three divided doses, until the results of the urine culture and sensitivity are available. At that time either oral ampicillin, 500 mg orally every 6 hours for 10 days or a first-generation cephalosporin may be substituted. Patients will usually benefit from symptomatic treatment, which includes hospitalization, bed rest, scrotal elevation, and ice packs to the scrotum to reduce swelling. If significant residual urine is detected, then a prostatectomy should be planned after the acute episode has resolved.

Men who develop acute epididymitis following sexual exposure are treated with ampicillin, 500 mg orally four times per day for 10 days, if *N. gonorrhoeae* has been cultured or found on Gram stain, or with tetracycline, 500 mg orally four times per day for 10 days if there is no evidence for gonorrhea. In addition, symptomatic relief is provided by bed rest and scrotal elevation. When epididymitis has been caused by sexual transmission, sexual partners must also be treated.

BALANOPOSTHITIS

Infection of the glans penis and foreskin occurs almost exclusively in the uncircumcised male. Usually the foreskin cannot be retracted; this allows smegma and secretions to accumulate and provides a warm, moist culture medium that predisposes to infection. Balanitis and balanoposthitis are commonest in children and may be associated with impaired urination because of a tight phimosis. It also occurs following sexual contact with an infected partner.

Diagnosis

The initial diagnosis is made from physical examination. The foreskin may be difficult to retract over the glans. Inflammation and swelling of the glans and/or prepuce are present. A Gram stain of the material under the foreskin will determine the class of organisms present. Sexually active patients who develop balanoposthitis give a history of sexual contact within 6 to 24 hours prior to the onset of symptoms. These patients may have erosive soreness and ulceration of the glans penis. Microscopic examination should reveal the presence of *Candida*.

Treatment

Most cases of balanoposthitis in children can be treated with soap and water cleansing, provided that the foreskin can be retracted over the glans. Acutely, this may not be possible, and a dorsal slit procedure must be performed. This will allow improved hygiene, which helps to rapidly resolve the inflammation and swelling. Once this has resolved, the patient should undergo a circumcision. Antibiotics are usually not required.

Patients who develop balanoposthitis following sexual exposure to women with candidal vaginitis are treated with topical nystatin ointment, 100,000 units per gram, twice a day for 10 days. If phimosis is present and discharge is discovered under the glans, the sexual partner also receives the same treatment. Figure 1 provides a flow chart that summarizes the content of the discussion in this chapter.

DISSEMINATED GONOCOCCAL INFECTION

PETER A. RICE, M.D.

INITIAL SYMPTOMS

Most patients with disseminated gonococcal infection (DGI) experience migratory or additive polyarthralgias as early symptoms. These symptoms may involve only a single joint, are usually transient, and may be associated with objective signs of synovitis or tenosynovitis. Constitutional features such as fever, chills, and headache are common. In about 25 percent of patients, skin lesions will be noted initially, and less than 20 percent will complain initially of local genitourinary symptoms. Dermatitis and cervicitis or urethritis are often asymptomatic throughout the course of DGI. Although most patients seek medical attention within 2 to 4 days of the onset of symptoms, some will be symptomatic for 1 week or longer prior to hospitalization.

Disseminated gonococcal infection predominates in women, and the initial manifestations of DGI are often temporally related to menstruation or pregnancy. Thus, most women note the onset of DGI within 1 week of their last menstruation.

PHYSICAL EXAMINATION

The musculoskeletal manifestations of DGI are the prominent feature. Whereas a single, hot, swollen joint is characteristic of nongonococcal bacterial arthritis, tenosynovitis and polyarthritis are more typical of DGI (Table 1).

In recent reports, tenosynovitis has been commoner than arthritis and is present in two-thirds of patients with DGI. It usually involves multiple joints, especially the wrists, fingers, toes, and ankles.

Monarthritis or polyarthritis, defined by the presence

TABLE 1 Differential Features of Disseminated Gonococcal Infection and Nongonococcal Bacterial Arthritis

DGI	*Nongonococcal Bacterial Arthritis*
Usually healthy, young adults	Often compromised host, often very young or aged
Tenosynovitis often	No tenosynovitis
Polyarthritis common	Monarthritis common
Skin lesions in two-thirds	No associated dermatitis
Wrists and small joints common sites	Large joints predominate
Migratory polyarthralgias	No prodomal joint symptoms
Synovial fluid culture positive in less than 50% of fluids that are cultured (only ⅓ of patients have a suppurative joint that yields synovial fluid for analysis)	Synovial fluid cultures are usually positive
Blood cultures are positive in less than 30% of all cases (50% in patients with tenosynovitis but no arthritis)	Blood cultures positive in 50% of patients
Rapid and complete response to antibiotics	Slower response to antibiotics (joint drainage important)

of purulent synovial fluid with more than 25,000 leukocytes per cubic millimeter is present in one third of patients. The knee is the most commonly affected joint, which may, in part, reflect the ease of diagnosis and aspiration of a knee joint effusion. However, other joints, including the hip and shoulder, may be affected. The sacroiliac joint, temporomandibular, and sternoclavicular joints are rarely involved.

The other common abnormality on physical examination is dermatitis, which is present in about two-thirds of patients, usually in those who have tenosynovitis. The skin lesions are usually multiple and are found most commonly on the arms and legs, sometimes on the trunk, hands, or feet, but rarely on the face. They are usually painless, and patients are often unaware of their presence. Commonest are small macules or papules. Occasionally, they may be painful and may even appear pustular or resemble vasculitis. Any form of skin lesion may be associated with DGI, however; this includes pustules, vesicles, bullae, erythema nodosum, or erythema multiforme. Sometimes new skin lesions develop despite the initiation of appropriate antibiotic therapy. The skin lesions are almost always sterile. Although most patients with DGI are febrile and often describe shaking chills, almost 40 percent of patients do not have any substantial fever once hospitalized. Most patients deny any local genitourinary, rectal, or throat symptoms, despite the fact that *Neisseria gonorrhoeae* is often recovered from these sites. Gonococcal meningitis and endocarditis are rare; immune-mediated glomerulonephritis secondary to DGI occasionally occurs.

RESULTS OF CULTURE

The genitourinary tract provides the best opportunity to recover *N. gonorrhoeae* despite the fact that localized genitourinary symptoms are infrequent. Eighty percent of patients with DGI will have cultures positive for *N. gonorrhoeae* from a genitourinary site. The organisms can be recovered from the synovial fluid in about 50 percent of patients with arthritis and are similarly recovered from the blood of patients with tenosynovitis. Concurrently positive blood and synovial fluid cultures are rare.

Any joint effusion should be aspirated and immediately plated onto chocolate agar as well as onto plain blood agar. A gram-stained smear of concentrated synovial fluid is useful, but will be positive in only approximately 25 percent of DGI joint effusions. The synovial fluid leukocyte count is usually 40,000 to 60,000 cells per cubic millimeter, although more variability exists than in nongonococcal bacterial effusions. Blood cultures should always be obtained as well as appropriate genitourinary cultures. The endocervix provides the highest culture yield in women. Urethral exudates from women should be obtained for culture if they are present, and a rectal culture should also be performed in women. In men a urethral specimen for culture should be taken with a thin, cotton-tipped swab or a Calgiswab. A pharyngeal culture should also be performed. The genitourinary, anal, and pharyngeal cultures should be plated onto selective media such as modified Thayer-Martin or modified New York City media to inhibit nonneisserial commensal organisms from overgrowing the culture plate.

DIFFERENTIAL DIAGNOSIS

DGI should be the leading diagnostic consideration in any sexually active patient who presents with polyarthritis or monarthritis. If tenosynovitis and/or dermatitis are the presenting signs or are present in conjunction with arthritis, the diagnosis is very likely to be DGI, and antimicrobial therapy should be initiated after appropriate cultures are performed.

The differential diagnosis of DGI includes hepatitis, Reiter's syndrome, acute rheumatic fever, bacteridal endocarditis, other bacteremic and viral illnesses, and other connective tissue diseases (Table 2).

Polyarthritis, as well as tenosynovitis, will occur commonly in the prodome of hepatitis B. A rash is also common, although the rash is more often urticarial. If synovial effusions can be aspirated, the characteristic leuko-

TABLE 2 Differential Diagnosis of Disseminated Gonococcal Infection

Illness	*Polyarthritis*	*Tenosynovitis*	*Dermatitis*	*Sex*	*Laboratory*	*Other Helpful Differential Features*
DGI	++	++	++ (Maculopapular vesicles pustules)	>Females	Positive cultures	Response to antibiotics
Hepatitis	++	++	+ (Urticaria, macules, papules)	Females and males	Abnormal hepatic function tests; HBsAg	Clinical evidence of hepatitis
Reiter's syndrome	++	+	+ (Nail lesions, keratodermia)	>Males	HLA B27	Conjunctivitis, sacroiliitis, oral lesions, balanitis
Acute rheumatic fever	++	+	Rare	Females and males	Positive throat culture or serologic evidence of *Streptococcus* B infection	Carditis, response to salicylates

Note: ++ = frequently; + = occasional.

cyte count is usually less than in DGI with arthritis, although variable counts have been reported. The major diagnostic clue will be the clinical and laboratory evidence of hepatitis. Positive serologic tests for hepatitis B and the absence of positive cultures for *N. gonorrhoeae* will help to confirm the diagnosis.

Acute rheumatic fever may present in young adults as a polyarthritis without evidence of carditis, chorea, or subcutaneous nodules; however, this disease is now uncommon in the United States. If a rash is present, it is usually evanescent and associated with fever. A recent streptococcal throat infection documented with appropriate cultural and serologic tests is necessary for a confirmatory diagnosis.

Bacterial endocarditis as well as other forms of bacteremia can also cause musculoskeletal and dermatologic manifestations that may mimic DGI. Positive blood cultures should establish the diagnosis. Similarly, viral illnesses such as rubella can cause an acute arthritis and a rash. Occasionally, Epstein-Barr viral or cytomegaloviral illness produce rashes and joint complaints, but other accompanying features usually distinguish these illnesses from DGI. Juvenile rheumatoid arthritis, rheumatoid arthritis, systemic lupus erythematosus, and other connective tissue disorders can also begin so explosively that they may suggest DGI. The subsequent clinical course will be necessary for the diagnosis of those more chronic conditions. The diagnostic response to antibiotics can be helfpul in DGI, and once all cultures have been obtained, a patient with suspected DGI should be treated with antibiotics.

TREATMENT OF DISSEMINATED GONOCOCCAL INFECTION

The outlook for patients with DGI is usually one of rapid and complete recovery. With appropriate antibiotic therapy, the fever and clinical symptoms are usually eradicated in a few days. Many different antibiotic regimens have been found to be equally effective. Hospitalization is usually indicated, especially for those who cannot

TABLE 3 Antimicrobial Management of Patients with Disseminated Gonococcal Infection

Purulent Arthritis: Hospitalize

First Choice	*Or*	*Or*	*Or*
Aqueous crystalline penicillin G: 10 million units IV per day for at least 3 days or longer if improvement (as judged by a decrease in quantity of joint fluid and decrease in the synovial fluid leukocyte count) has not occurred by 3 days; followed by amoxicillin 500 mg or ampicillin 500 mg by mouth, 4 times/day to complete 7-10 days of antibiotic treatment	If the patient is allergic to penicillin: Tetracycline HCl: 500 mg PO 4 times/day for 7-10 days (tetracycline should not be used for complicated gonococcal infection in pregnant women) *or* Erythromycin: 500 mg PO 4 times/day for 7-10 days	If the infecting strain is a PPNG:[*] Cefoxitin 1.0 g *or* Cefotaxime 500 mg, either given 4 times a day IV for 7-10 days	If the infecting strain is a PPNG and the patient is allergic to β-lactam antibiotics: Spectinomycin:[†] 4-8 g daily for 7-10 days

Tenosynovitis: if the patient is hospitalized (see text for possible exclusions)

First Choice	*Or*	*Or*	*Or*
Aqueous penicillin G: 10 million units IV per day for 3 days followed by amoxicillin 500 mg or ampicillin 500 mg 4 times/day to complete 7 days of antimicrobial treatment	If the patient is allergic to penicillin: Tetracycline HCl: 500 mg PO 4 times/day for 7 days (tetracycline should not be used for complicated gonococcal infection in pregnant women) *or* Erythromycin: 500 mg PO 4 times/day for 7 days	If the infecting strain is a PPNG: Cefoxitin 1.0 g *or* Cefotaximine 500 mg, either given 4 times/day IV for 7 days	If the infecting strain is a PPNG and the patient is allergic to β-lactam antibiotics: Spectinomycin: 4 to 8 g daily for 7 days

Outpatient Therapy (not infected with a PPNG strain)

First Choice	*Or*
Amoxicillin 3.0 g *or* ampicillin 3.5 g; either with 1 g probenecid PO followed by amoxicillin 500 mg or ampicillin 500 mg 4 times/day to complete 7 days of antimicrobial treatment	If the patient is allergic to penicillin: Tetracycline HCl: 500 mg PO 4 times/day for 7 days (tetracycline should not be used for complicated gonococcal infection in pregnant women) *or* Erythromycin: 500 mg PO 4 times/day for 7 days

Note: within categories, regimens are therapeutically equivalent.

* PPNG = penicillinase-producing *N. gonorrhoeae.*

† Spectinomycin resistance has not been reported for *N. gonorrhoeae* in the U.S. nor have DGI strains with spectinomycin resistance been yet reported anywhere in the world.

reliably comply with treatment, have uncertain diagnosis, or have purulent joint effusions or other complications. In the few instances where signs and symptoms of tenosynovitis are minimal, where the diagnosis is secure in a compliant patient, and where the patient does not have purulent arthritis, an oral regimen administered on an outpatient basis may be considered.

The therapeutic response is so dramatic that it has often served as a diagnostic guide. In contrast to patients with nongonococcal bacterial arthritis, patients with DGI usually do not require repeated mechanical joint drainage and almost never require open surgical drainage, even when hips or shoulders are infected.

Table 3 is a flow diagram of therapy of DGI that takes into consideration a variety of circumstances surrounding therapy.

Occasionally, patients will not respond to treatment rapidly and completely. For example, those with large, purulent joint effusions may require prolonged hospitalization, and their effusions may not clear for days or even for weeks. Indeed, the presence of a large, purulent joint effusion is the single most important factor that determines the length of hospitalization in patients with DGI. Seven days of antimicrobial therapy administered parenterally are usually sufficient to sterilize the joint even in patients with effusions that persist beyond that period.

Recently, there have been a few reports of penicillinase-producing strains of *N. gonorrhoeae* (PPNG) that have been isolated from patients with DGI. These strains will obviously not respond quickly or completely to the usual antibiotic regimen and clearly a diagnostic trial of penicillin will not be useful in such a circumstance. Newer cephalosporins and spectinomycin (see Table 3) have been effective in treating such resistant strains.

Most patients with DGI will require hospitalization. Two or 3 days of hospitalization are usually adequate to assess the response to treatment and allow enough time for all cultural results to return. Patients with a purulent joint effusion should be hospitalized, and after there has been an objective improvement in joint fluid parameters, an additional 7 days of antimicrobial therapy will be required with repeated mechanical joint drainage and non-weight bearing. Hospitalization is mandatory when the diagnosis is not certain or when the patient is not reliable. The strains that cause DGI are, in general, more sensitive to penicillin than are strains that cause local genitourinary infection; therefore, massive doses of antibiotics for prolonged periods are usually not needed. Since the recovery of *N. gonorrhoeae* from synovial fluid, blood, or skin is possible in less than 50 percent of patients, a therapeutic trial of antibiotics that results in a rapid response will often be very helpful for diagnostic purposes.

SYPHILIS

ROBERT R. TIGHT, M.D.

Syphilis is an infectious disease of great chronicity caused by *Treponema pallidum*. It is systemic from the outset, usually sexually transmitted, capable of involving practically every organ and system of the body and of mimicking a large number of other disease entities, and is distinguished by florid manifestations in some cases and years of completely asymptomatic latency in others.

ETIOLOGY

Certain characteristics of *Treponema pallidum* have diagnostic and therapeutic relevance. The delicate spiral-shaped organism is relatively thin (0.25 μ) and is not stained readily by ordinary laboratory methods necessitating indirect, darkfield microscopy for optimal visualization in the outpatient setting. *T. pallidum* cannot at present be cultured in vitro. Thus, less direct serologic methods are usually needed for diagnosis. *T. pallidum* is exquisitely sensitive to penicillin (and many other antibiotics), for which the minimal inhibitory concentration is less than 0.03 units per milliliter. To date, there has been no evidence of increasing antibiotic resistance as has occurred with *Neisseria gonorrhoeae*. Finally, *T. pallidum* multiplies much more slowly than many pathogenic bacteria, having a generation time of about 30 to 33 hours early in the course of infection and longer after the development of (partial) host immunity. This is thought to account for the relatively prolonged duration of therapy needed for the cure of syphilis. It appears that treponemacidal serum penicillin levels must be present for at least 1 to 2 days to cure incubating syphilis, for at least 7 days to cure early syphilis, and for at least 3 weeks to cure infections of more than 1 year's duration. This is sometimes referred to as the time-dose relationship in syphilis therapy, that is, low doses of penicillin are adequate, but only if continuously present for a relatively prolonged duration.

CLINICALLY USEFUL CLASSIFICATIONS OF SYPHILIS

Three different ways of classifying syphilis are shown in Table 1. The second is particularly important epidemiologically and therapeutically, since only early syphilis is considered infectious (with a few exceptions, e.g., pregnant females) and late syphilis requires a longer duration of therapy. Some authorities define early syphilis as syphilis of either less than 2 or less than 4 years' duration; I prefer to define early syphilis as being of less than 1 years' duration. It is important to emphasize that when syphilis is clinically latent, a reactive serologic test for syphilis (STS) is, by definition, the only indication of disease.

TABLE 1 Classifications of Syphilis

1.	Primary:	chancre at site of *T. pallidum* invasion
	Secondary:	mucocutaneous, hepatitis, meningitis, others
	Tertiary:	CNS, cardiovascular, gummatous, other
	Congenital:	early ($\leq$2 years of life), late
	Incubating:	very early syphilis prior to development of a chancre or reactive serologic test for syphilis
2.	Early: (infectious)	infection with *T. pallidum* of less than 1 year (including primary, secondary, incubating, early latent)
	Late:	infection of more than 1 year's duration (includes tertiary, asymptomatic neurosyphilis, late latent)
3.	Latent:	only evidence of syphilis is reactive treponemal STS
	Active:	primary, secondary, tertiary, or congenital

CLINICAL MANIFESTATIONS OF SYPHILIS

T. pallidum is capable of penetrating intact mucous membranes and cracked or abraded skin. Within a few hours after infection, spread to regional lymph nodes occurs, followed by bacteremic dissemination to metastatic systemic foci, long before the appearance of a chancre. An incubation period averaging about 3 weeks and varying inversely with the treponemal inoculum is followed by the appearance of the primary lesion of syphilis, the chancre. This is a painless shallow ulcer at the site of inoculation, genital or extragenital, and is accompanied by firm, nonsuppurative, nontender regional (typically bilateral inguinal) lymphadenopathy. Chancres heal spontaneously in a few weeks even without therapy.

Several weeks to several months later, secondary syphilis may ensue or the disease may remain latent. Secondary syphilis is characterized by highly variable mucocutaneous and systemic findings, including nonpruritic macules on the palmar and plantar skin and elsewhere, highly infectious mucous membrane lesions (mucous patches, condyloma lata), generalized lymphadenopathy, anorexia, fever, aseptic meningitis, hepatitis, nephrotic syndrome, and others. Relapses of secondary syphilis may occur; these generally become progressively milder clinically and usually cease within the first year after infection.

Following the secondary syphilis stage, a period of latency develops, which probably is lifelong in the majority of patients, even without specific antibiotic therapy. However, a minority, perhaps 30 percent, of untreated patients may develop central nervous system, cardiovascular, or gummatous tertiary syphilis.

Classic neurologic syndromes include general paresis and tabes dorsalis. In recent years, cases of classic neurosyphilis have become quite uncommon, presumably due to the widespread use of antibiotics. The Argyll-Robertson pupil—an irregular pupil that does not react to light but does accommodate—is virtually pathognomonic of tertiary syphilis, but is rarely seen now.

In addition, the entity of asymptomatic neurosyphilis is often a clinical concern. Such patients may have nonspecific or no clinical symptoms. The only evidence of neurosyphilis may be a positive serum and cerebrospinal fluid (CSF) serologic test for syphilis (STS) together with CSF pleocytosis and elevation of CSF protein.

Cardiovascular syphilis typically is manifested by development of aneurysmal dilatation of the ascending aorta, resulting in aortic valvular insufficiency. The most significant morbidity and mortality attributable to syphilis is related to cardiovascular and central nervous system syphilis.

The essential lesion of late benign syphilis is the gumma. Gummas result from hypersensitivity reactions, are characterized by granulomatous inflammation with central necrosis, and occur in any organ (and hence are not always "benign"), most commonly in skin, bone, and the liver.

Congenital syphilis, consisting of early and late stages much like those of acquired syphilis, occurs if an untreated mother with syphilis transmits the infection transplacentally to the fetus. In general, the longer the duration of untreated infection in the mother, the less likely the fetus will be infected. The spectrum of illness ranges from a fulminating fetal congenital syphilis to an uninfected child.

EPIDEMIOLOGIC CONSIDERATIONS

Most new cases of syphilis are seen in sexually active persons between the ages of 15 and 30 years. In recent years in the United States, nearly half the cases of early syphilis have occurred in homosexual men. Because of the wide variety of clinical manifestations of syphilis, diagnostic studies are indicated in any sexually active patient with findings consistent with syphilis or suggestive of any sexually transmitted disease (STD) or with a history of contact to a patient with syphilis.

DIFFERENTIAL DIAGNOSIS

Differential diagnosis of primary syphilis includes several other causes of ulcerative genital lesions including trauma, chancroid, lymphogranuloma venereum, and genital herpes simplex virus (HSV) infections. Genital HSV infections are currently much commoner than syphilitic chancres. The situation is further complicated by the possibility that syphilis may coexist with other ulcerative genital lesions and/or other STDs. Any newly developed oral, anal, or genital ulcer in a sexually active person requires that the diagnosis of syphilis be considered and diagnostic studies done.

The differential diagnosis of secondary syphilis is varied, but the diagnosis can be confirmed readily because the STS is virtually always reactive in secondary syphilis. Thus, the main requirement is an appropriate index of suspicion of the diagnosis. Any sexually active patient, especially a male homosexual with new skin lesions, constitutional symptoms, or an undiagnosed illness, should have an STS.

The differential diagnosis of late syphilis most importantly includes cardiovascular diseases resulting in aortic valvular insufficiency and ascending aortic aneurysm and causes of neurologic illness such as the stroke syndrome, seizure disorders, and dementia. Diagnostic studies should be undertaken in any patient with compatible cardiovascular or neurologic illness or possible gummatous lesions for which an alternative etiology is not clearly established. Since nontreponemal STS may be nonreactive in some cases of late syphilis, STS utilizing treponemal antigens (see below) are needed and should be ordered for any patient suspected of having late syphilis, even if a screening, nontreponemal STS is nonreactive.

Syphilis acquired during pregnancy may be subclinical in the mother while frequently causing severe fetal infection. Thus, routine STS at the time of the first prenatal visit is justified in pregnant females. In high-risk patients, an STS should be repeated in the third trimester. In addition, if manifestations of early syphilis develop in pregnancy, prompt diagnostic studies are imperative. Adequate treatment of the mother before the 16th week of pregnancy should prevent fetal damage. Treatment after that time should minimize the damage.

DIAGNOSIS OF SYPHILIS

The diagnosis of syphilis may be made by darkfield (DF) microscopy or serologically. *T. pallidum* may be demonstrated by DF microscopy of an appropriate cutaneous lesion, such as the chancre of primary syphilis or condyloma of secondary syphilis, and is identified by its characteristic morphology and motility. This requires some experience in interpretation since saprophytic nonpathogenic spirochetes morphologically similar to *T. pallidum* may also inhabit moist genital regions and the mouth. Thus, great care must be exercised in interpretation of DF preparations from oral or cervical lesions. Unfortunately, DF microscopy by an experienced microscopist often is not readily available.

There are two main types of STS: nontreponemal tests, such as the Rapid Plasma Reagin (RPR) card test and the Venereal Disease Research Laboratory (VDRL) test; and treponemal tests such as the fluorescent treponemal antibody absorption (FTA-ABS) test or the microhemagglutination test for *T. pallidum* antibodies (MHA-TP, TPHA). Nontreponemal tests utilize a nonspecific (cardiolipin) antigen extracted from beef heart and are technically simple and inexpensive, but have higher incidences of false-positive and false-negative results than treponemal tests. The treponemal tests are more demanding technically (particularly the FTA-ABS test) and more expensive, but utilize specific antigenic material derived from *T. pallidum*. They are more sensitive and specific, though false-positive reactions may occur in pregnancy and collagen-vascular disorders, and false-negative results may occur, particularly in very early syphilis. Nontreponemal tests generally are used for screening purposes and for treatment follow-up. Treponemal tests are used to confirm the diagnosis of syphilis (e.g., +VDRL, +FTA-ABS), to define a "biologic false-positive" nontreponemal STS (e.g., +RPR, −FTA-ABS), or in circumstances where a nontreponemal test is thought to be falsely negative, such as in suspected late syphilis. Treponemal tests tend to remain positive for life regardless of therapy, generally are not quantitated (i.e., titered), and are not useful for follow-up purposes or for assessing adequacy of therapy.

The FTA-ABS, MHA-TP, and RPR tests have not been standardized for testing CSF. The laboratory diagnosis of neurosyphilis is most clear in the setting of a reactive serum treponemal STS, CSF pleocytosis, elevated CSF protein, and a reactive CSF VDRL. Occasionally, the situation is not so clear. Nonreactive CSF test results with nontreponemal STS were well known in a small minority, perhaps 10 percent, of patients with classic neurosyphilis. Whether or not CSF FTA-ABS testing would improve sensitivity of CSF serologic testing has not been determined. Thus routine FTA-ABS testing of CSF is not currently recommended. However, in unusual, carefully selected cases (such as in the evaluation of a patient with an undiagnosed neurologic disorder compatible with neurosyphilis, a reactive serum FTA-ABS, and a nonreactive CSF VDRL), the CSF FTA-ABS test might be worth performing, particularly if a decision to hospitalize for intravenous therapy was a consideration. Consultation with an STD or infectious diseases specialist would probably be appropriate in such cases.

A suggested approach for the use of DF microscopy and STS in primary and secondary syphilis is as follows:

Suspected primary syphilis: Perform DF examination if facilities are available. Consider lesion nonsyphilitic only if three daily DF examinations are negative and nontreponemal STS is persistently negative for a month. If DF is positive, diagnose and treat primary syphilis. Obtain nontreponemal STS. If positive, confirm with serum FTA-ABS test. Otherwise, do not use FTA-ABS test in suspected primary syphilis. A negative nontreponemal STS should be repeated in 1 week and, if still negative, 1 month after the first STS. Unless DF microscopy is positive, a negative nontreponemal test after a month excludes the diagnosis. Most (more than 70%) DF-positive patients with primary syphilis have a reactive STS, but a few—if treated very early—may never develop a reactive STS.

Suspected secondary syphilis: Obtain nontreponemal STS. If positive, confirm with a treponemal STS. If nontreponemal STS is negative the diagnosis of secondary syphilis, for practical purposes, is excluded.

The diagnosis of tertiary syphilis is made in patients with clinical findings suggestive of central nervous system or cardiovascular syphilis or a gumma who have a positive serum treponemal STS with or without a positive serum nontreponemal STS. Most, but not all, patients with tertiary syphilis have a reactive serum nontreponemal STS. Patients with no clinical findings of syphilis, but with a reactive treponemal STS, such as elective surgical patients found to have a reactive screening STS, need to have

TABLE 2 Treatment of Syphilis

Stage of Syphilis	*Patients Without Penicillin Allergy*	*Penicillin-Allergic Patients*
Possible incubating* (epidemiologic treatment)	Benzathine penicillin G (BPG) 2.4 million units IM	----
Primary, secondary, or early latent	BPG 2.4 million units IM	Tetracycline HCl 2.0 g/day × 15 days or erythromycin base or stearate 2.0 g/day × 15 days
Late latent or latent of uncertain duration	CSF normal: BPG 2.4 million units weekly for 3 doses CSF abnormal: treat as neurosyphilis	Treat as neurosyphilis
Late neurosyphilis	Aqueous crystalline penicillin G (ACPG), 4 million units IV every 4 hours × 10 days followed by BPG 2.4 million units IM weekly for 3 doses *or* Aqueous procaine penicillin G (APPG) 2.4 million units IM daily plus probenecid 500 mg PO 4 times/day, both for 10 days, followed by BPG 2.4 million units IM weekly for 3 doses *or* BPG 2.4 million units IM weekly for 3 doses	Tetracycline HCl 2.0 g daily for 30 days
Congenital (treat all neonates with either proved or suspected congenital syphilis)	Symptomatic infants or asymptomatic infants with abnormal CSF: ACPG 25,000 units/kg IM or IV every 12 hours (i.e., 50,000 units/kg/day) for at least 10 days *or* APPG 50,000 units/kg IM daily for at least 10 days *or* Asymptomatic infants with normal CSF: BPG 50,000 units IM in a single dose	Antibiotics other than penicillin should not be used to treat neonates; after the neonatal period, penicillin-allergic patients less than 8 years of age should receive erythromycin in individualized doses, not to exceed daily adult doses, for 30 days; more than 8 years of age, treat with tetracycline in individualized doses, not to exceed daily adult doses, for 30 days
Syphilis in pregnancy	Penicillin, use dosage schedules appropriate for stage of syphilis as recommended for treatment of nonpregnant patients (see above)	Erythromycin stearate or base 2.0 g/day × 15 (early syphilis, and also treat infant with penicillin) or 30 (late syphilis) days

Note: Source: derived from Centers for Disease Control *STD Treatment Guidelines*, revised 1982.
* Patients exposed to infectious syphilis and felt to be at high risk of developing syphilis.

asymptomatic neurosyphilis carefully excluded. Diagnosis of neurosyphilis should be confirmed, in most cases, with a CSF VDRL. As noted above, the FTA-ABS test should not be done routinely on CSF, but might be considered in carefully selected problem cases after consultation with a specialist.

THERAPY OF SYPHILIS

Penicillin is the drug of choice for syphilis therapy. Suggested treatment regimens are summarized in Table 2. Patients with penicillin allergy should be treated with tetracycline. Pregnant women and children under the age of 8 years with congenital or acquired syphilis who are allergic to penicillin should be treated with erythromycin. Patients treated with tetracycline or erythromycin should receive particularly close follow-up since the efficacy of these drugs in syphilis therapy is not well established. There have been a few reports of infants born with congenital syphilis to mothers treated for syphilis during pregnancy with erythromycin.

ADDITIONAL THERAPEUTIC CONSIDERATIONS

There is some difference of opinion regarding the management of patients with neurosyphilis. Although treatment with benzathine penicillin, as outlined in Table 2, probably is effective in many cases of neurosyphilis, some clinicians prefer to hospitalize patients with neurosyphilis for treatment with 4 million units of aqueous crystalline penicillin G given intravenously every 4 hours each day for 10 days.

Treatment of primary and secondary syphilis with penicillin may be followed by a Jarisch-Herxheimer reaction, characterized by chills, fever, myalgia, headache, and other constitutional symptoms. This reaction is not to be confused with an allergic reaction to penicillin. Patients should be forewarned of this reaction, which is best managed with bedrest and aspirin or acetaminophen.

Patients may contract syphilis and another STD (e.g., gonorrhea) with a shorter incubation time than syphilis. These patients often seek medical evaluation while syphilis is still incubating. The effect on incubating syphilis of treatment for other STDs is therefore of interest. The penicillin regimen currently recommended for gonorrhea therapy has been shown to eradicate incubating syphilis. Spectinomycin, as used for gonorrhea therapy, and metronidazole, as used for treating vaginitis, are considered ineffective therapy for incubating syphilis, on the basis of experimental studies. All other regimens (ampicillin, amoxicillin, tetracycline, doxycycline) currently recommended for gonorrhea therapy and tetracycline regimens recommended for therapy of nongonococcal urethritis and lymphogranuloma venereum probably eradicate incubating syphilis, though this is unproved.

FOLLOW-UP AND RETREATMENT OF SYPHILIS

Quantitative nontreponemal STS results are of value in the follow-up of patients treated for syphilis. A decreasing titer or a stable, low titer typically follows satisfactory therapy. Most patients treated for primary syphilis experience reversion of nontreponemal STS to nonreactive within 12 months following treatment. Reversion takes longer after treatment for reinfection, secondary, or early latent syphilis, but usually occurs within 24 months. After treatment for late syphilis, reversion occurs in some cases, whereas a stable, low titer, so-called serofast syphilis, is the result in other patients. A rising titer (fourfold or more) suggests reinfection or inadequacy of therapy. It is worth pointing out that RPR titers typically are reactive to one or two dilutions higher than VDRL titers. Thus, the same test should be used in following up patients treated for syphilis in order to avoid misdiagnosing relapse or reinfection (as might occur, for example, if a VDRL test is done at the time of diagnosis but follow-up is with RPR tests).

All patients with early syphilis and congenital syphilis should be encouraged to return for repeat quantitative nontreponemal STS 3, 6, and 12 months after treatment. Patients with syphilis for more than 1 year's duration should also have a nontreponemal STS 24 months after treatment. Careful follow-up serologic testing is particularly important in patients treated with antibiotics other than penicillin. Examination of CSF should be planned as part of the last follow-up visit after treatment with alternative antibiotics. All patients with neurosyphilis should be carefully followed up with serologic testing for at least 3 years. Such patients should also be reevaluated clinically at 6 month intervals. Repeat CSF examinations should be considered at these times, unless the spinal fluid becomes completely normal with respect to VDRL testing, protein, and white cell count.

Retreatment should be considered when clinical signs or symptoms of syphilis recur or fail to resolve with therapy, when an increasing (fourfold or greater) titer of a nontreponemal STS occurs, or when an initially high-titer nontreponemal STS fails to decrease at least fourfold after a year. The possibility of reinfection should always be considered when retreating patients with early syphilis. A CSF examination should be performed before retreatment unless reinfection and a diagnosis of early syphilis can be established.

As with any STD, it is imperative for public health and disease control purposes that contacts be identified and treated. Thus, the assistance of public health authorities needs to be requested whenever syphilis is diagnosed. Such cooperation is essential for breaking the chain of infection. It may, for example, be possible to identify persons exposed to syphilis in the incubating stage, before symptoms develop. These individuals should be offered "epidemiologic" treatment even though perhaps only 20 to 30 percent of them have actually contracted the disease.

"MINOR" SEXUALLY TRANSMITTED DISEASE

STEPHEN J. KRAUS, M.D.

Syphilis and gonorrhea have traditionally been referred to as "major" venereal diseases, whereas chancroid, granuloma inguinale, and lymphogranuloma venereum have been known as "minor" venereal diseases. Syphilis and gonorrhea are considered major because they are among the commonest reportable infectious diseases and because they may result in serious sequelae. Sequelae of gonorrhea include pelvic inflammatory disease, epididymitis, septic arthritis, endocarditis, and meningitis. Untreated syphilis can result in devastating cardiovascular or central nervous system manifestations. The only "minor" aspect of the minor venereal diseases is their relative rarity in developed countries. Major sequelae occur with the minor venereal diseases. Genital lymphedema (elephantiasis) and destruction of genital tissue can be seen when chancroid, lymphogranuloma venereum, and granuloma inguinale are not treated in their early stages. This chapter reviews the clinical manifestations and diagnosis and therapy of these three sexually transmitted diseases, as well as the same aspects of genital warts. (Pediculosis pubis and scabies are covered in the chapter *Ectoparasitic Infection.*) Management of these infections must include examination of recent sexual contacts for the suspected pathogen and clinical syndrome as well as for other sexually transmitted diseases. These contacts should receive epidemiologic antibiotic treatment for the suspected pathogen when clinical manifestations are absent.

CHANCROID

Patients with chancroid present with one or several painful, purulent, deep, nonindurated, genital ulcers with ragged and undermined edges. Tender, often fluctuant, inguinal lymphadenopathy may be present. *Hemophilus ducreyi* is chancroid's etiology, and it produces lesions after a 3- to 14-day incubation period. Chancroid is commoner among men and, when present in women, is less painful and less likely to have inguinal lymphadenopathy. Chancroid is a common cause of genital ulcer disease in Africa, Central and South America, and Southeast Asia. Recent epidemics have been reported in Winnipeg, Ontario, and more than 500 cases occurred in Orange County, California, over a 2-year period.

Chancroid must be differentiated from other etiologies of genital ulcer disease in sexually active individuals. This differential includes syphilis, genital herpes, lymphogranuloma venereum, granuloma inguinale, fixed drug reactions, and trauma-induced ulcers. Deep ulcers with undermined edges and associated with suppurative inguinal lymphadenopathy are likely to be chancroid, but chancroid-like genital herpes has been described. Laboratory confirmation is essential for accurate diagnosis. Blood clot cultures, autoinoculation to induce similar lesions, and the Ito-Reenstierna skin tests are all outdated confirmatory tests. A gram stain of ulcer exudate has poor sensitivity and specificity. Chancroid diagnosis was revolutionized by the discovery that vancomycin (2 to 3 μg per milliliter) in an appropriate medium (such as chocolate or sheep blood agar) will adequately suppress contaminating bacteria and facilitate growth of the fastidious *H. ducreyi*. Cleaning the ulcer prior to culture is unnecessary. Ulcer exudate is plated directly onto the medium, which is then cross-streaked and incubated for several days in a humid, enriched (5% to 10%) carbon dioxide environment at 35 °C to 36 °C. Bubo aspirate can also be cultured, although *H. ducreyi* is more likely to be isolated from the ulcer.

All Nairobi, California, Winnipeg, and Atlanta isolates are susceptible to erythromycin and ceftriaxone. Cure rates with either of these antimicrobials exceeds 97 percent. Controlled trials found effective regimens to be erythromycin, in a dose of 500 mg by mouth four times a day for 7 days or ceftriaxone 250 mg IM in a single dose. Sulfamethoxazole-trimethoprim, 800 mg and 160 mg (2 regular or 1 double-strength tablet) twice a day by mouth for 7 days is an alternative regimen which can be used in areas where *H. ducreyi* is susceptible to this regimen.

Sulfonamides and tetracyclines are no longer used for treatment of chancroid because widespread resistance has emerged.

Fluctuant lymph nodes should be aspirated to reduce pain and to prevent spontaneous rupture with possible subsequent fibrosis, sinus tract formation, and lymphedema. Aspiration is accomplished by inserting a large-bore needle (16- or 18-gauge) through adjacent normal-appearing skin and then into the abscess. The purulent exudate is aspirated with a 30- to 50-ml syringe. More than one aspiration may be needed.

LYMPHOGRANULOMA VENEREUM

The primary lesion of lymphogranuloma venereum (LGV), a small papule or ulcer, usually goes unnoticed and heals rapidly without scar formation. It is the secondary stage for which patients seek medical care: the inguinal lymphadenitis or hemorrhagic proctitis. Failure to treat the secondary stage results in progression to the tertiary stage—granulomatous ulcers, fistulas, strictures, lymphedema, and elephantiasis. Special serotypes of *Chlamydia trachomatis* (L_1, L_2, L_3) cause LGV. The sporadic cases in North America and Europe are sometimes acquired in endemic areas of Africa, India, or the Caribbean. In contrast to LGV, where patients present only with inguinal nodes and no genital ulcer, other STD etiologies of inguinal adenopathy, such as genital herpes and syphilis, usually have genital ulcers at the time the patient presents with inguinal adenopathy. The differential of LGV's tertiary stage includes late granuloma inguinale and filariasis.

Although *C. trachomatis* can be isolated from LGV lesions and nodes, chlamydial culture is not universally available, and its sensitivity in LGV may be as low as 25 to 30 percent. The antigen used in the Frei skin test is no longer available. Serologic tests are, therefore, the most readily available avenue for the laboratory confirmation of LGV. The LGV complement fixation test is the serology offered by many laboratories. This test is not specific for LGV because the test's antigen cross-reacts with a variety of chlamydial types including the etiology of psittacosis. Therefore, the diagnosis of LGV is based on the combination of clinical signs and an elevated LGV fixation titer. Patients with LGV usually have titers greater than or equal to 1:64; indeed, the diagnosis of LGV should be suspect when the titer is less than 1:64. A twofold titer increase between acute and convalescent sera may occur, but the titer is usually high when the patient first presents in the secondary, or bubo, phase of the disease. A more sensitive, but less available, antibody detection system is the microimmunofluorescent antibody test. This test is also more specific for LGV, and it is frequently possible to detect antibody against the infecting serotype.

Statistically valid, controlled comparison studies of antimicrobial therapy for LGV are lacking. Uncontrolled studies report the following regimens to be effective: tetracycline, 500 mg four times a day; doxycycline, 100 mg twice a day; erythromycin, 500 mg four times a day; or a sulfonamide such as sulfamethoxazole, 2 g initially, then 1 g twice a day. Tetracycline is the preferred drug on the basis of effectiveness and cost; doxycycline is equally effective, but more expensive, erythromycin and sulfonamides are second-line therapy. Each antimicrobial agent is administered for at least 2 weeks and continued until the active manifestations (adenopathy, proctitis, or granulomatous ulcers) have resolved. Fluctuant inguinal lymph nodes should be aspirated by inserting a large-bore needle through adjacent normal-appearing skin and then into the exudate. Sinus tracts and strictures will not respond to antimicrobial therapy and may require surgical intervention. Systemic antimicrobial therapy should precede and accompany such surgery.

GRANULOMA INGUINALE

The genital ulcerations of granuloma inguinale have a beefy-red, "cobblestone" base and an elevated, pearly, glistening border. The ulcers are indurated and painless unless secondarily infected. A similar clinical picture can occur as a variant of chancroid: pseudogranuloma inguinale chancroid. Enlarged inguinal lymph nodes seen with chancroid, herpes, and syphilis are absent with granuloma linguinale, but subcutaneous granulomas in the inguinal area may mimic inguinal adenopathy. If allowed to go untreated, the end stage of granuloma inguinale can be destruction of genital tissue, phimosis, fibrosis, and lymphedema. The diagnosis of granuloma inguinale is confirmed by the cytologic or histologic identification of the etiologic *Calymmatobacterium granulomatis*. These bacteria stain in a bipolar manner and may be encapsulated. They are usually clustered in large monocytes and are referred to as Donovan bodies. Lesions appearing to be granuloma inguinale should also be cultured for *H. ducreyi* to exclude pseudogranuloma inguinale chancroid. Controlled studies of granuloma inguinale therapy are lacking, but tetracycline, 500 mg by mouth four times a day and continued for 2 weeks or until the lesions have healed, has been reported to be effective. Erythromycin or lincomycin have been used to treat granuloma inguinale in pregnancy. Chloramphenicol, 500 mg by mouth three times a day, or gentamicin, 1 mg per kilogram twice a day have been reported to be beneficial in resistant cases.

GENITAL WARTS

Small papules with verrucous (cauliflower-like) surfaces is the usual clinical appearance of genital warts. Variants include similar, but massive, lesions (the giant condyloma acuminatum of Buschke and Loewenstein) and flat warts—slightly elevated plaques with an even surface. Genital warts must be differentiated from molluscum contagiosum (which has an umbilicated apex), condyloma lata of secondary syphils (the darkfield of which should team with *Treponema pallidum*), pearly penile papules (small papules that circumscribe the penile corona), and genital Bowen's disease and carcinoma. Warts on the cervix are usually flat rather than verrucous and are often detected only by colposcopy. Genital warts may not be clinically evident for several months after viral transmission. Genital warts are an STD: two-thirds of sexual contacts of patients with genital warts have or will develop clinically evident genital warts. Anal warts without genital warts correlates with anal intercourse. Neonatal and childhood laryngeal papillomatosis is associated with maternal genital warts.

Genital warts are caused by papillomavirus, a member of the papovavirus family, which also includes the suspected cause of progressive multifocal leukoencephalopathy. More than 25 papillomavirus types have been identified in human warts, some of which are characteristic of genital warts, and some of these have a high association with cervical dysplastic and neoplastic changes.

Genital warts are usually diagnosed by clinical inspection and the exclusion of lesions similar in appearance. Histology of biopsy of currette scrapings can aid in the diagnosis. Colposcopy is needed to adequately evaluate cervical warts. The presence of koiolocytes on Pap smear is a readily available laboratory test to detect cervical papillomaviral infection as well as possible coexisting dysplastic/neoplastic changes.

The traditional and still the most widely employed therapy for genital warts is the topical application of a 10 to 25 percent solution of podophyllin in alcohol of tincture of benzoin. Allowing the applied solution to dry on the wart reduces irritation of the adjacent areas. The medication is thoroughly washed off 3 hours later and reapplied at weekly or twice weekly intervals until the wart is no longer clinically evident. The time between podophyllin application and removal can be gradually extended, depending upon patient tolerance to podophyllin irritation. Podophyllin can have systemic toxic effects when large volumes are used. Toxicities include neurotoxicity and abortion. This form of therapy is therefore contraindicated during pregnancy. Cervical and urethral papillomaviral infections should also not be treated with podophyllin.

Three months after starting podophyllin therapy, only 22 percent of patients are free of genital warts. This compares with 62 percent and 92 percent "cures" 3 months after cryotherapy with liquid nitrogen and electrosurgery, respectively. Cryotherapy, if available, is the recommended therapy for genital warts, and electrosurgery, which is more painful, is the second choice. However, podophyllin is most widely available. Surgical removal is usually needed for the giant condyloma acuminatum of Buschke and Loewenstein. Genital wart therapies attempt to eradicate clinically evident lesions. Sites of subclinical papillomaviral infection would ordinarily be missed, and, therefore, follow-up examinations are needed to treat newly detectable lesions.

SKIN AND SOFT TISSUE INFECTIONS

ACNE VULGARIS

RUTH K. FREINKEL, M.D.

Although almost everyone has acne vulgaris at some time, expression of the clinical picture and the course are extremely variable. The various types of lesions (comedones, papules, pustules, nodules, cysts) may be present alone or in combination. The entire acne area (face, neck, upper trunk) may be involved or just one part. Onset may be at puberty or much later in the late teens or early twenties. The disease may be present for a few years or may endure into midlife. The course may be progressive in its evolution or undergo cycles of exacerbation and remission. Inevitably, however, acne resolves spontaneously, leaving in its wake scars, which do not necessarily correlate with the severity of the preceding lesions. Resolution of acne does not appear to be accompanied by any changes in the known pathogenic factors such as hormonal stimulation, levels of sebum production, or follicular bacterial population.

Despite the unpredictability of the clinical picture, basic factors impinging upon pathogenesis are quite well understood. Acne is an inflammatory process centering upon those pilosebaceous organs of the face, neck, and upper trunk in which the patulous ducts of very large sebaceous glands open into the follicular canal of small, relatively inactive hairs. Two necessary but insufficient factors impinge upon this anatomic site in the production of acne lesions. One is the production of large amounts of sebum by the sebaceous gland under stimulation by androgens. The presence of sebum allows colonizaiton of the lower pilosebaceous follicle by microaerobic *Propionibacterium acnes*. Accompanying these changes is the development of the primary lesion of acne: abnormal keratinization of the follicle resulting in obstruction of the duct. Although the precise cause of the dyskeratosis remains unknown, once the flow of sebum is obstructed, both comedones and inflammatory lesions are triggered by bacterial products such as lytic enzymes and their products—specifically, those of the action of bacterial lipases on sebum lipids. The inflammatory response is not directed against *P. acnes* initially. However, when follicular rupture occurs it is followed by a chronic granulomatous response involving the contents of the follicle, including both bacteria and cellular debris. This process produces chronic, often self-perpetuating, nodules and cysts.

The above considerations provide the basis for principles of therapy in acne vulgaris.

1. Since there is, to date, no cure of the primary causes, treatment can only be suppressive until the disease resolves spontaneously.
2. In most cases of acne, excepting the most severe ones, suppression of the inflammatory reaction suffices to produce clinical remission, and, in mild cases, relieving follicular obstruction (comedolysis) may be all that is needed.
3. The unpredictability of the extent and course dictates that treatment be tailored to fit the clinical picture presented by each patient at various points in time.
4. Direct delivery of pharmacologic agents to the skin (i.e., topical applications) is preferable to systemic therapy if the efficacy is equivalent.
5. Acne usually occurs in otherwise healthy young people, and the treatment should not produce iatrogenic diseases.

Using these principles, it is possible to plan effective therapeutic regimens employing currently available agents which (*1*) alleviate blockage of the follicle, (*2*) decrease the follicular population of *P. acnes*, and (*3*) suppress sebum production.

THERAPY

Comedolytic Agents

Vitamin A and its analogues, the retinoids, reverse the follicular hyperkeratosis and thus act as comedolytic agents. Vitamin A acid is the topically active form, and 13-*cis* retinoic acid is the agent used for oral administration. The latter has profound effects on the skin. In addition to comedolysis, it suppresses sebum production and hair growth, and increases skin fragility. It appears to cure severe nodulocystic acne, but ordinary acne recurs after treatment is stopped.

Anti-Inflammatory Agents

A variety of nonspecific and specific topical antimicrobial agents provide effective treatment for mild to moderate inflammatory acne. Lotions containing broad-spectrum antibiotics and formulations containing benzoyl peroxide are the most effective preparations. The latter are available in many nonprescription preparations as are a number of less effective antiseptic creams, lotions, and gels. Systemic administration of broad-spectrum antibiotics tends to be more effective and may afford direct inhibition of chemotaxis in addition to antimicrobial actions. The anti-inflammatory effects of glucocorticoids may be employed advantageously in intralesional injections of chronic nodules and cysts. However, both topically applied and systemically administered fluorinated glucocorticoids are acnegenic and are rarely indicated for the treatment of acne.

Suppression of Sebum Production

Cyclic administration of estrogen-progestin combinations (oral contraceptive agents) induces suppression of sebum production and ameliorates acne. This effect is due to suppression of ovarian function and to some peripheral competition with the actions of androgens on the sebaceous gland. If excess production of adrenal androgens has been documented to provide a major source of androgenic hormones in female patients, oral contraceptives may not suffice. In these cases, low suppressive doses of glucocorticoids with or without oral contraceptives may provide relief for patients with otherwise recalcitrant nodular cystic acne.

Other Modalities

Although moderate attention to normal hygiene need not be discouraged, there is no evidence that cleansing the skin improves acne. On the other hand, cosmetics containing oil, including moisturizing lotions, are comedogenic and should be avoided. Ultraviolet light, either in the form of natural sunlight or artificial ultraviolet radiation, appears to be beneficial. Dietary factors do not have a consistent, documented role in acne, and dietary injunctions should not be imposed.

DOSAGES AND COMPLICATIONS

Vitamin A acid (isotretinoin) in strengths of 0.01 to 0.05 percent in lotions, gels, or creams is usually applied once a day. Irritating effects can be minimized by starting at a low concentration every other day; creams are less irritating than gels at the same concentration. Because topical isotretinoin has been reported to promote ultraviolet-induced skin cancer in animals, it is reasonable to limit its use during heavy sun exposure.

Oral administration of 13-*cis* retinoic acid in doses ranging from 0.1 to 2 mg per kilogram per day is effective in most patients in the range of 0.5 to 1.0 mg per kilogram. Courses of treatment for 4 months are followed by a rest period of several months or longer until the disease recurs. Because of the potentially serious adverse reactions, this drug should be reserved for patients with severe, nodular, recalcitrant cystic acne who have reached sexual maturity. Most patients experience dryness of the mouth, lips, and eyes at higher doses. Nausea, fatigue, myalgias, arthralgias, and alopecia are not uncommon. Serious effects include hyperostosis of bones, calcification of spinal ligaments, and early closure of the epiphysis. 13-*cis* retinoic acid is teratogenic, and severe congenital anomalies occur with alarming frequency when the drug is administered to pregnant women. Therefore, the drug should not be administered to women in the childbearing age in the absence of documented compliance with the most effective methods of birth control. Its use is not recommended as a substitute for other treatment.

Topical preparations of erythromycin, tetracycline, and clindamycin are available as 1 to 2 percent solutions and are applied one to two times daily. They appear to be safe and moderately effective especially when used in conjunction with other topical preparations.

Benzoyl peroxide in concentrations of 2.5 to 10 percent is formulated in lotions, gels, and creams. Irritating effects parallel therapeutic effects and occur least often with lotions and most frequently with gels; however, the irritation decreases with prolonged use, and a regimen of gradual increases in concentration and more efficient vehicles is advisable.

Broad-spectrum antibiotics administered orally remain the mainstay of acne therapy. Tetracycline is the first drug of choice, followed by erythromycin and minocycline.

Most patients respond to moderate or low doses of tetracycline or erythromycin. Treatment may be begun with as little as 500 mg given in a single dose, although large or heavy patients may require 750 mg divided into two doses. It is important to instruct patients to take the drugs on an empty stomach; tetracycline should always be taken at least 1.5 hours after or before ingestion of milk or milk products to insure good absorption. There is no need to prime the patient with a large dose of 1,000 mg per day; although this may slightly accelerate a favorable response, it has the disadvantage of increasing the appearance of gastrointestinal adverse effects and vaginal candidiasis. If response is not satisfactory after 4 weeks, the dose may be increased. Maximal improvement usually requires 2 to 3 months of treatment with the initial dose. After that time, patients can often be maintained on as little as 250 mg given daily or every other day. Treatment should be continued while the disease is active, although rest periods of 2 to 3 months each year are advisable.

Bacterial resistance often develops after prolonged administration of a given antibiotic and requires change to a different agent. In this situation, minocycline (starting at 100 mg per day) is very useful; minocycline is perhaps more effective than either tetracycline or erythromycin, but its use is limited because of its far greater costliness. Trimethoprim-sulfamethoxazole given once a day is also helpful for short-term use when other antibiotics fail or cannot be tolerated.

Gastrointestinal effects are common with all broad-spectrum antibiotics. They should not be ignored because of the danger of pseudomembranous colitis. Vaginitis due to candida albicans is a frequent complication and may prevent the use of oral antibiotics. Tetracyclines can cause phototoxicity and patients need to be careful to avoid excessive sun exposure. Tetracycline should never be used in pregnant women and should be discontinued several months prior to efforts to conceive since the drug deposits in fetal bones and teeth. In addition to other side effects, minocycline causes reversible vestibular dysfunction and may cause hyperpigmentation.

Oral contraceptives are helpful in women when other agents fail to control the disease. Those with very low estrogen content may not be as effective, and, occasionally, sebotrophic effects of certain progestins may worsen acne. In addition, the many other complications of cyclic hormone therapy interdicts their use as a routine treatment for acne, and risk-benefit ratios should be carefully considered before instituting their use.

ECTOPARASITIC INFECTION

HARLEY A. HAYNES, M.D.

Ectoparasites that affect humans include the following: (1) *Demodex folliculorum*; (2) sucking lice of the order Anoplura, including *Phthirus pubis* and *Pediculus humanis*, (*P. humanis capitis, P. humanis corporis*); (3) mites of the suborder Sarcoptiformes, family Sarcoptidae, including *Sarcoptes scabiei* var. *hominis, Sarcoptes scabiei* var. *canis, Notoedres cati*, and *Knemidokoptes mutans* and *K. laevis*; and (4) Sarcoptiformes, family Psoroptidae. In addition, a variety of house mites, food mites, grain mites, harvest mites, and bird and rodent mites either bite or temporarily infest man or cause allergic reactions upon contact, but these are not truly parasitic in man.

DERMODICIDOSIS

Demodex folliculorum is a small mite that is an obligate parasite of the human pilosebaceous follicle but may not be the cause of any disease. Infestation involves nearly all people over the age of 5. The mite may be seen on scrapings of stratum corneum from time to time and is clearly increased in some cases of acne rosacea. However, treatment directed at the mite seems not to be required. Acne rosacea is usually treated with low doses of tetracycline (250–500 mg orally per day). Occasionally individuals, usually female, who never use soap and water on the face have large populations of *Demodex folliculorum*, which may contribute to inflammation. Cleansing with soap and water appears to be all that is required to restore the situation to normal.

PHTHIRIASIS PUBIS

Phthirus pubis is widespread and fairly common. Infestation is usually sexually transmitted but may be acquired from contact with clothing or towels or shed hairs on which adult lice or nits are attached. The clinical presentation is generally that of moderate to severe pruritus of infested areas. The pubic area is usually involved, but the body hair, such as on the axillae, eyebrows, and eyelashes, may be involved. The patient is often unaware of any infestation, but with good lighting the examiner should be able to spot the shiny white nits, which are the egg cases, attached to the hairs in the infested area, and on closer inspection the adult lice, looking somewhat the color of freckles, will be seen on the surface of the skin, usually holding on to one or two hairs. Occasionally skin lesions representing a hypersensitivity reaction to the bite may be seen as blue-gray macules. Severe scratching and secondary infection are not common.

Treatment

The patient and sexual and household contacts should all be treated.

One percent gamma benzene hexachloride lotion (lindane, Kwell, Gammene) applied to the affected area (except eyelashes), washed off in no longer than 8 hours, and possibly as soon as 10 minutes, is usually effective in a single application. Retreatment in one week may be advised if indicated. This treatment is ovicidal, but the nits will remain attached to the hairs unless they are removed with a fine-tooth comb.

An over-the-counter treatment that is apparently as effective as gamma benzene hexachloride is a pyrethrum preparation, RID, which is available without prescription and includes a fine-tooth comb for nit removal.

Eyelash infestations are most easily treated by manual removal of nits and lice using forceps. Alternatively, an application of 0.025 percent physostigmine ophthalmic ointment will cause the lice to drop off. Smothering the lice with plain petrolatum jelly twice daily for 8 days also is effective.

Treatment of fomites is usually not necessary, but if desired, it can be accomplished by a spray of pyrethrum or gamma benzene hexachloride. Aerosol sprays should not be used for application on patients.

Consider obtaining cultures for gonorrhea and serologic testing for syphilis.

General facts about the life cycle of lice are important in the education and therapy of patients. The life cycle is similar for *Phthirus pubis* pediculosis and *Pediculosis humanis*; it is about 1 month, during which time the female lays 7 to 10 eggs each day. The eggs hatch in about 8 days, but may be delayed up to a month if away from body heat. The nits require an additional 8 days to reach maturity. A newly hatched louse must feed within 24 hours or die, and mature lice can survive no longer than 10 days without a blood meal. Even at the optimal temperature of 15 °C, they usually survive only 2 to 3 days away from the host. The eggs are attached to hairs near their exit point from the skin in the case of the pubic louse and the head louse. The length of time an infestation has been present may be estimated by how far out on the hairs nits can be seen. The poorly named body louse feeds on the host but lays the eggs on threads on the clothing in close contact with the skin, mostly on the inside seams. Nits may occasionally be attached to body hairs. All of these lice are about 3 to 4 mm long. The pediculi are longer than their width, the phthirus is wider than its length.

PEDICULOSIS CAPITIS

The head louse is seen worldwide and is fairly common in elementary school populations, even in affluent communities. Infestation is transmitted by very close contact and by shared hats, caps, brushes, and combs. The head louse is usually confined to the scalp but occasionally invades the beard. The number of nits greatly exceeds the number of adult lice, as patients have only 10 or fewer lice at any time. Pruritis is a major symptom, leading to scratching and frequent secondary infection. Occipital and cervical lymphadenopathy frequently develop and may be presenting signs.

Treatment

Identify and treat all affected individuals and, possibly, other close contacts as simultaneously as possible. Discontinue the sharing of hats, caps, towels, brushes, and combs.

Shampoo with 1 percent gamma benzene hexachloride shampoo, leaving the shampoo on for 10 minutes before rinsing. This may not be adequate contact time to kill the eggs; therefore, removal of as many nits as possible with a fine-tooth comb, or even clipping the hair to a shorter length in the case of an extremely long-lasting infestation, will reduce the possibility of viable eggs producing reinfection. A second shampoo treatment 10 days after the first is good insurance. Adverse side effects from gamma benzene hexachloride, particularly neurotoxicity, should not be a problem when it is used for pubic lice or head lice as described above, owing to the brief contact time and the small surface area treated.

The pyrethrum preparation RID, which is available without prescription, may be used in a 10-minute application and comes complete with a fine-tooth comb. Retreatment in 10 days seems reasonable for this preparation as well.

In the unlikely event that one of the two above treatments is ineffective due to resistance to the insecticide, malathion lotion, 0.5 percent (Prioderm Lotion, the Purdue Frederick Co, Norwalk, CT) has been shown to be effective when permitted to remain on the hair and scalp for approximately 12 hours, followed by shampooing with a neutral shampoo. Ten percent crotamiton lotion (Eurax, Westwood Pharmaceutical Co) has been reported effective in almost all patients after a single 24-hour application. A few patients required retreatment in 8 days.

If pyoderma is present, oral erythromycin or cloxacillin (in order of preference) and topical chlorhexidine (Hibiclens) washes are indicated.

PEDICULOSIS CORPORIS

Diagnosis of body lice usually requires finding nits in the seams of the inner garments, as examination of the skin surface generally shows nothing other than excoriations and possible secondary infection. Occasionally a nit or so may be found on body hair. Individuals with this infestation are generally exceedingly ill kempt. Differential diagnosis would include consideration of scabies—which should be sought by examining the skin for burrows and scraping the skin to see whether microscopic evidence of scabies can be found—and other metabolic causes of pruritus unrelated to infestation, such as liver or kidney dysfunction, lymphoma, polycythemia vera, and so on.

Treatment

Impound all infested clothing, place it in a plastic bag, spray with either gamma benzene hexachloride or pyrethrum, and close the bag tightly. Other effective pediculicides with which to treat the clothing are 1 percent malathion powder or 100 percent DDT powder. Alternatively, storing the clothes in the bag for 1 month without a chemical pediculicide will render them safe. Also, sending them to be cleaned and pressed or laundered and ironed is an effective way of killing the lice and their eggs.

If lice or nits are found on the skin or hair of the patient, treat with an overnight application of 1 percent gamma benzene hexachloride lotion, followed by bathing in soap and water.

SCABIES

The mite family *Sarcoptes* causes scabies in man and mange in other mammals. The mites are variants of a single species, *Sarcoptes scabiei*. While the host specificity is not complete, the mites survive for only a short period on another host. *Notoedres* is primarily responsible for infestation of cats and rabbits, but rarely of man. *Knemidokoptes* infests poultry but rarely man. Mites of the family *Psoroptidae* cause mange in many domestic animals and can be transmitted to man. *Sarcoptes scabiei* var. *hominis* is morphologically indistinguishable from the other races of this mite species. The female mite measures about 0.4 × 0.3 mm and when fertilized excavates a burrow in the stratum corneum. Each day she burrows an additional 2 mm or so and deposits 2 or 3 eggs to a total of 10 to 25 eggs and then dies in the burrow unless excoriation by the host removes her. The larvae emerge from the eggs after 3 to 4 days and migrate to the skin surface, where they reach maturity about 2 to 2-½ weeks after the eggs were laid. Copulation occurs on the skin surface; shortly thereafter the male dies and the impregnated female burrows into the stratum corneum to repeat the life cycle described above. The infestation may be spread by sexual contact or close personal contact. It is common for an entire household to become infested.

The mite tends to infest certain areas of the skin. The fingers, particularly the lateral aspects and the web spaces, and the flexor surfaces of the wrists are involved most frequently. In men the penis and scrotum and in women the region of the nipple are frequently involved. In children palms and soles are often infested. In a variation known as Norwegian scabies, there is massive infestation of the individual; erythema and scaling occur initially on the palms, soles, face, neck, scalp, and trunk and may become generalized. The diagnostic skin lesion is a burrow in the stratum corneum measuring about 0.5 mm in diameter and several millimeters in length. It has a wavy, linear shape. Upon close inspection using a hand lens, a grayish dot may be seen at the leading end of the burrow which is the location of the adult female mite. Burrows may be revealed by applying ink to the skin and then washing it off, staining the burrow track, but this is not usually necessary. The typical diagnostic burrows are produced only by *Sarcoptes scabiei* var. *hominis* and not by the animal mites. Microscopic identification of the mite, the larvae, or the fecal pellets is desirable before committing the patient and contacts to total cutaneous applications of gamma benzene hexachloride. The easiest technique is to take a # 15 scalpel blade and shave off a whole burrow, place it upon a microscope slide, apply some 10 percent potassium hydroxide (but do not heat the slide), place a cover slip on top, and examine it directly under the microscope. Alternatively, scraping of the surface of the burrow may be done either dry or using a drop of mineral oil to collect the mite and ova and larvae. The whole droplet is then moved to the microscope slide and examined with a cover slip on top without the addition of KOH. A very pruritic patient will have many excoriations and few typical lesions will be available for ready microscopic demonstration of the organism. Several tries to demonstrate the organism are desirable, but, if necessary, treatment on suspicion may be instituted.

Treatment

Treat all affected individuals and all close contacts as simultaneously as possible. Since the pruritus and most of the skin lesions seem to be hypersensitivity reactions occurring only after 3 to 4 weeks of infestation, it is not possible to rule out infestation because of lack of symptoms or easily visible signs. Great care must be used in treating premature infants, normal neonates, and pregnant women because of the concern about neurotoxicity from gamma benzene hexachloride.

Apply 1 percent gamma benzene hexachloride lotion to the entire skin surface, giving special attention to web spaces and heavily infested areas. *Do not* recommend a hot bath or shower prior to the application. After 6 to 8 hours have the patient bathe thoroughly in soap and water. If this preparation is used on infants or pregnant women the bathing is recommended after 4 hours. In general, a single such application will be effective, provided reinfestation from contacts does not occur. If necessary, preferably only if infestation can still be confirmed microscopically, retreatment in 10 to 14 days can be recommended.

Concomitant therapy for the hypersensitivity dermatitis is desirable in many cases. Anti-histamines, such as chlorpheniramine maleate, 4–12 mg every 4 to 6 hours as necessary and as tolerated, combined with a midpotency topical steroid such as triamcinolone cream 0.1 percent, and applications of 0.25 percent menthol lotion for itching as needed, to be continued for 2 weeks and extended as required are usually sufficient.

Patients should be warned about unnecessary overtreatment and retreatment with gamma benzene hexachloride, with emphasis on seizures as a major consequence. The physician should be prepared to encounter a certain amount of parasitophobia or other neurotic reaction to this infestation, which can result in pruritus and a belief that infestation is still active long after it has been objectively cleared.

Alternative therapies are either less efficacious or cosmetically unpleasant. The most reasonable alternative to gamma benzene hexachloride lotion is crotamiton cream or lotion (Eurax) applied once daily for 2 days. There are no reports of toxicity, but there have been no studies of its toxicity in infants and pregnant women. Six to 10 percent precipitated sulfur in a water-washable base or in petrolatum applied daily for 3 days is effective but messy. It is probably the safest treatment for infants and pregnant women. Another regimen that has been reported to be effective, but which I have never used, is 20 to 25 percent benzyl benzoate applied daily for 2 to 3 days, and 10 percent thiabendazole suspension applied twice daily for 5 days or taken orally in a dose of 25 mg per kilogram daily for 10 days. In the case of severe Norwegian scabies resistant to topical therapy, systemic methotrexate has been reported to be effective.

Treatment of fomites is not generally necessary, as fomite transmission is not as important as direct contact. Simple laundering of items is sufficient.

Consider obtaining cultures for gonorrhea and serologic tests for syphilis.

CELLULITIS AND SOFT TISSUE INFECTION

THOMAS T. YOSHIKAWA, M.D.

Infections of the skin and soft tissue may involve all layers of the integument, fascia, and muscle and may be complicated by necrosis or sepsis. This discussion will be limited to infections involving the skin that are not usually associated with crepitus and gangrene: impetigo, erysipelas, cellulitis, folliculitis, furuncle, and carbuncle.

Several general principles should be considered when managing patients with these particular dermatologic infections:

1. Determine clinically whether the patient can be managed as an outpatient or requires hospitalization. Factors that weigh in favor of inpatient therapy include the presence of systemic toxicity (e.g., fever, chills); the presence of significant underlying conditions such as insulin-dependent diabetes mellitus, neutropenia, or immunosuppression; involvement of the facial region, hands, or adjacent joint space; and the presence of surrounding edema or cutaneous necrosis.
2. Most of these skin infections are caused by group A beta-hemolytic streptococci and/or coagulase-positive *Staphylococcus aureus*.
3. Most strains of *S. aureus* produce penicillinase (i.e., are penicillin-resistant), and therefore this bacterium is best treated with a beta-lactamase-resistant antibiotic.

IMPETIGO

Impetigo is the commonest cutaneous bacterial infection. It presents clinically as two distinct types—crusted impetigo and bullous impetigo.

Crusted Impetigo

This form of impetigo occurs predominantly in preschool-aged children, with a peak seasonal incidence in the late summer and early fall. The commonest etiology is group A beta-hemolytic streptococci with *S. aureus* coisolated in 50 to 60 percent of patients. However, it is thought that the role of *S. aureus* under these circumstances is a subsidiary one. *S. aureus* may be isolated alone in crusted impetigo in 5 to 10 percent of cases. The lesion of crusted impetigo is an inflammation of the superficial skin layer between the stratum corneum and stratum granulosum.

The cutaneous lesions begin as small, thin-roofed vesicles that rapidly become pustular and easily rupture. The purulent drainage then dries, leaving a thick, soft, honey-colored crust. The lesion may vary in size from 1 to 3 cm and may be spread to other parts of the body by autoinoculation. The extremities and face are most commonly infected. The lesions are painless and heal without scarring. Regional lymphadenopathy commonly occurs, but systemic symptoms are generally absent.

The diagnosis is made clinically and generally is not difficult. Early vesicles or weeping lesions can be gram-stained or cultured, but this is not necessary in most patients unless staphylococci are suspected or the initial antibiotic therapy fails.

The treatment of choice for streptococcal impetigo is penicillin. Either oral or intramuscular preparations can be prescribed. Phenoxymethyl penicillin should be given orally for 10 days in doses of 50 mg per kilogram per day (in four equal doses) and 2 g per day (in four equal doses) to children and adults, respectively. Benzathine penicillin as a single intramuscular injection may be given as an alternative drug. The doses for children and adults are 50,000 units per kilogram and 2.4 million units, respectively. Patients allergic to penicillin should be treated with oral erythromycin (50 mg per kilogram per day, divided in four equal doses, for children; 2 g per day, in four equal doses, for adults). Topical treatment using warm soap and water compresses is valuable in removing crusts, debris, and dirt.

Bullous Impetigo

Bullous impetigo occurs less frequently than crusted impetigo. Newborn and older children are particularly susceptible. The infection is caused by *S. aureus*, which liberates a toxin, epidermolysin. These strains generally belong to *S. aureus* phage group II and can cause staphylococcal scalded-skin syndrome. The histopathology of bullous impetigo is similar to that for crusted impetigo.

The lesion of bullous impetigo starts as a vesicle that rapidly evolves to a bulla, 2 to 5 cm in diameter. The bulla is flaccid and has no peripheral erythema. It generally ruptures, leaving a raw, red base, which will eventually dry and form a thin, light brown, lacquer-like crust. Systemic symptoms are generally absent.

The diagnosis of bullous impetigo is made clinically by its typical appearance. *S. aureus* may be isolated from the lesions by culture.

Treatment should be initiated with an oral penicillinase-resistant penicillin, i.e., cloxacillin or dicloxacillin, for 10 days. The doses of cloxacillin or dicloxacillin for childen are 50 mg per kilogram per day (not to exceed the adult dose) and 25 mg per kilogram per day, both given in four equally divided doses. Adults should receive 2 g of cloxacillin or 1 g of dicloxacillin in four equally divided doses daily.

ERYSIPELAS

Erysipelas is a relatively uncommon cutaneous infection that occurs in the very young, the elderly, the debilitated, and individuals with chronic ulcers or lymphedema of the skin. Although it is a form of cellulitis, the distinct characteristics of erysipelas warrant a separate discussion.

The etiology of erysipelas is almost always group A beta-hemolytic streptococci. Group B streptococci may be isolated in newborns with this infection. Occasionally, other streptococci or, rarely, *S. aureus* may cause erysipelas. The histopathology of the skin shows intense edema, vascular dilation, abundant streptococci in tissue spaces and lymphatic channels, and leukocytic cellular infiltration. The dermis is primarily involved, with the epidermis only secondarily affected.

The cutaneous lesion of erysipelas is characteristically on the face, but may also be found on the scalp, extremities, and abdominal wall (especially with neonates with umbilical stump infections). The dermopathy is an erythematous, hot, raised (edema), indurated, tender, circumscribed lesion with a distinct advancing and elevated border. The margins are often irregular and serpiginous. Occasionally, vesicles and bullae develop. Patients are generally systemically ill with fever, chills, malaise, and headache.

Erysipelas is diagnosed by the typical clinical features of the lesion in association with constitutional symptoms. Patients may have bacteremia, and, therefore, blood cultures should be obtained. Culture of the skin, including the advancing edge, is of little microbiologic value and is not recommended. A brisk leukocytosis is common.

All patients should be hospitalized, and treatment should be begun with intravenous aqueous penicillin G. Children should receive 25,000 units per kilogram of penicillin per day in four divided doses, and adults should be treated with 8 million units per day in four divided doses. After the patient clinically improves, oral phenoxymethyl penicillin may be prescribed (dose is the same as for impetigo) to complete a 10-day treatment course. Patients with serious penicillin allergy may be treated with parenteral clindamycin (children, 20 mg per kilogram per day in three divided doses; adults, 1,800 mg per kilogram per day in three divided doses or vancomycin (children, 30 mg per kilogram per day in four divided doses; adults, 2 g per day in four divided doses).

CELLULITIS

Cellulitis is an acute inflammatory lesion of the skin that initially involves the epidermis and dermis and later spreads to the deeper subcutaneous tissues. It can occur in all age groups and usually is antedated by some type of skin injury, trauma, or decubitus ulcer.

The etiology of cellulitis is most frequently group A beta-hemolytic streptococci or *S. aureus*. However, in neonates or young children, group B streptococci or *Hemophilus influenzae*, respectively, may also be a cause of this infection. In leukopenic immunocompromised patients, gram-negative bacilli, especially *Pseudomonas aeruginosa*, should be considered as a potential etiology of cellulitis. With long-standing decubitus or diabetic ulcers, anaerobic bacteria, including *Bacteroides fragilis*, may be associated with cellulitis.

Cellulitis is typically erythematous, tender, warm and edematous. The borders are not elevated or sharply defined. Lymphangitic spread may occur proximally; tender, regional lymphadenopathy is found in one-half of the patients. Local abscesses with tissue necrosis may develop. The infection may occur anywhere on the body, but common sites are the extremities, sacrum, and surgical wound. Depending on the severity of the cellulitis or the patient's underlying illness, systemic symptoms—including shock, fever, chills, delirium, malaise, or weakness—may be prominent.

The diagnosis of cellulitis is not difficult and is based on its appearance. Patients who are otherwise healthy and do not have clinical features requiring hospitalization do not require special diagnostic studies. However, inpatients should have blood cultures performed, open wounds or drainage cultured and gram-stained, and the leading edge of the cellulitis aspirated for microbiologic studies.

Outpatient treatment for cellulitis should be with cloxacillin or dicloxacillin (see Impetigo section for doses) for 10 days. Patients with serious penicillin allergies may be treated with oral clindamycin (children, 10 mg per kilogram per day in four divided doses; adults, 600 mg per day in four divided doses) or erythromycin (see Impetigo section for doses). In young children, *H. influenzae* should be considered as a possible etiology if therapy with cloxacillin or dicloxacillin fails to result in clinical improvement or if the cellulitis involves the facial region and the child is ill. The antibiotic recommended for serious *H. influenzae* infection is chloramphenicol, 75 to 100 mg per kilogram per day in four divided doses. If the organism is ampicillin-sensitive, the drug may be given in doses of 200 mg per kilogram per day in six divided doses. Immunocompromised patients with cellulitis should be hospitalized and empirically treated with combination chemotherapy chosen from an aminoglycoside, broad-spectrum penicillin (e.g., piperacillin), or cephalosporin. Patients thought to have anaerobic bacteria (particularly *B. fragilis*) as a component of the cellulitis require therapy with such parenteral antibiotics as clindamycin, metronidazole, chloramphenicol, or cefoxitin.

FOLLICULITIS

Folliculitis is an infection within hair follicles. Damage or traction of the hair, maceration or occlusion of the skin, blockage of a pilosebaceous unit, or exposure to certain chemicals predisposes to folliculitis. The pyoderma may be superficial or deep.

The etiology of folliculitis is usually *S. aureus*, but occasionally streptococci and gram-negative bacilli may be causative. With superficial folliculitis there is an acute inflammatory reaction in the follicle area. With more chronic and deep folliculitis, lymphocytes, plasma cells, granulomatous reaction, destruction of sebaceous gland, or fibrosis may occur.

The skin lesion begins as a small pustule near the hair-follicle opening and is associated with redness and mild tenderness. Crusting forms later as the pustule ages or ruptures. Deep folliculitis is associated with greater inflammatory reaction. Folliculitis occurs in hairy parts of

TABLE 1 Summary of Cellulitis and Soft Tissue Infection

Type of Infection	*Skin Involvement*	*Etiology*	*Clinical Characteristics*	*Site of Infection*	*Treatment*
Crusted impetigo	Epidermis	Streptococci	Vesiculae; pustules; yellow-brown crusts	Face; extremities	Oral penicillin
Bullous impetigo	Epidermis	Staphylococci	Bullae; raw base	Extremities; trunk	Oral cloxacillin or dicloxacillin
Erysipelas	Epidermis; dermis	Streptococci	Red, hot, tender plaque with elevated borders	Face; extremities	Hospitalization; parenteral penicillin
Cellulitis	Epidermis; dermis; subcutaneous	Streptococci; staphylococci; others	Red, warm, tender, with irregular, flat borders	Anywhere	Oral cloxacillin or dicloxacillin; hospitalization in select patients
Folliculitis	Epidermis; dermis	Staphylococci	Inflammation near hair follicle	Head, neck, groin, axilla, thigh	Local compresses
Furuncle and carbuncle	Epidermis; dermis; subcutaneous	Staphylococci	Abscess around follicle	Same as folliculitis	Local compresses; oral cloxacillin or dicloxacillin; hospitalize select patients, drainage of large lesions

the body, i.e., face, scalp, axilla, groin, and thigh. A form of deep folliculitis of the bearded area is called sycosis barbae.

Therapy is primarily topical care. Cleansing of the involved skin with hexachlorophene-containing soaps is generally adequate for most cases of folliculitis. Occasionally, antibiotics (e.g., cloxacillin or dicloxacillin) may be needed for extensive or deep lesions.

FURUNCLE AND CARBUNCLE

A furuncle (''boil'') is caused by perifolliculitis progressing to a localized abscess of the skin and subcutaneous tissue. A carbuncle is a larger furuncle or several interconnecting furuncles located in deep tissues. Furunculosis occurs frequently in persons with nasal carriage of staphylococci, severe acne, blood dyscrasias, defect in neutrophil function, diabetes mellitus, and immunoglobulinopathy and in patients on corticosteroid therapy. However, most cases of furuncles or recurrent furunculosis occur in healthy persons.

The etiology of furuncles and carbuncles is usually *S. aureus*, although streptococci and, rarely, gram-negative bacilli have been isolated from these lesions. The lesion is an abscess consisting of neutrophils and staphylococci in the vicinity of the hair follicles. There is tissue necrosis and perivascular infiltrate. The abscess and inflammatory reaction infiltrate the subcutaneous tissue. With carbuncles, there are multiple abscesses that may coalesce or remain interconnected by channels; these may then drain through the skin. Surrounding cellulitis generally accompanies furuncles and carbuncles. Healing may leave scarring.

Furuncles occur most commonly in the same areas as folliculitis, i.e., head, neck, face, perineum, thigh, axilla, and groin. Carbuncles are found in the back of the neck, shoulders, buttocks, and thighs. Furuncles begin as a small, painful induration of the skin and subcutaneous tissue adjacent to a hair follicle. The lesion enlarges and becomes red, elevated, and more painful. Fluctuance develops and the lesion may rupture spontaneously because of central necrosis. Pain relief occurs immediately and healing is rapid. If the lesion progresses without rupture, then fever, chills, malaise, extensive cellulitis, and carbuncle formation are common complications.

Diagnosis of furuncles and carbuncles is not difficult. Large lesions can be drained for therapeutic reasons and the fluid collected for Gram stain and culture. Patients with systemic symptoms or carbuncles should have blood specimens drawn for culture.

For small furuncles, local warm compresses may be sufficient to promote healing and spontaneous drainage. Patients with facial lesions, significant cellulitis, carbuncles, or systemic symptoms require systemic antibiotics. If patients are deemed appropriate for outpatient therapy, cloxacillin or dicloxacillin (see Impetigo section for doses) is the drug of choice for 10 days. Patients allergic to penicillin may be given erythromycin or clindamycin. Severely ill patients require parenteral antibiotics, e.g., nafcillin, oxacillin, methicillin, or first-generation cephalosporins (dose of 200 mg per kilogram per day in six divided doses for children and adults), bed rest, and surgical drainage (when lesions mature and localize).

Patients with recurrent furuncles should be advised on good skin hygiene and avoidance of trauma; early therapy should be initiated at the first sign of a recurrence. Evaluation of the patient for nasal carriage of *S. aureus* is epidemiologically important, but recent approaches to eliminate the organism permanently have been unsuccessful. Tests to uncover any underlying predisposing factors (e.g., diabetes) may be unrewarding.

For a summary of treatment and characteristics of cellulitis and soft tissue infections see Table 1.

CREPITUS AND GANGRENE

W. LANCE GEORGE, M.D.

The presence of gas in or necrosis of the soft tissues during infection is a relatively common phenomenon; when present, these findings require that the clinician decide whether the disease process is one of several potentially rapidly fatal entities that require emergency medical and surgical management. The presence of gas or of tissue necrosis should suggest that anaerobes are likely to be involved.

Crepitation is a crackling sensation noted upon palpation of soft tissues that contain entrapped gas and is a distinctly uncommon finding. Gas in soft tissue is usually evident on radiographs of the affected area before being detectable on physical examination. The presence of gas in tissues is due to either metabolic production of various gases by bacteria; to mechanical introduction during debridement, irrigation, or surgery; or to accidental injection of air under pressure into the tissues. *Gangrene* simply means "death of the tissue." Although certain potentially lethal anaerobic infections may actually cause tissue necrosis or gangrene, there is a marked propensity for anaerobes (usually in association with facultative or aerobic bacteria) to infect previously devitalized tissue.

A variety of soft tissue infections are associated with either crepitations or gangrene and are listed in Table 1. Although all of these infections may be extremely serious and require aggressive debridement, those that require the most urgent management and have the poorest prognosis are necrotizing fasciitis, Fournier's gangrene, clostridial myonecrosis, and synergistic nonclostridial anaerobic myonecrosis.

NOMA

Noma is a rarely seen, spontaneous, progressive gangrene involving mucous membranes or mucocutaneous orifices that appears to be due to anaerobic bacteria. Major predisposing factors are severe malnutrition and poor oral hygiene. Treatment with high doses of penicillin G (approximately 20 million units per day) is the therapy of choice.

TABLE 1 Soft Tissue Infections Often Associated with Crepitations or Gangrene

Noma (cancrum oris)
Bacterial synergistic gangrene
Anaerobic cellulitis, gas abscess, and clostridial cellulitis*
Necrotizing fasciitis†
Fournier's gangrene†
Clostridial myonecrosis (gas gangrene)†
Streptococcal myonecrosis
Synergistic nonclostridial anaerobic myonecrosis (synergistic necrotizing cellulitis)†
Infected vascular gangrene*
Miscellaneous other infections involving anaerobes

* Indicates that abundant gas is usually present in the soft tissue early in disease.
† Indicates that the infection may have a rapidly lethal course.

BACTERIAL SYNERGISTIC GANGRENE

This chronic gangrene of the skin and superficial subcutaneous fat usually follows an operation (particularly one involving the abdomen or chest) and is characterized by extreme pain and redness, swelling, and tenderness of the wound. There is little systemic toxicity. Within several days the central area becomes purplish and then frankly gangrenous. There is slow, progressive enlargement of the lesion, such that there may be a central area of granulation tissue surrounded by gangrenous skin. The infection classically involves *Staphylococcus aureus* and a microaerophilic *Streptococcus*; however, facultative gram-negative bacilli, particularly *Proteus*, can also be involved. Treatment consists of debridement of devitalized tissue and antimicrobial therapy, the type of which depends on the organisms isolated.

ANAEROBIC CELLULITIS

Although the term *anaerobic cellulitis* is not properly descriptive—the process is more than just a cellulitis—the appellation persists in common usage. It is synonymous with *gas abscess* and is sometimes known as *clostridial cellulitis*, although the clinical picture for that condition is not necessarily different from those involving non-spore-forming anaerobes. The process involves the epifascial, retroperitoneal, or other connective tissues of the extremities, perineum, abdominal wall, buttock, hip, thorax, or neck. The lesion may exhibit necrotizing features and may spread rapidly but does not usually do so.

Pathologically, the lesion is basically a wet inflammation of the subcutaneous tissues that progresses to necrosis with crepitation within 2 to 5 days of onset; muscle involvement is nil. Pain may be the first symptom, but it is mild; subsequently, there is swelling of the overlying skin, and there may be erythema as well. Tenderness may develop, and soon crepitation becomes evident. Gas is commonly detected by palpation or by radiography; it is important to keep in mind, however, that the extent of infection cannot be judged by the extent of crepitation. Examination of the wound (if it has not been incised previously) at the time of surgery will, in most instances, reveal a foul odor, gas, and variable quantities of pus, along with shreds of devitalized soft tissues. The wound may be lined with a shaggy, gray-white pseudomembrane.

A variety of anaerobic bacteria, including clostridia on occasion, have been recovered from this type of process. The majority of anaerobes recovered are gram-positive cocci and *Bacteroides* species. Coliform bacilli, streptococci, and staphylococci may also be present. Debridement of devitalized tissue and initial empiric antimicrobial therapy are indicated.

NECROTIZING FASCIITIS

This acute, potentially life-threatening condition commonly originates in musculoskeletal wounds, but may also appear in an operative wound or even after trivial injury. A pathognomonic feature is subcutaneous and fascial necrosis, with undermining of the skin. There is sudden onset of pain and swelling; within 24 hours there may be considerable subcutaneous phlegmon, usually with cutaneous erythema or cellulitis. Blue-to-brown ecchymotic skin discoloration commonly develops, and pain is gradually replaced by numbness or anesthesia as a result of compression and destruction of cutaneous nerves at their site of passage through the edematous fascia. Fluid-filled vesicles later appear in the area of cellulitis, following which, the skin becomes necrotic. Local edema is present in most patients and may be massive. The extensive subcutaneous and fascial necrosis can be demonstrated by passing a sterile instrument along the tissue plane just superficial to the deep fascia; this cannot be done in ordinary cellulitis. Soft tissue gas is usually present, but may be demonstrable only on radiographs. This disease is a mixed infection that usually involves anaerobes (*Bacteroides* and *Peptostreptococcus* species), *S. aureus*, streptococci, and aerobic or facultative gram-negative bacilli.

Therapy is by emergency radical surgical debridement of all devitalized tissues; empiric broad-spectrum antimicrobial therapy is indicated.

FOURNIER'S GANGRENE

This is a life-threatening, necrotizing infection that begins in the scrotum or perineum and then spreads along fascial planes to involve the perineum, penis, abdominal wall, and thighs. It is a syndrome with variable involvement of deeper structures. Most cases represent a form of necrotizing fasciitis, but some are in the category of anaerobic cellulitis. On occasion, muscle may be involved also. Treatment involves emergency radical debridement and initial empiric broad-spectrum antimicrobial therapy directed against anaerobes and facultative bacteria.

CLOSTRIDIAL MYONECROSIS

Clostridial myonecrosis (gas gangrene) is a rapidly advancing, and sometimes rapidly lethal, infection that typically manifests with the sudden appearance of pain in a wound. Major predisposing causes of clostridial myonecrosis are extensive laceration or devitalization of muscles (particularly large muscle groups of the extremities), impairment of the blood supply to a limb or muscle group, contamination by foreign bodies, and delay in prompt surgical management of such injuries. Compound fractures predispose to gas gangrene because of the damage to muscles and their blood supply and, frequently, contamination of the wound. Surgery involving the gallbladder or bowel and surgery or manipulation of the upper female genital tract may precede clostridial myonecrosis of the abdominal wall and uterus, respectively. In addition, a number of cases have been reported to be associated with injections of various types. ''Spontaneous'' clostridial myonecrosis often involves *Clostridium septicum* and usually develops as a consequence of hematogenous seeding of a muscle or muscle group. This association is highly suggestive of an underlying colonic malignancy or other colonic disease.

Soon after the onset of pain, there is localized swelling, edema, and a thin, hemorrhagic exudate. Classically, a marked rise in the pulse rate—out of proportion to the slight elevation of temperature—is noted. The edematous area is very tender; the skin is tense and white, often with areas of blue discoloration. The swelling, edema, and toxemia increase rapidly, the serous discharge becomes more profuse, the skin becomes more dusky or bronzed, and bullae filled with dark red or purplish fluid often appear. Gas is usually present, but is not abundant in the early stages.

Certain peculiar mental changes have been described; these may consist of intellectual clarity with a full appreciation of the gravity of the disease, such that there is a profound terror or sense of impending doom. The toxic delirium may precede any visible changes in the wound.

The involvement of the underlying muscle is much more marked than is the skin involvement; although gas is usually present, it is not a prominent feature early in the course of infection. Changes in the muscle may be noted only at operation; hence it is imperative that prompt surgical exploration be carried out whenever gas gangrene is a clinical consideration. Early changes in the muscle consist primarily of edema and pallor, but later there is change in the color of the muscle, its blood supply is lost, contractility disappears, and gas may be demonstrable. In later stages of muscle involvement, there is progressive reddening, purple mottling, and change to a pasty or mucoid consistency of the muscle; eventually the muscle becomes diffusely gangrenous and even liquefied. Jaundice is rarely seen in clostridial myonecrosis of wounds, in contrast to uterine infection; when it does appear, it is associated with clostridial bacteremia and intravascular hemolysis. The most frequent causes of civilian clostridial myonecrosis are *Clostridium perfringens, Clostridium novyi*, and *C. septicum*; 80 to 95 percent of cases are caused by *C. perfringens*.

Diagnosis

The diagnosis of clostridial myonecrosis is made clinically. Detection of clostridia in a wound is not in itself of diagnostic value, because up to 88 percent of traumatic wounds may become colonized with clostridia in the absence of infection. In cases of myonecrosis, microscopic examination of muscle fragments or exudate may reveal clostridia, usually as large, gram-positive bacilli with square ends and no spores. Radiographs taken at intervals may help to detect early or incipient gas gangrene.

There are no satisfactory laboratory tests for diagnosis of gas gangrene, and one should not lose valuable time awaiting results of diagnostic tests. Rapid spread of the infection may occur within 2 to 4 hours, and irreversible changes may develop extremely rapidly. Accordingly, immediate surgical exploration is indicated when there is clinical suspicion of the possibility of clostridial myonecrosis.

Treatment

The cornerstone of treatment is early and radical surgical debridement of all involved tissues. This will often mean amputation in the case of myonecrosis in an extremity. Reoperation may be often necessary to ensure viability of the remaining tissues. Antibiotic therapy should include high doses of penicillin G (approximately 20 million units per day if renal function is normal). Either chloramphenicol or metronidazole is an acceptable substitute in the patient with a history of an anaphylactic-type reaction to penicillin. Hyperbaric oxygen is not of clear value, but should be considered in the desperate case or when complete resection of infected tissues is not possible (as in involvement of paravertebral muscles). It may also help to demarcate the area of disease and thus facilitate amputation at an appropriate level. Therapy with antitoxin (where it is still available) has not been shown to be beneficial and poses significant risks, because it is a horse-serum preparation.

STREPTOCOCCAL MYONECROSIS

Myositis or myonecrosis may also be caused by organisms other than clostridia, particularly the streptococci. Streptococcal myonecrosis is a fairly uncommon infection that may closely resemble clostridial myonecrosis, but has a less acute course. The incubation period is usually 3 to 4 days, and the presenting signs are swelling, edema, and a purulent or seropurulent wound exudate. Pain comes later in the course of illness (a distinct difference from gas gangrene), but may then be severe. Once pain becomes established as a symptom the progress of the illness is relatively rapid, although not so rapid as with clostridial myonecrosis. Gas is present both inter- and intramuscularly, but is not extensive. Involved muscles are at first pale and soft and later become bright red, with typical regular purple barring. Subsequently, the muscles become dark purple, swollen, friable, and, eventually, gangrenous. There is a peculiar sour odor to both the wound and to the large quantities of seropurulent discharge.

Patients with fatal disease die after one week or longer; toxemia, disorientation or mild delirium, and shock are preterminal events. Although the condition is often called anaerobic streptococcal myonecrosis, the anaerobic streptococci are almost always found in association with other organisms, particularly *Streptococcus pyogenes* and *S. aureus*. The character and course of the disease depend to some extent on the nature of the infecting organisms.

Management requires adequate incision, drainage and debridement of infected tissues, and high-dose penicillin G therapy plus the use of an antistaphylococcal agent if indicated.

SYNERGISTIC NONCLOSTRIDIAL ANAEROBIC MYONECROSIS

Another infection involving muscle has been described by various names, including synergistic necrotizing cellulitis, gram-negative anaerobic cutaneous gangrene, and necrotizing cutaneous myositis. A more appropriate name might be synergistic nonclostridial anaerobic myonecrosis, because this is a highly virulent soft tissue infection involving skin, subcutaneous tissue, fascia, and muscle; this infection occurs predominantly in the lower extremities and perineal areas.

Unique to this infection are discrete, large areas of blue-gray necrotic skin separated by areas of normal skin, with much more extensive involvement of underlying tissues than is evidenced upon superficial examination. There is extensive confluent necrotic liquefaction or dry gangrene of underlying muscle and fascia and subcutaneous tissues. Foul-smelling "dishwater" pus may drain from skin ulcers. Although severe systemic toxicity is usual and may appear suddently, there is usually extensive local necrosis before systemic toxicity occurs; there is also exquisite local tenderness and severe pain. Gas formation, present in 25 percent of cases, is usually not pronounced. Three-fourths of patients have diabetes mellitus; other associated or predisposing factors include advanced age, renal disease, and either obesity or malnutrition. The infecting flora includes aerobic or facultative gram-negative bacilli, anaerobic streptococci, and *Bacteroides*; there is a high incidence (approximately 30%) of bacteremia involving both anaerobes and nonanaerobes. Therapy requires emergency radical debridement and appropriate antimicrobial agents. Best results are seen in patients in whom amputation of the infected area is possible. Mortality is as high as 75 percent.

INFECTED VASCULAR GANGRENE

Infected vascular gangrene is another condition in which both soft tissue gas and gangrene may commonly be found. In this situation the muscle, and frequently the entire limb, has already died as a result of circulatory insufficiency, and the bacteria act primarily as saprophytes. There is little tendency for them to spread beyond the dead tissue into intact, healthy muscle, and there is seldom acute toxemia. There may be an extremely foul odor and considerable gas production, but little systemic toxicity. However, if neglected, infection may spread proximally, and various serious complications may develop. Therapy obviously consists of amputation of the affected extremity; antimicrobial therapy is indicated to protect the patient from bacteremia or proximal spread of the infection.

ANTIMICROBIAL THERAPY

Appropriate antimicrobial therapy of the above infections requires both an appreciation that they are usually polymicrobial and a knowledge of the infecting flora. Initial (empiric) therapy should be selected to cover organisms that are likely to be present; Gram stain of the exudate or infected material usually provides excellent information in this regard. Culture for anaerobes and nonanaerobes is always indicated for evaluation of the types of infection being considered here.

As mentioned above, penicillin G (approximately 20 million units per day—less if renal function is impaired) is the drug of choice for treatment of serious clostridial infections. Chloramphenicol (maximum, 2 g per day in divided doses), clindamycin (maximum, 2.4 g per day in divided doses), and metronidazole (maximum, 30 mg per kilogram per day in divided doses) have traditionally been the agents most active against all anaerobic pathogens; the dosage of these may need to be reduced if hepatic function is impaired. Because a low incidence (approximately 5%) of clindamycin-resistant *Bacteroides fragilis* has recently been noted in many centers, this agent should probably not be used to treat potentially life-threatening infections involving *B. fragilis* unless susceptibility of the isolate to clindamycin has been demonstrated by the laboratory. When either clindamycin or metronidazole is given for a serious or life-threatening anaerobic infection, penicillin should also be administered to ensure adequate coverage of fastidious microaerophilic streptococci and anaerobic gram-positive cocci. Whenever facultative (enteric or coliform) or aerobic gram-negative bacilli are suspected, an aminoglycoside should be administered. Antistaphylococcal therapy (e.g., nafcillin or oxacillin, 9 g per day in divided doses) may also be indicated on occasion. Therapy should, of course, be revised as results of culture and susceptibility testing become available.

OCULAR AND PERIORBITAL INFECTIONS

ENDOPHTHALMITIS

ANN S. BAKER, M.D.

Endophthalmitis is one of the catastrophic complications of ocular surgery, penetrating ocular trauma, and systemic infection. Until recently, infectious endophthalmitis was associated with an almost uniformly poor prognosis; in one large series between 1950 and 1977, 67 percent of patients with postoperative endophthalmitis lost all light perception. Both experimental and clinical evidence indicates that the expeditious use of intraocular antibiotics and therapeutic vitrectomy favorably alters the outcome of endophthalmitis.

Endophthalmitis is defined as inflammation of intraocular structures, typically severe in character and often associated with pain, decreased vision, inflammatory cells in the anterior or posterior chamber, hypopyon in many instances, lid swelling, chemosis and loss of the red reflex. In infectious or bacterial endophthalmitis one or more microorganisms are recovered from vitreous or aqueous fluids on at least two culture media (see below).

Most cases of bacterial endophthalmitis follow cataract extractions, with onset typically in the immediate postoperative period. Others that occur more than 3 months after surgery are termed late postoperative infections; these are most often infections of blebs raised for therapy of glaucoma. Endophthalmitis may rarely follow penetrating ocular trauma, after which multiple organisms may be found. Finally, endophthalmitis may follow bacteremic infections.

Symptoms of endophthalmitis include headache over the infected eye, eye pain, and decreased vision. Signs include swelling or chemosis of the conjunctiva and upper lid, hypopyon (or cells in the anterior chamber), and a decreased red reflex. Visual acuity may also be decreased.

Ultrasound of the orbit may be helpful in identifying a vitreous infiltrate as well as establishing the status of the retina.

To confirm the diagnosis of endophthalmitis, fluid should be aspirated from the anterior chamber and always from the vitreous, or the material from vitrectomy washings (which may be a total of more than 200 ml) should be collected on a 0.45-micron filter. The tiny drop of aspirate (or the filter paper) is then placed on brucella agar and chocolate agar plates, anerobic media and a Sabouraud's slant. Because the specimen is so tiny, the drop should be placed in the center of the plate.

The criteria for infectious endophthalmitis includes eyes from which organisms are cultured from a specimen of aqueous or vitreous fluid on at least two media. The area of growth on the culture plate may be so small that growth is required on at least two media to rule out contamination.

Organisms cultured from most postoperative cataract infections include coagulase-negative staphylococci, streptococci, and *Staphylococcus aureus*. In traumatic endophthalmitis, multiple organisms may be cultured; in these patients, the incidence of anerobic and gram-negative infections is high.

TREATMENT

There are several tenets of therapy for endophthalmitis. Treatment within 24 hours of diagnosis improves the outcome considerably. A delay of more than 24 hours in the performance of therapeutic vitrectomy has been associated with a dismal outcome; 50 percent of patients with late vitrectomy had no light perception in one series. Vitreous sampling is crucial in establishing a bacteriologic diagnosis. Coagulase-negative *Staphylococcus* is the commonest pathogen in postoperative endophthalmitis. Visual outcome is poor in the late-onset (or more than 3 months' onset) endophthalmitis. It is also poor in the patient with gram-negative or anerobic infection.

VITRECTOMY

There is presently a debate about the need for a vitrectomy and/or intravitreal antibiotics versus medical therapy alone. It is our clinical impression that vitrectomy and intravitreal antibiotics improve the outcome of endophthalmitis. A vitrectomy includes removal of all or part of the 3.9 ml of material in the vitreous.

Advantages include drainage of the abscess; this is a tiny closed space and drainage is imperative. The gel matrix of the vitreous is also removed so that diffusion for antibiotic delivery is better. Disadvantages include the risk of retinal tear or detachment and new fibrovascular ingrowths. The vitrectomy must be performed early to be of any value.

Indications for vitrectomy include gram-negative organisms on Gram stain or vitreous sample, fungal infection, or a gram-positive organism in a patient with visual acuity of 20/400 or less. In severe, progressive cases, repeat vitrectomy and reinstillation of antibiotics may be necessary.

ANTIBIOTIC THERAPY

There are four suggested approaches to antibiotic therapy in endophthalmitis:

Intravitreal Injection

Diffusion of the antibiotic occurs readily in the vitreous. Loss of the drug from the vitreous occurs through two routes: anteriorly to the posterior chamber and out through the aqueous drainage system (aminoglycosides); or by active transport across the retina (e.g., beta-lactam drugs or clindamycin). Competitive inhibitors such as probenicid inhibit this pump and may prolong the vitreous concentration of beta-lactams.

There is a concern about toxicity of intravitreal antibiotics, and thus several precautions should be taken. The intravitreal antibiotics should be given in the anterior part of the vitreous as a slow injection. A rapid-fire stream toward the back of the retina may tear the retina.

Suggested initial doses for endophthalmitis of unknown etiology include: a cephalosporin such as cefazolin (1 mg) and an aminoglycoside such as gentamicin (400 μg). Table 1 lists antibiotics and dosages used after the organism has been identified.

TABLE 1 Endophthalmitis: Intravitreal Doses (Total Volume, 0.1–0.2 ml)*

Antibiotic	*Dosage*
Aminoglycosides	
Gentamicin	0.4 mg
Tobramycin	0.5 mg
Amikacin	0.4 mg
Penicillins	
Methicillin	2.0 mg
Oxacillin	0.5 mg
Ampicillin	5.0 mg
Carbenicillin	2.0 mg
Miscellaneous	
Cefazolin	1.0 mg
Erythromycin	0.5 mg
Clindamycin	1.0 mg
Vancomycin	1.0 mg
Chloramphenicol	2.0 mg
Antifungal antibiotic	
Amphotericin B	5–10 μg

Note: Choice of antibiotic is determined by the organism isolated.
* Adapted from Peyman and Sanders

Subconjunctival Therapy

Subconjunctival therapy has been recommended (for one or two doses) if there are no bleeding or pressure complications. Doses of cefazolin (50 mg) and tobramycin (50 mg) result in good concentrations in the cornea that exceed the aqueous concentration by severalfolds; the vitreous levels are usually less than 1 μg per milliliter, however. Thus, the usefulness of this approach in endophthalmitis is still debated.

Topical Therapy

Topical therapy should be combined with other modes of therapy especially in the patient with a draining wound. One to two drops of antibiotic every 1 to 4 hours are usually sufficient. Cefazolin, 33 mg per milliliter, and gentamicin, 14 mg per milliliter are useful initial antibiotics.

Systemic Therapy

Systemic intravenous administration of antibiotics results in poor penetration of the vitreous barriers. Peak levels in the vitreous are typically only 1 percent of the serum level; penetration of the aqueous is slightly better, i.e., 2 to 10 percent of the peak level.

Preferred intravenous antibiotics in order of choice are cephalothin 12 g per day or vancomycin, 2 g per day. In patients from whom methicillin-resistant *S. epidermidis* has been isolated, vancomycin may be substituted. The role of intravenous antibiotics remains to be defined and must await studies of vitreal levels obtained after intravenous administration. Specific antibiotic therapy is adjusted when cultural and sensitivity data become available. Most cases due to coagulase-negative staphylococci respond well to a 7- to 10-day course of parenteral antibiotics, vitrectomy, and topical therapy; complicated cases involving *S. aureus*, gram-negative bacteria, or fungal endophthalmitis require a longer (14-day or more) course of parenteral therapy until the vitreous clears.

Close follow-up is mandatory to detect posttreatment complications including glaucoma, retinal detachment, and sterile uveitis.

STEROIDS

Systemic steroids may be used in the severely inflamed and infected eye to decrease inflammation in this tight, small space. Prednisone, 60 mg a day tapered rapidly after 5 days, may be used.

DIFFERENTIAL DIAGNOSIS

The differential diagnosis of endophthalmitis following cataract extraction should include sterile inflammation as well as bacterial and fungal infection. Sterile uveitis has been reported to occur in 2–3 percent of patients following intraocular lens implantation. Like bacterial infections, sterile endophthalmitis generally develops during the first week following the lens implantation.

PSEUDOPHAKIC ENDOPHTHALMITIS

Bacterial pseudophakic endophthalmitis (intraocular lens) is a postoperative complication of intraocular lens implantation. The presentation is similar to postcataract endophthalmitis. Most commonly, the bacteria are coagulase-negative staphylococci and *Staphylococcus aureus*, but a wide variety of gram-positive and gram-negative organisms have been isolated. The therapy should be similar to that for the patient with routine postoperative cataract endophthalmitis. Although it has been suggested that in cases of pseudophakic endophthalmitis the intraocular lens should be removed, this may be a difficult procedure with high morbidity. Most patients can be cured without removal of lens; in fact is removal may lead to a poorer visual outcome.

FUNGAL ENDOPHTHALMITIS

Fungal endophthalmitis may occur as an indolent infection, with the first symptoms often occurring days to weeks after the initial surgery. Pain in the involved eye, headache, and lid edema may be less pronounced than in bacterial infections. The commonest symptom is decreased vision. Fluffy exudates or nodules on examination frequently suggest fungal endophthalmitis. Intravitreal and systemic amphotericin B are the usual modes of therapy.

ANTIBIOTIC PROPHYLAXIS

For topical prophylaxis before cataract surgery we suggest polymixin B sulfate and bacitracin ophthalmic ointment (Polysporin) in the evening before surgery and in the postoperative period.

We use systemic antibiotics prophylactically for vitreal or retinal surgery. It is our impression that the patient with some type of immunosuppression such as steroid use or chemotherapy as well as patients with intraoperative complications such as vitreous loss during cataract surgery have a higher incidence of endophthalmitis than would be expected. Unplanned extracapsular extraction or vitreous loss had occurred in one-third of our reported cases of endophthalmitis. In the case of vitreous loss, one may speculate that the intact hyaloid face has some barrier function against intraocular penetration of microorganisms. Thus, a heightened index of suspicion for infectious endophthalmitis is warranted in cases of complicated cataract extraction. Subconjunctival and/or systemic antibiotics as well as topical antibiotics should be considered in the immunocompromised patient before cataract surgery.

Speed is of the essence in the evaluation and therapy of endophthalmitis. The goal should be to salvage vision rather than to perform enucleation, an all too common outcome of bacterial endophthalmitis.

INFECTION OF THE CONJUNCTIVA, EYELIDS, AND LACRIMAL APPARATUS

RHOADS E. STEVENS, M.D.

CONJUNCTIVITIS

Conjunctivitis denotes inflammation of the mucous membrane covering the eyelids and sclera. Regardless of etiology, signs and symptoms of conjunctivitis may include hyperemia, lid swelling, discharge, irritation or foreign body sensation, mild photophobia, and intermittent blurred vision. Crusting or mattering, which tends to stick the eyelids together, especially in the morning, is common and should not be confused with true purulent discharge. The vascular dilatation involves vessels of the conjunctival tissues that are freely movable over the scleral surface (thereby distinguishing conjunctivitis from episcleritis or scleritis). If injection involves the deeper vessels in the limbal zone, especially in the presence of a poorly reactive pupil and photophobia, the clinician should suspect uveitis. Local reactive lymphoid hyperplasia may appear on the tarsal conjunctiva as small fleshy elevations called follicles, or as larger vascularized "cobblestones" called papillae. Lymphatic drainage from the conjunctival sac is to the submandibular and preauricular nodes, where reactive lymphadenopathy may be noted. Infrequently, fibrin and inflammatory debris collect on the conjunctival surface in severe cases to form "membranes" or "pseudomembranes."

Acute conjunctivitis (developing over several days and lasting several weeks) is almost always a self-limited disease. A presumptive diagnosis can usually be made and appropriate therapy initiated on purely clinical findings. Cases of hyperacute conjunctivitis (develops in a matter of hours and rapidly worsens), ophthalmia neonatorum

---

The author would like to thank Drs. Deborah Pavan-Langston and Kenneth R. Kenyon for reviewing this manuscript.

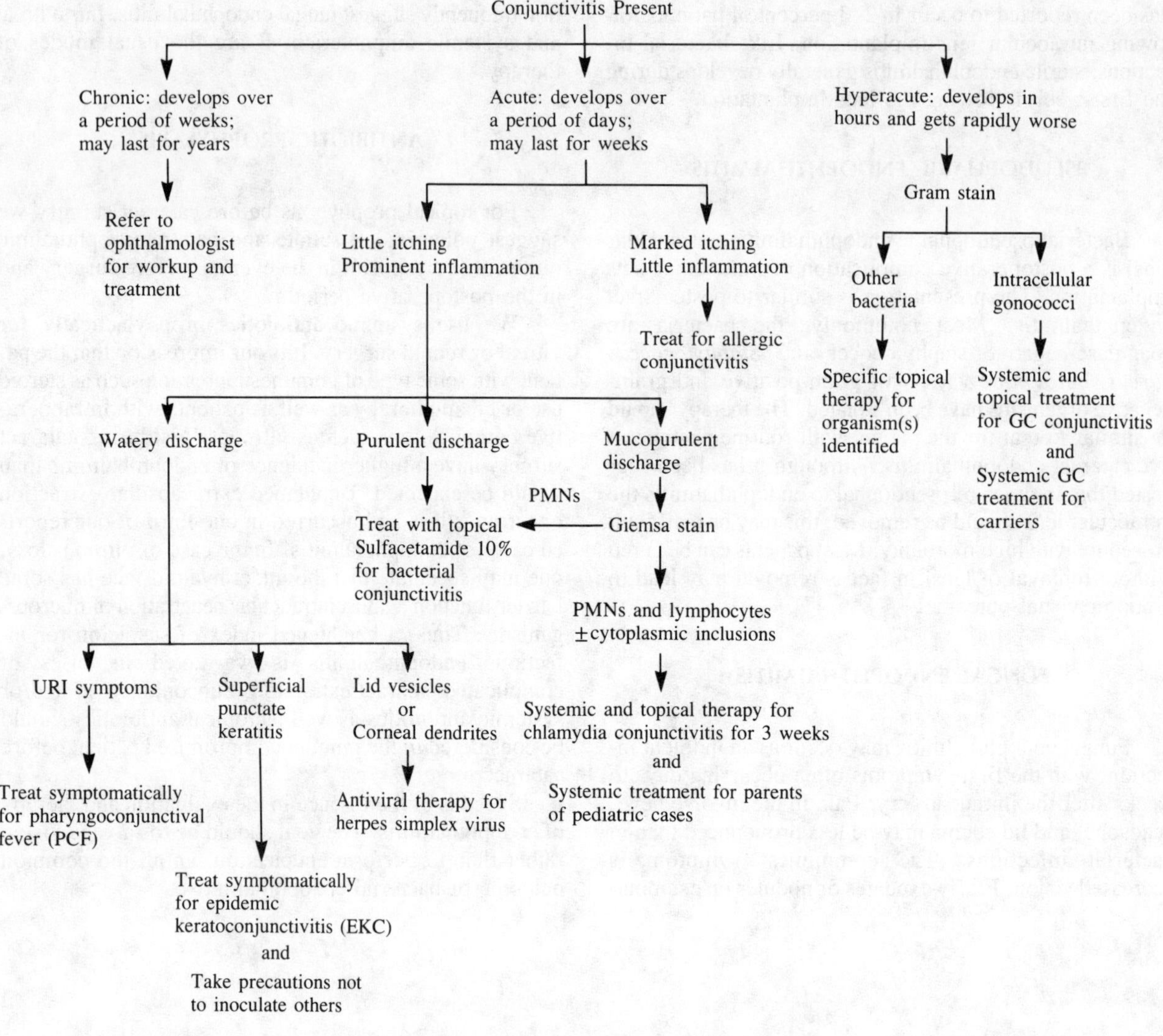

Figure 1 Diagnosis and management of conjunctivitis

(conjunctivitis in infants), conjunctivitis after ocular surgery or in association with other ocular disease (e.g., corneal ulcer), and chronic or unresponsive conjunctivitis all require microbiologic and pathologic investigation. Laboratory testing usually consists of cultures and scrapings. A sterile, cotton-tip applicator is used to sweep the conjunctival fornices and to inoculate a blood agar plate, a chocolate agar plate (for *Hemophilus* and *Neisseria*), a brain-heart infusion tube, and, possibly, thioglycolate broth (for anaerobes). Scrapings of the tarsal conjunctiva should be stained with Gram stain and Giemsa stain. Bacteria can be identified on Gram stain. However, correlation with cultural results is not always good. Giemsa stain (or, if not available, Wright stain) reveals cellular morphology. In general, polymorphonuclear leukocytes indicate an acute bacterial conjunctivitis. A monocytic response suggests viral or drug-induced disease. Eosinophils and basophils are prominent in allergic conjunctivitis. A mixed lymphocytic and polymorphonuclear response is highly suggestive of a chlamydial infection, which is confirmed by the presence of basophilic paranuclear cytoplasmic inclusion bodies within epithelial cells.

One should not overlook general palliative measures in the treatment of any conjunctivitis. Hot compresses help clean the lids of crust and speed resolution of the inflammation. Cool compresses may provide relief from irritative symptoms, especially itching. Aspirin is useful for the discomfort of conjunctivitis as it is for any inflammation.

Figure 1 provides a scheme for diagnosis and management of acute, hyperacute, and chronic conjunctivitis.

Acute Conjunctivitis

Acute bacterial conjunctivitis is distinguished by a purulent ocular discharge. *Staphylococcus aureus* is the commonest cause. Infection usually originates from the patient's own hands, face, or anterior nares. This gram-positive coccus is usually not invasive, but produces exotoxins that can additionally cause epithelial keratitis, peripheral corneal infiltration and ulceration, phlyctenulosis, eczematous blepharitis, and angular blepharoconjunctivitis. *S. aureus* is rarely observed in clusters in ocular exudates, tending instead to form short chains. *Staphylococcus epidermidis* is part of the normal ocular flora in a majority of humans. It can produce exotoxins as does *S. aureus* and, if present in sufficient numbers, can cause acute conjunctivitis or blepharoconjunctivitis. *S. epidermidis* has been known to contaminate eye cosmetics, which in turn may be the source of a pathogenic inoculum.

Streptococcus pneumoniae, the pneumococcus, is an aerobic, lancet-shaped, encapsulated gram-positive diplococcus. *Hemophilus influenzae* (same as *Hemophilus aegyptius* and Koch-Weeks bacillus) is an aerobic, pleomorphic, gram-negative organism that may appear as a coccobacillus or as a slender rod in conjunctival scrapings. Both organisms are found in the upper respiratory tract of healthy carriers, especially in children. For this reason, acute conjunctivitis from these isolates is commoner in children and in adults frequently exposed to children. Environmental crowding, such as can occur during the winter months of northern states, enhances pneumococcal carrier rates and infections. Both the pneumococcus and *H. influenzae* are prone to producing patchy subconjunctival hemorrhaging with the conjunctivitis.

Streptococcus pyogenes (beta-hemolytic streptococci) is an aerobic, invasive, gram-positive, toxigenic coccus. Fortunately, it is a relatively uncommon cause of conjunctivitis, because the disease is often severe with inflammatory membrane formation. Viridans streptococci are much less virulent and usually only produce clinical infection in the setting of antecedent ocular surface disease.

Other bacteria that may produce acute conjunctivitis include *Moraxella* species, *Neisseria* species, gram-negative rods, and anaerobes. *Moraxella lacunata* (diplobacillus of Morax-Axenfeld) is a large, aerobic, gram-negative diplobacillus that rarely causes acute conjunctivitis. More commonly, it incites a chronic conjunctivitis with excoriation of the canthal area, producing so-called angular blepharoconjunctivitis. Chronic infection in younger patients may manifest as a follicular conjunctivitis. Between *Neisseria gonorrhoeae* and *Neisseria meningitidis*, the former is by far the commoner cause of conjunctivitis. Any hyperacute conjunctivitis in adults must receive work-up to rule out gonococcal infection. Its diagnosis and therapy will be discussed under Ophthalmia Neonatorum (below). Although conjunctivitis may be caused by any of the gram-negative enteric bacilli, such infections are relatively uncommon. Disease usually occurs in chronically debilitated patients, alcoholics, and those with very poor hygiene. Soft contact lens wear may be a predisposing factor to gram-negative rod (especially *Pseudomonas* species) infection. The anaerobes *Peptostreptococcus* and *Propionibacterium acnes* are more frequently recovered from eyes with conjunctivitis than without. They are usually found in mixed culture with aerobes, and their significance in the pathogenesis of conjunctivitis is undetermined.

The average case of acute bacterial mucopurulent conjunctivitis, once diagnosed, can be treated effectively with topical antibiotic solutions or ointments alone. Sodium sulfacetamide is a good broad-spectrum antibiotic with activity against staphylococci, pneumococci, *H. influenzae*, and the moraxellas. It has little ocular toxicity. Sodium sulfacetamide 10 percent drops are instilled four times a day for 7 to 10 days, depending on clinical response. More clinically severe cases can be managed by increasing the drops to every hour during the day and adding sulfacetamide 10 percent ointment at bedtime; or by switching to 10 percent ointment 4 times daily and at bedtime. Chloramphenicol in 0.5 percent drops or 1.0 percent ointment is an excellent broad-spectrum antibiotic with very low ocular toxicity. However, its use should be avoided if possible because of reports of rare bone marrow toxicity from topical chloramphenicol therapy. Antibiotic combinations such as polymyxin B (10,000 units per milliliter), neomycin (2.5 mg per milliliter), gramicidin (0.025 mg per milliliter) drops (Neosporin), and similar ointment preparations, are quite effective against ocular pathogens. However, use of any preparation that includes neomycin runs the not uncommon risk of hypersensitivity to that agent. If the clinical status has not begun to improve after 3 days on the therapy initiated, the patient should be reevaluated. If gram-negative rods are seen on smear or recovered on culture, therapy may be switched to gentamicin or tobramycin 0.3 percent drops, every 4 hours, or ointment, four times daily.

Acute viral conjunctivitis is characterized by diffuse conjunctival hyperemia with watery discharge and a follicular response. It may be seen as a transient, benign feature in association with systemic RNA viral infections such as mumps, rubeola, or rubella. Conjunctivitis from systemic or local DNA viral infections such as herpes simplex, herpes zoster/varicella (chicken pox), adenovirus, and vaccinia, on the other hand, can be associated with much more severe ocular consequences.

Adenoviral conjunctivitis, commonly known as pink eye, is one of the most frequent and severe forms of conjunctivitis. After an incubation period of 5 to 12 days, the patient experiences the onset of conjunctivitis, usually unilateral, with preauricular lymphadenopathy. The other eye frequently becomes involved, but to a lesser degree, several days later. The conjunctivitis runs a 7- to 16-day course with associated symptoms that may linger a month or more. The infectious, contagious period is 10 to 14 days, but the virus may be present in the eye up to 30 days after the onset of illness. Because of this, patients should be cautioned not to expose others to their ocular secretions. Special care should be taken by health care professionals not to initiate an epidemic from contaminated hands and instruments.

If the adenoviral infection is accompanied by pharyngitis and fever up to 104 °F, it is classified as pharyngoconjunctival fever (PCF). Although adenovirus 3 is the commonest cause of PCF, practically any of the adenoviral types can produce this syndrome. If the adenoviral conjunctivitis is associated with foreign body sensation, photophobia, and a superificial epithelial keratitis on examination, the syndrome is termed epidemic keratoconjunctivitis (EKC). EKC can follow a fulminant course, with inflammatory membrane formation and late symblepharon. At 11 to 15 days into the disease, when the active epithelial lesions and conjunctivitis are resolving, focal subepithelial infiltrates may form to blur vision and produce night glare for weeks to come. Adenovirus type 8 is the commonest etiologic agent for EKC, but epidemics have also resulted from types 19 and 37 as well. Less than 5 percent of the general population in the United States has antibody to adenovirus type 8. Thus, susceptibility to EKC is great.

Therapy for adenoviral conjunctivitis is basically symptomatic. Antipyretics for fever, cool compresses for comfort, and, in severe cases, drops or ointment may be used for 1 to 2 weeks to help the patient through the most uncomfortable period. Although drops are not curative, patients sometimes find relief from 0.125 percent prednisolone drops or from a bland antibiotic preparation such as erythromycin or bacitracin. Although these are usually self-limited infections, an occasional patient may end up with a chronically red and irritated eye that is poorly responsive to any form of therapy. The corneal infiltrates usually resolve without therapy over weeks to months. Steroids are effective in suppressing or resolving the infiltrates, but are not generally recommended because of possible complications of treatment and rebound inflammation once therapy is terminated.

Acute hemorrhagic conjunctivitis (AHC) first appeared in West Africa in 1970. Since that time many epidemics of AHC have occurred in the densely populated humid areas of the world, including a recent outbreak in southern Florida. This infection by enterovirus type 70 is characterized by the sudden onset of ocular pain, itching, photophobia, eyelid edema, and watery discharge. Both eyes soon become involved. Subconjunctival hemorrhage and, usually, a follicular response appear. Improvement in this self-limited disease occurs over 2 to 4 days and is usually complete by 7 days. Crowded populations of low socioeconomic status are more commonly affected. The infection is often spread by school children who introduce it to other family members. Transmission of ACH to family members at risk can be reduced by simple hygienic measures such as hand washing and use of separate towels.

Herpes simplex virus conjunctivitis can occur with or without vesicles on the eyelids from primary or recurrent infection. If it is highly suspected or is confirmed by epithelial giant cells and eosinophilic intranuclear inclusion bodies on Giemsa stain, antiviral therpay is indicated. Idoxuridine 0.5 percent or vidarabine 3 percent ointment five times a day for 10 days or until resolution, idoxuridine 0.1 percent drops every hour by day and ointment at bedtime, or trifluoridine 1 percent drops nine times a day for 14 days may be used. These provide equivalent therapy, but failure to improve may require change to another drug—or discontinuation if toxicity is suspected. Treatment is longer if keratitis is present. Acyclovir is equally effective and less toxic, but is not commercially available in an ocular preparation.

Conjunctivitis associated with varicella may be manifested by diffuse involvement, by focal limbal lesions, and, rarely, by pox on the bulbar conjunctiva. Antiviral therapy is similar to that for herpes simplex conjunctivitis, but is usually not required for this self-limited condition. It is felt that the varicella virus is less responsive to antiviral therapy than is herpes simplex. In contrast to primary infection, secondary involvement of the eye with varicella as in herpes zoster, can be devastating. The conjunctivitis is diffuse and is unresponsive to antiviral therapy. Treatment is supportive, with ocular lubrication and warm compresses. Periocular scarring may result regardless of therapy. More importantly, intraocular involvement, which may lead to severe uveitis, glaucoma, and cataract, should be excluded by ophthalmic exam.

Fortunately, vaccinial conjunctivitis should be a disease of the past now that smallpox is apparently eradicated from the globe.

Acute conjunctivitis from *Chlamydia* will be discussed under Chronic Conjunctivitis.

When itching is the most prominent symptom of acute conjunctivitis, allergy is by far the commonest etiology. The patient is usually more symptomatic than the clinical appearance suggests. The signs of acute allergic conjunctivitis include a milky edema of the bulbar conjunctiva, mild conjunctival injection, a ropy mucoid discharge, and papillae on the tarsal conjunctiva. Treatment modalities include avoidance of the allergen, cool compresses, and, if necessary, an ocular astringent-decongestant-antihistamine drop (such as Vasocon A) up to four times a day for a limited period of time.

Chronic Conjunctivitis

Many cases of a chronic red eye will be of apparent etiology. A red eye persisting after acute adenoviral conjunctivitis, follicular conjunctivitis from the lesions of molluscum contagiosum, drug- or eyedrop-induced conjunctivitis, and conjunctivitis from eye makeup are examples. Other causes such as dry eye, ocular pemphigoid, chronic lacrimal obstruction, and sebaceous gland carcinoma are not as readily apparent and may require extensive work-up by an ophthalmologist to confirm.

Chronic bacterial conjunctivitis is most commonly caused by *S. aureus*, but can be produced by a variety of organisms. Especially in the presence of rosacea (rhinophyma and facial telangiectasis), chronic staphylococcal colonization of the eye can produce blepharoconjunctivitis, as evidenced by greasy debris on the lashes, dilated meibomian openings, microchalazia, and thickened telangiectatic lid margins. Therapy should be started by scrubbing the lid margins with a warm, moist cloth twice daily. This lid hygiene may be necessary on a chronic basis. Topical treatment for staphylococcal blepharoconjunctivitis consists of sulfacetamide 10 percent, bacitracin 500 units per gram, or erythromycin 0.5

percent ointment two to three times a day for 21 days. Prednisolone 0.125 percent with sulfacetamide 10 percent in drop or ointment form to the lid margins and conjunctiva twice a day for 2 to 3 weeks, or until a response is seen, is particularly good for quieting the acutely inflamed eye. Chronic steroid use is rarely indicated. Patients with rosacea may require tetracycline, 250 mg orally four times per day (tapered as allowed) chronically to control the abnormal meibomian gland secretions that irritate the eyes and enhance staphylococcal colonization.

Chlamydia are obligate intracellular parasites that infect conjunctival epithelial cells. They produce an acute follicular conjunctivitis that may evolve into a chronic mucopurulent conjunctivitis. The chronic form, termed adult inclusion conjunctivitis, is characterized by tarsal follicles and a mixed lymphocytic and polymorphonculear inflammatory response. On occasion, the organisms can be seen on Giemsa stain of conjunctival scrapings as basophilic paranuclear cytoplasmic inclusions within epithelial cells. Corneal involvement with epithelial keratitis, stromal infiltrates, and superficial vascularization may develop in association with the conjunctivitis. Sustained reinfection from *Chlamydia*, which is exceedingly uncommon in the United States, leads to trachoma. In this country the infection is usually acquired by young adults from the urethral or vaginal discharge of recent sexual partners. Patients with adult inclusion conjunctivitis and their sexual partners should be treated with oral tetracycline (preferred) or erythromycin, 1.0 g per day for at least 21 days. Oral sulfacetamide (6 to 8 [on the basis of body size] g per day) for 3 weeks is also effective. Children and breast-feeding mothers should not be given tetracycline because the child's developing permanent teeth will be discolored.

Ophthalmia Neonatorum

Ophthalmia neonatorum is arbitrarily defined to be inflammation of the conjunctiva in the first month of life. The newborn, with its underdeveloped immune system, is prone to infection from certain organisms that can cause hyperacute conjunctivitis in other age groups as well. Another common feature is that this conjunctivitis may represent simply one manifestation of a systemic infection. Diagnosis of neonatal conjunctivitis by time course of onset is unreliable. All cases should receive cytologic and microbiologic work-up.

Passage through the birth canal exposes the neonate to all of the organisms that live there. The Centers for Disease Control (CDC) recommends culture of all pregnant women for gonococcus. Women with positive cultures must be treated. Women with active or recurrent herpes simplex type 2 viral infection are usually delivered by cesarean section, but even this does not totally eliminate neonatal exposure.

Chemical conjunctivitis from Crede's prophylaxis (2% silver nitrate at birth) develops a few hours after instillation and lasts 24 to 36 hours. The ocular discharge is usually mucoid in this self-limited disorder.

Although *S. aureus* is the most frequent cause of bacterial ophthalmia neonatorum, conjunctivitis may result from any of the bacterial species that can be cultured from the endocervix. It may occur at any time postpartum and is characterized by purulent discharge. Septicemia may occur in severe cases, especially in premature infants. Conjunctival scrapings and cultures are mandatory. Initial therapy for gram-positive organisms and *Hemophilus* species is erythromycin ointment 0.5 percent four to six times daily. Gram-negative bacilli are treated with gentamicin 0.3 percent drops four to six times daily (depending on severity and response) (hourly for *P. aeruginosa)* for 2 weeks. If the organism is resistant to gentamicin, tobramycin can be used at the same dosage. Evidence of systemic disease suggests additional systemic antibiotic coverage.

Neisseria gonorrhoeae bacterial infection produces the severest form of ophthalmia neonatorum, which, if untreated, may result in corneal perforation. Despite a dramatic reduction due to silver nitrate prophylaxis, its incidence is still 0.6 percent. Classically, it presents as a hyperacute conjunctivitis beginning 2 to 4 days after birth with grossly purulent exudate, chemosis, and lid swelling. Partial treatment or inadequate prophylaxis may delay its onset and reduce its severity. Diagnosis of gonococcal conjunctivitis is made by microscopic examination of smears and by cultures with Thayer-Martin medium or chocolate agar. On Gram stain, the gonococci appear as gram-negative diplococci present in polymorphonuclear leukocytes. Their adjacent surfaces are flattened like a coffee bean.

Systemic involvement in gonococcal ophthalmia neonatorum is common. As such, concurrent topical and parenteral therapy are recommended. All patients with gonococcal conjunctivitis regardless of age should be admitted to hospital. Topical therapy is with aqueous penicillin G drops (20,000 units per milliliter) instilled every hour until improvement is seen, and then gradually tapered. Tetracycline 1.0 percent ointment every 2 hours is an alternative. Frequent cleaning of the conjunctival cul-de-sac with saline is also useful. Neonates and children should receive intravenous crystalline penicillin G, 50,000 units per kilogram per day in two divided doses for 7 days. Pregnant or breast-feeding women and children allergic to penicillin should receive erythromycin, 500 mg orally four times a day for at least 7 days. Parenteral therapy for adults is intravenous aqueous crystalline penicillin G, 10 million units daily for 5 days. Patients with penicillinase-producing gonococcal infection should receive cefoxitin sodium, 1.0 g or cefotaxime sodium, 0.5 g, intravenously four times a day. These are therapeutically equivalent and the choice is based on sensitivity of the organism. Penicillin-allergic adults are treated with oral tetracycline 500 mg four times a day for at least 7 days.

All adults involved in transmitting gonococcal conjunctivitis to neonates, children, or other adults should receive therapy as noted in the chapter on dysuria.

Chlamydia are presently the leading cause of ophthalmia neonatorum. This infection has also been termed inclusion conjunctivitis of the newborn or inclusion blenorrhea. In some population groups, 12 percent of pregnant women shed *Chlamydia* in the third trimester, so neonatal exposure is common. The conjunctivitis may appear from 1 day to 4 weeks after birth. Although it usually presents as a mild unilateral or bilateral mucopurulent conjunctivitis, it may also present as a hyperacute conjunctivitis. Infants prior to 4 months of age do not develop follicles in response to chlamydial infection as adults do. Systemic chlamydial involvement, such as pneumonitis, otitis media, rhinitis, and vaginitis, is common and may or may not occur concurrently with the conjunctivitis. Diagnosis is made by scrapings (as described under Conjunctivitis) and culture. Immunofluorescent detection of the organism with monoclonal antibodies may speed and increase the accuracy of diagnosis in the future. Treatment is by oral erythromycin, 10 mg per kilogram per day in four divided doses for 3 to 4 weeks. Additional topical treatment is with tetracycline 1 percent or sulfacetamide 10 percent ointment four times daily for 3 to 4 weeks. The mother and her sexual partner should also be treated for *Chlamydia*.

INFECTIONS OF THE EYELIDS

Eyelid skin is extremely thin and elastic. Deeper within the lids are layers of loose areolar tissue. As a result, large amounts of fluid can accumulate within these layers of the lid. Dense fibrous tissue prevents spread of this swelling to the forehead or cheek. However, inflammatory swelling of one lid can readily spread to the other lid of the same eye and sometimes across the bridge of the nose to involve the lids of the fellow eye. The fibrous connective tissue of the orbital septum separates the eyelids (preseptal) from the orbit.

Orbital inflammation can almost always be separated from preseptal involvement on the basis of clinical findings. Acute orbital inflammation is characterized by proptosis, restricted ocular motility, and pain on attempted extraocular movement. Furthermore, marked chemosis, reduced corneal sensation, and blurred vision may be present. These signs are rarely found in preseptal processes.

Chronic blepharoconjunctivitis has been previously discussed.

Bacterial preseptal cellulitis results from trauma around the orbit, especially around the superior orbital rim. The trauma may or may not have broken the skin. The upper lid is tense and inflamed. Some degree of fluctuation is usually present. The patient does not appear extremely ill, nor are there any signs of orbital cellulitis. *S. aureus* is the usual cause of preseptal cellulitis, although occasionally streptococci, *H. influenzae, Peptococcus* species, *Peptostreptococcus* species, *Bacteroides* species, and clostridia may be found in pure or mixed culture. *H. influenzae* produces a characteristic and rather atypical preseptal cellulitis in children 6 to 36 months of age. This preseptal cellulitis has the additional features of purple discoloration of the involved area, mucopurulent ocular discharge, signs of systemic toxicity, and sometimes orbital inflammation as evidenced by chemosis, proptosis, and limited extraocular motion.

Therapy of preseptal bacterial cellulitis includes incision and drainage (except in cases due to *H. influenzae*), microbiologic work-up, and systemic antibiotics. The lid should be incised for 2 to 3 cm over the area of fluctuation, preferably along the lateral one-third of the orbital rim. A foul-smelling discharge, necrotic tissue, and gas formation should alert the clinician to probable anaerobic infection. Drainage is aided by blunt spreading of the tissues and by constant moist or dry heat. The drainage fluid should be examined by Gram stain and cultured for aerobes and anaerobes. Intravenous antibiotic therapy in full systemic dosage is initiated and modified on the basis of microbiologic findings. Penicillin G is the mainstay of treatment and is used alone if gram-positive rods are found. Nafcillin is added for gram-positive cocci, and gentamicin is added for gram-negative rods. Finally, nafcillin and gentamicin are combined with penicillin G if no organisms are seen on Gram stain. Oral antibiotics may be substituted for intravenous therapy after 48 to 72 hours if clinical improvement is sufficient. Antibiotic therapy should be continued for 7 days or until resolution of purulent drainage. Streptococcal cellulitis is always treated for 10 days to prevent subsequent glomerulonephritis. In the event of *H. influenzae* preseptal cellulitis, intravenous ampicillin combined with topical chloramphenicol is the treatment of choice. Tetanus toxoid and tetanus immune globulin should be administered if necessary in cases of preseptal cellulitis.

Impetigo is a highly contagious, rapidly spreading, superficial primary pyoderma that may involve the eyelids. It is commoner among children and begins as small red macules that rapidly progress to thin-walled vesicles that rupture, ooze, and crust. Peripheral spreading occurs, sometimes with satellite lesion formation. The conjunctiva and globe remain quiet. Lid swelling develops beneath the surface infection. Impetigo is caused by *S. aureus* and group A. *Streptococcus pyogenes*, perhaps by mutually promoting each other's growth. Laboratory work-up should include Gram stain and culture of the vesicle fluid. Treatment consists of oral cloxacillin for 10 days and topical bacitracin ointment (500 units per gram) three to four times daily. Cephalexin can be substituted for cloxacillin in penicillin-sensitive patients. Ideally, the ointment is applied after scrubbing the infected skin with soap and water. Intravenous nafcillin therapy may be necessary in severely afflicted or in extremely young patients. (Also see chapter *Cellulitis and Soft Tissue Infection.*)

Erysipelas is a superficial form of streptococcal cellulitis that uncommonly affects the lid. The group A beta-hemolytic streptococci gain access to the dermis via any break in the skin and incite a spreading, acute inflammatory response. The involved area is bright red, hot, tender, indurated, and well defined. The overlying surface skin may exfoliate. Signs of systemic toxicity and orbital inflammation may be present. Microbiologic confirmation of the infection is often difficult. Needle aspiration of the lesion should not be attempted because the infection may be spread. Blood cultures may be positive for streptococci. Erysipelas of the eyelid is treated by intravenous penicillin G until there is clinical improvement, followed by penicillin VK for a total of 10 days.

INFECTIONS OF THE LACRIMAL SYSTEM

The lacrimal system is the passageway for tear flow from the conjunctival sac to the nose. It consists of puncta, near the inner canthus of each lid, which are continuous with canaliculi. The canaliculi course medially and usually join near the lacrimal sac to form a common canaliculus. This common canaliculus enters the lacrimal sac 3 to 4 mm below its domed fundus. Tears flow from the tear sac down the nasolacrimal duct to enter the nose beneath the inferior turbinate.

Patients with infection of the canalicular system present with a complaint of epiphora and swelling of the lower lid medially. The punctum may be red and swollen, often described as "pouting." Canaliculitis may be secondary to dacryocystitis and the wide variety of bacteria causing it. Isolated canaliculitis, on the other hand, is characteristically due to *Actinomyces. Actinomyces* is an anaerobic, gram-positive, weakly acid-fast organism that appears histologically as fine, branching filaments. *Nocardia*, a similar organism, can also cause isolated canaliculitis. Diagnosis of actinomyces canaliculitis is made by expression of typical "sulfur granules" from the involved canaliculus through the punctum. *Actinomyces* is sensitive to penicillin and sulfa drugs, but infection recurs when therapy is discontinued; therefore, treatment consists of evacuating the canaliculus by expression, curettage, or, rarely, incision.

Dacryocystitis, or inflammation of the tear sac, is almost always secondary to stasis and subsequent infection as a result of nasolacrimal duct obstruction. The chronic form presents as epiphora, medial canthal mucopurulent discharge, and a nontender swelling on the side of the nose. Reflux of mucus or pus from the puncta on massage of the swollen sac is confirmatory evidence of chronic dacryosystitis. Acute dacryocystitis presents as a red, tender, sometimes fluctuant swelling inferomedial to the eye. Spontaneous drainage may occur.

Acute dacryocystitis is most commonly caused by *S. pneumoniae*, but streptococci, staphylococci, diphtheroids, *Klebsiella pneumoniae, H. influenzae, P. aeruginosa, Actinomyces, Candida*, and other fungi have also been cultured from patients with cases of dacryocystitis.

Treatment of acute dacryocystitis in adults consists of oral dicloxacillin and hot compresses to quiet the infection until normal drainage of the lacrimal sac can be reestablished by surgical dacryocystorhinostomy (DCR). Transcutaneous incision and drainage of the tear sac in acute dacryocystitis can temporarily improve the clinical picture. However, it produces scarring and is not curative. DCR is also the treatment of choice for chronic adult dacryocystitis. Topical sulfacetamide or tobramycin drops are frequently tried in acute and chronic dacryocystitis. However, drops simply change the organisms producing the infection and do not address lacrimal sac stasis, which is the underlying etiology.

Cases of acute and chronic dacryocystitis in young children may be due to congenital dacryostenosis, which is amenable to probing. However, recurrent lacrimal probing is fruitless and possibly damaging.

KERATITIS

C. STEPHEN FOSTER, M.D.

The avascularity and extreme thinness of the cornea set the stage for rapid destruction of this tissue as a result of infection and/or intense inflammation. Many well-documented examples exist of small, "innocent" or "benign" superficial corneal ulcers progressing to perforation in 24 to 48 hours. Corneal ulcers must be considered emergencies, and all ophthalmologists should have a well-thought-out plan for rapid diagnosis and therapy. Too often the cause and hence the proper course of therapy for corneal ulcers is unclear. Confounding variables are rapidly compounded when broad-spectrum antimicrobial therapy is instituted without an adequate diagnostic evaluation or capture of the offending organisms. Therapy with agents to which the organism is only partially sensitive invariably results in progression of the ulceration and usually thwarts later attempts at organism isolation. Laboratory studies should be executed much more often than they currently appear to be, and the ophthalmologist should personally execute the harvesting and planting of the material for culture. Scrapings for smears and cultures are absolutely mandatory in any case of neonatal conjunctivitis, hyperacute conjunctivitis, membranous conjunctivitis, and in any case of corneal ulceration. Any postoperative infection, intraocular or otherwise, and any case of chronic conjunctivitis, blepharitis, or keratitis, for example, should similarly be studied carefully with extensive laboratory studies.

Progressive corneal ulceration in patients without significant systemic disease may be caused by herpes simplex keratitis, adenoviral keratitis, bacterial keratitis, fungal keratitis, parasitic keratitis, medicamentosa keratitis, factitious keratitis, or trophic keratitis. The major defense against confusion about the cause of progressive corneal ulceration is a systematic approach to diagnosis and therapy.

It is essential to obtain a complete ophthalmic and systemic history from a patient with corneal ulceration since the presence of diabetes mellitus, rheumatoid arthritis, diseases associated with a compromised immune status or sicca syndrome, among others, may significantly alter the diagnostic likelihoods and therapy. The usual thorough execution and recording of a complete ophthalmic examination is similarly essential, with special attention being paid to corneal sensation, Bell's phenomenon, lid eversion for retained foreign body, lagophthalmos, and lid/lash/globe relationships.

SIGNS AND SYMPTOMS

The symptoms of corneal infection include foreign-body sensation, photophobia, and decreased vision. Signs include blepharospasm, conjunctival vascular injection, profuse tearing, and the presence of a dulled corneal reflex or possibly the appearance of a white infiltrate in the corneal stroma. If the process has existed for a substantial period, corneal neovascularization may have begun in the corneal periphery.

Signs observable by slit-lamp biomicroscopy include a corneal epithelial defect, which stains with fluorescein; perhaps loss of corneal stromal substance with excavation; white cell infiltration into the corneal stroma; inflammatory cells in the anterior chamber, possibly to the extent that frank hypopyon develops; and ciliary spasm with reactive meiosis.

DIAGNOSIS

The diagnosis of corneal infections is based first on clinical findings as described above, followed by appropriate microbiologic studies.

The responsibility for obtaining material for smears and cultures and for planting the cultures themselves rests with the ophthalmologist. Culture should never be obtained and sent in transport media to a microbiology laboratory for plating. The culture plates should be no older than 2 weeks. Since most fungi grow well at room temperature on blood agar, we routinely employ two blood agar plates for ocular cultures—one placed in the incubator for isolation of bacteria and one kept at room temperature for fungus isolation. The Sabouraud's agar plate is also used for fungus isolation. Thioglycolate broth or cooked meat broth may be used for isolation of anaerobic organisms. An alternative approach for the isolation of these delicate organisms is to plate the culture on blood agar and/or on chocolate agar and immediately place the plates in a Gaspak jar or in an anaerobic incubator. We use an anaerobic incubator.

A sterile cotton-tipped swab moistened with cooked meat broth or a calcium alginate swab may be used for lid and conjunctival cultures. Conjunctival swabbing of both the inferior and the superior fornix of each eye is performed with a separate swab for each eye. Lid margin and conjunctival swabs are plated on blood agar plates; one economical technique is to plant both lid and conjunctival cultures from each eye on a single blood agar plate in the pattern shown in Figure 1. The swabs are then plunged to the bottom of cooked meat tubes for anaerobic organism isolation.

A dry, sterile swab is used to remove mucus and loose, purulent material from any corneal ulcer; this is cultured on blood agar plates, on chocolate agar, on Sabouraud's agar, and in cooked meat broth. Then, for specific diagnosis of the ulcer, a number 15 Bard-Parker scalpel blade or a Kimura spatula with sharpened edges are suitable instruments for obtaining the corneal material for smears and cultures. The commonest cause of negative results from slides and cultures of corneal ulcers is inadequate scrapings of the ulcer margins and base. Scraping should be obtained with great vigor, under the operating microscope or by slit-lamp biomicroscopy, and multiple scrapings should be done. Three precleaned glass slides are prepared from scrapings by spreading a small amount of material thinly over a very small area of each slide. The slides are fixed in absolute methanol for 5 minutes. One slide is then stained with Gram stain, one with Giemsa stain, and one kept as a spare. Brief, very mild heat fixation is acceptable for the Gram stain. "C" streaks are made on the culture plates from each corneal scraping (Fig. 2). One of the blood agar plates and the Sabouraud's agar plate are kept at room temperature; the other blood agar plate, the chocolate agar plate, and the cooked meat tube are incubated at 35 °C. One additional technique for examination of smears that is probably slightly more sensitive than the traditional Gram and Giemsa staining procedure employs acridine orange stain

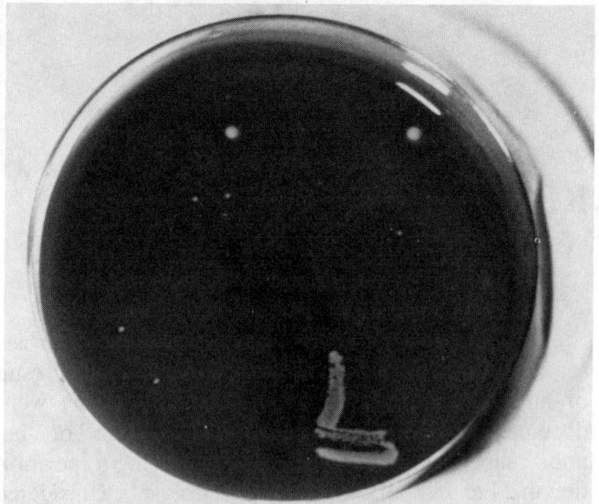

Figure 1 Lid and conjunctival culture plate. Separate moistened swabs for the right conjunctiva, the right lid margin, the left conjunctiva, and the left lid margin have been used to make streaks on a single blood agar plate. The conjunctival swabs were streaked in small streaks on the superior part of the plate. These cultures are negative. The lid swabs were used to make the initial R and L on the bottom part of the plate. The lid swab from the left eye is positive, showing colonies of *Staphylococcus aureus.*

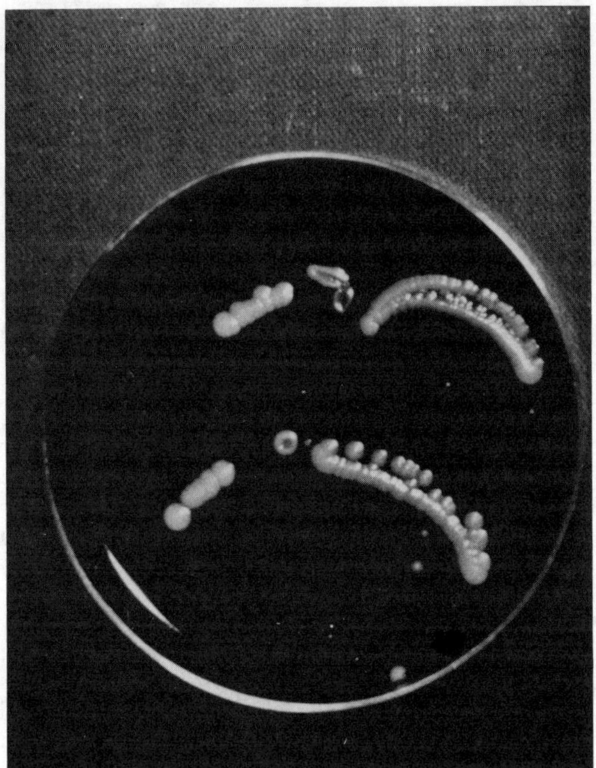

Figure 2 "C" streaks from a bacterial corneal ulcer. Note that the bacterial colonies are growing on the "C" streaks assuring that the microorganisms are from the corneal scraping and not from contaminant.

with subsequent fluorescent microscopy of the stained smear. The modified Ziehl-Neelsen acid-fast stain should be performed in any case where *Mycobacterium* or *Actinomycetes*, including *Nocardia*, is suspected. The Gomori methenamine-silver stain and/or the periodic acid–Schiff (PAS) stain and the Schwartz stain should be used if fungus is suspected. Diagnostic taps of the anterior chamber are not indicated, even if hypopyon is present, as long as Descemet's membrane has remained intact. A single exception to this rule may occur in fungal keratitis, and this will be discussed subsequently.

BACTERIAL KERATITIS

Except in the mildest cases of gram-positive bacterial keratitis, it is probably wisest to hospitalize patients with central bacterial corneal ulcers. Subconjunctival antibiotics (preferably chosen on the basis of results from smear; see below) may be administered every 12 to 24 hours for 3 to 7 days, along with fortified antibiotic topical drops every 15 to 30 minutes around the clock. Aggressive topical antibiotic therapy is usually sufficient; if there is any question about the ability of nursing personnel to comply with around-the-clock-every-15-minute orders, subconjunctival antibiotics are recommended. Before the subconjunctival injections and for diagnostic scrapings, children should be anesthetized briefly with general anesthetic. Patients should receive topical anesthetic and a small amount (0.1 to 0.2 ml) of subconjunctival anesthetic (2% lidocaine [Xylocaine]), prior to any subconjunctival injection. Most of the pain from subconjunctival antibiotic injections appears to result from the irritating qualities of the drugs themselves. I have had some experience with longer-acting anesthetics (e.g., bupivacaine hydrochloride [Marcaine]) used subconjunctivally before antibiotic injection. These seem to work well at alleviating patient discomfort after the usual 2-hour wear-off period of lidocaine. Since we often inject two antibiotics subconjunctivally, we usually inject them at separate sites. Recommended dosages of selected antibiotics are listed in Table 1.

Fortified topical antibiotics may be prepared aseptically by mixing parenteral preparations and artificial tears or by simple dilution of parenteral preparations (Table 1). A typical regimen of topical fortified antibiotic drops for a patient with a bacterial corneal ulcer might include one such antibiotic administered every hour on the hour and another administered every hour on the half hour.

For initial therapy for bacterial keratitis, some advocate broad-spectrum antibacterial agents (e.g., subconjunctival and topical gentamicin and cefazolin) regardless of the results of the Gram stain. Others choose to be guided to slightly more specific therapy by the gram-stained smear from the ulcer. I advocate the latter approach. A regimen for initial antibiotic therapy, based on the findings on the gram-stained smear from the ulcer, are shown in Table 2. I advocate checking the bacterial and fungal cultures early each morning and at the end of each day. Antibiotic therapy is then modified on the basis of the culture results and the sensitivities of the organisms isolated. I favor debriding the surface of the corneal ulcer each day; this aids in penetration of the topical and subconjunctival antibiotics. After adequate antibiotic therapy, both the concentration and frequency of administration of the topical antibiotics is reduced and eventually discontinued. A continuous-wear bandage soft

TABLE 1 Recommended Doses of Selected Antibiotics

	Route	
Antibiotic	*Subconjunctival*	*Topical*
Amikacin	250 mg	25–50 mg/ml
Ampicillin	100 mg	---
Bacitracin	10,000 units	10,000 units/ml
Carbenicillin	100 mg	4 mg/ml
Cefazolin	100 mg	33–100 mg/ml
Cephaloridine	100 mg	---
Clindamycin	150 mg	---
Colistin	25 mg	5–10 mg/ml
Gentamicin	40 mg	15 mg/ml
Kanamycin	30 mg	---
Methicillin	100 mg	---
Neomycin	250 mg	30 mg/ml
Oxacillin	100 mg	100 mg/ml
Penicillin G	0.5–1 million units	100,000 units/ml
Polymyxin B	5–10 mg	10,000 units/ml
Ticarcillin	250 mg	25 mg/ml
Tobramycin	40 mg	15 mg/ml
Vancomycin	25 mg	50 mg/ml

TABLE 2 Initial Antibiotic Therapy for Bacterial Keratitis

Results of Gram Stain	Antibiotic, Dose	
	Subconjunctival	*Topical*
Gram-positive cocci	Cefazolin, 100 mg Gentamicin, 40 mg	Cefazolin Gentamicin
Gram-positive bacilli	Penicillin G, 1 million units	Cefazolin Bacitracin
Gram-negative bacilli	Tobramycin, 40 mg Ticarcillin, 250 mg	Tobramycin Ticarcillin
Gram-negative cocci	Penicillin G, 1 million units	Cefazolin Bacitracin
Equivocal or negative smear	Tobramycin, 40 mg Cefazolin, 100 mg	Tobramycin Cefazolin

contact lens may be added for treatment of persistent epithelial defects after the infection has been adequately treated. Other forms of adjunctive therapy include (*1*) cycloplegics, (*2*) collagenase inhibitors (e.g., 20% N-acetylcysteine [Mucomyst], or 1% medroxyprogesterone [Provera]) for progressive stromal ulceration, and (*3*) topical corticosteroids for excessive inflammatory reaction after the causative organism has been isolated and is being correctly treated.

FUNGAL KERATITIS

Although fungal keratitis may exhibit certain highly characteristic signs, many investigators believe that it is rarely advisable to treat a "presumptive fungal corneal ulcer" with antifungal agents for corneal ulcer therapy unless fungal elements are seen on smear from the corneal scrapings or fungi grow from such scrapings in culture. Certain rare exceptions to this generalization exist, but in general it is far better to administer antibacterial therapy, repeating the corneal scrapings and performing corneal biopsy in an effort to isolate a causative organism than to add yet another agent to the therapeutic regimen. The following is an example of unfortunate results of antifungal therapy given before fungi were seen or isolated.

Case report. A 38-year-old white woman was treated by a physician in her hometown in the Bahamas with an intramuscular penicillin injection and steroid eye drops for red eye. The patient had no known history of ocular trauma or ocular infections. Ten days after the penicillin injection, the patient went to an ophthalmologist because her ocular status had not improved. The visual acuity was 20/400 in the affected right eye at that time, and the ophthalmologist noted a central corneal infiltrate in the right cornea. Therapy consisted of dexamethasone/neomycin sulfate/polymyxin B sulfate (Maxitrol) drops, atropine drops, and sulfacetamide ointment at bedtime. Two weeks of this regimen had no beneficial effect; the corneal infiltrate became slightly larger and more dense.

The woman consulted a second ophthalmologist; by now, the visual acuity in the right eye was limited to hand movements. The eye was extremely injected. Slit-lamp biomicroscopy revealed a very large central corneal stromal infiltrate—dense, white, with multiple round, dense snowball-like satellite infiltrates; a hypopyon; and dense plaque of fibrin-like material on the corneal endothelium. A dense coagulum of fibrinous material filled most of the anterior chamber (Fig. 3). Scrapings of the corneal infiltrate were plated on blood agar (at 35 °C and 20 °C), on Sabouraud agar, and in meat broth; specimens were taken for Gram stain. The Gram stain of the smear revealed only neutrophils.

The patient was admitted to the hospital and treated with subconjunctival gentamicin and cephalothin sodium (Keflin), topical bacitracin and gentamicin, and topical pimaricin (Natamycin). The initial impression was of fungal keratitis. The patient also received oral flucytosine, 2 g four times a day. Over the next 4 days, the ocular status seemed to be improving. The cultures were negative.

The clinical picture then began to deteriorate, with further progression of ulceration (Fig. 4). Corneal scrapings and a superficial corneal biopsy were performed; histopathologic analysis (including study for fungal elements) and culturing of this material were unrevealing. The clinical picture continued to worsen (Fig. 5); 17 days after the patient's admission to the hospital by the second ophthalmologist, penetrating keratoplasty was performed for diagnosis and therapy. The excised corneal button was processed immediately for microbiologic examination. Vast numbers of septate hyphae were easily found in the excised material. *Fusarium* species grew on blood agar and Sabouraud agar.

The classic clinical characteristics of fungal keratitis were present in this patient: feathery borders of stromal infiltrate, satellite lesions, hypopyon, endothelial plaque. Indeed, the patient had fungal keratitis, but the organism was not captured in initial diagnostic efforts. Inadequate therapy hindered further attemps at isolation of the organism while allowing the infection to proceed deeper. Therapy with pimaricin should not have been initiated. If the clinician's suspicion of fungal keratitis was strong enough to warrant antifungal therapy, it was strong enough to warrant diagnostic keratectomy. I wish to emphasize the importance of making the maximal initial di-

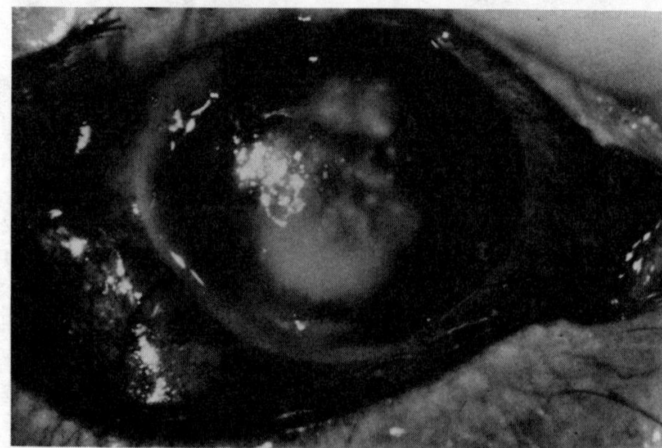

Figure 3 Fungal corneal ulcer with characteristic endothelial plaque, hypopyon, and satellite lesions.

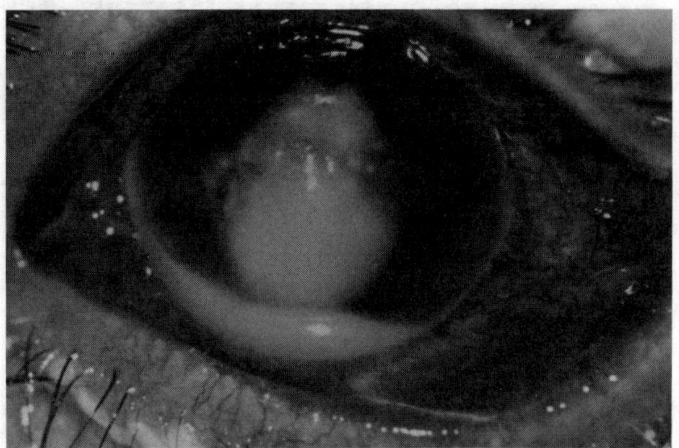

Figure 4 Same eye as in Fig. 3. Note progression with increasing hypopyon and increasing density in stromal infiltration.

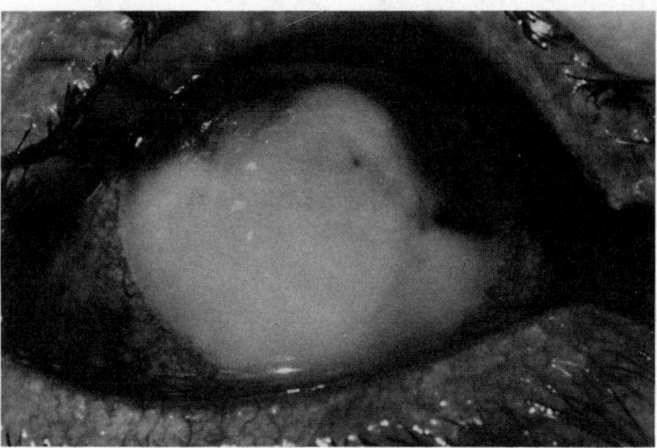

Figure 5 Same eye as in Figs. 3 and 4. Note the progression, with the anterior chamber now virtually full of pus and the cornea nearly completely opacified from the progression of the fuscarian keratitis.

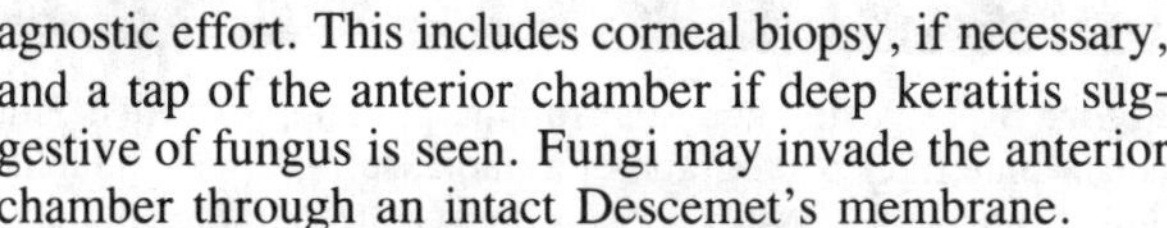

agnostic effort. This includes corneal biopsy, if necessary, and a tap of the anterior chamber if deep keratitis suggestive of fungus is seen. Fungi may invade the anterior chamber through an intact Descemet's membrane.

My current therapeutic approach to fungal keratitis is shown in Table 3. Ideal antifungal agents for treatment of keratomycosis are not available. Amphotericin B does not penetrate the deeper corneal layers well, and at high doses it is very toxic to the cornea. We currently use 0.3 percent amphotericin B topically. Pimaricin, 5 percent suspension, is well tolerated by the cornea, but its spectrum is limited, and it does not penetrate well. It is the drug of choice for superficial corneal infections caused by fungi susceptible to it (most notably *Fusarium*). Flucytosine, 1 percent, and miconazole, 1 percent, are the drugs of choice for treatment of candidal keratomycosis. These drugs penetrate the cornea well and are well tolerated by the eye.

In my opinion, miconazole is the initial drug of choice for keratomycosis caused by filamentous fungi, at least in geographic areas where *Fusarium* is not the predominant cause of fungal keratitis (it is a common cause of fungal keratitis in southern climates, including the Caribbean). Miconazole is safe and effective used topically and subconjunctivally (10 mg) for keratomycosis. We have shown that it is well tolerated topically and subconjunctivally in an experimental model, and I have reported on its safety and efficacy when given topically and subconjunctivally to patients with candidal or aspergillus keratitis. Amphotericin B, 0.3 percent topically, can also be highly useful in keratomycosis with overlying epithelial defect, allowing adequate penetration of this drug.

Initial antifungal therapy should be modified on the basis of clinical response and sensitivity testing of the fungal isolate. Additional therapy for ulcerative keratitis usually includes cycloplegic agents and may include collagenase inhibitors such as EDTA, N-acetylcysteine, or medroxyprogesterone. Corticosteroid therapy is controversial. If the causative agent has been isolated and specific therapy begun, it is probably reasonable to employ steroidal and nonsteroidal anti-inflammatory agents

TABLE 3 Therapeutic Approach to Fungal Keratitis

		Antibiotic		
Result of Smear	*Further Diagnostic Procedures*	*Topical*	*Subconjunctival*	*Oral*
Yeast or pseudohyphae	----	Flucytosine *and* Miconazole	Miconazole	Flucytosine Ketoconazole
Hyphal fragments	----	Miconazole *or* Pimaricin* *or* Amphotericin B	Miconazole	Ketoconazole
No hyphal fragments or yeasts; mild to moderate clinical picture	Repeat scrapings; biopsy cornea; if clinical picture is stable, delay therapy until cultures or histopathologic tests confirm diagnosis			
Severe clinical picture	Biopsy cornea	Miconazole *or* Amphotericin B	Miconazole	Flucytosine

* In geographic areas where *Fusarium* is common, treat superficial ulcers with pimaricin.

judiciously to minimize tissue destruction from excessive host response. Surgical intervention in the form of conjunctival flap or penetrating keratoplasty may occasionally be necessary.

HERPES SIMPLEX KERATITIS

When considering therapy for herpes simplex keratitis (HSK), the clinician must determine the pathophysiologic form of herpetic infection involved. At least six major forms exist, and therapy is different for each. In this section, I will discuss infectious (dendritic) epithelial keratitis, noninfectious (trophic, metaherpetic) epithelial keratitis, and infectious stromal (interstitial) keratitis. I will not discuss the other pathophysiologic forms (immune [disciform] edema, limbitis, and uveitis) since these forms should never be confused with frank corneal ulceration.

Infectious (Dendritic) Epithelial Keratitis

Infectious epithelial keratitis is usually associated with the dendrite, the hallmark of HSK. The earliest lesions may be punctate focal elevations of swollen epithelial cells that are infected with live virus. These lesions stain with rose bengal; fluorescein pools around them, but does not stain them. Within a day, the cells are destroyed, and the area stains with fluorescein in a stellate or dendritic configuration. The basis of this configuration is not known, but it is probably due to the cell-to-cell spread of virus. Geographic ulcers may develop. These larger epithelial defects with serpiginous borders are also caused by live virus, may be associated with stromal infiltration, and may be confused with ulcers of bacterial keratitis. Rose bengal brightly stains the virus-infected cells at the edge of the stellate, dendritic lesions or geographic lesions of infectious epithelial HSK; fluorescein stains the entire epithelial defect and spreads out beneath the loosely adherent, adjacent epithelial cells. The rose bengal staining pattern is quite typical, with palisading punctate rose bengal-stained cells lining the periphery of the fluorescein-stained defect (Fig. 6). Corneal sensation may be decreased; this decrease may be focal. Corneal hypoesthesia may be permanent.

The patient with dendritic keratitis presents with a red eye associated with various amounts of ocular irritation and blurred vision. Treatment consists of antiviral therapy, usually after debridement. My first-choice antiviral agent currently is trifluorothymidine (Viroptic) drops, used every 2 hours throughout the day. Idoxuridine or vidarabine ointment or, when available, acyclovir ointment, five times a day for 10 to 14 days, may be used instead. Idoxuridine drops can be used hourly while the patient is awake and every 2 hours during sleep. Antibiotic ointment at bedtime and drops four times daily, along with cycloplegics as needed for iritis, are indicated. The dendrite should begin to heal within 2 to 3 days; fluorescein staining is broken up into islands. Treatment should continue for 5 to 7 days after the epithelial defect heals. Lack of response may mean that the medication is not being administered reliably or that the virus is resistant to the antiviral drug.

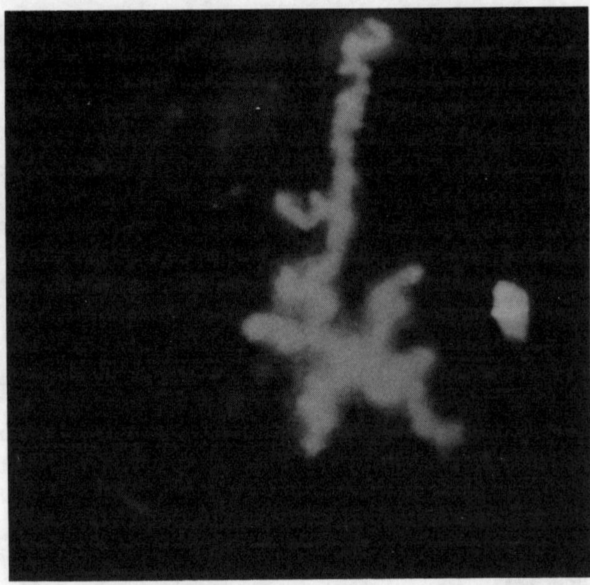

Figure 6 Dendritic keratitis from herpes simplex virus. This cobalt blue filter photograph of a fluorescein-stained epithelial defect shows the classic dendritic-form pattern of the epithelial defect created by the herpes simplex virus of this cornea.

Gentle mechanical debridement (after topical anesthesic) is done with a cotton-tipped applicator, blunt-tipped foreign-body spatula, chalazion curette, Kimura spatula, or scalpel blade. This can be done initially (which is preferable) or, if the patient does not respond to antivirals, in 2 to 3 days. Mechanical debridement has the advantage of rapidly removing viral antigen that probably contributes to immune disciform HSK. Mechanical debridement is followed by antiviral treatment and, if the defect is large, patching. Chemical debridement, using iodine for example, is contraindicated; it damages the basement membrane and predisposes the patient to trophic epithelial defects. Careful follow-up is necessary to be certain that the anticipated clinical response has begun within 2 to 3 days and to observe for drug toxicity or allergy. Complete healing is expected by 10 to 14 days.

It must be emphasized that steroids are contraindicated in infectious epithelial HSK. Although topical steroids do not provoke reactivation of latent virus and clinical recurrence, they make the recurrent disease, when it occurs spontaneously, more severe. In these circumstances, epithelial defects enlarge; stromal ulceration may occur with astonishing rapidity and progress to perforation. This is an important reason that patients with red eyes should not receive steroids without a careful biomicroscopic examination to rule out HSK.

Noninfectious (Trophic, Metaherpetic) Epithelial Keratitis

Trophic epithelial defects occur in some patients with a history of HSK. The defect is not caused by active viral

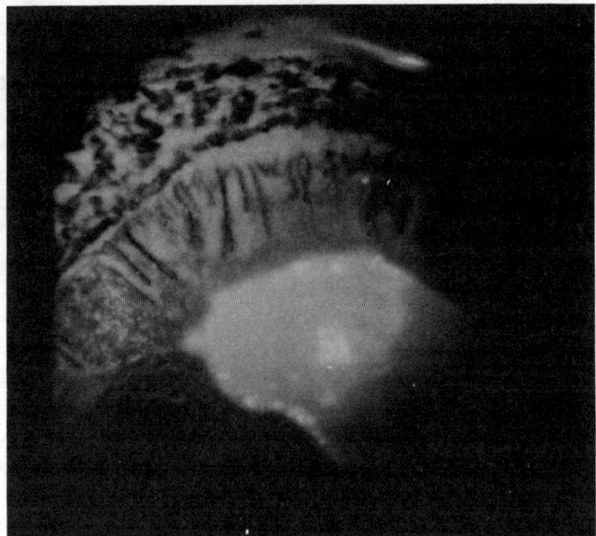

Figure 7 Metaherpetic herpes keratitis. This is a nondescript epithelial defect staining with fluorescein. No infectious viral particles are present, though this patient has previously had herpes and the epithelial basement membrane has been damaged.

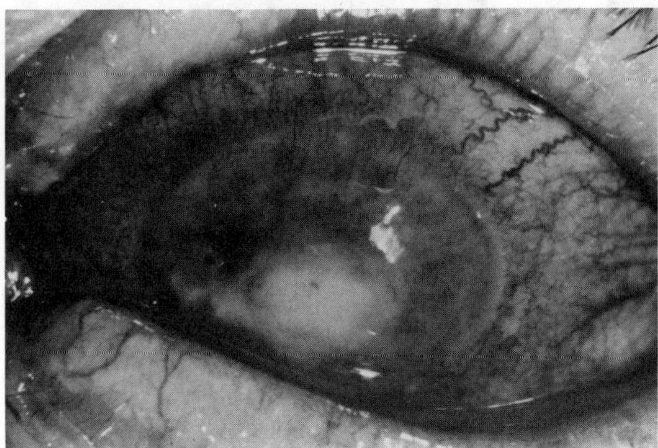

Figure 8 Interstitial herpes stromal keratitis. Note the intrastromal infiltrate with the cheesy-white character of the stromal inflammatory response. Note also the associated ''limbitis'' superiorly.

infection; rather, it is due to basement membrane damage by past infection. It is comparable to recurrent erosion syndrome in that the pathogenesis for both diseases involves basement membrane damage and failure of normal hemidesmosome attachment complexes to form. Typically, trophic defects have smooth, rolled edges of heaped-up epithelium that do not stain with rose bengal in the bright, palisading punctate arrangement seen in infectious HSK (Fig. 7). Often they persist after antiviral treatment would have been expected to heal a geographic ulcer. Trophic defects must be distinguished from active geographic ulcers because treatment of the two differs.

Bandage soft contact lenses and pressure patching are the main treatments for trophic epithelial defects. An antibiotic of comparatively low epithelial toxicity, such as chloramphenicol drops, should be used with the bandage lens. Erythromycin ointment and pressure patching constitute another acceptable approach. Some authors recommend freshening the edges of the defect and debriding the base prior to patching or applying a bandage lens. The bandage lens protects the cornea from lid movements, which can pull off loosely adherent epithelium. Artificial tears given every 2 hours keep the surface well lubricated during the period of bandage lens wear and after healing, when the lens is removed. I usually leave soft lenses in position for 4 to 6 months regardless of the origin of the defect.

Stromal melting is a serious sequela of persistent trophic epithelial defects, and its treatment is difficult. If corticosteroids have been used for inflammation, they must be tapered off and managed with extreme caution; abrupt discontinuation may not be wise. N-Acetylcysteine (20% drops every 2 hours), a collagenase inhibitor, or medroxyprogesterone (1% drops every 6 hours), an inhibitor of collagenase synthesis, may help. Cyanoacrylate adhesive can be applied to the defect and covered by a bandage lens. Conjunctival flap may be extremely effective in arresting progressive stromal ulceration. Lamellar keratoplasty patch grafting is useful for impending or frank perforation.

Infectious Stromal (Interstitial) Keratitis

Interstitial keratitis is a necrotic process associated with white stromal infiltrates and subsequent neovascularization that usually occurs in patients with a history of infectious epithelial HSK (Fig. 8). Differential diagnosis must rule out bacterial or fungal keratitis. Live virus and an immune response are believed to contribute to this disease state. Opinion concerning the use of steroids is similar to that involved in the treatment of immune disciform keratitis. If the lesions do not involve the visual axis, then antivirals, cycloplegics, and artificial tears may suffice. If the corneal and anterior chamber reactions are severe and the infiltrates involve the visual axis, steroids should be used along with antivirals and antibiotics. The minimal steroid dose required to control the immune reaction should be used. The disease follows a protracted course, and steroids must be tapered off very gradually for weeks or months. Fortunately, this is a relatively uncommon manifestation of HSK. Trifluorothymidine may penetrate into corneal stroma more effectively than idoxuridine or vidarabine and thus may be the antiviral of choice for infectious stromal HSK.

TRACHOMA

MOHSEN ZIAI, M.D.

Trachoma is the leading cause of blindness throughout the world. It is estimated that 400 million individuals suffer from this disease. The overwhelming majority of affected persons live in endemic areas of Southeast Asia, the Middle East, and Africa, where environmental and personal standards of hygiene are suboptimal and where virtually every child under 2 years of age is affected.

The infection produces a chronic form of conjunctivitis with bacterial superinfections that lead to scarring if the cycle is not broken. These conjunctival scars result in trichiasis and entropion with consequent damage to the cornea causing ulcerations, opacity, and loss of vision.

The causative agent of trachoma is *Chlamydia trachomatis* and in endemic areas the disease is associated with the serotypes A, B, and Ba, in contrast to other serotypes causing inclusion conjunctivitis and urethritis in nonendemic areas. The mode of transmission is eye to eye spread by contaminated hands or objects. In the uncomplicated form the disease has a relatively self-limited natural history and eventual recovery is expected. Initial symptoms consist of photophobia and lacrimation, with a clear or purulent discharge. The course of the disease is chronic, and even in the absence of reinfection there are frequently remissions and exacerbations.

In the early stages a chronic follicular conjunctivitis is observed, manifested by follicles on the upper tarsal plate and papillary hypertrophy as well as by inflammatory infiltration of the conjunctiva of varying degrees. Linear scars follow, and if they are severe they may lead to tear deficiency syndromes, dacryostenosis, and trichiasis with entropion which usually affects the upper lid, causing corneal ulceration and scarring. The vascular pannus (neovascularization) is superficial, more marked in the area of the superior limbus. Other forms of scars as well as inflammatory processes are found in chronic cases.

In the United States the disease is seen mainly in Mexican Americans and American Indians as well as some other minorities. Older individuals who have lived in the area known formerly as the Trachoma Belt of Oklahoma and Texas may manifest recurrences of the disease, with some active infection found in their children.

The diagnostic features of the disease are its insidious onset, the presence of upper tarsal follicles, limbal follicles, corneal infiltration, and scars. In addition, one can observe vascular pannus developing early over the cornea where epithelial keratitis and marginal infiltrates are also seen. Laboratory diagnosis of trachoma in the initial stages can be made by direct immunofluorescence or Giemsa stain of conjunctival scrapings as well as by detection of tear microimmunofluorescent antibody or isolation of the organism in culture. Tear or serum antibody is probably the method of choice in chronic cases.

Treatment of trachoma must be considered in the context of two separate objectives. First and foremost is the organization of campaigns for the control of the disease or at least prevention of blindness. Second is the treatment of individual patients with the best possible method, notwithstanding the usual obstacles encountered in campaigns and public health efforts directed at the masses.

In mass treatment campaigns systemic use of antimicrobials often results in serious complications. Sulfonamide drugs, although effective against trachoma, are associated with undesirable side effects, particularly allergic skin and systemic reactions. The use of tetracyclines is risky for children as well as pregnant or lactating women. The expense involved in the use of rifampin and certain serious effects associated with the use of some forms of erythromycin are examples of difficulties that could be encountered with the use of systemic drugs in such campaigns. Therefore, the procedure of choice in these mass treatment campaigns is to emphasize the promotion of hygiene as well as prolonged use of topical antimicrobials in the form of ointments. For the latter purpose ointments of either 1 percent tetracycline or 1 percent erythromycin are reasonable choices. I recommend the intermittent administration of the drug topically for 5 consecutive days every month for 6 months or periodic community-wide treatment (5 days per week for 6 weeks). In case sensitivity or superinfection by resistant organisms develops, the drug should be discontinued. Effective vaccines against trachoma are not available.

As far as the treatment of individual patients is concerned it must be remembered that systemic use of antimicrobials is preferable, as topical treatment will usually not eradicate the organism even though it may greatly improve the signs of infection. I recommend any of the three drugs: tetracycline, 2 g per day in four divided doses, or doxycycline, 100 mg twice daily for 3 weeks in adults (tetracyclines should not be given to children or pregnant women); sulfonamides, for example, sulfisoxazole, 6 g per day in four divided doses for adults, 150 mg per kg per day for children in four divided doses; or erythromycin, for example, erythromycin ethyl succinate, 30 mg per kg per day in four divided doses for children, 2 g per day in four divided doses for adults. Effective treatment of the disease and eradication of the organisms require 3 weeks of systemic drug administration. Clinical improvement may not become apparent for 2 weeks or more after the initiation of systemic therapy. The patient should be under supervision and the necessary precautions concerning the side effects should be kept in mind. In infants and young children erythromycin is probably preferable to sulfonamides.

Trichiasis and cicatricial entropion resulting from chronic trachoma can be treated surgically. Cryotherapy is useful in certain cases. When corneal damage is occurring, corrective therapy must be considered a matter of emergency.

CARDIOVASCULAR AND RELATED INFECTIONS

INFECTIVE ENDOCARDITIS AND MYCOTIC ANEURYSM

LAWRENCE R. FREEDMAN, M.D.

Infective endocarditis (IE) refers to infection established within a platelet-fibrin vegetation on the endocardial surface of the heart. The disease is curable and the risk to the patient small when the infection is diagnosed immediately after it is established and the correct antibiotics are administered in a fashion to ensure their proper delivery to the site of infection for a sufficient period of time.

On the other hand, if the patient delays seeking the help of a physician or if the physician does not establish the diagnosis promptly, the risks to the patient may result in permanent incapacity or death. In these instances even proper treatment may not prevent these devastating complications. If the proper therapy is not instituted, death is the rule.

The establishment of infection depends upon the existence of a platelet-fibrin vegetation on the endocardium and the delivery to this vegetation of bacteria capable of sticking and multiplying. In about half the patients who develop IE, the patient and his physician are aware of lesions in the heart that are known to induce the formation of endocardial vegetations. In a similar proportion of patients, an explanation for bacteremia that establishes infection in the vegetations is apparent. Thus, IE is theoretically preventable in only about one-fourth of the patients who develop the disease, i.e., those known to be susceptible prior to the occurrence of bacteremia from an identifiable source. Even this figure is, however, overoptimistic, since prevention depends on administering antibiotics known to be effective in preventing the establishment of infection, and this depends on the interaction between the specific microorganisms circulating in the bloodstream and the antibiotic administered. In most instances (e.g., after tooth extractions) the likelihood of particular microorganisms being disseminated with predictable antibiotic sensitivities is a matter of statistical probability. For example, endocarditis due to enterococci or staphylococci has been reported (albeit rarely) after tooth extraction, a procedure for which antibiotics are advised that are not predictably effective against these bacteria.

So it is that, despite our theoretical capacity to interfere with the establishment of bacterial infection of the endocardium, practically speaking, we can hope to prevent but a small proportion of these infections.

In the preantibiotic era IE was considered to be virtually uniformly fatal. today, despite the availability of a potent antimicrobial armamentarium, the disease still carries significant risks of incapacity (embolic lesions to the central nervous system, cardiac malfunction, glomerulonephritis) and death even though sterilization of the infection may have been accomplished.

The challenge then is twofold: to prevent as many instances of IE as possible, and in cases where prophylaxis failed or was not employed, to promptly diagnose and effectively treat the patient.

PROPHYLAXIS

Evidence is lacking demonstrating the efficacy of antibiotic prophylaxis of infective endocarditis in humans. The studies that have tested the effectiveness of antibiotics in preventing IE in the rabbit model have, on the other hand, shown unequivocally that antibiotics are able to prevent endocarditis in the presence of transient bacteremia. There is general acceptance of the view that prophylactic antibiotics are indicated in patients with heart (and other intravascular) lesions known to be at risk of becoming infected when subjected to procedures that induce bacteremia. Furthermore, careful testing in the rabbit model has provided important guidelines to gauge the quantities of antibiotics necessary in humans to prevent infection by specific bacteria.

Detailed recommendations have been published by the American Heart Association and, although these cannot be subjected to experimental investigation in humans, a recent review of prophylaxis failures affirms the general validity of these recommendations.

There are many areas of uncertainty and controversy. For example, it is evident that prophylaxis may fail (probably rarely) even when the AHA recommendations are followed and the microorganism responsible for infection is sensitive to the antibiotics used. On the other hand, there are known to be different degrees of effectiveness of antibiotic regimens, but to date there are no recorded instances of patients developing streptococcal endocarditis when parenteral penicillin and streptomycin (as recommended by the AHA) were employed.

Other causes of failure of prophylaxis include infection with bacteria not anticipated to result from a procedure, for example, staphylococcal or enterococcal endocarditis after dental procedures. The most significant problems in the field of prophylaxis are, however, that dentists often do not adhere to the AHA recommendations, and patients are often unaware of having an intracardiac (or other intravascular) abnormality that requires prophylaxis prior to, for example, dental procedures.

The following tables list the bacteria likely to be disseminated by procedures, giving rise to consideration of antibiotic prophylaxis (Table 1), a classification of patients into risk categories according to the likelihood of development of endocarditis following a procedure (Table 2), and, finally, a set of recommendations (Table 3) taken from those of the American Heart Association. Table 4 lists the different antibiotic regimens and, in addition, includes the recommendations of a working party of the British Society for Antimicrobial Chemotherapy (BSAC).

The BSAC developed recommendations that are somewhat different from those of the AHA on the basis of their concern regarding the known frequency of lack of compliance with the AHA recommendations. It will be of considerable interest to see if compliance is any better with the BSAC proposals.

The original BSAC recommendation B (Table 4) does not call for a repetition of the dose of amoxicillin in 6 hours, but studies of the prophylaxis of IE in rabbits have shown the relative ineffectiveness of a single dose and the effectiveness of amoxicillin when repeated. In patients undergoing general anesthesia, the BSAC recommends regimen D parenterally, without gentamicin in all but the very high-risk patient group.

Since the frequency with which streptomycin resistance is recognized in enterococci is rising, it is the recommendation of several workers that gentamicin be regularly employed in regimens D and F. In view of recent experimental studies demonstrating the superiority of vancomycin and gentamicin over ampicillin and gentamicin for the prevention of streptomycin-resistant enterococcal endocarditis in animals, careful consideration must be given to preferring regimen F with gentamicin over regimen D for clinical use.

For the prevention of staphylococcal IE, as for example, in the placement of prosthetic heart valves, the use of beta-lactamase-resistant penicillin or cephalosporin antibiotics is recommended (see chapter on prosthetic valve endocarditis). In some communities there is a high prevalence of methicillin-resistant staphylococci. In these areas, I recommend vancomycin and gentamicin (regimen F).

Finally, although prosthetic valve endocarditis is discussed in another chapter, it is important to emphasize here that patients who have undergone the insertion of prosthetic heart valves for preexisting valvular disease are often unaware of the continued need to consider taking prophylactic antibiotics prior to procedures that induce bacteremia. Curiously, patients frequently have the impression that when prosthetic valves have been inserted to replace previously damaged natural valves, they are no longer susceptible to developing endocarditis. Upon leaving the hospital following prosthetic valve surgery,

TABLE 1 Target Bacteria for the Establishment of Antibiotic Regimens to Prevent Infective Endocarditis and Procedures Giving Rise to Their Bloodstream Dissemination

- Streptococci (nonenterococcal, non-group A)
  - Arising from:
    - Dental procedures likely to result in gingival bleeding
    - Surgery or instrumentation of the respiratory tract, including bronchoscopy
- Penicillin-resistent streptococci (nonenterococcal, non-group A)
  - Arising from:
    - Dental and respiratory tract procedures in patients receiving oral penicillin for rheumatic fever prophylaxis or parenteral carbenicillin
- Enterococci
  - Likely to arise from:
    - Surgery or instrumentation of the urinary tract
    - Surgery of the lower digestive tract or gallbladder
    - Gynecological infections or vaginal hysterectomy
    - Esophageal dilatation, sclerotherapy of esophageal varices
    - Upper gastrointestinal endoscopy with biopsy
  - Less likely to arise from:
    - Upper gastrointestinal endoscopy
    - Percutaneous liver biopsy
    - Proctoscopy, sigmoidoscopy, barium enema
    - Pelvic examination, uterine dilatation and curettage
    - Uncomplicated insertion or removal of an intrauterine device
- Staphylococci
  - Arising from:
    - Contamination during cardiac surgery
    - Drainage of staphylococcal abscesses

Note: Adapted with permission from: Freedman LR. *Infective endocarditis and other intravascular infections*. Plenum Medical Book Company, 1982.

TABLE 2 Classification of Patient as Candidate for Antibiotic Prophylaxis by Reason of Risk of Developing Infective Endocarditis

Very high risk
- Previous infective endocarditis (even without current evidence of heart disease)
- Heart valve prosthesis
- Coarctation of the aorta
- Indwelling vascular catheter (left side of the heart)

High risk
- Rheumatic and other acquired valvular heart disease
- Congenital heart disease: ventricular septal defect, tetrology of Fallot, aortic stenosis, complex cyanotic heart disease, patent ductus arteriosis
- Systemic pulmonary arterial shunts
- Idiopathic hypertrophic subaortic stenosis
- Mitral valve prolapse with mitral insuffiency
- Marfan's syndrome
- Indwelling vascular catheters (right side of the heart)
- Renal dialysis with A-V shunt appliance
- Ventriculoatrial shunts for hydrocephalus

Low risk
- Indwelling transvenous cardiac pacemakers
- Congenital pulmonary stenosis
- Mitral valve prolapse without mitral insufficiency

Note: Adapted with permission from: Freedman LR. *Infective endocarditis and other intravascular infections.* Plenum Medical Book Company, 1982.

it may not have been explained to the patient that he or she is at least as susceptible to developing IE as before surgery and that, as far as we know at this time, this susceptibility lasts forever.

DIAGNOSIS

Despite the attention that has been directed to the prevention of IE, and because of the occurrence of infection in drug addicts and in patients on chronic hemodialysis, patients with intravenous catheters, and patients with prosthetic heart valves, the overall frequency of infection has not declined and may even be increasing. It is essential, therefore, that attention be directed to the prompt diagnosis of infection in order to institute proper therapy in the hope of minimizing the devastating consequences of these infections.

The signs and symptoms of infective endocarditis may be entirely nonspecific and vary considerably from one patient to the next, depending upon the patient (e.g., drug addict, hemodialysis patient, patient previously in excellent health with no known susceptibility), the length of time infection has been present before the patient sees a physician, and whether the patient has been taking antibiotics.

In the preantibiotic era, as today, the initial complaints of the patient might be vague-fatigue, backache, nausea, and headache for example. In some instances, the patient might notice nothing other than fever. Some patients might deny symptoms completely and be unaware of the extent to which their symptoms have become accepted as normal feelings until successful treatment of IE reveals to them how much better they feel compared with how they felt before the institution of antibiotic therapy.

In hospital practice patients are often seen after having been admitted to specialty services and found not to have responded satisfactorily. For example, some patients have been admitted to neuropsychiatric services and treated with electroshock therapy before the diagnosis of IE was established. Other patients have been treated with steroids for skin lesions that were compatible with vasculitis. The diagnosis of temporal arteritis and polymyalgia rheumatica has also been applied to patients later found

TABLE 3 Recommendations for Antibiotic Prophylaxis of Infective Endocarditis According to Predicted Infecting Bacterium and Patient's Relative Risk

	Nonenterococcal, Non-Group A Streptococci Likely			
Patient Risk	*Penicillin-Sensitive*	*Penicillin-Resistent?*	*Enterococci Likely*	*Staphylococci Likely*
Very High	D/F	D/F	D/F	F
High	A or B/C or E	D/C or E or F	D/F	E or F
Low*	B/C or E	D/C or E	D/F	E

Note: Adapted with permission from: Freedman LR. *Infective endocarditis and other intravascular infections.* Plenum Medical Book Company, 1982.
The capital letters A–F denote the antibiotic regimens described in Table 4. Slash = recommended in case of penicillin allergy.
* There is considerable uncertainty concerning the need to recommend antibiotic prophylaxis in low-risk patients (Table 2).

TABLE 4 Antibiotic Regimens for the Prophylaxis of Infective Endocarditis

	Recommendation of the American Heart Association			*British Society for Antimicrobial Chemotherapy (Recommendation of a Working Party)*		
Regimen	*Antibiotic*	*Dose*	*Schedule*	*Antibiotic*	*Dose*	*Schedule*
A	Aqueous crystalline penicillin G	2,000,000 U IV or IM	½ to 1 hour prior to procedure	---	---	----
		then 1,000,000 U IV or IM	6 hours later			
B	Penicillin V	2.0 g PO	1 hour prior to procedure	Amoxicillin	3.0 g PO	1 hour before operation, taken in the presence of the dentist or dental nurse (then repeat 6 hours later*)
		then 1.0 g PO	6 hours later			
C	Erythromycin	1.0 g PO	1 hour prior to procedure	Erythromycin	1.5 g PO	1–2 hours before procedure under supervision
		then 500 mg PO	6 hours later			
D	Ampicillin	2.0 g } IM or IV	½ hour prior to procedure	Amoxicillin *plus*	1.0 g IM in 2.5 ml of 1% lignocaine	Immediately before induction of general anesthesia or 15 minutes before procedure
	Gentamicin	1.5 mg/kg } IM or IV		Gentamicin	120 mg IM	
		then Repeat once	8 hours later	*then*		
				Amoxicillin	0.5 g PO	6 hours later
E	Vancomycin	1.0 g IV during 1 hour	1 hour prior to procedure	---	---	---
F	Vancomycin	1.0 g IV during 1 hour	1 hour prior to procedure	Vancomycin	1.0 g IV	During 20–30 minutes before induction of anesthesia
	plus			*followed by*		
	Gentamicin	1.5 mg/kg (not to exceed 80 mg IM or IV)		Gentamicin	120 mg IV	
		then	Repeat 8 hours later			

Note: Adapted with permission from: Freedman LR. *Infective endocarditis and other intravascular infections.* Plenum Medical Book Company, 1982.
* Author's recommendation

to have IE as the underlying illness. Some patients have been found to have IE only after an extensive search for gastrointestinal carcinoma was negative.

The diagnosis of infection is particularly difficult in the elderly, in whom it has been noted in some series that the majority of cases were diagnosed at autopsy without having been suspected during life.

In summary, the diagnosis of IE should not be delayed because it was not considered. Once considered, the diagnosis is pursued by performing cultures of venous blood (cultured aerobically, anaerobically, and for fungi). Rarely, arterial blood cultures may be useful to recover fungi. Although IE is characterized by persistent bacteremia, it is rare that the duration of bacteremia is useful as a diagnostic criterion. Certain bacteria are rarely detected in the blood in patients without IE (e.g., alpha-hemolytic streptococci, at time intervals distant from oral-dental procedures), whereas other bacteria (e.g., staphylococci, gram-negative rods) may be found in the blood in patients with or without endocarditis. Some microorganisms (e.g., *Candida* species) may raise strong suspicions of IE even when evidence is lacking at the time that the positive blood culture is performed. Blood cultures may, of course, be negative in patients with IE who have been given antibiotics inadequate to treat the infection properly.

Attention has been directed to the finding that the frequency of IE in patients with staphylococcal bacteremia was higher when there was no obvious primary focus of infection than when such a primary focus was evident. Although this difference has been confirmed by other investigators, the frequency of IE in patients with an obvious primary focus of infection was sufficiently high to seriously limit the usefulness of this finding in arriving at a therapeutic decision. In the presence of staphylococcal bacteremia in a patient with a primary focus of infection, diabetics were more likely to have endocardial vegetations by echocardiography than nondiabetics. Thus, even when a primary focus of infection is evident, the finding of staphylococci in the bloodstream should always suggest the possibility that the patient has infective endocarditis.

Up to this point, I have emphasized the nonspecificity of symptoms of IE and the difficulty in bringing this diagnosis to mind when faced with a patient who does not feel well. It must be emphasized, however, that there are clinical findings strongly suggestive of IE, so suggestive in fact, that they may be sufficient to have the physician decide to begin treatment for IE irrespective of the microorganism recovered from the bloodstream or before blood cultures become positive or despite being unable to culture bacteria from the blood. These findings are those that have a strong likelihood of being detected in patients with IE who are seen after the infection has been present for some time or who have been treated inadequately. Since both of these conditions existed for all patients with IE in the preantibiotic era, they came to be known then as the classic signs of IE.

Patients with a heart murmur (and evidence of vegetations by echocardiography), fever, petechiae, Osler nodes, Janeway lesions, an enlarged spleen, hematuria, and evidence of emboli to the skin or major organs are likely to have IE. Of course, other explanations for these findings must be sought and the presence of some, but not all, of these findings lessens the likelihood that IE is present.

There are no strict criteria as to when a patient with or without a positive blood culture has clinical findings sufficient to start treatment for IE. This decision requires a careful evaluation of the patient and is a matter requiring the best judgement. Delay in starting treatment may be fatal, and yet treatment started before obtaining bacteriologic proof of infection may seriously interfere with later efforts to culture bacteria from the blood and with proper treatment, thus permitting the development of major debilitating complications.

THERAPY

The evaluation of antibiotic regimens for the treatment of IE is constantly undergoing refinement and revision. Although it is easier to gather data regarding the effectiveness of antibiotics in rabbits than it is in humans, it must be carefully borne in mind that rabbits differ from humans and that the final judgment on the effectiveness of different recommendations must await the outcome of sufficient clinical trials in humans. Although single case reports may be useful guides to treatment, the fact that certain antibiotics may be effective does not address the question of how regularly they are effective.

This word of caution is particularly applicable to the use of antibiotics given orally. The variation in absorption from one patient to another is sufficiently unpredictable to urge that parenteral antibiotics be utilized whenever possible, particularly in circumstances where it has not been possible to document the continued effective absorption of oral agents.

Prior to Knowlege of the Responsible Microorganism

The decision to treat a patient for IE is often made before the infecting agent has been identified. In these instances most authors recommend a treatment as for penicillin-resistant streptococci (discussed below). In the case of penicillin allergy, vancomycin is substituted for pencillin.

If there is a response to treatment and causative microorganisms remain unidentified, treatment is usually continued for 6 weeks.

In cases where there is reason, on the basis of previous bacteriologic evidence, to suspect that other microorganisms (e.g., staphylococci) might be responsible, antibiotic coverage would, of course, have to take these previous observations into consideration.

When the Infecting Agent is Identified

Careful bacteriologic studies are essential to determine optimal antibiotic therapy. It is particularly important to determine the minimal inhibitory concentration and minimal bactericidal concentration of various antibiotics to the test microorganism. Selected studies of antibiotic synergy may also be useful. When antibiotics are administered it is useful also to know what dilution of serum will kill the microorganisms in the blood. Recent studies suggest that the rate of bacterial killing by serum may be a better indicator of in vivo efficacy of the test agent than the conventional test, which measures the killing effect of serum after a fixed time of incubation.

Whenever possible, therapy should be undertaken with antibiotics that are bactericidal to the infecting organism. The location of bacteria within a vegetation effectively blocks the access of polymorphonuclear leukocytes, so bactericidal antibiotics are mandatory for effective antibacterial effect.

Infection Caused by Penicillin-Sensitive Viridans Streptococci and *Streptococcus bovis* (MIC of 0.2 μg/ml or less)

There are three regimens recommended by the American Heart Association, the choice depending on the patient's age, VIIIth nerve function, renal functional complications of IE, and the finding of nutritionally-deficient variants of streptococci. In addition, certain authors also gauge their therapy according to the duration of symptoms prior to therapy and whether vegetations are detected by echocardiography.

REGIMEN 1

Aqueous crystalline penicillin G	10–20 million units continuously or in equally divided doses every 4 hours intravenously for 4 weeks

This is the AHA regimen preferred in patients 65 years of age or more, in patients with VIIIth nerve dysfunction, or in patients with reduced renal function (adjusting dose according to level of renal function). The quantity of penicillin necessary to achieve a serum bactericidal effect at a dilution of at least 1:8 is considered highly desirable.

REGIMEN 2

Aqueous crystalline penicillin G	As in regimen 1
or	
Procaine penicillin G	1.2 million units every 6 hours intramuscularly for 4 weeks
plus	

Streptomycin 10 mg per kilogram (not to exceed 500 mg) every 12 hours during the first 2 weeks of penicillin.

The use of streptomycin is relatively contraindicated in patients over age 65 or in patients with VIIIth nerve or renal impairment. This regimen is preferred by many for patients who have had symptoms for more than 2 months and for those with echocardiographic evidence of vegetations. Although this regimen has not been shown clinically to be better than regimen 1, the data in rabbit endocarditis indicate more rapid sterilization of vegetations when penicillin is combined with streptomycin. Whether 2 weeks of streptomycin in humans is necessary for this effect is not known. In rabbits the synergistic effect of streptomycin is seen within 3 days. These observations lead me to believe that even 3 to 5 days of streptomycin would be useful to add to regimen 1.

REGIMEN 3

Aqueous crystalline penicillin G	As in regimen 2 but for 2 weeks
or	
Procaine penicillin G	
plus	As in regimen 2
Streptomycin	

This regimen is considered acceptable for patients with histories of symptoms for less than 2 months and no visible vegetations by echocardiography. It is not recommended for patients with shock, extracardiac foci of infection, prosthetic valve endocarditis, or for patients infected with nutritionally deficient variants of viridans streptococci.

The major reason to search for short-term therapy in endocarditis is the desire to minimize the discomfort and the risks of treatment as well as to effect considerable savings in the cost of treatment. One way to accomplish most of these goals is to administer the therapy described in regimen 3 and follow it with 2 additional weeks of oral penicillin to be taken at home. In order to feel confident about intestinal absorption of oral medication it is important to measure serum bactericidal levels and compare them with those obtained following intravenous administration of drug. In theory, this modification should make regimen 3 as effective as regimen 2.

About 20 percent of viridans streptococci cultured from the gingivae of children and from their blood after dental extracton have been found to be tolerant to penicillin (MBC, 10 or more times greater than MIC). It has been demonstrated in IE in rabbits that tolerant strains are less rapidly killed than nontolerant strains. Both were more rapidly killed when penicillin was added to streptomycin for the therapy of IE in rabbits. This constitutes yet another argument for treating penicillin-sensitive IE with penicillin and streptomycin.

The isolation of *Streptococcus bovis* from the blood of a patient indicates a high probability of an associated gastrointestinal disease with significant risk of colon carcinoma. Although the nature of this association is not yet clarified, the importance of searching for gastrointestinal disease should not be neglected. Some authors suggest that the isolation of any unusual streptococcus (e.g., group F streptococci, *S. milleri*) from the bloodstream may offer an important clue to the presence of occult intestinal disease. These infections are not common; I recommend the complete investigation of the gastrointestinal tract in these patients.

Endocarditis Due To Streptococci Resistant to Penicillin (MIC more than 0.2 μg/ml) and Enterococci

The combination of penicillin G (20 million units intravenously per day) plus streptomycin (7.5 mg per kilogram body weight intramuscularly every 12 hours, maximum, 500 mg per dose) is recommended for the treatment of infection due to enterococci that are sensitive to streptomycin (MIC less than 2,000 μg per milliliter). For enterococci resistant to streptomycin (MIC, 2,000 or more μg per milliliter), it is recommended that gentamicin (1.0 mg per kilogram body weight intramuscularly or intravenously every 8 hours be substituted for streptomycin. Trough serum concentrations of streptomycin should not exceed 5 μg per milliliter. Trough gentamicin levels should not exceed 1 μg per milliliter. Peak streptomycin levels of 15 to 30 μg per milliliter are considered optimal and vestibular toxicity is diminished by avoiding levels in excess of 30 μg per milliliter. Gentamicin peak levels of at least 3 μg per milliliter have been reported to be necessary for adequate bactericidal activity but, of course, the risks of renal and auditory toxicity rise as the serum levels increase.

Treatment is generally recommended for 6 weeks; however, recent data suggest that if the infection is on the aortic valve (and not on the mitral valve) and if the patient has had symptoms for less than 3 months, 4 weeks of treatment may be sufficient.

Although ampicillin is more active than penicillin in vitro for enterococci, sufficient experience has not yet been reported to enable this drug to be recommended for routine therapy. When ampicillin has been employed, it has been administered intravenously 12.0 g per day and may be associated with rash.

Endocarditis Due To Staphylococci

For cases with staphylococci resistant to 0.1 μg per milliliter or more of penicillin G, the usual therapy is with a semisynthetic penicillinase-resistant penicillin such as nafcillin or oxacillin at a dosage level of 12 g per day intravenously for a period of 6 weeks.

Staphylococci sensitive to as little as 0.1 μg per milliliter of penicillin G may be treated with this antibiotic at a dosage of 20 million units intravenously per day.

There is debate as to whether an aminoglycoside, shown to increase the rate of killing of staphylococci treated with (and sensitive to oxacillin) in the rabbit, have a place in treatment in humans. Clinical studies of this issue have confirmed the more rapid eradication of staphylococci from the bloodstream of patients treated with the penicillin-aminoglycoside combination, although the overall mortality in the two groups was equal.

In view of this positive effect of adding an aminoglycoside in humans and animals, my preference is to include gentamicin (3 mg per kilogram per day intramuscularly or intravenously) for the first 5 to 7 days of treatment.

Methicillin-Resistant Staphylococci

There is an ever-increasing frequency of methicillin-resistant staphylococci, both hospital- and community-acquired. IE due to bacteria that are resistant to methicillin are best treated with vancomycin (1.0 g intravenously every 12 hours) in combination with rifampin (900 to 1,200 mg PO in 2 or 3 divided doses) for a period of 6 weeks. It is unresolved whether gentamicin is a useful adjunct to this therapy. The isolation of such bacteria requires careful laboratory studies of antibiotic sensitivity. Combinations of rifampin with beta-lactamase-resistant penicillins have not been found to be predictably effective in treating these infections.

The increasing frequency of methicillin-resistant staphylococci in the community has led some experts to recommend vancomycin (with or without rifampin) as the initial drugs to be used for suspected staphylococcal infections until laboratory sensitivity testing is accomplished. The decision to use this approach will obviously vary with the prevalence of these bacteria in the community and the potential consequences of increasing use of vancomycin on the ability of bacteria to develop resistance to it.

Penicillin Allergy

In patients with IE due to streptococci, enterococci, or staphylococci, the presence of hypersensitivity sufficient to preclude the use of a penicillin (including semisynthetic varieties) is an indication for the substitution with vancomycin for penicillin.

Endocarditis Due To Pseudomonas Aeruginosa

The treatment of this particularly lethal form of IE has become complicated by the recent emergence of beta-lactamase-positive strains, suggesting the induction of these enzymes. A. M. Lerner and his colleagues, who have the greatest experience with this infection, have most recently recommended the use of ticarcillin (18 g per day intravenously) and tobramycin (8 mg per kilogram intravenously per day in three divided doses) for 6 weeks. The risk of significant renal and ototoxicity is high with such doses of aminoglycoside and serum levels must be carefully monitored, peak levels of 12–20 μg per milliliter being the range desired, depending on the sensitivity of the bacterial strain being treated.

In patients with right-sided infection, surgery is recommended if bacteremia persists after 2 weeks of therapy or if it recurs after 6 weeks of therapy. For left-sided infection, immediate valve replacement is indicated. Antibiotic therapy is, of course, carried out even when valve removal or replacement is necessary.

Infection Due To Bacteria Rarely Responsible for IE

There are many bacteria that have been identified as uncommon causes of IE. The bacteria are often fastidious and slow growing, making it difficult to determine antibiotic sensitivities. In addition, there may be differences in antibiotic sensitivities among isolates from different patients. Although treatment will depend on the outcome of laboratory sensitivities and clinical response, Table 5 lists a broad guide to antibiotics that might be useful until the laboratory sensitivity data become available. Effective antibiotic therapy is generally carried out for 6 weeks (see Table 5).

TABLE 5 Initial Therapy for Endocarditis Due to Unusual Bacteria

Bacterium	*Possible Initial Therapy*
Cardiobacterium hominis *Actinobacillus actinomycetemcomitans* *Hemophilus* species Non-typhoidal salmonellae *Escherichia coli, proteus* species *Klebsiella* species, *Providencia* *Eikenella corrodens* *Listeria, Erysipelothrix* Lactobacilli *Rothia dentocariosa* *Moraxella nonliquefaciens* *Moraxella kingii* *Pasturella multocida* *Pasturella pneumotropica* *Pasturella haemolytica* *Streptobacillus moniliformus* *Bordetella bronchiseptica*	*A penicillin (ampicillin)* *plus* An aminoglycoside (gentamicin)
Alcaligenes faecalis *Pseudomonas* cepacia *Pseudomonas* maltophilia *Serratia marcescens* Brucella species *Campylobacter* Chlamydiae *Aeromonas hydrophila* *Acinetobacter*	Tetracycline *or* Trimethoprim sulfamethoxazole *or* (perhaps) chloramphenicol *plus* An aminoglycoside
Diphtheroids Corynebacteria	Vancomycin
Anaerobes	Penicillin G (if not *B. fragilis*) or metronidazole

Fungal Endocarditis

It is difficult to evaluate the effectiveness of the treatment of fungal IE, since relapse has been documented as long as 20 months after treatment of infection. A patient who developed transient fungemia during hyperalimentation was found to have definite evidence of fungal IE 18 months later. Most cures of candidal endocarditis have not been followed serially for more than 6 to 12 months.

Fungal IE is due mostly to *Candida* species, with a minority of cases due to *Aspergillus* and *Histoplasma capsulatum*. There is always an identifiable route by which fungi gained access to the circulation, e.g., intravenous drug use, indwelling IV catheters, hyperalimentation, cardiac surgery.

Therapy is generally considered to require amphotericin B and 5-fluorocytosine (5-FC) combined with surgery in definite cases of IE. Amphotericin B is given in a test dose of 1.0 mg (or 0.1 mg if necessary), gradually building to 100 mg per day over 3 to 4 days. The drug may produce chills, fever, and hypotension, sometimes requiring 25 to 50 mg hydrocortisone in the infusion in order for the patient to be able to tolerate the drug. Therapy (whether or not surgery is performed) should continue for 6 to 8 weeks.

Oral 5-FC may be added to amphotericin B in doses of 150 mg per kilogram per day (to a maximum of 12.0 g per day). Although side effects are mild, intestinal perforation has been noted and the dosage must be reduced in the presence of renal insufficiency. 5-FC is not recommended as single-drug therapy.

MYCOTIC ANEURYSM

Aneurysmal dilatation of an artery associated with bacterial infection of the vessel wall is referred to as mycotic aneurysm. Such aneurysms may result from trauma, direct extension of adjacent infection, and malformations of the aorta (coarctation, patent ductus arteriosus), in the latter case the pathogenesis being similar to that of IE.

Infections occur spontaneously in the lower abdominal aorta and iliac vessels and are due, it is believed, to delivery of bacteria to nonbacterial thrombotic vegetations associated with atherosclerosis. It is of some interest that although a variety of different bacteria may be responsible, the commonest infecting agent is a *Salmonella* species, accounting for about one-half of these infections. The second most frequent infecting agent is *Escherichia coli*. The onset of these infections is usually insidious, and the symptoms may be those of pain, tenderness, a palpable mass, and arterial embolization.

Diagnosis depends on recovering the responsible agent in the bloodstream (in about 50% of cases) and a high index of suspicion based on symptoms and physical findings. Therapy consists of a combination of surgical repair and antibiotic therapy directed at the offending agent. Surgical repair should avoid the use of prosthetic devices because of the obvious risk of infection.

It is of particular interest that bacteria that so rarely infect vegetations within the heart and produce IE (*Salmonella* species, *E. coli*) are the commonest causes of infection of vegetations in the lower abdominal aorta. The explanation for this difference in bacterial localization is not apparent.

Mycotic aneurysms arising as a complication of bacterial endocarditis are most often detected in the central nervous system even though emboli elsewhere are common when searched for. When aneurysms are detected outside of the CNS they should be treated surgically as well as with antibiotic therapy.

The frequency of mycotic aneurysms in the CNS in patients with IE is not known. Symptomatic lesions are detected in 2 to 10 percent of patients. With the use of CT scan and angiography to investigate symptomatic patients, lesions that are identified and are susceptible to removal are managed surgically. The problem arises when the aneurysms are located in an area that is difficult to approach surgically and when aneurysms are detected that are asymptomatic. The surgical management of such patients requires the closest collaboration with a neurosurgeon since the risk of fatal rupture of an aneurysm is high. There is a significant likelihood of healing of mycotic aneurysms with effective antibiotic therapy directed at the underlying IE. The difficulty is in establishing the risk of rupture of any aneurysm detected and balancing this risk with that of the neurosurgical procedure necessary to treat the aneurysm effectively. Some authors go so far as to recommend cerebral angiography in all patients with IE even in the absence of symptoms. My own preference is to undertake CNS investigations only in patients with findings or symptoms referable to CNS.

If it is necessary to insert a prosthetic heart valve in a patient with a mycotic aneurysm, it will be necessary to correct the arterial lesion first since anticoagulants are contraindicated in patients with mycotic aneurysm.

PROSTHETIC VALVE ENDOCARDITIS

PHILLIP I. LERNER, M.D.

The burgeoning use of prosthetic heart valves over the past quarter century has created an important new disease of medical progress, prosthetic valve endocarditis (PVE). The unique characteristics of PVE demand recognition if the incidence, morbidity, and mortality of this infection are to be controlled. At major medical centers with active cardiac surgical programs, PVE accounts for 15 to 30 percent of all cases of endocarditis. Mortality rates ranged for 50 to 60 percent during the period 1965–1975; although more recent experiences offer encouragement, overall case-fatality rates remain discouragingly high for certain organisms. During the past decade, both the risk of infection and the types of infecting organisms have changed. These changes result from improved surgical techniques and equipment, a better understanding and application of antibiotic prophylaxis, increased use of bioprosthetic devices (combining cloth-covered supporting struts with homologous or heterologous tissue, especially porcine valves) as opposed to completely mechanical valves, and newer definitions of PVE itself, including culture-negative cases that histologically, pathologically, or clinically behave precisely like culture-positive PVE.

INCIDENCE

Early PVE begins within 60 days of surgery; in late PVE, endocarditis develops more than 60 days after valve insertion. Sixty days is chosen arbitrarily in the hope of separating those infections related to the operation from those not related to surgery and/or the immediate postoperative period. This distinction may not hold true for all organisms. The incidence of early PVE was considerably higher prior to 1969 (2.5%) compared with an average risk of 0.75 percent among reports published during 1969–1976. Before 1975 there were few good prospective studies of the risk of late PVE. Clinical experience and retrospective studies before 1969 suggested that the risk of late PVE was higher for aortic valve than for mitral valve prostheses.

Since 1975, prospective studies have provided more detailed and accurate data. A prospective analysis of 1,465 consecutive valve replacement survivors at the University of Alabama Medical Center from 1975 to July 1979 found the cumulative actuarial risk per person to be 4.1 percent at 48 months. The risk for PVE was greatest at 5 weeks, but subsequently declined to a stable level 12 months after operation. Original surgery for natural valve endocarditis (NVE) resulted in a fivefold incremental risk for subsequent PVE, whether the NVE was active or inactive at the time of valve replacement. PVE following NVE usually became evident within the first 6 months after surgery; organisms causing PVE in patients operated on for NVE were often different from those that caused the NVE. Black race was a risk factor (fourfold increment), and male gender doubled the risk, the latter also being more important in the first few months after surgery. Patients with a mechanical prosthesis had a threefold higher risk of PVE, especially in the early months after operation than did persons with bioprostheses. There was no higher risk of PVE associated with aortic valve prostheses compared with mitral valve replacements. Thirty-four (64%) of the 53 patients with PVE died; most deaths occurred within 3 months of the onset of PVE.

MICROBIOLOGY

Microorganisms responsible for PVE differ significantly from those producing NVE, with clear-cut differences in the relative importance of certain pathogens in early and late PVE (Table 1). *Staphylococcus epidermidis* is the single most common organism in both groups, accounting for 30 to 40 percent of all cases; in NVE, it is responsible only 1 to 3 percent of the time (rarely, other coagulase-negative staphylococci are involved). *Staphylococcus aureus* is no longer a dominant organism, probably because of proper use of prophylactic antibiotics, but the case-fatality rate remains high. Streptococci tend not to cause early infections. Gram-negative bacilli, infrequent pathogens in NVE, account for 20 to 25 percent of early and 10 percent of late PVE cases. Case-fatality rates are high, especially in early PVE. The range of enteric and nonfermentative gram-negative bacilli associated with PVE is extensive and includes *Escherichia coli*, *Klebsiella* species, *Enterobacter* species, *Proteus* species, *Pseudomonas* species, *Serratia* species, and Mima/Herellea/Acinetobacter. Increasingly, especially in late PVE, fastidious gram-negative coccobacilli (*Hemophilus* species *Cardiobacterium hominis*, *Actinobacillus actinomycetemcomitans*) are responsible, in addition to occasional anaerobic isolates such as *Eikenella corrodens* and *Bacteroides fragilis*.

Fungal PVE is not uncommon and is consistently associated with a poor prognosis. *Candida* species are the commonest isolates followed by *Aspergillus* species, but *Histoplasma capsulatum*, *Cryptococcus neoformans*, *Mucorales*, and even saprophytes such as *Penicillium*, *Curvularia*, *Phialophora*, and *Paecilomyces* have been reported. Contaminated gluteraldehyde-fixed porcine prostheses caused several cases of PVE with *Mycobacterium chelonei*. Even *Legionella* species, other *Mycobacteria*, *Corynebacterium diphtheriae*, *Listeria*, *Rickettsia*, *Chlamydia*, and *Mycoplasma* have been implicated. Culture-negative cases account for 5 to 15 percent of cases in large series, particularly in patients recently exposed to antibiotics or in those with fungal PVE.

The fact that many cases of late PVE are caused by microbes similar to those causing early PVE such as *S. epidermidis*, fungi, and diphtheroids suggests that persistent perioperative contamination with these weakly pathogenic organisms (possibly suppressed by prophylac-

TABLE 1 Bacteriology of Prosthetic Valve Endocarditis

	Onset Following Surgery			
	Cases Prior to 1975*		Cases 1976–1979†	
Organism	<2 months	>2 months	<2 months	>2 months
S. epidermidis	41	36	26	16
S. aureus	30	22	1	6
Gram-negative bacilli	30	19‡	1	8‡
Streptococci (viridans and other nonenterococci)	9	41	1	14
Enterococci	6	14	0	5
Pneumococci	2	0	0	1
Diphtheroids	12	6	7	7
Fungi	18	9	1	3
Others	---	---	1	3
None (culture-negative)	3	7	1	3
Total	151	154	39	66

* From Karchmer AW, Swartz MN. Infective endocarditis in patients with prosthetic heart valves. In: Kaplan EL, Taranta AV, eds. *Infective Endocarditis.* An American Heart Association Symposium monograph no. 52. Dallas: American Heart Association, 1977.

† From Dismukes WE. Prosthetic valve endocarditis: factors influencing outcome and recommendations for therapy. In: Bisno AL, ed. *Treatment of Infective Endocarditis.* New York: Grune & Stratton, 1981.

‡ Numbers not specified, but largely fastidious gram-negative coccobacilli.

tic and/or postoperative antibiotics) may not become clinically apparent until many months have passed. This observation challenges the validity of an arbitrary 2-month distinction between early and late PVE. A year may be a more appropriate cutoff point for these organisms, particularly *S. epidermidis*. Excluding the organisms just mentioned, the microbiology of late PVE, particularly beyond the first year, increasingly resembles that seen in subacute NVE, with a predominance of streptococci, presumably from the transient bacteremias associated with dental, genitourinary or gastrointestinal sources.

PATHOGENESIS AND DIAGNOSIS

Endocarditis occurring early after valve insertion is due either to contamination during (open heart) surgery or to noncardiac infections in the immediate postoperative period. Specimens of valve prostheses and native cardiac tissues obtained during surgery frequently (70%) yield skin organisms (*S. epidermidis*, diphtheroids); the same bacteria may be found in blood from the heart-lung machine and extracorporeal circulation and even from air in the operating room. Perioperative and postoperative sources of infection include arterial lines, intravenous catheters, cardiac pacing wires, chest tubes, urethral catheters and endotracheal tubes, all vital but invasive elements in the intensive care setting. Pneumonia and/or an infected pleural space, sternal/mediastinal wound infections, phlebitis, urinary infections, and infected decubitus ulcers add to the risk of bacteremia in this vulnerable period.

The signs and symptoms of early PVE are neither sensitive nor specific and the occurrence of fever and leukocytosis in the immediate postoperative period provokes a lengthy differential diagnosis. Splinter hemorrhages are of little diagnostic value in early PVE, as they occur commonly in uninfected patients following cardiopulmonary bypass. Pulmonary emboli and the postpericardiotomy syndrome may mimic infectious complications. Some patients develop a febrile mononucleosis-like illness (postperfusion syndrome) 4 to 6 weeks after surgery, probably due to blood transfusions which transmit cytomegalovirus or, rarely, Epstein-Barr virus.

Although bacteremia is its hallmark, fortunately not all early bacteremias in prosthetic valve recipients result in PVE. Some patients, in the early postoperative period, have obvious extracardiac sources of bacteremia without signs of endocarditis; providing that none develop during treatment, such patients can be managed with short (2 to 3 weeks) courses of antibiotic therapy. Others have persistent bacteremia (often with gram-negative organisms) even after elimination of the extracardiac sources of infection. Bacteremia that persists for 24 or more hours suggests PVE when there is no proven extracardiac source or after extracardiac sources have been eliminated, or when bacteremia is associated with murmurs of prosthetic incompetence or stenosis, evidence of excessive or abnormal prosthetic motion, systemic embolization (particularly to large vessels), and new or progressive atrioventricular or bundle branch conduction disturbances. Splenomegaly is often absent in early PVE, and 40 percent of patients have a normal white blood cell count. Petechiae, particularly conjunctival, are the commonest peripheral manifestations of PVE and occur in 30 to 60 percent of patients. Roth's spots, Osler's nodes, and Janeway's lesions–common peripheral stigmata of subacute NVE–are more likely to be found in late PVE than in early PVE. Anemia, microscopic hematuria, and an elevated erythrocyte sedimentation rate are useful findings, although much less so in the early postoperative period; increased concentrations of circulating immune complexes offer additional support to the diagnosis of PVE, regardless of the timing. Systemic emboli to the central nervous system, kidneys, spleen, and major peripheral vessels occur in 7 to 28 percent of patients, and splenomegaly occurs in approximately one-third of later cases. Daily auscultaton of the heart is essential to detect new or changing murmurs (particularly those of a regurgitant nature), changes in valve sounds in patients with a mechanical prosthesis, and the appearance of new sounds such as gallops or friction rubs. In contrast to NVE, where infection is usually confined primarily to the valve leaflet(s), PVE more commonly occurs at the interface of the prosthesis and the valve annulus, with extension to adjacent cardiac tissues occurring in up to 60 percent of cases and frank intraseptal or myocardial abscess, in almost 40 percent of cases. The murmurs of mitral and/or aortic insufficiency often indicate paravalvular leaks from dehiscence of the seat of the prosthesis from the periannular tissue. The absence of a regurgitant murmur does not, however, exclude the presence of paravalvular leak. In 15 percent of cases, more commonly at the mitral site than at the aortic, infection involves primarily the central structures of the mechanical valve (i.e., the disc or ball), producing obstruction and thus muffling or obliterating the prosthetic heart sounds or causing other new or unusual murmurs. Purulent pericarditis occurs in approximately 10 percent of autopsy cases (more commonly in staphylococcal infections), but mycotic aneurysms and diffuse myocarditis are uncommon complications. In patients with aortic valve PVE, pulse pressure changes usually herald important developments; narrowing of the pulse pressure may accompany worsening heart failure or signal valve obstruction or thrombosis due to vegetations. Serial electrocardiograms may detect heart block or other arrhythmias, indicating conduction system involvement by an intraseptal abscess extending from paravalvular infection. New murmurs or congestive heart failure also can result purely from mechanical complications, such as tears along the annular suture line, without PVE. After the first 2 months, the features of PVE more closely resemble the picture of NVE.

Late PVE caused by *S. epidermidis* may be quite indolent, with few classic signs. Valve dysfunction, arrhythmia or a major embolus may be the first clue. Not all blood cultures grow the organism, and it may be difficult to differentiate infection from contamination. Complicated *S. epidermidis* PVE, defined as a case with annulus involvement or valve dehiscence or obstruction, is more likely to involve a methicillin-resistant organism and to require surgery for cure. Complicated *S. epidermidis* PVE accounts for 84 percent of all such cases and is characterized by death or treatment failure 44 percent of the time. Uncomplicated cases more nearly resemble NVE with this organism: a higher percentage of methicillin-sensitive organisms and a 55 percent cure rate with antibiotics alone.

Early reports suggested infection involving porcine bioprosthetic valves was usually confined to the central leaflets and not notably invasive; more recent experiences document invasion of paravalvular tissues in up to 50 percent of such cases, particularly when infection begins during the initial postoperative year, less frequently when porcine PVE begins more than a year after implantation. Occasionally the tissue leaflets themselves are destroyed by the infection, producing significant valvular incompetence.

M-mode echocardiography is not always useful in the diagnosis of PVE, since intense echos generated by mechanical prostheses can distort images and subtle changes that might detect a vegetation or abnormal valve motion. Two-dimensional studies may be more helpful in detecting vegetations, documenting prosthetic dehiscence and paravalvular leaks, and assessing left ventricular function. Echocardiography may be more useful for monitoring patients with bioprosthetic valves since there is less interference from the hardware. Cinefluoroscopy may demonstrate abnormal rocking motion of the valve because of disruption of the suture line, but unless a vegetation is demonstrated, it is difficult to distinguish infectious complications from purely mechanical difficulties. Finding incomplete excursion of radiopaque elements of the prosthetic valve may suggest invasion by clot or vegetation. Cardiac catheterization and angiography have also been employed to assess prosthetic function, left ventricular performance, detect dysfunction of a second valve, examine the coronary circulation, and detect fistulae, aneurysms, and/or filling defects. Although there is some concern about dislodging thrombi and vegetations at the time of catheterization and angiography in patients with PVE, the risk is extremely small.

ANTIMICROBIAL THERAPY

The same principles guiding successful antimicrobial treatment of NVE pertain, including the use of parenteral bactericidal antibiotics, singly or in combination, given over extended periods of time. Precise in vitro susceptibility testing of the infecting organism (including studies for possible synergy) and assessment of the in vivo effectiveness of the antibiotics selected (serum bactericidal levels) are absolutely essential. Most patients with PVE receive at least 6 weeks of antibiotic therapy, but infection with more virulent or resistant organisms may extend treatment for an 8-week period.

Withholding antimicrobial therapy pending isolation and identification of an etiologic agent in a suspected case of PVE can pose a therapeutic dilemma. The clinical status of the patient dictates the degree of urgency regarding the initiation of therapy, but since the range of pathogens is so great in the presence of an intravascular foreign body, every effort must be made to recover and identify the infecting organism before initiating therapy to insure optimal antimicrobial treatment and monitoring. When signs and symptoms suggest acute PVE, especially in the early postoperative period, empiric therapy (as described below for culture-negative PVE) should be instituted immediately after a series of blood cultures is performed. Likewise, when the patient is critically ill with congestive heart failure secondary to a recent onset of valvular insufficiency or a paravalvular leak with suspected valve ring abscesses, immediate empiric antimicrobial therapy is necessary. When the history suggests a more indolent process without evidence of hemodynamic deterioration, antibiotics may be withheld for 24 to 48 hours, pending recovery of an organism from the blood cultures. In the early postoperative period, when prophylactic or other antibiotics (employed for the treatment of specific extracardiac infections) are being used, blood samples should probably also be inoculated into culture media containing antibiotic-binding resins. Organisms usually considered contaminants, such as *S. epidermidis*, micrococcus, and diphtheroids, should raise one's index of suspicion for PVE and prompt the drawing of additional cultures. Diphtheroids and other fastidious bacteria often do not provoke a high-grade bacteremia; consequenty not all blood cultures will be positive, and several days may elapse before a positive culture is recognized.

A combination of vancomycin, gentamicin, and ampicillin usually initiates treatment for suspected or culture-negative PVE. Ampicillin is included because of the increasingly prominent role of fastidious gram-negative coccobocilli. Doses are similar to those given for proven *S. aureus* PVE. Blood cultures are often negative in fungal endocarditis, especially those not due to *Candida* species (e.g., *Aspergillus*), and this possibility must be carefully considered when undertaking antibiotic therapy for "culture-negative" PVE. In some patients with negative blood cultures, careful bacteriologic and histologic study of surgically extracted peripheral arterial emboli may yield an etiologic diagnosis.

Antibiotic therapy is usually initiated with two bactericidal antibiotics potentially synergistic for the suspected or proven pathogen (a penicillin or cephalosporin plus an aminoglycoside). A trough serum bactericidal level of 1:8 should be the minimal goal of therapy in these patients. In experimental animal models of endocarditis, antibiotics exhibiting in vitro synergy (checkerboard technique) sterilize vegetations more rapidly than do single-drug regimens. While the clinical benefits of this phenomenon remain uncertain in the treatment of NVE, most investigators generally employ such combinations when treating PVE.

In all cases of suspected or proven PVE due to *Staphylococcus aureus*, therapy should be initiated with a penicillinase-resistant penicillin, provided that the patient has no history of penicillin allergy. Parenteral nafcillin or oxacillin (2 g every 4 hours), given for at least 6 weeks, is generally recommended. High-dose penicillin G therapy, in the range of 20 to 30 million units per day, can be substituted if the MIC of the organism is less than 0.1 μg per milliliter. Gentamicin or tobramycin (1.5 mg per kilogram every 8 hours) is usually combined with the penicillinase-resistant penicillin or penicillin G in the treatment of *S. aureus* PVE, at least for the first 2 to 4 weeks of therapy, with careful renal and audiometric monitoring. In patients with a history of penicillin allergy, either a first-generation cephalosporin (e.g., cefazolin 1 g every 6 to 8 hours) or vancomycin alone (500 mg every 6 hours) can be substituted. In patients with PVE caused by methicillin-resistant strains of *S. aureus*, vancomycin is the antibiotic of choice; an aminoglycoside (gentamicin preferred or tobramycin) is added only with extreme caution if the response is incomplete or the blood culture still positive. Vancomycin or a combinaton of nafcillin (or oxacillin) plus gentamicin (or tobramycin) has been advocated for patients whose *S. aureus* isolate is determined to be "tolerant" in vitro (as indicated by Schlicter studies). For patients failing conventional therapy, or in those where bacteremia persists, adding rifampin (300 mg orally every 8 hours in adults; 18 mg per kilogram per day in three divided doses in children) may produce a striking clinical and laboratory response.

Antimicrobial therapy for *S. epidermidis* and diphtheroid PVE requires a more detailed discussion. To treat *S. epidermidis* PVE properly, methicillin-resistant strains must not be overlooked. The microbiology laboratory can mistakenly designate *S. epidermidis* strains methicillin-susceptible when they are actually methicillin-resistant, since only a small portion of the total bacterial population (one resistant cell in 10^5 to 10^7 susceptible cells) expresses resistance in the absence of exposure to that antibiotic. Although every cell in the methicillin-resistant subpopulation is genetically capable of expressing resistance, only a small number do so under nonselective growth conditions (i.e., absence of methicillin). When exposed to methicillin, the resistant subpopulation declares phenotypic resistance, but takes 48 to 72 hours to do so. Therefore, antibiotic susceptibility test systems employing low inocula (agar or microtiter broth dilution), those relying on measurements of rapid turbidimetric growth (Autobac I or MS-2), or those requiring rapid confluent growth around a paper disk (agar diffusion) usually fail to detect the slow-growing resistant subpopulation. Methicillin-resistance can be reliably identified (Table 2) by testing higher inocula incubated for 72 hours, easily performed if the laboratory is properly alerted. Kirby-Bauer plates containing a methicillin disc incubated for 24 hours at 30 °C may isolate resistant colonies in the clear zone around the disc, but the preferred method is described in Table 2. More than 75 percent of *S. epidermidis* strains isolated from patients with PVE within 12 months of valve implantation are methicillin-resistant, but more than 12 months after surgery less than 25 percent of these strains are methicillin-resistant. Methicillin-resistant strains are also resistant to other semisynthetic penicillins and to all cephalosporins, but are susceptible to vancomycin and usually to rifampin and gentamicin. A recent prospective randomized multicenter trial compared two 6-week regimens: (*1*) vancomycin, 7.5 mg per kilogram intravenously every 6 hours, plus rifampin, 300 mg orally every 8 hours; or (*2*) vancomycin and rifampin as noted plus gentamicin, 1 mg per kilogram intravenously every 8 hours during the initial 2 weeks of therapy. Preliminary analysis indicates a 75 to 80 percent cure rate with either regimen (combined with surgical intervention in 64% of cases), but rifampin-resistant

TABLE 2 Staphylococcus Epidermidis: Tests for Methicillin Susceptibility

Pick four or five colonies of strain and grow overnight in brain heart infusion broth (organisms = 5×10^8 CFU*/ml)

Inoculate with 0.1 ml (5×10^7 CFU) by spreading on surface:
Mueller-Hinton agar with 20 μg methicillin/ml
Mueller-Hinton agar with 12.5 μg methicillin/ml

Incubate agar plates for 72 hours at 37°C

Read:
Colonies on agar with 20 μg methicillin/ml = methicillin-resistant strain
No colonies on agar with 20 μg or 12.5 μg methicillin/ml = methicillin-susceptible strain

Note: Modified from Archer GL. Antimicrobial Agents and Chemotherapy 1978; 14:353–359.
* Colony forming unit

S. epidermidis strains were isolated from surgical specimens or blood cultures at the time of relapse in 40 percent of patients receiving the first regimen, whereas none were recovered from the group that received 2 weeks of gentamicin therapy. Therefore, the three-drug regimen, which minimizes the risk of nephrotoxicity by utilizing only 2 weeks of gentamicin, appears to be the current regimen of choice. When PVE is due to a methicillin-susceptible strain of coagulase-negative staphylococcus (*S. epidermidis* or otherwise) a semisynthetic penicillin or a first-generation cephalosporin is appropriate therapy; many investigators add either gentamicin and/or rifampiin as second or third drugs. Absent data to the contrary, and considering the possible consequences of this infection, a three-drug regimen seems a reasonable recommendation.

Determining appropriate antimicrobial therapy for diphtheroid PVE can be a problem, as these fastidious gram-positive coccobacilli may be difficult to isolate and maintain in culture, and the microbiology laboratory may have difficulty performing MICs, MBCs, and serum bactericidal studies. When the isolate is sensitive to penicillin, a combination of penicillin G (4 million units every 4 hours) plus gentamicin (1.5 mg per kilogram every 8 hours) is administered for 6 weeks because 90 percent of diphtheroid strains from PVE patients are synergistically killed by this combination. Isolates with MICs for penicillin as high as 256 μg per milliliter will yield to the synergistic influence of gentamicin, so long as the isolate is susceptible to gentamicin. Others recommend vancomycin in this situation. For patients allergic to penicillin or those whose diphtheroid isolates are resistant to gentamicin, vancomycin, 7.5 mg per kilogram every 6 hours for 6 weeks, is recommended, alone or with the addition of gentamicin and rifampin. Renal function must be monitored closely.

Fungal PVE requires combined medical and early surgical treatment. For candidal endocarditis, intravenous amphotericin B (up to 1 mg per kilogram per day) is combined with oral flucytosine (dose adjusted for renal function, which is monitored).

Prolonged parenteral therapy is the optimal way to treat PVE. Oral therapy has little or no role here, certainly not during the early stages of treatment. The average duration of treatment is 5 weeks, but patients infected with staphylococci or enteric and nonfermentative gram-negative bacilli or fungi often receive 6 or 8 weeks of therapy, respectively, because of the severe consequences of relapse in these patients. Streptococcal infections (particularly those occurring after the first year) respond to shorter courses of therapy (4 weeks). Certain patients are cured with antibiotic therapy alone, usually those developing PVE a year or more after surgery and infected with relatively avirulent organisms that are highly susceptible to antibiotics: streptococci, fastidious gram-negative coccobacilli, and methicillin-susceptible *S. epidermidis*. Such patients are usually hemodynamically stable wth no evidence of an invasive infection.

SURGERY

Surgery plays an increasingly important role in managing these patients since it is now possible to replace an infected prosthesis during active endocarditis without developing recurrent infection. During the past 10 to 15 years, debridement of infected tissues and restoration of valvular function by placing a new prosthesis has become standard therapy for almost 50 percent of patients during their initial period of antibiotic therapy. Some even consider early surgery the primary treatment for PVE, preferring not to wait for complications. One would like to suppress the infection with appropriate antibiotic therapy for 10 to 14 days prior to surgery, but, as is true in NVE, survival is inversely related to the severity of heart failure at the time of surgery, so it is essential to operate before hemodynamic deterioration becomes severe and irreversible. Surgical intervention must be considered an option in all patients with PVE. The question of if and when is often difficult to resolve. Earlier concerns that reoperation posed formidable technical problems have largely been allayed as cardiac surgical expertise has improved dramatically, while fatality rates for patients treated only medically remain substantial, in the range of 60 percent. In patients who undergo valve replacement as part of therapy for PVE, this figure drops to 40 percent. Circumstances warranting possible or definite surgical intervention are listed in Table 3. The goals of prompt valve replacement are to curtail the extension of infection into vital or inaccessible cardiac structures, prevent abscess formation, and diminish the possibility of paravalvular leaks, dehiscence, or thrombotic (occlusive) stenosis. In general, aortic PVE carries a worse prognosis than mitral PVE, porcine heterografts fare better than mechanical valves, and early PVE consistently demonstrates more risk factors than does late PVE. When the tissues removed at surgery harbor viable organisms or evidence of active inflammation, an additional 6 weeks of antibiotic therapy (dating from the time of surgery) is usually recommended; otherwise 4 additional weeks of therapy is sufficient.

ANTICOAGULATION

Systemic emboli occur in 15 to 30 percent of patients with infected mechanical or porcine prosthetic valves.

TABLE 3 Indications for Considering Surgical Intervention in PVE

Hemodynamic complications
1. Moderate to severe or rapidly progressive heart failure (N.Y. Heart Association Class III or IV) caused by valvular insufficiency (tissue valves) or valve dehiscence with paravalvular leak (mechanical valves)
2. Acute decrease in cardiac output, caused by valve obstruction

Evidence of extending valve infection (annular abscess, myocardial abscess, mycotic aneurysm) suggested by new or progressing conduction system disturbances or purulent pericarditis; fever persisting >10 days in spite of appropriate antibiotic therapy

Antibiotic failure
Persistent fever and/or bacteremia, relapse following apparently successful antibiotic therapy, or ineffective or unavailable antimicrobial therapy

Selected organisms associated with increased mortality:
Fungi (definitely)
S. aureus (debated; consider case by case)
S. epidermidis (with any feature(s) noted above)

Emboli: recurrent or single major (e.g., coronary, cerebral) or new echocardiographic evidence of vegetations; emboli associated with any of the features noted above

Note: Adapted from Dismukes WE. Management of infective endocarditis. In: *Cardiovascular Clinics*, 11/3, Critical Care Cardiology. Philadelphia: F.A. Davis Co. 1981:189–208.

Hemorrhagic central nervous system events also complicate PVE, particularly when anticoagulation has been excessive. The management of anticoagulation in patients with PVE is thus controversial. In one study, mortality was similar for patients maintained on careful warfarin anticoagulation and those not anticoagulated, but morbidity due to systemic emboli, particularly to the central nervous system, was increased in the non-anticoagulated group. Current guidelines suggest continuing anticoagulation (1.5 times control) during treatment of PVE, but discontinuing warfarin if any cerebrovascular event occurs. If evidence of hemorrhage or a hemorrhagic infarct is absent, cautious anticoagulation can be resumed after 72 hours.

PROPHYLAXIS

Since the infecting organism in most cases of early PVE gains access to the prosthesis during surgery, perioperative antibiotic prophylaxis is routinely employed. To date there is no well-designed, prospective, double-blinded study conclusively proving the benefits of this practice. However, two properly designed studies have demonstrated that short-term (48 hours) use of prophylactic antibiotic during the perioperative period is as effective in preventing PVE as is the use of a prophylactic antibiotic given for a longer period of time. One typical schedule is 1 g of cephalothin intramuscularly on call to the operating room, 2 g intravenously at the start of the operation, and 2 g intravenously every 6 hours for seven doses. Since it is not possible to provide prophylaxis against all potential pathogens, the agent used should at least be effective against staphylococci.

Persons with prosthetic heart valves are analogous to patients with an abnormal native endocardium and so remain forever at risk for colonizing their prosthesis during the transient bacteremias that accompany certain procedures, particularly dental, gastrointestinal, and genitourinary manipulations. Prophylactic regimens derived from in vitro data and the rabbit model of experimental endocarditis suggest that bactericidal antibiotics (penicillin[s], cephalosporin[s], vancomycin) administered prior to the induction of bacteremia can prevent or suppress bactermia and thus avoid prosthetic infection. Although no trials in humans as yet document the efficacy of prophylactic antibiotics in patients with prosthetic valves who undergo bacteremia-associated procedures, their use is justified on theoretical grounds, carries minimal risk, and they should be employed according to the guidelines of the American Heart Association (see chapter, *Infective Endocarditis and Mycotic Aneurysm*).

STERNAL WOUND INFECTION AND MEDIASTINITIS

TEMPLE W. WILLIAMS, Jr., M.D.
RICHARD HARRIS, M.D.

During the past 30 years, median sternotomy has become the standard incision for most cardiac procedures requiring cardiopulmonary bypass. Advantages of this procedure include speed, exposure, patient comfort, and a low incidence of infection. Good surgical technique, appropriate prophylactic antibiotics, and good postoperative wound care are all important in minimizing infection at the operative site. In spite of this, however, sternal wound infections and mediastinitis continue to be serious, though fortunately uncommon, complications of cardiovascular surgery.

Predisposing factors for development of infection include prolonged operative time, early reoperation, use of extracorporeal circulation–assist devices, closed chest massage, and excessive bleeding during and after the surgery. Patients with chronic obstructive pulmonary disease with or without concomitant infection, diabetes mellitus, and obesity are predisposed to the development of this complication.

DIAGNOSIS

Diagnosis is not difficult, but relies upon suspicion by the physician. Continued unexplained postoperative fever is often the first sign. Persistent drainage from the incision is a useful finding as is the presence of an unstable sternum, an audible or palpable mediastinal crunch or click, a sternal wound that sucks air during inspiration, or wound dehiscence. It is important to note that the first indication of deep sternal wound infection is often an innocuous-appearing sinus that may mimic a pustule or stitch abscess.

Positive cultures of wound drainage as well as leukocytosis are usually present. Blood culture specimens obtained during chills or with fever may also be positive. Cultures of wound drainage yielding *Staphylococcus epidermidis* should be confirmed by consecutive culture and then treated accordingly.

Radiographic corroboration of the diagnosis can be accomplished by an upright chest film that reveals mediastinal widening or air or air-fluid levels in the mediastinum. Other diagnostic studies helpful in delineating the extent of the infection in the mediastinum include computed tomographic (CT) scans or sinograms (in those patients with an established draining sinus tract).

TREATMENT

As soon as infection of the sternum and/or mediastinum is recognized, the entire incision should be reopened. The mediastinum should be debrided and irrigated to remove bone wax, fibrin, blood clots, and bone fragments that might serve as a nidus for continuing infection. Specimens for culture should be taken from the retrosternal area so that postoperative antibiotic treatment can be delineated. Anaerobic cultures are mandatory. The edges of the sternum must be debrided, and the sternal margin should be reapproximated with wire. Circumferential and longitudinal wires may be necessary in patients with a fragmented sternum. Substernal chest tubes are inserted to allow drainage of the mediastinum and left in place until drainage ceases. On occasion, the entire sternum will need to be removed because of extensive destruction by the infection. In these patients, the wound should be packed open until adequate granulation tissue is present for skin grafting. In patients with a large defect, a composite graft (vascularized pectoralis major or rectus abdominus muscle flaps) may be used to fill this space.

Appropriate parenteral antibiotics determined by culture and sensitivity data, should be continued for a minimum of 4 to 6 weeks, followed by appropriate oral antibiotics for an additional 4 to 6 months in all patients in whom there is evidence of osteomyelitis of the sternum at reoperation. Local irrigation of the mediastinum using inflow and outflow catheters may be useful in patients with extensive involvement of the mediastinum. The antibiotics used for irrigation are the aminoglycosides effective for the patient's gram-negative bacilli or neomycin (0.5 g per liter of normal saline) and bacitracin (50,000 units per liter) for staphylococci. The aminoglycoside is chosen on the basis of the sensitivity of the organism: tobramycin or gentamicin (80–160 mg per liter of normal saline); amikacin or kanamycin (0.5 g per liter). Dilute iodophor compounds also have been used successfully in this setting.

Hospitalization prior to surgery, the antibiotic prophylaxis for the surgery (often a cephalosporin), and the postoperative period in an intensive care unit all increase the hazard of more resistant organisms, including aerobic gram-negative bacilli and staphylococci, being the etiology of these infections. Therefore, it is mandatory to obtain appropriate cultures so that optimal treatment can be designed for each patient. Parenteral bactericidal antibiotics alone or in combination are indicated. The combination of a beta-lactam and an aminoglycoside seems particularly efficacious for gram-negative bacilli. Remember that staphylococci resistant to methicillin and/or oxacillin will be resistant to all beta-lactam agents (including cephalosporins), and vancomycin becomes the treatment of choice in that patient. Please refer to the chapter *Bacterial Osteomyelitis* for the details of the choice of antibiotics and appropriate doses for use in adults.

MYOCARDITIS AND PERICARDITIS

JAMES W. BROOKS, Jr., M.D.
C. GLENN COBBS, M.D.

Inflammation of the myocardium, myocarditis, and inflammation of the pericardium, pericarditis, may result from a wide variety of infectious and noninfectious processes. Since the myocardium and visceral pericardium are adjacent structures, inflammatory disorders have the potential to involve them concomitantly, resulting in so-called myopericarditis. Disease of the myocardium and pericardium caused by infectious agents may produce a dramatic, potentially life-threatening illness. Prompt recognition and treatment is often essential for a successful outcome.

ETIOLOGY AND PATHOGENESIS

Viral Myopericarditis

Viral myopericarditis is usually caused by members of the enterovirus group. Group B coxsackieviruses, types 1–6, have been most frequently implicated as causative organisms. Group A coxsackieviruses and echoviruses have less frequently been incriminated. Other viruses that have been associated with myopericarditis include poliovirus, influenza A and B, adenovirus, Epstein-Barr, mumps, rubella, and herpes simplex types 1 and 2. The association of viruses with myopericarditis comes largely from a limited number of epidemiologic and serologic studies. Actual isolation of virus from myocardium or pericardium has rarely been accomplished. Attempts at viral isolation and appropriate serologic studies are frequently not performed in patients with pericarditis whose disorder resolves without complication. Therefore, the true incidence of viral myopericarditis is unknown.

Infections caused by coxsackieviruses and echoviruses are relatively common in children and adults and may produce a variety of clinical syndromes. Most often, disease is characterized by signs and symptoms of an upper respiratory tract infection or acute gastroenteritis. It is estimated that approximately 5 percent of symptomatic coxsackievirus infections are complicated by myopericarditis. Viral replication in the myocardium and pericardium results in cell necrosis and an acute inflammatory reaction. This acute phase usually resolves over several weeks. Some patients may progress to a chronic inflammatory phase characterized by persistent evidence of myocardial dysfunction or pericardial involvement. Although antecedent viral infection is often suspected in some patients with chronic inflammatory congestive cardiomyopathy, a clear association has rarely been proved.

Bacterial Pericarditis

In the preantibiotic era, purulent bacterial pericarditis occurred almost entirely as a complication of pleuropulmonary disease, usually caused by gram-positive cocci. *Streptococcus pneumoniae* accounted for 50 percent of the cases of bacterial pericarditis, whereas staphylococcal and other streptococcal species accounted for 20 percent and 10 percent of cases, respectively. Pericarditis due to gram-negative aerobic bacilli was distinctly uncommon.

In recent years, however, primary pleuropulmonary disease has accounted for only 20 percent of cases of purulent bacterial pericarditis (Table 1). There has been a corresponding decrease in the incidence of pneumococcal pericarditis, so that this organism now accounts for only about 15 percent of cases (Table 2). Presently most patients either have a predisposing, debilitating illness and develop pericarditis as a complication of disease at another site (30%) or develop bacterial pericarditis following cardiovascular, thoracic, or esophageal surgery (25%). In the latter situation, wound infection is usually obvious, but signs of pericardial involvement may be subtle. Another 20 percent of cases of bacterial pericarditis are associated with infective endocarditis. Finally, patients with antecedent noninfectious pericarditis (uremic, malignant, postoperative) have an increased susceptibility to bacterial superinfection, presumably because pericardial effusion compromises pericardial host defenses.

These changes over the past 40 years in the underlying disease processes leading to bacterial pericarditis and the trend toward an older patient population with a greater number of chronic illnesses have resulted in bacterial pericarditis becoming predominantly a nosocomial infection. There has been a dramatic increase in the number of cases caused by gram-negative bacilli. These organisms now account for about 30 percent of all cases of purulent bacterial pericarditis, whereas *Staphylococcus aureus* is responsible for another 30 percent of cases.

TABLE 1 Bacterial Pericarditis: Site of Primary Infection and Patients at Risk

Site	*Frequency (%)*
Pleuropulmonary disease	20
Bacteremia	30
Postoperative wound infection and mediastinitis	25
Endocarditis, myocardial abscess	20
Subdiaphragmatic abscess	5
Other risk factors: burns, antecedent aseptic pericarditis	

Tuberculous Pericarditis

Mycobacterium tuberculosis is an important cause of acute and chronic pericardial disease. Tuberculous pericarditis occurs most frequently in men, especially blacks. Fewer than 1 percent of all patients with tuberculosis have involvement of the pericardium.

Tuberculous pericarditis is thought to result from reactivation of disease in mediastinal lymph nodes and subsequent spread to the pericardium. Less commonly, it may occur from direct extension of adjacent parenchymal lung disease or from bacteremia. Early on, tuberculous pericarditis is associated with an exudative pericardial effusion. After several weeks or months, resorption of this fluid begins, and fibrous deposition and pericardial thickening occurs. Tamponade may occur early with constriction usually a later complication.

Fungal Pericarditis

In debilitated patients with cancer, pericarditis is occasionally caused by *Candida* species or *Aspergillus*.

TABLE 2 Organisms Causing Bacterial Pericarditis

	Frequency (%)
Staphylococcus aureus	30
Gram-negative bacilli (*Proteus, Escherichia coli, Pseudomonas, Klebsiella*)	30
Streptococcus pneumoniae	15
Other streptococci	10
Hemophilus influenzae	5
Anaerobes	5
Others	5

Aspergillus pericarditis occurs only in association with invasive pulmonary aspergillosis. Histoplasmosis may occasionally cause acute or chronic pericarditis in nonimmunocompromised individuals, often in association with the syndrome of sclerosing mediastinitis.

Parasitic Pericarditis

Pericarditis caused by parasites is rare, but may be seen in association with infection by *Entamoeba histolytica, Echinococcus, Trypanosoma, Toxoplasma gondii*, microfilariae, and *Trichinella spiralis*.

CLINICAL MANIFESTATIONS

Significant overlap exists in the clinical manifestations of viral, bacterial, and tuberculous pericarditis, and, in fact, it is frequently difficult to distinguish a noninfectious from an infectious etiology.

Viral Myopericarditis

Viral myopericarditis usually presents as an acute illness. The commonest symptoms at presentation are fever and pleuritic chest pain. Other less common complaints are cough, dyspnea, myalgia, and arthralgias. About 60 percent of patients relate symptoms of a viral upper respiratory tract infection 2 to 3 weeks before pericarditis develops. Occasionally, patients experience symptoms of gastroenteritis prior to the onset of pericarditis. Fever and tachycardia are common. A pericardial friction rub is the hallmark of pericarditis, but is present in only 40 to 50 percent of patients and may be intermittent. Congestive cardiomyopathy may be present in 20 percent of patients hospitalized for viral myopericarditis. Evidence for pericardial tamponade is unusual in viral myopericarditis, but may occur.

Bacterial Pericarditis

Since purulent bacterial pericarditis is almost always a complication of disease at an adjacent or distant site, the signs and symptoms of the primary infectious process often overshadow the pericardial involvement. Therefore, a high index of suspicion in those patients at risk for bacterial pericarditis is necessary. Bacterial pericarditis presents in an acute fashion, and clinical deterioration may be rapid. Although fever, chills, and tachycardia are common, chest pain is often absent. Since bacterial pericarditis often progresses to produce cardiovascular decompensation from pericardial tamponade, the development of hypotension, narrowed pulse pressure, paradoxical pulse, jugular venous distention, and muffled heart sounds in the setting of a primary bacterial infection should prompt an immediate search for pericardial involvement and tamponade.

Tuberculous Pericarditis

As opposed to viral and bacterial pericarditis, tuberculous pericarditis begins in an insidious fashion in 75 percent of patients. Symptoms are nonspecific, with cough, dyspnea, chest pain, and weight loss predominating. Night sweats are present in only one-third of patients. The initial clinical presentation often does not suggest pericardial disease. Fever and tachycardia are seen in more than 90 percent of patients, but fewer than one-half of patients have a pericardial rub, distant heart sounds, or a paradoxical pulse. Often the diagnosis is only suspected in the evaluation of cryptogenic right-sided heart failure or when pericardial effusion is detected in patients presenting with cardiomegaly.

EVALUATION

Laboratory data (Table 3) are usually quite nonspecific. Most patients with infectious pericarditis have a leukocytosis, but a marked increase in immature forms is more typical of a bacterial etiology. Levels of cardiac enzymes may be mildly elevated in patients with viral myopericarditis and reflect ongoing myocardial necrosis. In evaluating patients for a noninfectious etiology, the assessment of thyroid functon tests, antinuclear antibody, and rheumatoid factor may be helpful.

Chest roentgenogram reveals cardiomegaly in most patients with viral, bacterial, or tuberculous pericarditis. Pleural effusion can be seen in all three types, but is commoner in tuberculous pericarditis. A pulmonary opacity is present in up to one-third of patients with bacterial or tuberculous pericarditis, but is rarely observed in patients with viral pericarditis. An apical pulmonary infiltrate typical of reactivation tuberculosis is uncommon in association with tuberculous pericarditis. Pericardial calcification is present in approximately one-half of patients with chronic tuberculous pericarditis.

The electrocardiogram is abnormal in most patients with infectious pericarditis, but only about 20 percent of patients have diffuse elevation of the ST segment considered classic for pericarditis. Most patients have only inversion of the T wave or nonspecific changes of the ST segment and T wave.

CONFIRMATION OF ETIOLOGY

Viral Myopericarditis

The definitive diagnosis of viral myopericarditis requires isolation of the virus from the myocardium or pericardium. Virus usually cannot be cultured from pericardial fluid. Most patients with viral myopericarditis recover without developing pericardial constriction or tamponade. Therefore, when a history compatible with viral myopericarditis is present, patients may be observed

TABLE 3 Laboratory and Clinical Findings in Infectious Pericarditis

Parameter	Etiology: Viral	Purulent Bacterial	Tuberculous
White blood cells			
Leukocytosis present	70%	100%	"Common"
Differential count	Increased PMNs, may have left shift	Marked left shift	Variable, occasionally shift to left, occasionally monocytosis
Cardiac enzymes (CPK, SGOT, LDH)	Elevated in 30%–60%, more common in first week	Normal	Normal
PPD	Negative	Negative	Positive in 90%
Arrhythmias	Common: atrial fibrillation, atrial flutter, ventricular ectopy	Uncommon	Occasional: atrial fibrillation, heart block
Roentgenogram			
Cardiomegaly	60%	75%	80%
Pleural effusion	40%	33%	70%
Lung infiltrate	Usually absent	30%–50%	33%
Pericardial fluid	Usually exudative, normal glucose	Exudative, PMNs usually >90%, glucose usually <35 mg dl	Exudative, serosanguineous in 75%, mononuclear predominance, glucose often low
Pericardial fluid culture	Negative	Positive in nearly 100%	Positive in 40%–50%
Risk of tamponade	Low	High	Moderate

without pericardiocentesis or more invasive surgical procedures. Since biopsy and culture of myocardium or pericardium is generally not warranted, a presumptive diagnosis is made by isolating virus from stool or the oropharynx and demonstrating a fourfold rise in type-specific antibody (Fig. 1). Viral isolation in conjunction with a single high titer (1:32 or greater) of type-specific antibody is also acceptable. When viral myopericarditis is suspected, the stool and oropharynx should be cultured for virus and a sample of acute serum obtained with a follow-up convalescent serum in 2 to 4 weeks. If a virus implicated as an etiologic agent of myopericarditis is recovered from the stool or oropharynx, the sera should be checked for the corresponding type-specific antibody. In the absence of a positive oropharyngeal or stool culture, screening the sera for antibodies against all of the possible viruses is impractical.

Bacterial Pericarditis

When the diagnosis of purulent bacterial pericarditis is considered, a search for an underlying primary infectious process should be made and an echocardiogram should be performed to confirm the presence of pericardial fluid. Early surgical intervention is crucial for successful therapy. A sample of pericardial fluid should be obtained at pericardiectomy for culture and appropriate stains. Fluid should be cultured anaerobically as well as aerobically; in the absence of previous antimicrobial therapy, this will usually confirm the diagnosis.

Tuberculous Pericarditis

The diagnosis of tuberculous pericarditis ultimately depends on identifying *M. tuberculosis* in pericardial fluid or pericardium. A presumptive diagnosis of tuberculous pericarditis may be made by culturing *M. tuberculosis* from extrapericardial sites, such as the lung, pleura, or bone marrow in a patient with inflammatory pericardial disease (Fig. 2). The intermediate-strength purified protein derivative (PPD) skin test may be helpful in suggesting the diagnosis since it is positive in approximately 90 percent of patients with tuberculous pericarditis. Two or three control skin tests should be applied to exclude anergy in patients with a negative PPD. The presence of hemodynamic compromise as a consequence of pericardial disease is an indication for prompt pericardiectomy. Empiric antituberculous therapy should be initiated until culture results are available. When patients have no evidence of hemodynamic compromise from pericardial disease, an extrapericardial site may be investigated initially. For example, pleural biopsy will provide the diagnosis of tuberculosis in about one-third of patients with an associated pleural effusion. If the investigation of extrapericardial sites is unhelpful, a pericardial biopsy is recommended for diagnostic purposes. Pericardial fluid is exudative, usually hemorrhagic, and demonstrates a predominance of mononuclear cells. The examination of pericardial fluid rarely yields a positive result for acid-fast bacilli and culture of pericardial fluid is positive in only 40 to 50 percent of patients. In contrast, pericardial biopsy will provide the diagnosis in more than 90 percent of patients.

TREATMENT AND PROGNOSIS

Viral Myopericarditis

Patients thought to have acute viral myopericarditis should be hospitalized and observed for the development

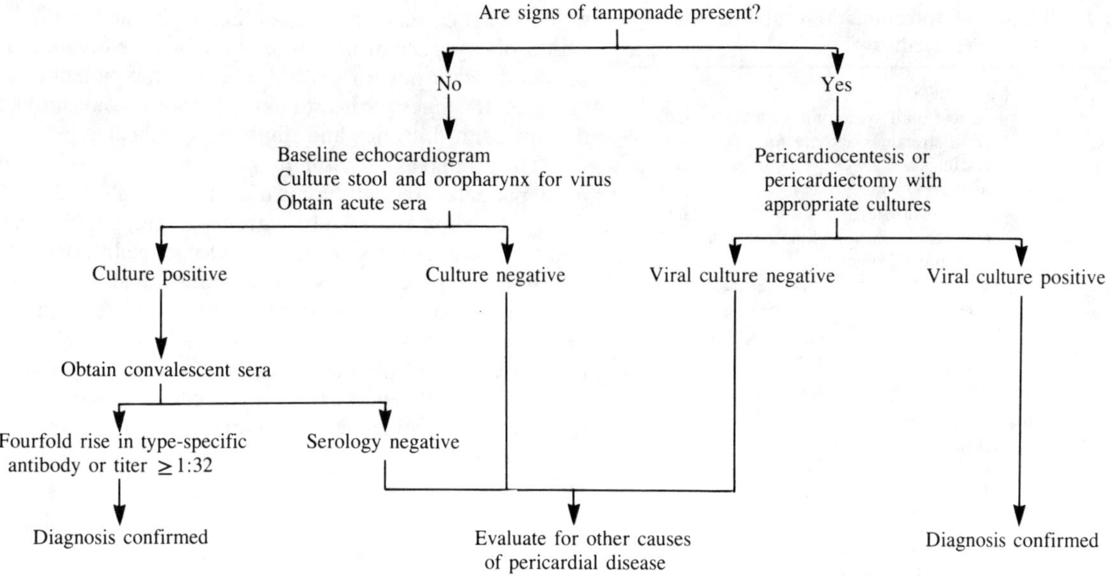

Figure 1 Confirmation of suspected viral myopericarditis.

Suspected tuberculous pericarditis

Are signs of tamponade or constriction present?

No

Yes

Apply PPD and three controls
Baseline roentgenogram and echocardiogram

Is there evidence of extrapericardial disease
(e.g., lung, pleura, bone marrow)?

Surgery: pericardial window or stripping;
send tissue for pathology and culture
Pericardial fluid analysis and AFB strains
Begin empiric anti-TB therapy

Yes

No

Biopsy and culture involved site
Begin empiric anti-TB therapy

Extrapericardial TB
identified

Extrapericardial TB
not found

Pericardial biopsy and culture
Begin empiric anti-TB therapy

Culture negative

Culture positive

Culture positive

Reassess for
other etiologies

Diagnosis confirmed
Treat for 9 months

Diagnosis confirmed
Treat for 9 months

Diagnosis confirmed
Treat for 9 months

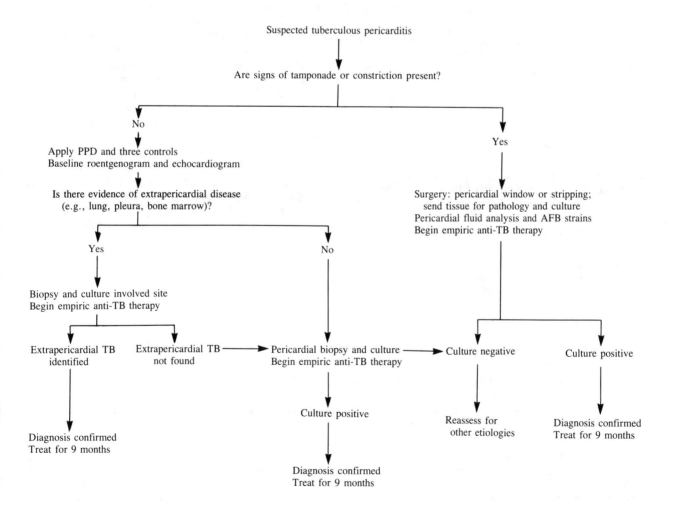

Figure 2 Confirmation of tuberculous pericarditis.

TABLE 4 Therapy of Infectious Myocarditis and Pericarditis

Viral	*Acute phase* Bed rest until symptoms resolve, then avoid strenuous activity for several weeks Aspirin 650 mg PO q.i.d. or indomethacin 50 mg PO t.i.d. Avoid corticosteroids and anticoagulants Treat heart failure and arrhythmias in conventional manner Pericardial window or pericardiectomy only if tamponade develops
	Chronic phase or relapses Prednisone 60 mg PO daily; gradual tapering over several weeks
Bacterial	*Initial empiric therapy* Surgical drainage *plus* Nafcillin 1.5 g IV q4h *plus* gentamicin, dose adjusted for renal insufficiency
	Subsequent therapy Adjust antibiotics according to cultures Continue therapy for 4–6 weeks
Tuberculous	Isoniazid 300 mg PO daily × 9 months *plus* Rifampin 600 mg PO daily × 9 months *plus* Prednisone 60–80 mg PO daily; gradual tapering after several weeks Add ethambutol 15 mg/kg/day PO if infection is acquired in area with high frequency of INH resistance Pericardiectomy: if tamponade or constrictive pericarditis is present; otherwise reserved for those failing medical therapy, indicated by persistent pericardial fluid, the development of constrictive pericarditis, or intractable pain
Fungal (*Candida, Aspergillus*)	Amphotericin B 0.4–0.6 mg/kg/day IV

of pericardial tamponade, congestive heart failure, and arrhythmias. When the clinical situation suggests tamponade, a catheterization of the right side of the heart can confirm the diagnosis. Since cultures of pericardial fluid for virus are rarely positive, pericardiocentesis is not indicated in the absence of tamponade. In fact, in our experience, pericardiocentesis is associated with an excessive risk and should be reserved for emergency situations. When clinically indicated, we recommend proceeding directly to open pericardial biopsy with pericardial stripping, if necessary.

There is presently no effective antiviral chemotherapy for enteroviral disease and treatment is largely supportive (Table 4). Aspirin or indomethacin will usually provide symptomatic relief of chest pain. Corticosteroids should be avoided in the acute phase of viral myopericarditis since there is some evidence in animal models that corticosteroids during the acute phase may exacerbate the myocarditis. Anticoagulants should also be avoided as they increase the risk of intrapericardial hemorrhage. Additional evidence in animal models of coxsackieviral myopericarditis suggests that exercise during the acute phase accelerates myocarditis and increases the risk of developing congestive cardiomyopathy. Therefore, it seems prudent to place patients at bed rest during the acute phase, especially if cardiac enzyme levels are elevated, an indication of myocardial necrosis. We advise avoidance of strenuous activities for several weeks as the patient convalesces. If congestive heart failure develops, conventional therapy with diuretics and digitalis is indicated.

The prognosis for viral myopericarditis is good, with most patients gradually returning to normal in 2 to 4 weeks. Cardiomegaly and electrocardiographic changes will resolve over the same period. Occasionally, patients develop chronic congestive heart failure, and a few will have a refractory, rapidly progressive course resulting in death. Constrictive pericarditis is a rare sequel of viral myopericarditis. Relapses of symptoms of acute viral myopericarditis are not unusual. If this occurs despite therapy with nonsteroidal anti-inflammatory agents, a trial of prednisone, 60 mg daily tapered over several weeks, is indicated.

Bacterial Pericarditis

In the absence of a previously identified primary infectious process, patients with bacterial pericarditis should be started on antibiotics to cover *S. aureus*, other gram-positive cocci, and gram-negative bacilli. Initial empiric therapy should include intravenous nafcillin, 1.5 g every 4 hours, and gentamicin at a dose appropriately adjusted for the patient's renal function. Additional gram-negative coverage may be added if the situation warrants. Intrapericardial administration of antibiotics is unnecessary since intravenous administration results in adequate penetration into the pericardial space.

Bacterial pericarditis represents a purulent process in a closed space, and prompt drainage is almost always necessary. In the preantibiotic era, surgical drainage alone was associated with a 50 percent survival rate. Early pericardiectomy is recommended and antibiotic therapy should be adjusted according to cultural results. Antibiotic therapy should be continued for 4 to 6 weeks.

The mortality rate of bacterial pericarditis remains at 40 to 50 percent. The high mortality is a reflection of the serious nature of this infection, the debilitating illnesses of many of the patients, and the usual delay in diagnosis. Successful outcomes are likelier with early aggressive surgical and medical intervention.

Tuberculous Pericarditis

The choice of therapy for tuberculous pericarditis remains somewhat controversial. Since this is an uncommon disease, large randomized therapeutic trials have not been possible. Triple-drug therapy was recommended in the past. We recommend therapy with two bactericidal drugs: isoniazid, 300 mg orally, and rifampin, 600 mg orally, each day. If the patient is from Southeast Asia or another area with a high frequency of resistance to isoniazid, ethambutol, 15 mg per kilogram per day orally, should be added until sensitivities return. Therapy should be continued for 9 months. There is evidence in uncontrolled trials that the addition of corticosteroids results in a more rapid resorption of pericardial fluid and suppresses the chronic inflammatory response. Therefore, if patients do not have constrictive pericarditis requiring early pericardiectomy at presentation, we recommend beginning 60 to 80 mg of prednisone daily, followed by a slow tapering of the medication after several weeks. Immediate pericardiectomy is indicated for patients presenting with pericardial tamponade or hemodynamic compromise from constrictive pericarditis. Otherwise, a trial of medical therapy with antituberculous drugs and corticosteroids is advised, with early surgical intervention for those patients failing to respond appropriately.

Mortality rates remain at 20 to 40 percent for tuberculous pericarditis. Death is usually a result of either inability to make the correct diagnosis and begin appropriate therapy or the complications of progressive hemodynamic compromise from the pericardial disease.

BONE AND JOINT INFECTIONS

BACTERIAL OSTEOMYELITIS

JACK L. LeFROCK, M.D.
BRUCE R. SMITH, Pharm. D.
ABDOLGHADER MOLAVI, M.D.

Osteomyelitis continues to pose both diagnostic and therapeutic dilemmas for the clinician, despite recent advances in radionuclide imaging, surgical techniques, and antimicrobial therapy. Intravenous drug abuse, radiation therapy for cancer, and newer orthopaedic procedures, such as total joint replacements, bone-grafting, and reconstructive surgery, have broadened the scope of this disease.

Osteomyelitis is an inflammatory process in bone and bone marrow. It is caused most often by pyogenic bacteria but may be caused by other microorganisms including mycobacteria and fungi. Osteomyelitis may be classified on the basis of its pathogenesis as of either hematogenous origin or contiguous focus (with or without peripheral vascular disease) (Table 1). These in turn may be classified as either acute or chronic forms of the disease.

In the past, osteomyelitis usually resulted from hematogenous spread of bacteria to bone and was mostly seen in children with *Staphylococcus aureus* as the causative agent in 80 to 90 percent of the cases. However, in recent years the disease has changed. Hematogenous osteomyelitis is decreasing in frequency while contiguous osteomyelitis and osteomyelitis in association with peripheral vascular disease is increasing. In addition to these changes, there also has been a shift in the age distribution to older patients as well as increasing frequency of unusual bacterial causes, including gram-negative bacilli, anaerobes, and mixed organisms.

HEMATOGENOUS OSTEOMYELITIS

This is generally caused by a single organism, with *S. aureus* being responsible for the majority of cases. However, the type of organism may vary with the age of the patient (Table 2). This disease generally occurs in children younger than 12 years, teenagers, and young adults who participate in strenuous physical activities. Bone infection follows bacteremia. The metaphyseal ends of long bones are the most frequent sites of involvement in children and the diaphysis of the long bones in adults.

S. aureus may also cause spinal osteomyelitis with paravertebral abscess formation. This syndrome generally occurs in older men who have had urinary tract manipulation and infection and in drug addicts.

CONTIGUOUS OSTEOMYELITIS

This type is secondary to an adjacent area of infection, as in postoperative infections, direct inoculation from

TABLE 1 Classification of Osteomyelitis and Associated Features

	Hematogenous	Secondary to Contiguous Focus of Infection	Due to vascular Insufficiency
Age distribution	1–20 and >50 years	25–50 years	≥50 years
Usual bones involved	Long bones, vertebrae	Long bones	Small bones of feet
Microbiology	Usually monomicrobial: *Staphylococcus aureus*, *Streptococcus* (group B) Gram-negative bacilli (*Hemophilus influenzae*)	Usually mixed infections: *Staphylococcus aureus* and *epidermidis*, gram-negative bacilli	Usually polymicrobial: *Staphylococcus aureus* and *epidermidis*, gram-negative bacilli Anaerobes
Associated factors	Trauma, bacteremia, IV drug abuse	Trauma and surgery, soft tissue infections, radiation therapy	Diabetes mellitus, peripheral vascular disease
Clinical features	Fever, local tension and swelling	Fever, swelling and erythema	Fever, swelling, ulceration and drainage

TABLE 2 Osteomyelitis: Commonly Isolated Organisms

Hematogenous osteomyelitis
- Infants <1 year
  - Group G *Streptococcus*
  - *Staphylococcus aureus*
  - *Escherichia coli*
- Children 1–16 years
  - *Staphylococcus aureus*
  - Group A *Streptococcus*
  - *Hemophilus influenzae*
- Adults >16 years
  - *Staphylococcus aureus*
  - *Staphylococcus epidermidis*
  - Gram-negative bacilli
    - *Pseudomonas aeruginosa*
    - *Serratia marcescens*
    - *Escherichia coli*

Contiguous focus osteomyelitis (polymicrobic infection) all ages
- *Staphylococcus aureus*
- *Staphylococcus epidermidis*
- Group A *Streptococcus*
- Enterococcus
- Gram-negative bacilli
- Anaerobes

trauma, or extension from an area of soft tissue infection. In contrast to hematogenous osteomyelitis, more than one pathogen is often isolated from the infected bone. *S. aureus* is the most commonly isolated pathogen, but aerobic gram-negative rods and anaerobes also are often isolated. In this form of osteomyelitis, one often finds bone necrosis, compromised soft tissue, and loss of bone stability, which make this type more difficult to treat than acute hematogenous osteomyelitis.

OSTEOMYELITIS ASSOCIATED WITH VASCULAR INSUFFICIENCY

This infection usually develops in a diabetic as an extension of a local infection either from cellulitis or a trophic skin ulcer. The small bones of the feet, generally the metatarsals and phalanges, are involved. These patients have impaired local inflammatory response that predisposes the involved tissues to infection and necrosis. Multiple aerobic and/or anaerobic pathogens often can be isolated from the infected bone.

CHRONIC OSTEOMYELITIS

Both of the above types of osteomyelitis can become chronic. There are no exact criteria as to when acute osteomyelitis becomes chronic.

DIAGNOSIS

In addition to the historical data and physical findings, cultures of infected material and hematologic and radiographic studies are helpful in making a clinical and etiologic diagnosis.

Blood cultures should be performed for all patients with suspected osteomyelitis. Approximately 50 percent of patients with acute hematogenous osteomyelitis will have positive blood cultures. Leukocytosis may occur with white cell counts exceeding 20,000 per cubic millimeter. However, normal or only slightly elevated WBC counts are not uncommon. The erythrocyte sedimentation rate (ESR) may be normal early in the disease, but usually increases with the duration of illness.

Radiographic changes are often difficult to interpret. Bone density must change at least 50 percent to be detected radiologically. Thus, there may be no definable radiologic changes in osteomyelitis for the first 10 to 14 days in spite of bone destruction or periosteal new bone formation. The initial radiologic findings may be simply soft tissue swelling and/or subperiosteal elevation. Roentgenograms may give misleading information in up to 16 percent of patients and are of no diagnostic value in an additional 23 percent of patients with osteomyelitis. Lytic changes are not seen until 2 to 6 weeks after the onset of disease. Sclerotic changes of periosteal new bone formation (involucrum) denote a more chronic process.

On the other hand, changes are seen on bone scintography as early as 24 hours after the onset of symptoms because of increased bone blood flow and early bone reaction. However, not all patients with acute osteomyelitis have abnormal bone scans. There are reports of normal bone scans, or "subtle" or "cold" defects. In some situations gallium scan shows increased uptake in areas of polymorphonuclear leukocyte infiltration. However, gallium scan does not show bone detail well so it is often difficult to distinguish between bone and soft tissue inflammation. Scanning the infected area with gallium 48 hours after injection and comparing with a ^{99m}Tc bone scan helps resolve this problem. Computed tomography (CT) is useful in identifying areas of dead bone (sequestrum). However, CT cannot be utilized when metal is present in or near the area of bone infection because of the scatter effect, with resultant loss of image resolution. Radiographic follow-up is important in assessing the effectiveness of drug therapy and the need for surgical intervention.

The bacteriologic diagnosis of osteomyelitis rests on isolation of the pathogenic bacteria from the bone or the blood. In chronic osteomyelitis, sinus tract cultures are not reliable in predicting which organism(s) will be isolated from the infected bone because there is a poor correlation between these cultures and those done on bone biopsy material. Bone biopsy specimens should be carefully cultured and stained for aerobes, anaerobes, mycobacteria, and fungi. The biopsied material should also be submitted for histopathologic evaluation.

THERAPY FOR HEMATOGENOUS OSTEOMYELITIS

In acute hematogenous osteomyelitis, a prolonged course of antimicrobial therapy (4 to 6 weeks). with a bactericidal agent should be directed toward specific causative bacteria isolated by bone biopsy and culture. Therapy based upon wound swab cultures of skin and skin structures above the infected bone is often inappropriate. These cultures usually reflect bacterial colonization without accurately identifying the organism in the underlying bone itself. Only the isolation of *S. aureus* from deep wound culture has correlated with its presence in bone.

Oral therapy has been used successfully after 2 weeks of parenteral therapy in the treatment of pediatric osteomyelitis. This method of therapy should be entertained where there is good laboratory backup and close patient monitoring to ensure compliance. Patients casually treated with oral antibiotics often receive inadequate dosage and inadequate monitoring, resulting in a failure rate of 19 percent. For successful therapy, the orally administered antibiotic should be monitored by the measurement of serum bactericidal activity against the causative pathogen. A peak bactericidal dilution of at least 1:8 or greater should be maintained. In children, this form of therapy offers advantages in convenience, comfort and cost. We treat adults with 6 weeks of intravenous therapy, and children, with 2 weeks of intravenous therapy followed by 4 weeks of oral therapy.

TREATMENT OF CHRONIC OSTEOMYELITIS

Chronic osteomyelitis secondary to surgery, trauma, or contiguous focal infection must be approached with combined medical and surgical therapy. Debridement should be done as soon as possible to remove all necrotic bone and sequestra. Abscesses or fistulous tracts must be eliminated. Material obtained at the time of surgery should be cultured for aerobes and anaerobes. Internal fixation devices, plates, pins, and screws should be removed. If bone stabilization is required, an external fixation device can be utilized. The wound may have to be debrided every 48 to 72 hours until all nonviable tissue has been removed.

Antimicrobial therapy should be initiated as early as possible, should be directed specifically against the offending pathogen(s), and should be administered intravenously in high doses for 6 weeks after the last debridement. Antimicrobial therapy prior to the time when debridement cultures are obtained should consist of broad-spectrum antibiotics to cover both aerobes and anaerobes. It is advisable to give antibiotics prior to debridement in order to reduce cellulitis or soft tissue swelling and reduce the risk of bacteremia.

THERAPY IN GENERAL

The consequences of inadequate therapy can be grave and lifelong. Knowing the types of organisms producing the osteomyelitis should lead to the use of a specific bactericidal agent except when multiple organisms are involved. Blind therapy is dangerous. Empiric choice of a narrow-spectrum agent not effective against the organism(s) within the bone may lead to treatment failure and chronic relapses. On the other hand, empiric broad-spectrum therapy may unnecessarily expose the patient to excessive or potentially toxic antimicrobial therapy and also inflate the cost of treatment.

The agents chosen for use should be demonstrated to be effective against the organism isolated from bone by in vitro sensitivity tests, such as the minimum inhibitory concentration (MIC) and minimum bactericidal con-

TABLE 3 Antibiotic Therapy for Osteomyelitis in Adults

Organism	*Antibiotics of First Choice**	*Alternative Antibiotics**
Staphylococcus aureus	Nafcillin or oxacillin 2 g q6h	Clindamycin 600 mg q8h, vancomycin 500 mg q6h, cefazolin 1 g q8h
Staphylococcus epidermidis	Nafcillin or oxacillin 2 g q6h	Vancomycin 500 mg q6h, cefazolin 1 g q8h
Non-enterococcal *Streptococcus*	Penicillin G 3 million units q6h	Clindamycin 600 mg q8h, cefazolin 1 g q8h
Enterococcal *Streptococcus*	Ampicillin 2 g q6h *plus* gentamicin 5 mg/kg per day q8h	Vancomycin 500 mg q6h *plus* gentamicin 5 mg/kg per day q12h
Enterobacter species	Cefotaxime 2 g q8h *plus* gentamicin 5 mg/kg per day q8h	Ceftazidime *or* ceftizoxime 2 g q8h *plus* gentamicin 5 mg/kg per day q12h
Escherichia coli	Ampicillin 2 g q6h	Cefazolin 1 g q8h, cefuroxime 1.5 g q8h
Proteus mirabilis	Ampicillin 2 g q6h	Cefazolin 1 g q8h, cefuroxime 1 g q8h
Proteus vulgaris	Cefotaxime 2 g q8h	Cefuroxime 1.5 g q8h, ceftizoxime 2 g q8h
Providencia rettgeri	Ceftazidime 2 g q8h	
Morganella morganii	Ceftazidime 2 g q8h	
Serratia marcescens	Cefotaxime 2 g q8h	Ceftazidime *or* ceftizoxime 2 g q8h, mezlocillin *or* piperacillin 4 g q6h, *plus* gentamicin 5 mg/kg per day q12h
Pseudomonas aeruginosa	Azlocillin 4 g q6h *or* piperacillin 3 g q4h *plus* tobramycin 5 mg/kg per day q8h (in order of choice)	Ceftazidime 2 g q8h *plus* tobramycin 5 mg/kg per day q12h
Bacteroides species	Clindamycin 900 mg q8h IV	Metronidazole 500 mg q8h, cefoxitin 2 g q6h

* Administered intravenously.

centration (MBC). Disk sensitivities have been used as the basis of therapy, but disks contain concentrations of drugs in excess of those achievable in bone, and results may not be directly applicable to the clinical situation. The antimicrobial agent chosen should penetrate the involved bone in concentrations greater than those required to be active against the organisms.

Soft tissue swelling, periosteal thickening, and periosteal elevation are the earliest changes but are subtle and may be missed. Lytic changes are not seen until 2 to 6 weeks after the onset of disease. Sclerotic changes of periosteal new bone formation (involvarum) denotes a longer process. Radionucleotide scanning (technetium plus gallium or indium) are most helpful in the course of acute disease prior to the development of radiologic changes. Positive scans may be seen as early as 24 hours after the onset of symptoms. CT is useful to identify areas of dead bone (sequestrum).

The bacteriologic diagnosis of osteomyelitis rests on the isolation of the pathogenic bacteria from the bone or the blood. In chronic osteomyelitis, sinus tract cultures are not reliable for predicting which organism(s) will be isolated from the infected bone. There is a poor correlation between sinus tract cultures with bone biopsy cultures. Bone biopsy material should be carefully cultured and stained for aerobes, anaerobes, mycobacterium and fungus. The bone should also be submitted for histopathological evaluation.

Antimicrobial therapy should be initiated as early as possible, should be directed specifically against the offending pathogen(s), and should be administered intravenously in high doses for 4 to 6 weeks. Surgical intervention, in the form of bone debridement, is usually required in addition to antibiotics in the therapy of osteomyelitis arising from a contiguous focus of infection, diabetic ulcers, and peripheral vascular disease. In addition, combination intravenous and oral antimicrobial therapy may need to be given for 3 to 6 months in forms of osteomyelitis where extensive bony changes and tissue damage have occurred.

The antimicrobial agent(s) chosen for use should be demonstrated effective against the organism isolated from bone by in vitro sensitivity tests—MIC and MBC. It is best to choose an antibiotic or antibiotic combination that has a low ratio of MIC to MBC relative to its expected serum concentration. We prefer the antibiotic chosen to be able to obtain serum levels at least eight times the MIC. Table 3 outlines the choice of antibiotics for the therapy of bacterial osteomyelitis in adults.

BACTERIAL ARTHRITIS

JACK L. LEFROCK, M.D.
DON WALTER KANNANGARA, M.D., Ph.D.

Bacterial arthritis is an inflammation of the joint space, synovial fluid, synovium, and articular cartilage caused by a variety of microorganisms. The process is generally acute and constitutes a medical emergency; if untreated for even 24 to 48 hours, permanent joint damage may result. The vast majority of episodes are caused by the common pyogenic bacteria, including *Staphylococcus aureus, Streptococcus* species, *Hemophilus influenzae,* and *Neisseria gonorrhoeae*. The aerobic gram-negative bacilli and anaerobes account for additional cases.

There are three modes by which a joint space may be seeded. For both children and adults, the commonest cause is hematogenous. Roughly 50 percent of patients with septic arthritis will have concomitant postive blood cultures. A primary source, such as otitis, endocarditis, and so on, should be sought. A small percentage of cases will be the result of direct inoculation of the joint space, either accidentally (atypical mycobacteria, actinomyces) or iatrogenically (arthrocentesis, instillation of corticosteroids). Rarely, septic arthritis may result from spread of contiguous infection (*Mycobacterium tuberculosis*).

Once the synovium is seeded, the resulting inflammatory reaction may result in rapid destruction of the articular cartilage. Since this cartilage is avascular and unable to regenerate, permanent damage results.

The specific etiologic agent in any given patient can be anticipated by identifying the patient's age, host factors and presence of prior disease (Table 1).

Patients with chronic underlying diseases, especially those with cirrhosis and diabetes mellitus, have impaired phagocytic defenses, more frequent bacteremias, and consequently a higher incidence of septic arthritis. The importance of underlying joint diseases, for example, rheumatoid arthritis or degenerative joint disease, cannot be overemphasized. Septic arthritis in patients with underlying chronic arthritis is often subacute and may mimic a flare-up in the underlying disease. Aspiration without culture and Gram stain of the material amounts to negligence. Septic arthritis in patients with rheumatoid arthritis is caused by *S. aureus* in 80 percent of cases.

Nearly half of the cases of septic arthritis in adults involve the knee joints, followed in descending order of frequency by hip, shoulder, elbow, sternoclavicular joint, ankle, sacroiliac joint, and small joints of the hands and

TABLE 1 Causative Organism in Septic Arthritis by Age in Years (Percentages)

	2	*2–15*	*16–50*	*>50*
Staphylococcus aureus	35	50	15	75
Streptococcus hemolyticus	15	20	5	5
Streptococcus pneumoniae	10	10	—	5
Hemophilus influenzae	35	2	—	—
Neisseria gonorrhoeae	—	5	75	—
Other	5	13	5	15

TABLE 2 Initial Synovial Fluid Findings in Infectious Arthritis

Disease	Mucin Clot	White Cell Count/mm^3	Cell Type	Synovial Fluid—Blood:Glucose Ratio	Stained Smear*	Culture
None	Good	200–600	Mononuclear	0.8–1.0	−	−
Acute bacterial arthritis	Poor	10,000–>100,000	>90% polymorphonuclear	<0.5	+	+
Fungal arthritis†	Good-Poor	3,000–30,000	>70% polymorphonuclear	0.5–1.0	±	+
Tuberculous arthritis	Fair-Poor	10,000–20,000	50%–70% polymorphonuclear	≤0.5	±	+

* Gram stain for bacteria; potassium hydroxide (KOH) wet mounts for fungi; Ziehl-Neelsen stain for mycobacteria
† Based on a small number of analyses reported in the literature

feet. Monoarticular arthritis is most common when the infecting agent is *S. aureus*, whereas with *N. gonorrhoeae*, polyarticular involvement is usual.

Joints involved in acute pyogenic arthritis are usually warm, tender, erythematous, and associated with general constitutional symptoms, such as malaise and fever. Roentgenographically, the joint capsule may be distended with fluid, accompanied by soft tissue swelling; less commonly, destructive changes in the bony structures will be evident. The latter may occur with pyogenic arthritis in which there has been delay in diagnosis or in mycobacterial infections or when infections complicate rheumatoid arthritis.

DIAGNOSIS

The diagnosis is established by examination and culture of synovial fluid. A positive Gram stain or culture is generally specific. Prior antibiotic therapy may result in a negative culture or Gram stain. It is important to do a Gram stain, acid-fast stain if the Gram stain is negative, and culture. Synovial fluid is analyzed for total and differential leukocyte count, crystals, glucose, and mucin clot (Table 2). Other parameters include protein, complement, pH, color, and turbidity. However, there is significant overlap of all these findings among different types of inflammatory arthritis, for example, septic, rheumatoid, gouty, and pseudogouty. In septic arthritis, the leukocyte count is usually greater than 50,000 per cubic millimeter with more than 90 percent of the cells being polymorphonuclear leukocytes. The glucose is less than 60 percent of simultaneous serum glocuse, mucin clot is poor, and protein is greater than 3 g. The appearance is cloudy or turbid with a yellow to green hue.

Roentgenograms taken in the first 7 to 10 days of infections are of little diagnostic help because they show only distention of the joint capsule and periarticular swelling. Initial films should nevertheless be obtained, because septic arthritis may be a consequence of preexisting osteomyelitis, which would be revealed on x-ray. Follow-up films are important in evaluating the extent of articular damage.

Skin lesions, particularly those that can be aspirated and examined on Gram-stained smears, can provide a clue as to the presence of bacteremia (meningococcal, gonococcal, or staphylococcal) and indicate a specific organism.

TREATMENT

Successful management consists of three elements: prompt diagnosis, appropriate antimicrobial therapy, and drainage of the joint space. Delaying therapy more than 7 days commonly results in incomplete recovery.

Antimicrobial Therapy

Selection of antibiotics is initially determined by the clinical setting, age of the patient, and results of the Gram stain of the joint fluid. Selection may later be modified based on bacteria isolated and their antibiotic susceptibility (Table 3). Parenteral antibiotics reach adequate levels in the joint fluid and intra-articular injection of antibiotics is not indicated for therapy of bacterial arthritis. In fact, intra-articular antibiotics may produce a chemical synovitis. The duration of parenteral antibiotics is generally 14 days or longer, the only exception being gonococcal arthritis, in which the organisms are usually very sensitive and 7 days will suffice. However, when the organism is difficult to eradicate (such as *S. aureus* or gram-negative bacilli) parenteral treatment should be given for 4 weeks.

Joint Drainage

The joint should be aspirated by needle as often as required to remove pus which contains enzymes that destroy cartilage. Repeated aspiration may be required for 7 to 10 days. Indications for open surgical drainage are (1) hip infections; (2) presence of loculations (incompletely removed by aspiration especially when *S. aureus* is the pathogen); and (3) persistently high neutrophil counts (>25,000 per cubic millimeter) in the joint fluid or positive cultures despite appropriate antibiotic treatment and multiple closed aspirations.

After open drainage the wound should be allowed to heal by secondary closure, and antibiotics are continued for 1 week after the procedure.

Other Measures

Weight bearing should be avoided until all signs of inflammation subside. The joint should be maintained in

TABLE 3 Choice of Antibiotics in Therapy of Septic Arthritis

Organism	*Drugs of First Choice*	*Alternative Drug*
Neisseria gonorrhoeae	Penicillin G, 2 million units IV q4h for 3 days, followed by penicillin V, 500 mg orally qid for 4 days	Cefotaxime, 1 g IV q4h for 1 week Cefoxitin, 2 g IV q6h for 1 week Doxycycline, 100 mg IV q12h for 1 week
Staphylococcus aureus	Nafcillin, 2 g IV q4h for 4 weeks	Oxacillin, 2 g IV q4h for 4 weeks Cephalothin, 2 g IV q4h for 4 weeks Vancomycin, 500 mg IV q6h for 4 weeks
Streptococcus pneumoniae, Streptococcus pyogenes	Penicillin G, 2 million units IV q6h for 2 weeks	Cefazolin, 1 g IV q8h for 2 weeks Vancomycin, 500 mg IV q6h for 2 weeks
Hemophilus influenzae	Ampicillin, 1 g IV q4h for 2 weeks	Cefotaxime, 2 g IV q4h for 2 weeks Cefamandole, 2 g IV q6h for 2 weeks Chloramphenicol, 1 g IV q6h for 2 weeks Cefuroxime 1.5 g IV q8h for 2 weeks
Presumed pygenic arthritis with no organism recovered	Nafcillin, 2 g IV q4h plus gentamicin, 3–5 mg/kg per day in divided doses q8h for 2 weeks	Cephalothin, 2 g IV q4h *or* vancomycin, 500 mg IV q6h plus an aminoglycoside, e.g., gentamicin, 3–5 mg/kg per day IV in divided doses q8h for 2 weeks
Escherichia coli, Proteus mirabilis	Ampicillin, 1 g IV q4h plus gentamicin, 3–5 mg/kg per day in divided doses q8h for 2 weeks	Cefazolin, 2 g IV q8h for 2 weeks Mezlocillin, 3 g IV q4h for 2 weeks Cefuroxime, 1.5 g IV q8h for 2 weeks Ceftriaxone, 1 g IV q24h for 2 weeks
Pseudomonas aeruginosa	Ticarcillin, 3 g IV q4h plus gentamicin 3–5 mg/kg per day in divided doses q8h for 3 weeks	Other anti-*Pseudomonas* penicillin, e.g., piperacillin or azlocillin, 3 g IV q4h plus an aminoglycoside, e.g., gentamicin, 3–5 mg/kg per day in divided doses q8h or amikacin, 15 mg/kg per day in divided doses q8h for 3 weeks Ceftazidime, 2 g IV q8h for 3 weeks

Note: The recommended durations are only approximate. The exact duration of therapy should be determined by the clinical response.

the position of maximal function but strict immobilization is not required. Once the joint is pain free, initially passive and subsequently active exercises are instituted. Weight bearing is allowed when all signs of inflammation have resolved and no effusion is present. Residual problems, such as limitation of movement, difficulty in ambulation, or shortening of an extremity, may occur in a few patients. Appropriate orthopedic measures or rehabilitation medicine is required in such cases. Chronic indolent forms of arthritis may need synovectomy in addition to chemotherapy to eliminate the infection.

NONBACTERIAL ARTHRITIS SYNDROME

CHARLES B. SMITH, M.D.

Although bacteria that are easily cultured in the laboratory are the commonest infectious agents associated with arthritis syndromes, infectious arthritis may also be caused by a wide variety of viruses, chlamydia, mycoplasmas, fungi, or bacteria that do not grow on the usual bacterial culture media. Culture-negative infectious arthritis may present either as acute polyarticular or as a chronic pauciarticular arthritis. Because different types of infectious agents are associated with acute and chronic arthritis, the following discussion will address the two syndromes separately.

ACUTE POLYARTICULAR ARTHRITIS

Acute polyarticular arthritis has been associated with a large variety of viral infections. The clinical clues to viral arthritis include symptoms suggestive of systemic viral illnesses such as acute onset of fever, malaise, and myalgias and an epidemiologic setting suggestive of a particular viral illness. Signs of involvement of other organ systems such as the skin or the liver are helpful clues to the viral etiology of arthritis. The arthritis is usually migratory and polyarticular, although pauciarticular arthritis involving a few large joints such as the knee may be prominent. Joint swelling, erythema and tenderness are present, but are not of the severity that is characteristic of acute arthritis due to pyogenic bacteria. Laboratory abnormalities are not usually helpful other than to indicate nonspecific inflammation (moderately elevated erythrocyte sedimentation rate and leukocytosis). The joint fluid contains leukocytes and mononuclear cells usually predominate, although early in the course, a polymorphonuclear leukocytosis may be seen. Definitive diagnosis is based on a classic clinical picture such as that of rubella or chickenpox, or the diagnosis may require demonstration of infection by isolation of the virus or by demonstration of a diagnostic rise in titer of antibodies.

Hepatitis B Virus

Acute symmetrical polyarthritis involving the small joints of the upper extremity and often the knees is a common finding in the prodrome before jaundice develops in patients with hepatitis B viral infection. The diagnosis is suggested when an individual at high risk of developing hepatitis B viral infection (drug abuse, male homosexuality, heavy exposure to blood products) develops fever, chills, malaise, arthralgias, and acute polyarthritis. Lymphadenopathy and the transient appearance of an urticarial or maculopapular rash should also suggest the diagnosis. The arthritis and rash are thought to be due to circulating virus-antibody immune complexes, and these may be associated with increased circulating cryoglobulins and decreased serum complement. Specific diagnosis is confirmed by a positive blood test for HBs antigen during the acute illness or by a rising titer of antibody to HBs later in the illness. The arthritis is usually self-limited to a period of a few weeks, although in some patients the arthritis has persisted for up to 6 months. Therapy for joint symptoms is usually successful with aspirin (600 mg orally four times a day). Because aspirin may interfere with blood clotting, this therapy should be stopped when jaundice or chemical evidence of hepatic disease appears.

Rubella Virus

Arthritis is a common finding in patients with rubella or in those who have received the live, attenuated rubella viral vaccine. It is commoner among adults than children and commoner among women than men. The arthritis is usually polyarticular, involving the fingers, wrists, elbows, and knees and is characterized by pain and stiffness rather than swelling and erythema. History of recent vaccination or the finding of the typical morbilliform rash, postcervical lymphadenopathy, fever, upper respiratory symptoms, and general malaise help to make the diagnosis. Joint fluid is usually difficult to obtain and reveals a moderate increase of mononuclear cells (1,000 to 2,000 per cubic millimeter). Definitive diagnosis is made by isolation of the virus from pharyngeal secretions or from the joint fluid and by demonstrating a diagnostic rise in titer of antibodies. Therapy for rubella virus arthritis is aspirin. The arthritis usually last for only 3 to 4 weeks; however a few patients have developed recurrent mild attacks of arthritis involving the knees that may persist for several years. No specific therapy for these recurrent attacks has been identified.

Other Viral Infections

Acute polyarticular arthritis syndromes have rarely been associated with other common childhood viral illnesses including mumps, varicella, erythema infectiosum, and infections with enteroviruses, adenoviruses, cytomegalovirus, Epstein-Barr virus, and herpes simplex virus. These have generally been self-limited in duration and, as with other forms of viral arthritis, it is important to reassure the patient and to limit therapy to relatively benign anti-inflammatory agents and analgesics.

Mycoplasmal Infections

Mycoplasma pneumoniae infections are occasionally associated with an acute migratory polyarticular arthritis that is usually self-limited to a course of a few weeks. Rarely, patients who are hypogammaglobulinemic or who are otherwise immunosuppressed have developed an acute purulent monoarticular arthritis from which *M. pneumoniae* has been isolated. *Ureaplasma urealyticum* and *Mycoplasma hominis* are other mycoplasmas that commonly inhabit the genitourinary tract and that may infect the joints in patients who are immunologically deficient. Diagnosis of these mycoplasmal infections is by isolation of the organism on special mycoplasmal media or by detection of rises in specific antibodies. A response to therapy with tetracycline (tetracycline hydrochloride, 500 mg orally four times a day for 10 days) has been described in patients with mycoplasmal joint infections.

Lyme Arthritis

An arthritis syndrome has recently been described that is characterized by onset with a red papule on the skin that expands into a contiguous spreading erythema (erythema chronicum migrans), and which is followed several days or weeks later by an oligo- or polyarticular arthritis lasting approximately 1 week. Cardiac involvement (AV block) or neurologic involvement, with meningitis, encephalitis, or peripheral neuropathy, may also complicate the illness. Originally described in Lyme, Connecticut, Lyme arthritis has been found in patients inhabiting both coasts of the United States and in Europe. The disease distribution follows that of the *Ixodes* tick, and the illness is due to infection with a spirochetal organism that infects these ticks. A response to penicillin therapy is consistent with the spirochetal infectious etiology. Penicillin (250 mg orally four times a day for 10 days) is the currently recommended therapy, and similar doses of tetracycline hydrochloride are used in patients allergic to penicillin.

Reiter's Syndrome

Reiter's syndrome is a reactive arthritis that occurs in genetically predisposed individuals (HLA type B27) following infection with enteric pathogens such as *Salmonella* or *Shigella* or following infection of the genitourinary tract with *Chlamydia trachomatis*. The sexually acquired form of Reiter's syndrome is particularly common in young sexually active men. The syndrome consists of urethritis, conjunctivitis, dermatitis, and arthritis, which is characterized by involvement of the fingers, plantar fasciitis, tenosynovitis, and spondyloarthropathy, as well as involvement of the major joints. Diagnosis is based on clinical identification of the syndrome. The symptoms are best controlled with nonsteroidal anti-inflammatory agents (indomethacin, 25 mg orally every 8 hours). Treatment of the chlamydial infection with tetracyline or erythromycin has not been associated with dramatic improvement in the symptoms of arthritis or urethritis; however, well-controlled studies have not been done. For this reason and because chronic chlamydial infection of the genitourinary tract can have serious complications in both men and women, I recommend treatment of the patient and the sexual partner with either tetracycline hydrochloride or erythromycin in doses of 500 mg orally four times a day for 14 days. If facilities are available for culturing *Chlamydia* from mucous membranes and joint fluids, it would be reasonable to limit this antimicrobial therapy to those who are culture-positive.

Noninfectious Causes of Acute Febrile Polyarticular Arthritis

It is important to remember that not all febrile patients with acute polyarticular arthritis have an infectious disease. Acute gout may present in this fashion, and, certainly, all inflammatory joint fluids should be examined for crystals. Adult and juvenile rheumatoid arthritis, systemic lupus erythematosus, acute rheumatic fever, sarcoidosis, and a large variety of other inflammatory arthritides need to be considered in the differential diagnosis.

CHRONIC MONO- OR OLIGOARTICULAR ARTHRITIS

Mycobacteria

M. tuberculosis involves the skeletal and synovial tissues in 1 percent of patients. Because extrapulmonary tuberculosis often progresses slowly and routine bacterial cultures are negative, the diagnosis of tuberculosis synovitis is often delayed for several months, resulting in permanent joint damage. The diagnosis should be suspected in any patient with chronic, slowly progressive, "sterile," mono- or oligoarticular arthritis who is tuberculin-positive. The organism is more readily cultured from biopsied synovial tissues than from joint fluids, and the associated histologic demonstration of granulomas and acid-fast bacilli is particularly helpful in leading to the correct diagnosis. Therapy is the same as that for pulmonary tuberculosis (INH, 300 mg per day, and rifampin, 600 mg per day) except that a course of 18 months is preferred. When extensive joint damage has occurred, surgical debridement and reconstruction may be useful after the infection is controlled by chemotherapy.

Atypical mycobacteria (e.g., *M. avium, M. kansasii, M. fortuitum*) are less pathogenic than *M. tuberculosis*; thus, they are less commonly a cause of joint infections. When joint involvement occurs, it is usually in a setting where host defenses have been severely depressed (corticosteroid therapy, cancer chemotherapy, AIDS) or when these saprophytic organisms are introduced into a joint during prosthetic surgery, trauma, or repeated corticosteroid injections into the joint. The arthritis is usually monoarticular and slowly progressive, so that permanent joint damage occurs by the time the clinician—in frustration—resorts to surgical exploration, and the diagnosis is made on the basis of the histologic examination and culture of biopsy tissues. Antimicrobial therapy is very difficult because the atypical mycobacteria are often multiply resistant. Three to four antimicrobial agents should be used, and their selection should be based on sensitivity testing. Because the response to chemotherapeutic agents is often very slow or unsatisfactory, surgical debridement of involved synovium is an important part of the therapeutic plan.

Fungi

A relatively acute polyarticular arthritis syndrome has been associated with intitial infections with *Coccidioides immitis* and *Histoplasma capsulatum*. The arthritis is often associated with erythema nodosum or erythema multiforme, and the course is usually benign, suggesting hypersensitivity reaction as the pathogenesis rather than direct seeding of the joint with infectious organisms. Acute septic arthritis commonly follows disseminated infection with *Blastomyces dermatididis* and may be seen in immunosuppressed patients as a manifestation of disseminated infection with *Candida albicans, Aspergillus fumigatus*, or *Cryptococcus neoformans*. These invasive infections are usually diagnosed by growing the fungus from synovial fluid and other organ tissues. Therapy is with amphotericin B, using doses appropriate for the serious systemic infection.

Chronic mono- or oligoarticular infection with fungi represents a much greater diagnostic and therapeutic problem for the practitioner. The course is usually indolent, resembling posttraumatic or osteoarthritis, and partial response of symptoms to anti-inflammatory agents often leads away from consideration of an infectious etiology. The course from onset of symptoms to diagnosis is often numbered in years, and all too often the diagnosis is made by accident when tissues are routinely examined by the pathologist during reconstructive surgery. As is the case with mycobacterial joint infections, culture of synovial tissues gives a much higher yield than does examination or culture of the synovial fluid. Therapy for most fungal infections is with amphotericin B (see chapter *Antifungal Chemotherapy*) and the duration of therapy is determined by the relative sensitivity of the organism and the rapidity of the clinical response. There are few data to indicate a therapeutic role for intra-articular amphotericin B. Because the diagnosis is often made long after permanent damage to the joint occurs, surgical debridement and reconstruction are helpful in obtaining the maximal functional result.

INFECTIONS AFFECTING MORE THAN ONE SYSTEM CAUSED BY BACTERIA OR VIRUS

TUBERCULOSIS

ASIM K. DUTT, M.D.
WILLIAM W. STEAD, M.D.

With the dramatic decline of tuberculosis in Western countries, physicians often fail to consider the disease in the differential diagnosis, sometimes with tragic results. The index of suspicion should be especially high when persons in certain groups manifest cough with persistent fever or loss of weight: the elderly, disadvantaged persons, and immigrants from developing countries. The clinical presentation may vary over a wide spectrum from virtually no symptoms through symptoms such as mild, persistent fever and loss of weight to severe symptoms including cough, malaise, fever, and even hemoptysis. Isolation of *Mycobacterium tuberculosis* is essential for a firm diagnosis, but a strong clinical suspicion may suffice as an indication for specific chemotherapy.

Once the possibility of tuberculosis is considered, the steps for diagnosis are rather simple. Most important is the collection of secretions and/or biopsy materials for microscopy and culture. Radiologic examination and tuberculin testing are also of importance, but are not diagnostic. A classic roentgenogram of the chest may strongly suggest the disease, but all too often the radiographic presentation is quite atypical, especially when the infection has been acquired recently.

A positive tuberculin reaction by Mantoux test (10 or more millimeters' induration) indicates infection with tubercle bacilli. A compatible clinical presentation and radiographic abnormality increase the possibility of the disease. However, a negative tuberculin test does not necessarily rule out the diagnosis, as 20 to 25 percent of patients who are clinically ill may have an initial negative test. A repeat of the test 2 weeks later may be positive. Some patients are anergic and may not be able to show enough T-cell activity to develop a positive tuberculin reaction.

DIAGNOSIS

Pulmonary Tuberculosis

Spontaneously produced sputum provides necessary material for smear and culture in diagnosis of pulmonary tuberculosis. At least three early-morning sputum specimens should be examined by microscopy (Fig. 1). If one of these is positive, no further collection is necessary. When all are negative on microscopy, at least five specimens should be submitted for culture.

If a patient is unable to produce sputum or is uncooperative, an alternative method is to induce sputum by inhalation of heated aerosol of saline. Other methods are early-morning gastric lavage and laryngeal swab or aspiration; these are not quite as productive.

When microscopy of sputum is negative on at least three specimens, bronchial washing through a fiberoptic bronchoscope may be indicated. In addition, postbronchoscopy sputum specimens should be collected because they often yield positive result. Transtracheal puncture may be necessary as a last resort in unconscious patients with a life-threatening illness. In occasional patients, transthoracic needle aspirate of the lung may be indicated for obtaining necessary material for bacteriology. In rare circumstances the diagnosis is made only by open lung biopsy.

Although fluorescent microscopy is much more sensitive, it is quite nonspecific and must be confirmed by Ziehl-Neelsen or Kenyoun staining. Positive microscopy never confirms the presence of *M. tuberculosis* because other mycobacteria may be present. Therefore, cultural examination is necessary for isolation and identification of *M. tuberculosis*. Furthermore, testing for susceptibility to antituberculosis drugs is useful for identifying the occasional case of primary drug resistance.

Extrapulmonary Tuberculosis

For the diagnosis of tuberculosis in extrapulmonary sites, secretions and/or biopsy material should be obtained for examination (Fig. 1). In the case of pleural and pericardial effusion, biopsy and/or fluid should be examined and cultured. The yield from culture of pleural fluid is small, presumably because of the relatively small population of organisms present. Cerebrospinal fluid smear and cultural examination are necessary in meningitis, but positive results are found in only 20 to 40 percent of the cases of tuberculous meningitis. Cultural examination of ascitic fluid in tuberculous peritonitis may confirm the diagnosis, but microscopy and culture of a percutaneous biopsy specimen is preferred.

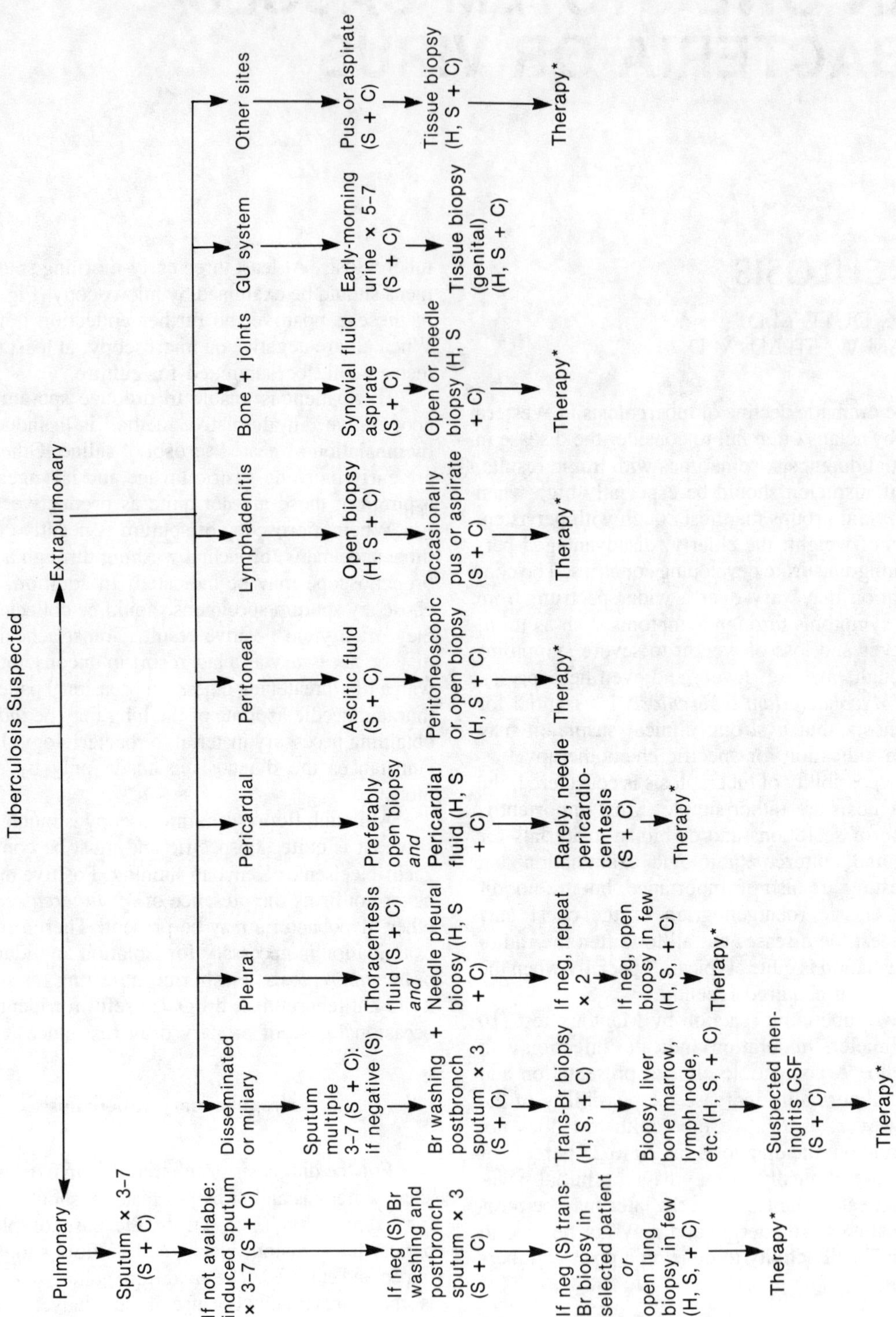

Figure 1 Diagnosis of suspected tuberculosis. Abbreviations: S = smear, C = culture for mycobacteria, H = histology, Br = bronchial, Bronch = bronchoscopy, CSF = cerebrospinal fluid, Bx = biopsy, neg = negative, GU = genitourinary; * therapy started in suspected cases, awaiting cultural results and/or clinical response.

The definitive diagnosis of genitourinary tuberculosis requires the isolation of *M. tuberculosis* by urine culture. An acid-fast stain of an early-morning specimen should be performed on 3 to 5 separate days.

In tuberculosis of joints, bacteriologic examination of synovial fluid is important. Positive synovial fluid culture may be found in approximately 80 percent of cases, and about one-fourth may show the organism in the smear examination. Pus and fluids from discharging sinuses from any site should be submitted for microscopy and culture.

If the microscopic examination of fluid is negative, a definitive diagnosis is delayed for 6 to 8 weeks while cultural results are awaited. Hence, biopsy of the involved tissue, either by needle or exploratory surgery, is often required for early diagnosis.

In cases of the pleural effusion, closed-needle biopsy should be performed to obtain three to four pieces of pleura to submit for both microscopy and culture. The tissue sections should also be stained for acid-fast bacilli. It is common to find a typical granulomatous pleuritis in which no organisms can be found by special staining. Culture of one or two tissue fragments greatly increases the diagnostic yield of the procedure. It is a common error to place all tissue fragments into formalin, which precludes culture. If the first set of biopsies is not diagnostic, at least one more attempt should be made before considering the results negative. Repeated biopsies increase the yield of positive results by 15 to 20 percent. In rare circumstances, surgical biopsy of pleura may be indicated.

Surgical biopsy is preferred for pericardial disease because it is usually a safer procedure and gives enough tissue for examination, while providing drainage of the fluid through a pericardial "window." In disseminated or miliary tuberculosis, needle biopsy of liver and bone marrow is recommended. Hepatic biopsy is positive in more than 80 percent of cases and bone marrow, in more than 50 percent if examined by both microscopy and culure. Miliary pulmonary disease with negative sputum smears is best approached by transbronchial biopsy through a fiberoptic bronchoscope. Rarely, open lung biopsy may be necessary for the diagnosis. Percutaneous biopsy of the peritoneum is generally productive, but open biopsy may be obtained at exploratory laporotomy. Lymph nodes generally require excision biopsy. A Craig-needle biopsy of bone, joint, or vertebra is quite productive if specimens are examined both by microscopy and culture. If results are unsatisfactory, an open surgical biopsy is the next step.

Clinical Diagnosis

A diagnosis of tuberculosis may be justified despite negative bacteriologic results when the clinical picture is strongly suggestive and the clinical situation calls for therapy. Patients with a positive tuberculin test, compatible abnormal radiographs with or without symptoms, and in whom other possible causes have been reasonably excluded should be given a trial of chemotherapy.

Chemotherapy is initiated only after necessary materials have been submitted for bacteriological studies.

Such patients are observed for the clinical response to therapy. If there is prompt improvement over a few weeks the diagnosis of tuberculosis is likely correct and therapy should be continued to completion. If there is no improvement or worsening over a few weeks, diagnostic efforts to find the correct diagnosis should be undertaken, because tuberculosis is not likely in those circumstances.

CHEMOTHERAPY

Until a few years ago, the standard therapy for tuberculosis consisted of isoniazid (INH) and ethambutol (EMB) with a supplement of 1 to 3 months of streptomycin (SM) in cavitary smear–positive cases. The therapy was effective provided that the drugs were taken for 18 to 24 months. During the past decade, the availability of another oral bactericidal agent, rifampin (RIF) has made it possible to complete therapy much more quickly. By using INH and RIF together, the duration of treatment has been reduced to 9 months. it can even be shortened to 6 months if SM plus pyrazinamide (PZA) or EMB plus PZA are added to the regimen for the first two months.

Bacteriologic Concept of Drug Therapy

Many in vitro and in vivo studies in animals have increased our understanding of the bacterial population in tuberculous lesions and the action of drugs on them. Tubercle bacilli are obligate aerobes and thrive best in an environment with high oxygen tension. There are at least three distinct bacterial populations in a tuberculous lesion: *(1)* the largest population (ranging from 10^7 to 10^9 organisms) is actively replicating in a neutral or slightly alkaline medium in cavitary lesions; *(2)* a much smaller population (ranging from 10^2 to 10^5 organisms) exists in a neutral or slightly alkaline milieu of closed caseous and noncaseous lesions where it is metabolically less active or even dormant; *(3)* a similar small population (ranging from 10^2 or 10^5 organisms) is slowly replicating in the acid medium inside macrophages.

The size and metabolic activity of these bacterial populations is important because tubercle bacilli mutate to drug-resistant forms at a predictable rate irrespective of the presence or absence of antituberculous drug. Mutants resistant to each drug develop independently of other mutations and at a rate of approximately one per 10^{-5} to 10^{-6} replications. Those resistant to two drugs develop rarely, approximately once per 10^{-10} to 10^{-12} replications. Hence, a cavitary lung disease with a bacterial population of 10^7 to 10^9 organisms may contain 100 to 10,000 mutants resistant to any effective drug, and small populations in closed caseous or noncaseous lesions and in macrophages may have few or none. Thus, all cavitary tuberculous lesions harbor a mixture of drug-sensitive and -resistant bacilli, making at least two drugs essential to success.

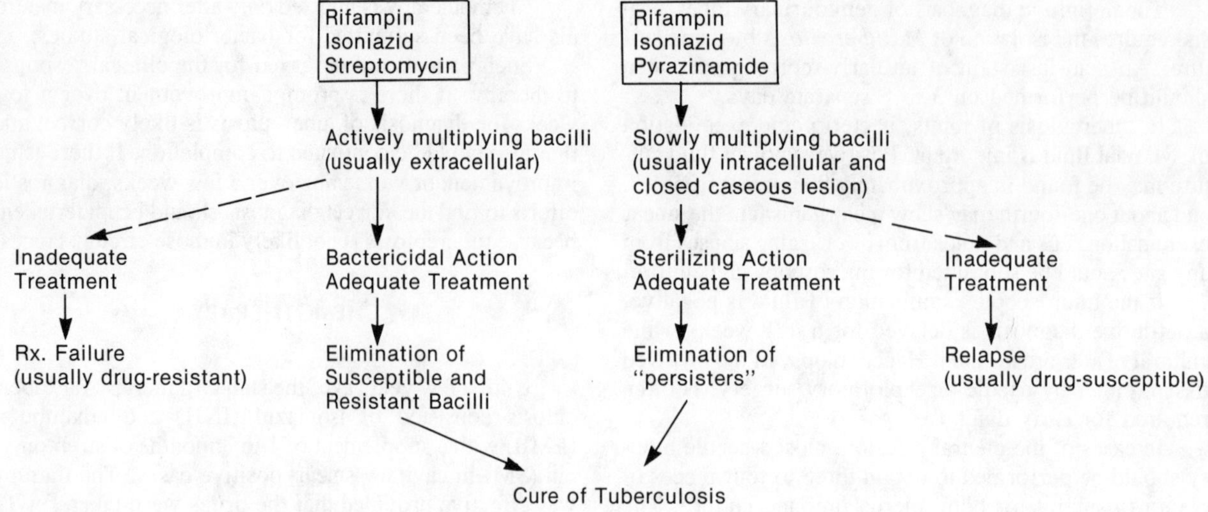

Figure 2 Current principles of tuberculosis chemotherapy.

Tubercle bacilli replicate rather slowly, about every 16 to 20 hours. The antituberculous drugs are effective in killing tubercle bacilli only when the organisms are replicating. Hence, antituberculous drugs are best given in a single daily dose, but must be given for a prolonged period to allow time to kill the entire population, including those that are semidormant and divide only intermittently.

Rapid elimination of the actively multiplying large population of bacilli is essential to prevent emergence of drug-resistant mutants, a process that results in treatment failure. Elimination of smaller populations of intermittently multiplying organisms by extended therapy is necessary to prevent late relapse due to replication of the "persisters."

Drug Action on the Bacilli

The antituberculous drugs are generally classified as bactericidal and bacteriostatic. SM/capreomycin (CAP), RIF, INH, and PZA are considered batericidal. The bacteriostatic drugs are EMB, ethionamide (ETA), cycloserine (CS), *para*-aminosalycylic acid (PAS). EMB in dosage of 25 mg per kilogram is considered by some to be bactericidal and certainly is more effective in eliminating bacilli than in the usually prescribed dose of 15 mg per kilogram.

Among the bactericidal drugs, SM, INH, and RIF are highly active against actively multiplying extracellular bacilli (Fig. 2). With intensive daily therapy, these organisms can be eliminated rapidly. Selection of drug-resistant mutants is avoided and conversion of sputum smears to negative is prompt. Inadequate dosage or irregular ingestion may lead to treatment failure, with emergence of drug resistance.

RIF, INH, and PZA are active against slowly replicating organisms located inside the macrophages or extracellularly (Fig. 2). PZA is particularly effective in the acid environment inside macrophages. RIF is capable of killing bacilli that show even the slightest metabolic activity and, hence, is a useful drug during the continuation phase. With adequate duration of therapy, even the persisters are eliminated, resulting in a permanent cure. Inadequate length of treatment may permit a late relapse due to late replication of the persisters. Such a relapse is usually due to drug-sensitive organisms. It has been shown that most antituberculous drugs are effective when given twice weekly after the initial period of intensive daily administration. The addition of SM or PZA is not generally necessary, but the bactericidal activity of RIF and INH can be intensified by a supplement of SM and PZA to the regimen for the first 2 months. Such a regimen can further reduce the total duration of therapy to 6 months, with an added advantage of being effective even in the presence of INH resistance.

Treatment of Newly Diagnosed Tuberculosis

Before initiation of therapy, four possible clues to the probability of INH resistance should be sought (Fig. 3): *(1)* Has the patient received antituberculous drugs anytime in the past? *(2)* Is the patient from a country with a high prevalence of disease and drug resistance, e.g., Southeast Asia, Africa, or Latin America? *(3)* Is it likely the patient acquired the infection from an individual with a drug-resistant case? *(4)* Does the patient live in an area where INH resistance is common (more than 5%)?

If the answers to all of these inquiries are "no," therapy may safely be initiated with INH, 300 mg, and RIF, 600 mg, daily. In the United States, the incidence of initial drug resistance is low except for a few areas—the Mexican border, large cities, parts of California—where the addition of SM/CAP and PZA should almost be routine. Drug susceptibility should be determined on the in-

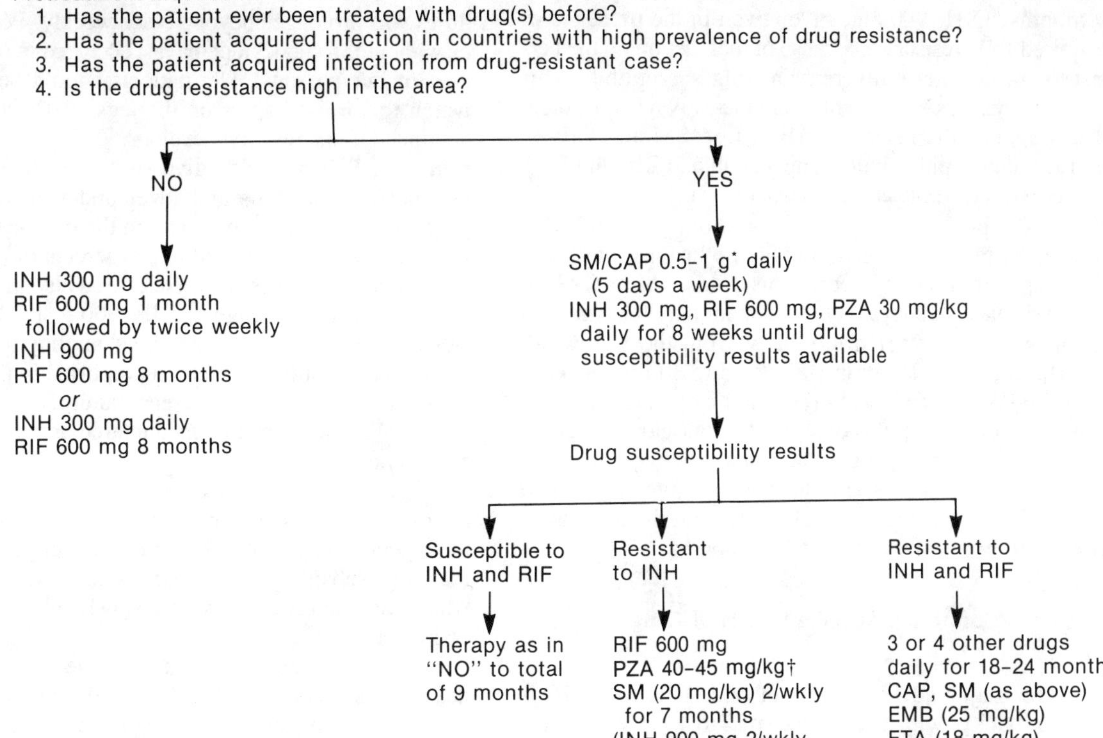

Figure 3 Chemotherapy of tuberculosis. * One gram is preferred; however, in patients who are elderly or weigh less than 100 pounds or have impaired renal function, the dose is revised downward. † Round off dose to tablet size.

tial sputum specimen in each case. We recommend that the drugs be given as combination capsules, e.g., Rifamate (Merrell-Dow) or Rimactizide (Ciba). Each capsule contains INH, 150 mg, and RIF, 300 mg, and thus, two capsules a day in the early morning furnishes the total daily dose. In addition to the convenience of the combination capsule, the patient is precluded from taking only one of the drugs. Both drugs are given daily for 9 months or daily for 1 month followed by INH, 900 mg, and RIF, 600 mg twice weekly, for another 8 months, i.e., two combination capsules and two INH 300-mg tablets twice a week.

Our experience in more than 2,500 patients with the latter regimen has proved successful in more than 95 percent of cases now followed up to 8 years. We have also treated more than 500 patients with various forms of extrapulmonary tuberculosis with similar results and less than 1 percent relapse. Our experience also indicates that the regimen is effective in patients whose tuberculosis is associated with various medical disorders, e.g., diabetes, alcoholism, corticosteroid therapy, malignancy, cytoxic chemotherapy.

The addition of a third drug, e.g., EMB or SM, does not add significantly to the bactericidal action of INH and RIF. Such a supplement is recommended by some to ensure against failure in the event of initial INH resistance. We do not routinely add a third drug to our regimen, but add both SM and PZA if we have a clue that there may be INH resistance (see above). Several recent studies have shown that initial intensive treatment with SM (0.5 to 0.75 g, or about 20 mg per kilogram); INH, 300 mg; RIF, 600 mg; and PZA, 25-30 mg per kilogram daily for 2 months, followed by INH, 300 mg, and RIF, 600 mg daily or twice weekly for another 4 months (i.e., total, 6 months), produces similar results. The regimen considerably reduces the duration of therapy for patients in whom more prolonged therapy would be difficult.

Drug Therapy in Suspected or Proven INH Resistance

If drug resistance (to INH) is suspected, therapy should be initiated with SM, INH, RIF, and PZA in the dosages mentioned above until the drug susceptibility results are known (usually 2 months) (Fig. 3). Therapy is then changed according to the results. If the organisms prove to be sensitive to INH and RIF, the treatment may be completed with INH, 300 mg, and RIF, 600 mg daily, or INH, 900 mg, and RIF, 600 mg, twice weekly for the remainder of the 9 months. When INH or RIF resistance is found, the therapy is changed to SM (1.0 to 1.5 g; approximately 20 mg per kilogram) PZA, 40 to 45 mg per kilogram; and INH, 900 mg, or RIF, 600 mg (depending on susceptibility) twice weekly for the remainder of the 9 months. INH, 900 mg, given even in the presence of acquired INH resistance because of their action on the persisters, which generally remain drug susceptible. This regimen ensures effectiveness of at least two bactericidal drugs against the resistant bacilli, i.e., SM and RIF on extracellular rapidly multiplying bacilli and RIF and PZA on the slowly replicating organisms.

In the presence of resistance to both INH and RIF, all drugs are discontinued, and therapy is instituted with three or four other antituberculous drugs. SM or CAP (if SM resistant) is given 5 days a week initially for 3 months along with two other drugs daily from the following: EMB, 25 mg per kilogram; PZA, 25 to 30 mg per kilogram; ETA, 500 to 750 mg (depending on tolerance; 750 mg is preferred, but this drug causes nausea); CS, about 18 mg per kilogram per day, accompanied by pyridoxine, 100 mg twice a day. The latter two are given in divided doses. As these drugs are not bactericidal, the total duration of therapy must be 18 to 24 months.

Monitoring Adverse Effects of Drugs

The major adverse effect of both INH and RIF is hepatotoxicity, with an incidence of 2 to 4 percent. There is no detectable increase when PZA, another potentially hepatotoxic drug, is included in the regimen. We have encountered hepatotoxicity in 2.5 percent of more than 2,000 patients treated with INH and RIF, even though the majority were elderly and there were many alcoholics. However, prudence dictates that two hepatotoxic drugs should not be used together in patient with active hepatitis. For such persons, we recommend starting treatment with INH and EMB with a supplement of SM if the sputum smear is positive. When the hepatitis subsides, RIF may safely be exchanged for EMB to obtain the advantage of short-course therapy.

Beyond routine baseline biochemical tests for hepatic function, regular biochemical monitoring leads to more confusion than enlightenment, since transient benign elevation of hepatic enzymes is common during therapy. We advise each patient to stop therapy immediately upon development of suspicious symptoms—e.g., anorexia, nausea, vomiting, or scleralicterus—and to report to the clinic for hepatic enzyme estimation. If symptoms are accompanied by elevation of hepatic enzymes of more than five times the base level, drug toxicity is likely. After symptoms have abated and the hepatic enzymes have returned to base line, drugs are reintroduced one at a time, starting with half dosage and monitoring of hepatic enzymes. In this manner, the offending drug can be identified and therapy changed appropriately. It is not uncommon that both drugs can be reintroduced without further adverse effect.

Twice weekly therapy with RIF may give rise to immunologic and hematologic side effects of petechiae and thrombocytopenia. This rarely occurs with a dosage of 600 mg RIF, but was a problem when the dosage 900 to 1,200 mg was used, particularly when the interval between doses was prolonged beyond twice weekly. Petechiae with or without thrombocytopenia has occurred in only 0.5 percent of our patients. The patients should be advised to watch for bruised spots on the legs. RIF should be discontinued if this reaction develops. Twice weekly administration of RIF may also give rise to flu-like syndrome, associated with chills and fever and with considerable aches and pains over the body on the day the medication is taken. This has occurred in 2.5 percent of our patients. The incidence of these adverse effects also increases with the use of higher dosage of RIF (900 to 1,200 mg). The side effect may be eliminated by changing to daily therapy. Other major adverse effects reported in the literature are hemolytic anemia, acute renal failure, and "shock syndrome," but we have not encountered any in our 9 years' experience.

The other side effects are minor, e.g., drug fever, allergies, skin rashes, and gastrointestinal intolerance—these occur in approximately 5 percent of patients. These reactions subside on temporary withdrawal of the drug, which can often be reintroduced slowly without recurrence of symptoms.

SM may cause vestibular damage, but only rarely, hearing loss. This adverse effect is dose related and may be reduced by injecting the drug only 5 days a week. Also, the dose of the drug should be cut to 0.5 g for persons older than 60 years of age and for patients with renal failure. Inquiry about dizziness and staggering may detect early toxicity. The drug may also cause allergic rashes and fever, which subside on withdrawal.

EMB is a well-tolerated drug and free from major adverse effects, but is of little value in short-course chemotherapy. The major side effect is optic neuritis (visual disturbances), which rarely occurs with the dose of 15 mg per kilogram, but may occur in 1 to 3 percent of patients receiving the more effective dose of 25 mg per kilogram. Monitoring of the side effect requires regular testing with reading and color charts and referral to an ophthalmologist for opinion in persons in whom toxicity is suspected.

PZA commonly causes flushing and, rarely, a skin rash. Hyperuricemia regularly occurs with PZA therapy, but rarely precipitates clinical gout. This is commoner during daily than during intermittent therapy. Arthralgia is frequent and occurs more often with daily treatment (7%) than with twice weekly administration (1% to 3%). Arthralgia is usually self-limiting and responds well to analgesics.

During therapy the health care team must remain in close contact with the patients because they may report suspicious symptoms. The patients should be informed about the symptoms of adverse effects and instructed to discontinue therapy if a problem is suspected and to report to the clinic promptly for clinical and laboratory assessment.

Surveillance of Patients During Therapy

Bacteriologic monitoring of patients during therapy is an important aspect in the management of tuberculosis. We suggest that three to five specimens of sputum be submitted for bacteriologic examination initially and that a drug susceptibility test be included. Then a sputum specimen should be submitted every 2 weeks until three specimens are reported to be negative. Thereafter, one specimen a month is adequate for the duration of therapy and for 6 months after completion. During follow-up one specimen every 3 months for another 6 months should be cultured after which the patient is discharged from supervision with the advice to return if symptoms recur.

A satisfactory response to treatment is observed by the gradual decline in the bacterial population of the sputum. Prolonged persistence of organisms in the sputum (more than 5 months) or reversion to positive bacteriology after conversion to negative should raise suspicion of treatment failure. Reevaluation of the patient's compliance and a repeat drug susceptibility test are then indicated in order to make the best choice of a retreatment four-drug regimen.

Frequent roentgenograms of chest are not indicated if bacteriologic studies are done as suggested. The health care team must evaluate whether the patient is taking the medications regularly as prescribed. This is carried out by frequent interviews with the patient, by checking attendance at clinic appointments and picking up of drugs, by surprise pill counts, and by random examination of urine for the color of RIF and for excretion of INH. In patients thought to be noncompliant, direct ingestion of drugs under supervision must be carried out. Twice weekly administration of drugs facilitates direct supervision.

Support by the Health Department

Most health departments provide facilities for collection of sputum specimens and bacteriologic examination. Monitoring of adverse effects of drugs and compliance of patients are provided through the able assistance of public health nurses. Expert advice is also provided by the personnel for difficult problems that may arise during management.

The public health nurses perform contact evaluation, with tuberculin testing and radiography when indicated, after receiving notification of an active case. Delay in notification of the health department may be catastrophic, particularly for children in whom the disease may progress rapidly with fatal results. Busy physicians who undertake to treat tuberculosis are well advised to take advantage of the facilities provided by local health departments in keeping up with patients for the 9 months of therapy.

NONTUBERCULOSIS ("ATYPICAL") MYCOBACTERIAL INFECTION

EDWARD H. KASS, M.D., Ph.D.

The "atypical" mycobacteria were so named at a time when *Mycobacterium tuberculosis* was a common cause of disease. When it was recognized that members of the genus *Mycobacterium* occurred in nature, sometimes caused disease, and could be confused with *M. tuberculosis* in smears, the confusing organisms were labeled "atypical." As the incidence of tuberculosis has declined, increasing attention has been paid to related microorganisms, and this has led to much clarification of their taxonomic characteristics and their relation to disease.

Because the nomenclature of the nontuberculosis mycobacteria has changed over the past decades and because many more species have been recognized, a table is appended listing some of the older nomenclatures along with the currently accepted names for this group of organisms.

Undoubtedly, more strains will be found as work with this group of organisms proceeds. The taxonomic details are best left to the experts in the field. The usual clinical laboratory will generally be able to identify the broad grouping of each organism by its chromogenic properties and by the rapidity of multiplication and may be able to add further information about the probable species.

Since the organisms are acquired largely from soil and water—and person-to-person transmission is rare—there is little risk to the attending staff and to other patients. Most therapy can be conducted in ambulatory patients or on an outpatient basis.

Although certain mycobacteria have traditionally been considered to be pathogenic and others nonpathogenic, this distinction has become less definitive as the number of immunocompromised individuals has grown. Isolation of any of these organisms in the presence of clinical evidence of disease, and without reasonable alternative diagnoses, should suggest infection due to these organisms and should indicate the need for diagnostic biopsy and culture when these are feasible.

Skin testing with extracts of these organisms has sometimes been used for diagnostic purposes. Such skin tests are of value in regions where these mycobacteria are not endemic in soil and water. In warmer climates, where these organisms are commonly found, cross-reactivity among strains and virtually universal exposure make the skin tests relatively unreliable. The organisms should be

TABLE 1 Nontuberculosis Mycobacterial Species

Present Name	*Former Name(s)*
M. kansasii	Runyon Gr. I, photochromogens, *M. luciflavum*
M. marinum	Runyon Gr. I, photochromogens, *M. balnei*
M. simiae	Runyon Gr. I, photochromogens, *M. habana*
M. scrofulaceum	Runyon Gr. II, scotochromogens, *M. marianum*
M. szulgai	Runyon Gr. II, scotochromogens
M. gordonae	Runyon Gr. II, scotochromogens, *M. aquae*
M. flavescens	Runyon Gr. II, scotochromogens
*M. avium–M. intracellulare**	Runyon Gr. III, nonchromogens, Batty bacillus
M. xenopi	Runyon Gr. III, nonchromogens, *M. littorale*
M. ulcerans	Runyon Gr. III, nonchromogens, *M. buruli*
M. gastri	Runyon Gr. III, nonchromogens
*M. terrae**	Runyon Gr. III, nonchromogens, Radish organism
M. triviale	Runyon Gr. III nonchromogens
*M. fortuitum**	Runyon Gr. IV, rapid growers, *M. ranae*
M. chelonei	Runyon Gr. IV, rapid growers, *M. abscessus*
M. smegmatis	Runyon Gr. IV, rapid growers, Smegma bacillus
M. phlei	Runyon Gr. IV, rapid growers, Timothy bacillus
M. vaccae	Runyon Gr. IV, rapid growers

* Complex of related organisms that will undoubtedly be subdivided further in the future.

sought in any unexplained lesions of the pulmonary organs or of the skin, particularly in individuals who have had occupational exposure to dust or whose skin has been exposed to abrasion or trauma, especially in tropical and subtropical climates. Dissemination from a primary focus is uncommon, except to regional lymph nodes.

Antimicrobial sensitivity data with these organisms must be viewed as no more than guides to effective therapy. Slow-growing strains undergoing only slight inhibition may nevertheless appear to be highly sensitive to a given drug. Conversely, therapeutic results indicate that satisfactory clinical responses may be experienced even when the in vitro sensitivity data suggest substantial resistance to the drugs used.

Because many of these organisms multiply slowly and are generally intracellular, treatment needs to be prolonged. Prolonged treatment, stretching over 2 years or more, is usually required, and although the following recommendations offer suggested guides to therapy, sustained follow-up, with repetition of treatment when recurrences are found, is necessary.

In giving recommendations for treatment, only those organisms that have been most often reported as causes of disease will be listed. For other organisms, if pathogenicity is expected, treatment such as that listed for infection due to *M. kansasii* is desirable, at least until sensitivity tests have shown that other drugs, such as tetracycline, may be used.

M. kansasii usually causes pulmonary lesions that are radiologically difficult to distinguish from tuberculosis. These are often accompanied by cavitation. The organism also may cause lesions of the skin and may disseminate in immunocompromised hosts. It is particularly common in the American Southwest, and in portions of the Middle West but may be found in all parts of the United States and in many other countries. Treatment consists of rifampin, 600 mg per day, plus INH, 300 mg per day, and ethambutol, 15 mg per kilogram per day for 24 months. If resistance to one or more of these drugs occurs, substitute streptomycin, 1 g three times weekly, intramuscularly, for 6 months and reevaluate for evidence of ototoxicity before continuing.

M. marinum, as the name implies, is found in water and particularly affects swimmers. Granulomas of the skin result and often heal spontaneously. Treatment is tetracycline, 2.0 g per day in divided doses. Alternatively, other tetracyclines such as minocycline (200 mg per day) may be used. Treatment is given for 2 months and is then reevaluated. If the lesion is responding, continue for 1 month and reevaluate as before. If there is no apparent response to treatment after 2 months, treat as for *M. kansasii* above, using only rifampin and ethambutol, and reevaluate after 12 months of treatment. Streptomycin, used as above, may be substituted if there is sensitivity to either of the above drugs.

M. avium—M. intracellulare is the name given to a diverse group of related organisms producing chronic pulmonary infection, particularly in middle-aged or older men. Treatment is as for *M. kansasii*. However, if sensitivity studies show sensitivity to streptomycin, this should be added as a fourth drug in doses of 1 g three times weekly for 6 months, as above. This infection is occasionally fatal, so multiple-drug therapy as soon as possible is important. If resistance to one or more drugs is encountered in vitro, cycloserine should be added. The latter drug is given as 250 mg per day for 10 days, and then the same dose, on alternate days thereafter. If the patient is found to be mentally dull or confused or complains of dizziness or blurring of vision, the dosage of cycloserine is reduced to 125 mg per day given every 2 days. Treatment is given for 2 years before reevaluation.

When there is persistent cavitation after therapy has been continued for at least 6 months—with no evidence that the cavity has been receding in size—or if the cavity has persisted despite diminution after 2 years of treatment, surgical removal of the affected area will often produce a cure. Of course, such surgery will depend upon the location of the lesion and the clinical condition of the patient.

M. ulcerans is the cause of the Buruli ulcer, an indolent ulcer of the skin encountered in many subtropical and tropical countries. The ulcer has best been treated by wide surgical incision followed by skin grafting.

M. scrofulaceum has been so named because of its tendency to produce cervical lymphadenitis in young children, thus mimicking the similar lesion produced by *M. tuberculosis*. However, in contrast to the tuberculous child, patients with infection due to *M. scrofulaceum* are generally nonreactive to the tuberculin standard 5-unit skin test dose of PPD. Treatment should be begun as for *M. kansasii*, but surgical excision of lymph nodes, where feasible, can be performed within 3 months after such chemotherapy if steady improvement has not occurred. Such surgical treatment is often curative.

For the other mycobacteria, as indicated above, treatment should be as outlined for *M. kansasii* infection, as a beginning. Surgical intervention is often useful when feasible. Treatment must be prolonged, must consist of multiple drugs, and requires close monitoring of the patient. Fortunately, these infections have little tendency to disseminate and are seldom fatal, so prolonged treatment becomes feasible.

Recently, an extensive experience with infections due to *M. chelonei* and *M. fortuitum* has been published. Although these findings have not yet been confirmed, they were extensive enough to cause changes in recommended treatment for these infections. The infections due to these two organisms commonly affect the skin and subcutaneous tissues rather than the lung, and such infections may lead to osteomyelitis. Treatment should consist of removal of foreign bodies (such as catheters) from the lesion, wherever possible, and the administration of amikacin (15 mg per kilogram per day) plus cefoxitin (200 mg per kilogram per day, with a maximum of 12 g per day). Susceptibility studies are necessary, and treatment should be continued for 12 weeks. If the isolate is susceptible to cefoxitin, amikacin can be discontinued after 8 weeks. Probenecid (0.5 g by mouth three times daily) should be given with the cefoxitin. If *M. fortuitum* is identified, rather than *M. chelonei*, the dose of cefoxitin can be reduced to 8 g per day.

Since therapy must often be prolonged, cultures during treatment are essential. If cultures are still positive after 12 weeks of treatment and the organism remains sensitive in vitro, treatment should be prolonged for 6 months.

Oral therapy is possible in milder instances of the infection—that is, infections that are not spreading rapidly and are localized to the skin and subcutaneous tissues. Data on oral therapy are scant for this group of infections; hence it is advisable to begin with parenteral therapy and then, if healing is proceeding, the cultures are free of the pathogens, and at least 6 weeks of parenteral therapy have been given, treatment can be changed to sulfadiazine (4 g per day) plus doxycycline (200 mg per day) in divided doses for 6 weeks further or until healing is complete.

It is obvious from the foregoing that there is much to be learned about this group of infections and that knowledge is accumulating slowly because of the relative rarity of these infections. Therefore, advice from an expert should be sought in all instances of severe and life-threatening infections in order to see if the above recommendations need revision in the light of newer knowledge.

LISTERIOSIS

NELSON M. GANTZ, M.D.

Reports of *Listeria* as a cause of infection appear to be increasing in frequency. The increased recognition of listeria infections in recent years is probably due to a number of factors, which include greater awareness of the organism by microbiologists and clinicians as well as the prolonged survival of susceptible hosts, such as renal transplant recipients and patients with malignancy.

Listeria monocytogenes is an aerobic gram-positive, non-spore-forming bacillus. The organism can appear similar to diphtheroids and may be reported as that by inexperienced laboratory personnel. Clinicians may interpret the isolation of a "diphtheroid" as a contaminant. The organism can also be confused on the interpretation of the gram-stained smear from a clinical specimen. The organism can appear as coccoid forms and be called a streptococcus or pneumococcus or appear as a gram-negative rod because of over-decolorization of the gram-stained smear and resemble *Hemophilus influenzae*.

EPIDEMIOLOGY

Infections caused by *Listeria* occur most often in neonates, immunosuppressed hosts, and elderly patients, but in epidemic outbreaks due to a common food source, all age groups may be affected. In certain areas of the world, such as France, most of the infections occur in neonates and pregnant women. In the United States, infection in the immunosuppressed host predominates, with illness occurring in renal transplant recipients, patients with hematologic malignancies, and other patients receiving high-dose corticosteroids or immunosuppressive therapy. Infection is also reported in the elderly, in patients with alcoholism and/or cirrhosis, and in the normal host. *Listeria* is an intracellular pathogen, and host defenses depend primarily on T-cell immunity. Corticosteroids depress cell-mediated immunity and are an important predisposing factor in the development of listeria infection.

The source of *Listeria* in most patients with the disease is unknown. Although animal carriage is common, direct transmission via this route is unusual except if the organisms have had an opportunity to multiply in a contaminated food. *Listeria* may be carried by cattle and may contaminate dairy foods. In addition to obscure environmental sources, transmission from mother to infant occurs via the transplacental route or during delivery. Most of the listeria infections occur sporadically, but epidemics have been described associated with eating raw vegetables contaminated with *Listeria*. However, persons at risk should not curtail their consumption of raw vegetables.

DIAGNOSIS

The diagnosis of listeriosis depends upon isolating the organism from a blood or cerebrospinal fluid (CSF) culture. The gram-stained smear of CSF is positive in only 25 percent of cases of listeria meningitis. Serologic tests for *Listeria* antibodies are not helpful in establishing a diagnosis. Determining the serotype of the *Listeria* organism isolated is useful in analyzing a cluster of listeria infections. In contrast to other bacterial causes of meningitis, a predominance of mononuclear cells occurs in one-third of patients.

CLINICAL FEATURES

Symptoms and signs of acute meningitis and/or parenchymal central nervous system disease are the commonest presentations of listeriosis. The findings may be subtle in an immunosuppressed host, with only fever and headache present. Bacteremia without a source is the second most frequent type of infection. All patients with listeria bacteremia should have a lumbar puncture to assess the possibility of meningitis. The presence of persistent listeria bacteremia should suggest the diagnosis of endocarditis. Neonates may present with meningitis, bacteremia, and/or disseminated infection.

TREATMENT

The treatment of listeria bacteremia and meningitis requires bactericidal drugs. Adults should be given ampicillin, 2 g intravenously every 4 hours (administered in 100 ml of normal saline or an equal volume of 5 percent dextrose and water given over a 30 minute period). The ampicillin should be combined with gentamicin at a dose of 1.5 mg per kilogram intravenously given every 8 hours in a patient with normal renal functin. Both drugs should be given intravenously for 3 weeks to prevent relapse. In a patient with listeria endocarditis, 4 weeks of therapy are required. The use of chloramphenicol, erythromycin, or tetracycline in combination with ampicillin may be antagonistic and should be avoided. In penicillin-allergic patients, trimethoprim-sulfamethoxazole should be given intravenously in a dose of 10 mg per kilogram per day of trimethoprim in three divided doses and sulfamethoxazole, 50 mg per kilogram per day in three divided doses. Each vial of trimethoprim-sulfamethoxazole contains 80 mg of trimethoprim and 400 mg of sulfamethoxazole. Thus, a 70-kg adult with listeria meningitis and a penicillin allergy should receive 3 vials of trimethoprim-sulfamethoxazole intravenously every 8 hours if there is normal renal function. Another alternative drug to trimethoprim-sulfamethoxazole is erythromycin, which is given intravenously in a dose of 1 g every 6 hours.

Neonatal meningitis caused by *Listeria* is treated with ampicillin intravenously, 50 mg per kilogram given every 6 hours for infants older than 7 days, with gentamicin, 2.5 mg per kilogram given every 8 hours. Fourteen days is usually adequate to treat neonatal listeria meningitis. Third-generation cephalosporins such as moxalactam have no activity against *Listeria*.

TETANUS

DONALD L. BORNSTEIN, M.D.

Tetanus, a potentially lethal neurotoxic illness characterized by intense muscular spasm and rigidity, is caused by the action of tetanospasmin, a potent neurotoxin released by *Clostridium tetani*. Spores of this organism are ubiquitous in soils and dust and can be introduced into the body by major trauma or by trivial or even inapparent penetrations of the skin. The disease is totally preventable by active immunization, and in the United States fewer than 100 cases have been reported annually for the last decade. However, tetanus is still rampant in developing countries, and it is estimated to cause from 160,000 to 900,000 deaths per year, primarily in newborns (tetanus neonatorum) whose mothers have not been immunized.

PATHOGENESIS

C. tetani is an obligate anaerobe and will not germinate after introduction in the human body unless there is accompanying tissue necrosis, anoxia, foreign material, or microorganisms. Spores have lain dormant months to years after the initial seeding only to be reactivated by trauma or surgery (latent tetanus). When conditions permit germination of the spores, tetanospasmin, a 150,000-dalton neurotoxin is released into the local tissues, where it is picked up by lymphatics and carried into the circulation. The toxin binds to motor nerve endings in local and distant muscle fibers and ascends within the axon or perineural sheath to the neuronal cell body in the spinal cord or the brain stem. There it blocks synaptic transmission of motor inhibitory stimuli from interneurons, which are required for coordination of agonistic and antigonistic signals into purposeful motor activity. The toxin appears able to ascend along sympathetic nerve fibers as well. It is no longer believed that the toxin reaches the CNS directly from the bloodstream or that the toxin exerts a significant direct effect on acetylcholine release at the neuromuscular junction. Like strychnine, tetanospasmin blocks inhibitory regulation of motor neurons; does not stimulate excitation directly.

The wounds that introduce tetanal spores are usually minor and occur around the home or in the garden. They include splinters, thornpricks, minor burns, abrasions, scratched dermatitis, and, especially in older persons, contaminated varicose ulcers, as well as sealed puncture wounds, crush injuries, major lacerations, gun-shot wounds, open fractures, and other major trauma accompanied by soil contamination—the so-called tetanus-prone wounds. Drug addiction has caused serious cases of tetanus, especially among ''skin-poppers'' who use subcutaneous rather than intravenous injection. In the United States, more than two-thirds of cases occur in persons over 50 years of age. In other parts of the world the umbilical stump, the postpartum uterus, and the middle ear (chronic otitis media with perforation of the tympanic membrane) represent major portals of entry. In more than 25 percent of cases in the United States, no wound or site of entry can be identified by examination or by history, which indicates how little inflammation or necrosis is required for the production of lethal amounts of this deadly toxin.

CLINICAL PRESENTATION

The first manifestations of tetanus appear from 3 days to 3 weeks after a known injury, usually between the fifth and tenth day. The commonest presenting symptom is tightness in jaw and facial muscles and in the neck, with or without malaise, headache, or other systemic complaints. Over the next 36 to 72 hours, these symptoms progress to trismus (spasm of the masseters, which prevents opening the mouth), spasm of the facial muscles, which produces a characteristic grimacing facies (risus sardonicus), pain and dysfunction on swallowing, and pain and spasm in the neck and back. In another day or two, the back and trunk muscles and the extremities are tense, rigid, extended, and the abdomen is board-like. Waves of uncoordinated tonic spasms follow, accompanied by great pain and anxiety, causing opisthotonos, an arching of the spine due to extensor spasm severe enough to fracture vertebvral bodies and to tear abdominal muscle fibers. Bowel and bladder function are impaired; swallowing is impossible; laryngeal spasm can occur. The unsedated patient is in terror of the recurrent spasms, exhausted, perspiring excessively, calling out in pain, unable to take fluids or nutrition, and; most important, in danger of asphyxia and anoxia because of aspiration, immobility, rigidity of the chest wall, constriction of the airway, and the more frequent spasms that cause long apneic periods. In the more severe cases, marked sympathetic overactivity is seen, with tachyarrhythmias, hyperthermia, hypertensive episodes, and sometimes refractory hypotension.

In most cases, symptoms and signs reach a plateau after the first 5 days or so and persist at that level until the effects of the fixed neurotoxin wear off, which usually takes from 4 to 6 weeks. Tetanus leaves no permanent neural injury, and if the serious complications accompanying 3 to 6 weeks of intensive hospital care are avoided, full recovery can be expected.

Trismus is an early and almost invariable finding (more than 90% of cases) because toxin carried to myoneural junctions in the masseters has a much shorter intra-axonal path to the CNS than is true for muscles of the arms or legs. Short incubation periods (fewer than 7 days) and rapid development from first symptoms to the first major spasms (less than 3 days) correlate with more severe illness and more complications.

More than 90 percent of cases seen in the United States are generalized. There are a few patients who have partial immunity or have a minor intoxication whose symptoms are limited to rigidity and spasm of the muscles around the site of injury. These patients with local tetanus generally do well, but the disease can become generalized later in its course if not recognized and treated effectively. Another group of patients acquire tetanus after an injury to the head, face, or neck or from a chronic eardrum perforation. In these cases the incubation period is short because the path to the CNS is shorter than from an extremity. Cephalic tetanus has a poorer prognosis, in part from a delay in recognition. Cranial nerve involvement is commonly seen along with trismus.

DIAGNOSIS

There is no laboratory test or pathologic finding that can establish the diagnosis of tetanus; diagnosis rests purely on clinical grounds. It is possible to recover spores of *C. tetani* from wounds in patients without the disease, and organisms are recovered from debrided wounds in only about 30 percent of cases. The clinical diagnosis is distinctive and, except in the earliest stages or in unusual mild cases in persons with partial immunity, is readily distinguishable from other causes of muscular rigidity and spasms. The differential diagnosis of trismus as an isolated finding includes local pathology such as dental abscess, subluxation of the temporomandibular joint, retropharyngeal abscess, and mumps. Painful spasms similar to those in tetanus are seen in strychnine poisoning, but here the muscles are relaxed and not rigid between spasm. There has been some confusion with patients receiving phenothiazine drugs, who may be somewhat rigid, but these patients tend to be dystonic to some degree, have a history of drug ingestion, and their muscular symptoms are rapidly reversible with diphenhydramine, 50 mg intravenously. Hysterical reactions can easily be distinguished by the lack of generalized rigidity, trismus, or true spasms.

TREATMENT

The goals of therapy are twofold: to neutralize unbound toxin while removing any residual nidus of *C. tetani* and to provide optimal physiologic support until the effects of the bound toxin dissipate. The first goal is easily accomplished; the second poses major problems for even the most skilled hospitals and intensive care facilities.

When the diagnosis of tetanus is first made, the patient should be transferred to an intensive care unit with full facilities for cardiovascular and pulmonary monitoring and ventilatory support because the disease progresses rapidly from the initial presentation and emergency intervention may be required.

Human tetanus immune globulin (TIG) should be administered, 3000 units intramuscularly, in several sites; infiltration of a portion of the TIG around the wound of entry is recommended for a particularly contaminated wound. It is customary to begin penicillin G (1 million units intravenously every 4 hours). If a site of entry is found, it should be thoroughly debrided 30 minutes or more after antitoxin has been injected, cultured, and left open. Manipulation may release more toxin into the blood, so it is important to wait until TIG is absorbed into the circulation. Penicillin should be continued for 7 days, if no site can be identified for debridement, to prevent further germination of *C. tetani*. Cefazolin, 1.0 g every 8 hours intravenously, or tetracycline, 0.5 g orally, every 6 hours can be used for those with hypersensitivity to penicillin. Antibiotics alone provide little protection from tetanus, however.

Since a lethal dose of tetanus toxin is much smaller than an immunizing dose, clinical tetanus does not confer protective immunity. It is therefore important to administer a first dose of alum-adsorbed tetanus toxoid, at a different site from the TIG. When the patient is ready to leave the hospital, the first booster dose is administered, and arrangements should be made for a second booster dose 6 months later.

The major cause of death in tetanus is respiratory compromise and failure. The chest wall is fixed and rigid, with low compliance and poor respiratory excursions. Recurrent spasms of chest wall, pharyngeal muscles, or the larynx can produce long apneic periods and hypoxia. Impaired swallowing and deep sedation lead to aspiration of mouth contents and risk of aspiration pneumonia. Immobility and prolonged bed rest favor atelectasis. The result is alveolar hypoventilation, hypoxemia, and respiratory acidosis.

At the first clinical or laboratory signs of respiratory compromise, a cuffed endotracheal tube or, preferably, a tracheostomy tube should be placed, with the patient under appropriate sedation and general anesthesia. This will protect against the dangers of laryngeal spasm and of aspiration and allow for effective suctioning. For most patients who require intubation the duration of need is such that an endotracheal tube would have to be replaced by a tracheostomy tube in any case. Because of the spasticity of the chest wall, protecting the patency of the airway may not be enough, and ventilating the lungs mechanically will be necessary. The stiffness of the chest usually requires total paralysis of skeletal muscle for adequate ventilator function. Paralysis is effected with the nondepolarizing neuromuscular blocker D-tubocurarine by intravenous drip or intramuscularly, about 15 mg per hour. This regimen—paralysis and mechanical ventilation—is the most effective and successful for serious cases, but carries with it grave monitoring responsibilities to ensure that the paralyzed patient is never accidentally disconnected from the respirator, an accident that would cause fatal or crippling anoxic brain damage. In addition, the quality of the nursing care, and especially of tracheostomy care, will determine the course of the recovery in most cases.

The patient will require medication to relieve anxiety, rigidity, and painful spasms, since these patients are mentally alert. Diazepam in the form of a continuous intravenous drip or intermittent intravenous bolus (5 to 20 mg every 3 to 4 hours, as required) has proved to be effective for these problems and for preventing the nightmares that paralyzed but inadequately sedated patients can suffer after recovery. Diazepam is very irritative if it infiltrates; only a secure intravenous line should be used. Painful spasms may require more powerful analgesia, and narcotics may be required. Chlorpromazine is sometimes helpful for its calmative effects, and it is sometimes alternated with diazepam, at doses of 25 to 50 mg (as required) every 6 hours intravenously or intramuscularly. Short-acting barbiturates such as pentobarbital, 50 mg to 100 mg intramuscularly every 6 hours, are generally used for sedation in addition to diazepam. The choice of sedatives and muscle relaxants will depend upon the overall strategy for dealing with respiratory support. If paralysis and ventilator support are required, as in most cases today, these choices may be less critical than when total control of spasm depends on these drugs. It is also important to limit unnecessary stimuli to the patient since minor stimulation can trigger a painful spasm in a lightly sedated patient.

With good control of ventilation and spasm by paralysis and sedation, successful management of the patient rests on avoiding the complications that attend immobility and paralysis in an intensive care setting for the 3- to 6-week period that will pass before the effects of tetanus toxin wear off adequately to allow a simpler regimen. Dedicated nursing care is required to prevent serious decubitus ulcers, atelectasis, contractures, infections around infusion sites, and to keep the tracheostomy stoma clean and the airway clear. Many complications known to occur in such patients can be prevented or recognized and treated promptly. Low-dose heparin is often used to prevent pulmonary embolism; it is appropriate especially in obese or elderly patients (5,000 units every 12 hours by deep subcutaneous injection with a 25-gauge needle using concentrated [10,000 units per milliliter] heparin). Antacids may prevent stress ulcers; daily weighings can help assess fluid losses (which are always much greater than is appreciated) thus avoiding a dangerous degree of hypovolemia; and enteral feeding via a nasogastric tube—or, if necessary, a gastrostomy or jejunostomy tube—can prevent the severe catabolic state and wasting that can otherwise occur. Frequent chest roentgenograms and urine examinations can help detect urinary tract and pulmonary infections at an early stage.

Autonomic dysregulation, a hallmark of the most serious cases, represents the major complication of tetanus after ventilation has been secured. Beginning about 7 to 10 days after admission, or sometimes even earlier, there are episodes of sympathetic hyperactivity with marked and rapid swings of blood pressure, signs of myocardial irritability, hyperthermia, and profuse sweating. Refractory hypotension, bradycardia and cardiac arrest are late and ominous signs. Propanolol (10 mg orally every 3 to 6 hours) or other beta-blockers can control the tachycardia and some other catechol effects. The hypertension may on occasion require phentolamine; the hypotension may respond to stimulating the patient and correcting for hypovolemia. Some patients have had several episodes of cardiac arrest and resuscitation. Aggressive cardiovascular monitoring is required to guide management.

Untreated, more than 80 percent of patients would die; overall, our mortality rates are about 40 percent. In intensive care units, however, this can be reduced to about 10 percent. The role for intrathecal human TIG in severe cases has been claimed, but not substantiated as yet. Hyperbaric oxygen, once advocated by some, is clearly useless and dangerous in this disease.

PREVENTION

Immunization prevents this lethal disease. Cases occur only in unimmunized or partially immunized persons. Yet despite the safety and the wide availability of tetanus toxoid, recent surveys in the United States reveal that 11 percent of young adults and 49 percent to 60 percent of persons over the age of 60 years lack protective levels of antibody. After an immunizing series of three DPT injections in infancy and a booster dose of DPT at age one and on entering school, a booster dose of tetanus toxoid should be administered every 10 years, at age 15, 25, 35, and so on. Since immunity to diphtheria is lost over time, the recommended form of tetanus toxoid for adults (Td) contains a small amount of diphtheria toxoid (2 flocculation units) as well. Whenever a patient is seen with a puncture wound or other penetrating wound or laceration and the possibility of introduction of tetanus spores is considered, the history of the patient's tetanus immunization must be carefully reviewed. If an immunizing course of three injections of toxoid has been received, as in persons with U.S. military service or with childhood immunizations, and if the last booster dose has been administered within 10 years, no further immunization is necessary for minor wounds. If the last booster dose was received within 5 years, no further toxoid is required for major wounds. Since a booster dose of toxoid is innocuous except in the very rare patient with marked hypersensitivity to previous toxoid doses, in most emergency rooms the practice is to boost for minor wounds and for major wounds if the interval since the previous booster dose has been 5 years or 1 year, respectively, although this is probably not necessary.

Persons with a wound who have not been immunized, or whose immunization history is partial or uncertain, require three doses of toxoid, the second following in a month and the third in 6 to 12 months. Since the first injection of Td will not offer protection for the current wound, passive immunization with TIG is additionally required for anything other than innocent, clean, minor wounds. The usual dose is 250 units intramuscularly, but for more serious tetanus-prone wounds, 500 units or as much as 1,000 units are sometimes used, depending on the severity of the wound. Arrangements to complete the immunization series should be made at this time. Infants born of unimmunized mothers should also receive a dose of TIG to prevent the rare and avoidable cases of tetanus neonatorum.

GRAM-NEGATIVE BACTEREMIA

DONALD E. CRAVEN, M.D.
WILLIAM R. McCABE, M.D.

Gram-negative bacteremia is defined as the isolation of gram-negative bacilli from blood cultures. This term is usually reserved for bacteremia caused by members of the families Enterobacteriaceae and Pseudomonadaceae; *Salmonella* and *Hemophilus* species are not included. By comparison, *gram-negative sepsis* is a term often used to describe a clinical condition characterized by fever, chills, and impaired tissue perfusion, irrespective of whether bacteremia has been documented.

Gram-negative bacteremia was uncommon in the preantibiotic era, but since 1950 it has become one of the commonest infectious disease problems in medical centers throughout the United States. An incidence of bacteremia as high as one episode per 100 hospital admissions has been reported in university teaching hospitals, but lower rates have been reported from smaller community hospitals. Common etiologic agents include *Escherichia coli*, species of *Klebsiella, Enterobacter, Serratia, Proteus*, and *Bacteroides*, as well as *Pseudomonas aeruginosa*. Fifteen to 20 percent of gram-negative bacteremias are mixed or polymicrobial. Fatality rates for gram-negative bacteremia vary depending on the patient's underlying disease, but overall fatality rates are in the range of 25 percent.

EPIDEMIOLOGY

Gram-negative bacillemia may be categorized as hospital-acquired (nosocomial), or community-acquired. Community-acquired bacteremia usually originates from the genitourinary or gastrointestinal tracts and is frequently caused by *E. coli* sensitive to many antibiotics. Some "community-acquired" bacteremias, acquired during earlier hospitalization or during residence in nursing homes, may be caused by bacteria that are more antibiotic resistant. Hospital-acquired infections that account for approximately 75 percent of cases, may originate from the urinary tract, gastrointestinal tract, respiratory tract, skin, or mucous membranes. Nosocomial bacteremia may be associated with prior surgery or the use of invasive devices and are generally caused by more antibiotic-resistant species of bacteria.

The increasing frequency of gram-negative bacteremia over the last three decades can be attributed to several factors. Enteric gram-negative bacilli are relatively avirulent and have limited invasive capacity in the normal host, but they comprise the major aerobic flora of the gastrointestinal and female urogenital tract and readily colonize the hospital environment. Nosocomial gram-negative bacilli are known for antibiotic resistance. *P. aeruginosa* is inherently resistant to many antibiotics, whereas other species of gram-negative bacilli acquire antimicrobial resistance from plasmids or R-factors. Plasmids are extrachromosomal fragments of DNA that may rapidly transmit resistance to several antibiotics. Gram-negative bacilli resistant to multiple antimicrobial agents are a continuous problem in hospitals.

The increasing incidence of gram-negative bacteremia over the last 30 years also reflects changes in medical management and the hospital population (Table 1). Patients are older and often have chronic disease. Radical surgery, immunosuppressive therapy, and extensive use of devices that violate natural host barriers have become an integral part of modern medical management.

TABLE 1 Factors that Predispose to Development of Gram-Negative Bacteremia

Underlying host diseases
Diabetes mellitus
Cancer
Congestive heart failure
Hepatic disease
Renal failure
Granulocytopenia
Thermal injury
Devices
Intravascular catheters (peripheral, central, tunneled, and arterial)
Indwelling bladder catheter
Tracheostomy
Endotracheal tube
Nebulization equipment
Prosthetic devices
Treatment Factors
Surgery
Steroids
Cytotoxic drugs
Irradiation

CLINICAL MANIFESTATIONS

The clinical manifestations of gram-negative bacteremia are protean and may vary from fulminant and lethal disease to infections that may go unrecognized for days. Clinical findings suggestive of gram-negative bacteremia are shown in Table 2. Many of these symptoms and clinical signs are nonspecific. Therefore, it is imperative to maintain a high index of suspicion and draw blood for cultures whenever bacteremia is suspected. The classic triad of shaking chills, high fever, and hypotension occurs only in approximately one-third of patients. Fever, although a nonspecific sign, is usually present unless the patient is elderly, uremic, or receiving treatment with corticosteroids. In patients with leukemia, gastrointestinal disease, or those who have had genitourinary tract manipulation, fever may be the only indication of bacteremia.

Approximately 40 to 50 percent of patients with bacteremia develop shock—defined as a decrease in blood pressure to 90/60 mm Hg or less. Shock usually occurs 4 to 10 hours after the initial signs of bacteremia caused by gram-negative bacilli. Because of the high frequency of shock associated with gram-negative bacteremia, it is essential that the etiology of any episode of shock be clearly elucidated and the possibility of bacteremia considered. The combination of hyperpnea, tachypnea, and respiratory alkalosis in the absence of pulmonary abnormalities is an important early clinical sign of bacteremia. In elderly patients, unexplained oliguria, increased confusion, or stupor also may be the only signs of sepsis.

Leukocytosis is common, although some patients may manifest normal or low leukocyte counts. Gram-negative bacteremia is a frequent complication of antineoplastic chemotherapy producing granulocytopenia (less than 1,000 neutrophils per cubic millimeter). Neutropenia secondary to bacteremia is an infrequent consequence in patients with normal hematopoietic function. Mild to moderate thrombocytopenia occurs in about 70 percent of patients. Disseminated intravascular coagulation (DIC), characterized by decreased levels of clotting factors II, V, and VIII, together with hypofibrinogenemia, thrombocytopenia and circulating fibrin split products is found in approximately 12 percent of patients but only about one-fourth of these patients exhibit clinical manifestations attributable to DIC.

PATHOPHYSIOLOGY

Endotoxin, or lipopolysaccharide (LPS), a major constituent of the gram-negative cell envelope, is generally thought to initiate the changes observed during bacteremia. However, several careful experimental and clinical studies have indicated that factors other than free endotoxin liberated from the bacterial cell wall contribute to the

TABLE 2 Clinical Manifestations of Gram-Negative Bacteremia

Fever, chills, hypotension
Fever alone (in a patient with a malignancy, hematologic disorder, urinary tract disease, or intravenous or urinary tract catheters)
Hypotension*
Tachypnea, hyperpnea, and respiratory alkalosis*
Change in mental status (confusion, stupor, agitation)*
Oliguria or anuria*
Acidosis*
Hypothermia*
Thrombocytopenia*
Disseminated intravascular coagulation*
Adult respiratory distress syndrome*
Evidence of a urinary tract or pulmonary infection

* Without an alternative cause.

manifestations of such infections. Irrespective of the role of endotoxin, a variety of vasoactive materials have been implicated as potential mediators of the circulatory changes observed in bacteremic shock. These include endogenous pyrogen (interleukin-1), Hageman factor, plasmin, complement components, kinins, serotonin, histamine, prostaglandins, endorphins, and catecholamines (epinephrine and norepinephrine). However, precise delineation of their role in human disease is limited by the lack of definitive data.

Available evidence suggests that the activation of the coagulation, fibrinolysis, kinin, and complement systems may contribute to the hemodynamic and other pathophysiologic alterations seen in gram-negative bacteremia. Activation of Hageman factor (Factor XII) by either intact bacilli or endotoxin results in sequential activation of the intrinsic coagulation system and the conversion of plasminogen to plasmin. Circulating gram-negative bacilli, endotoxin, and plasmin are all capable of activating the complement system through the classical or alternate (properedin) pathways. Anaphylatoxins (C3a and C5a) cause peripheral vasodilation and increased vascular permeability. Plasmin and activated Hageman factor also activate the kinin pathway, resulting in vascular permeability and early peripheral vasodilatation in shock. Bradykinin, in turn, increases the release of prostaglandins PGE2 and PGF2.

More recent studies have suggested that prostaglandins and endorphins may contribute to the pathogenesis of septic sock. Endotoxin may also release prostaglandins, prostacycline, or thromboxane. Inhibitors of prostaglandin synthesis such as ibuprofen and indomethacin have ameliorated endotoxin-induced hypotension in experimental animals. One uncontrolled clinical study of patients in shock reported improvement in blood pressure following the intravenous administration of 1.2 mg of the endorphin inhibitor naloxone, but a recent, randomized, placebo-controlled clinical study of patients in septic shock at our institution was unable to confirm any beneficial effect of naloxone in septic shock.

Shock in patients with gram-negative bacteremia is associated with a sevenfold increase in fatality. Therefore, goals for treating patients with gram-negative bacteremia include early diagnosis and therapy to prevent shock and rapid correction of any hemodynamic alterations that occur.

Two types of hemodynamic alterations have been noted in patients with gram-negative bacteremia. ''Warm shock'' is characterized by evidence of a hyperdynamic circulation. Increased cardiac output with decreased peripheral resistance is characteristically associated with a high or normal central venous pressure, hyperventilation, and lactate accumulation in the initial phase of sepsis. Patients in ''cold shock'' are usually pale, cyanotic, and have cold and clammy extremities. Cold shock tends to occur late in the course of septic shock. Physiologic alterations in cold shock include decreased cardiac output, increased peripheral vascular resistance associated with decreased central venous pressure, hyperventilation, and lactate accumulation. Respiratory alkalosis usually occurs early and may evolve to a metabolic acidosis, which carries a poorer prognosis.

ANTIBIOTIC TREATMENT

Due to the nature of the disease, therapy for gram-negative bacteremia is usually initiated before the etiologic agent and antibiotic sensitiviities are known. Initial treatment should be based on the type of infection (community-acquired or nosocomial), the probable site of infection, and the bacterial flora residing at that site. Basic principles of management include prompt recognition of the clinical signs and symptoms of bacteremia and identification of the source of infection. Blood cultures, gram stains, and cultures of infected sites should be performed to identify the etiologic agent and determine antibiotic sensitivity. Fluids, oxygen, and adequate doses of an appropriate antibiotic should be administered promptly. In addition, management of complications such as shock, hypoxia, and hemorrhage is of paramount importance. Any abscess should be drained and infected foreign bodies removed as soon as possible.

Once the source of infection is identified, appropriate antimicrobial therapy designed to cover all the pathogenic flora at that site should be instituted (Table 3). Aminoglycosides, such as gentamicin, tobramycin, or amikacin have a broad spectrum of activity against aerobic gram-negative bacilli, including *P. aeruginosa*. The type of aminoglycoside selected (Table 4) will depend on the condition of the patient, the type and location of infection, and the specific antibiotic resistance pattern of the hospital flora. At Boston City Hospital we presently recommend gentamicin for initial coverage of gram-negative rods because it is less expensive and the number of gentamicin-resistant gram-negative bacilli is low. Initial therapy with tobramycin or amikacin may be more appropriate in other hospitals, depending on the general patterns of bacterial resistance. Doses of aminoglycosides should be altered for patients with renal failure and blood

TABLE 3 The Choice of Antibiotics for Suspected Gram-Negative Bacteremia by Site of Infection

Site of Infection	Likely Etiologic Agent	Initial Antibiotic of Choice
Urinary tract (community-acquired)	*E. coli* *K. pneumoniae* *P. mirabilis*	Aminoglycoside* *or* Cefoxitin†‡
Urinary tract (hospital-acquired)	*K. pneumoniae* *Proteus* species *P. aeruginosa*	Aminoglycoside* *or* Cefoxitin‡ *or* Third-generation cephalosporin‡
Gastrointestinal tract		
Bowel	*E. coli* *Bacteroides* species *K. pneumoniae* *Proteus* species *P. aeruginosa*	Aminoglycoside* *plus* Clindamycin *or* Cefoxitin
Biliary tract	*E. coli* *K. pneumoniae* *Proteus* species	Aminoglycoside* *plus* Ampicillin
Reproductive tract	*E. coli* *K. pneumoniae* *Bacteroides* species	Aminoglycoside* *plus* Clindamycin *or* Cefoxitin alone
Respiratory tract (patient with tracheostomy or endotracheal tube)	*P. aeruginosa* *Acinetobacter* species *Serratia* species *E. coli* *K. pneumoniae*	Aminoglycoside* *or* Aminoglycoside* *plus either* Carbenicillin§ *or* Cefoxitin‡ *or* Third-generation cephalosporin‡

Aspiration (in hospital)	*E. coli* *Bacteroides* species *Fusobacterium* species *K. pneumoniae* *Acinetobacter* species *Serratia* species	Aminoglycoside* *plus* Penicillin *or* Clindamycin
Decubitus ulcers	*E. coli* *Bacteroides* species *K. pneumoniae* *Proteus* species *P. aeruginosa* *Enterobacter* species	Aminoglycoside* *plus* Clindamycin *or* Cefoxitin *or* Third-generation cephalosporin‡
Burns	*P. aeruginosa* *Enterobacter* species	Aminoglycoside* *or* Aminoglycoside* *plus* Carbenicillin§
Intravascular device	*P. aeruginosa* *Acinetobacter* species *Serratia* species	Aminoglycoside* *or* Cefoxitin *or* Third-generation cephalosporin‡
Neutropenic patient (<100 PMN/mm³)	*E. coli* *Klebsiella* species *P. aeruginosa*	Aminoglycoside* *plus* Carbenicillin§

* Because of their toxicity, aminoglycosides may soon be replaced by newer agents such as aztreonam or Imipenem-cilastatin. An initial loading dose for amikacin = 8 mg/kg, gentamicin = 2 mg/kg, or tobramycin = 2 mg/kg. Modify dosage in patients with renal insufficiency. Revaluate antibiotic regimen after culture and sensitivity data are available and treat with least toxic drug to which the organism is sensitive.

† Patients having a recent hospitalization, indwelling bladder catheters, or residents of nursing homes should initially receive an aminoglycoside.

‡ If the organism is sensitive. Resistant nosocomial gram-negative bacilli or *P. aeruginosa* bacteremia should be treated with an aminoglycoside. Third-generation cephalosporins include cefotaxime, cefoperazone, ceftazidine, moxalactam, ceftriaxone.

§ Ticarcillin, mezlocillin, azlocillin, or piperacillin may be used interchangeably with carbenicillin. Monitor bleeding parameters when these agents are used.

TABLE 4 Antibiotics Frequently Prescribed for the Treatment of Gram-Negative Rod Bacteremia

Antibiotic	*Dose**	*Comments*
Aminoglycosides		
Gentamicin	1.7 mg/kg IM or IV q8h	Aminoglycosides have excellent spectrum against aerobic gram-negative bacilli, including *P. aeruginosa*
Tobramycin	1.7 mg/kg IM or IV q8h	
Amikacin	7.5 mg/kg IM or IV q12h	
Extended-spectrum penicillins		
Carbenicillin	5 g IV q4h	Useful in combination with an aminoglycoside for treating *P. aeruginosa* bacteremia or for treating patients with neutropenia
Ticarcillin	3 g IV q4h	
Piperacillin	3 g IV q4h	
Mezlocillin	3 g IV q4h	
Azlocillin	3 g IV q4h	
Cephalosporins		
First-generation		
Cephalothin	2 g IV q4h	Activity limited to *E. coli, K. pneumoniae,* and *P. mirabilus*; should should not be used unless sensitivity of organism is known
Cefazolin	2 g IV q8h	
Cephradine	2 g IV q6h	
Cephapirin	2 g IV q4h	
Second-generation		
Cefoxitin	2 g IV q4h	Cefoxitin provides good coverage against *B. fragilis* and most aerobic gram-negative bacilli except *P. aeruginosa*
Cefamandole	2 g IV q4h	
Third-generation		
Moxalactam	4 g IV q8h	Third-generation cephalosporins have limited activity against *P. aeruginosa*; bleeding is a reported adverse effect of moxalactam that is corrected by the use of vitamin K
Cefotaxime	2 g IV q4h	
Cefoperazone	3 g IV q6h	
Ceftriaxone	1 g IV q12h	
Other beta-lactams		
Imipenem-cilastatin	500 mg of each drug IV q6h	Good coverage for aerobic gram-negative bacilli and *B. fragilis*
Monobactams		
Aztreoman	2 g IV q8h	Good coverage for aerobic gram-negative bacilli
Trimethoprim-Sulfamethoxazole	2 ampules IV q8h	Effective against many resistant nosocomial gram-negative bacilli

* Doses are the maximum for patients with bacteremia and normal renal flow. Doses should be adjusted after organism and antibiotic activity are known or if patient has impaired renal function.

levels should be monitored in individuals who have impaired renal function, no response to therapy, or in whom long-term therapy is required. Because of their well-known ototoxicity and nephrotoxicity, aminoglycosides may soon be replaced by newer less toxic antibiotics such as aztreonam or imipenem-cilastatin. A cephalosporin is also less nephrotoxic than an aminoglycoside and may be used if the organism is sensitive.

Infections originating from the gastrointestinal tract or the female reproductive tract may involve aerobic gram-negative bacilli and anaerobic organisms such as *Bacteroides fragilis*. For this reason, combinations of antibiotics such as an aminoglycoside (chosen as indicated above) and clindamycin would be indicated for initial therapy.

A cephalosporin may be used for initial therapy only if the organism is likely to be susceptible. First-generation cephalosporins—such as cephalothin, cephapirin, or cephradine—have activity against community strains of *E. coli, Klebsiella pneumoniae*, and *Proteus mirabilis*, but some strains are resistant and activity is lacking against many of the nosocomial gram-negative bacilli making this group of agents inappropriate for initial therapy of suspected gram-negative bacteremia. Second-generation cephalosporins, such as cefoxitin, have a greater spectrum of activity against aerobic gram-negative bacilli. Cefoxitin also has activity against *B. fragilis*, but second-generation cephalosporins have no activity against *P. aeruginosa*. Third-generation cephalosporins—such as moxalactam, cefotaxime, ceftriaxone, ceftazidime, and cefoperazone—have activity against a variety of enteric gram-negative bacilli including some activity against *P. aeruginosa*. These antibiotics have a high therapeutic-toxicity ratio and serum blood levels do not need to be monitored. Consequently, they are easier to use and are less toxic than aminoglycosides for patients with impaired renal function.

Extended-spectrum penicillins—such as ticarcillin, carbenicillin, azlocillin, mezlocillin, and piperacillin—are generally used in combination with an aminoglycoside for treating patients with neutropenia or serious infections caused by *P. aeruginosa*. It should be emphasized that once the sensitivities of the offending organism are known, the least toxic and least expensive antibiotic to which the organism is sensitive should be prescribed. The duration of therapy depends on the source of infection. In general, antibiotics should be continued for a minimum of five afebrile days or longer if a local source of infecton persists.

MANAGEMENT OF SHOCK

Shock is the most frequent complicaton of gram-negative bacteremia. Optimal care requires the prompt institution of appropriate antibiotics as well as maintenance of an adequate intravascular volume. A central venous pressure (CVP) catheter or a Swan-Ganz catheter inserted to measure pulmonary artery wedge pressure (PAWP) are valuable aids for monitoring intravascular fluid expansion. Furthermore, an indwelling bladder catheter (using sterile precautions and a closed drainage system) is usually inserted to measure urinary output and renal perfusion.

Initially fluid (5% dextrose in normal saline) should be infused at a rate of 10 to 20 ml per minute for 10 to 15 minutes. If the CVP or PAWP do not increase by a level of 5 cm of water or 2 mm Hg, respectively, further fluid should be administered. If the need for further fluid volume is established, either colloid or crystalloid may be used at a rate of 10 to 20 ml per minute. Signs of fluid overload and cardiac decompensation include a sudden progressive increase in the CVP of more than 5 cm of water, a CVP of more than 12 to 14 cm of water, or an increase of PAWP of more than 8 mm Hg or an absolute level of more than 20 mm Hg.

If volume expansion does not produce prompt improvement, vasoactive agents should be added to increase cardiac output further. Dopamine is usually given by constant infusion in a dose of 2 to 20 μg per kilogram per minute. If there is no response to dopamine, isoproterenol in a dose of 2 to 8 μg per minute or dobutamine in a dose of 2 to 15 μg per kilogram per minute should be instituted to enhance cardiac output and increase urine output.

The role of corticosteroids in the treatment of shock caused by gram-negative bacilli remains controversial. Based on the available data, we do not recommend the use of steroids for patients in shock. If they are used, doses equivalent to 2 g of methylprednisolone should be administered within the first 24 hours of shock. Although some experts recommend the use of naloxone, a beta-endorphin antagonist for the treatment of septic shock, data from a randomized, placebo-controlled trial at our institution indicate that naloxone (1.2 mg IV) was no more effective than placebo.

Clinical evidence of disseminated intravascular coagulation (DIC) occurs in less than 5 percent of patients with gram-negative bacteremia, and these patients are invariably in shock. Heparin has been suggested for treatment, but enthusiasm for heparin therapy must be tempered by evidence that such treatment failed to reduce fatalities in either experimental models or humans despite improvement in coagulation factors. For treatment of DIC, we suggest that maximal efforts be directed at replacing blood products and reversing the cause of shock.

Hypoxia occurs frequently in septic shock, and monitoring of arterial blood gases is essential to maintain proper tissue oxygenation. Patients who develop adult respiratory distress syndrome (ARDS) often require mechanical ventilation with a volume-cycled ventilator. Patients who have a progressive decrease in their arterial PaO_2 despite the use of increasing oxygen concentrations, may benefit from positive end expiratory pressure (PEEP).

Oliguric renal failure is another complication of septic shock. If the urine flow is less than 30 ml per hour, the patient should be treated with an intravenous infusion of 12.5 g of mannitol over 5 minutes. If there is no response, this dose should be repeated in 2 hours. Individuals failing to respond to mannitol can be given furosemide (240 mg) intravenously.

IMMUNIZATION AND PREVENTION

The search for an effective vaccine against gram-negative bacteremia has been limited by the large number of organisms causing disease. However, it is now known that gram-negative bacilli share common antigens present in the core region of the lipopolysaccharide. Although there is no program for actively vaccinating individuals at risk for gram-negative bacteremia, vaccination of individuals with rough bacterial mutants containing these core antigens is being evaluated, and hyperimmune serum obtained from patients following immunization has been shown to significantly increase the survival rates of patients in septic shock compared with a control group of patients given preimmune serum. Although more research is needed, there appears to be a role for immunotherapy in the treatment of gram-negative sepsis.

In the meantime, major efforts should be directed at preventing gram-negative bacteremia. Since the majority of gram-negative bacteremias are nosocomial in origin, the use of proper handwashing along with careful evaluation of the need for and care of invasive devices such as the indwelling bladder catheter, endotracheal tube, central venous and intravenous catheters will reduce the frequency of local infections and subsequent bacteremia. Additional measures should include the rational use of antibiotics and the appropriate collection and feedback of surveillance data used to monitor nosocomial infection.

RICKETTSIAL INFECTION

THEODORE E. WOODWARD, M.D.

Rickettsiae cause three major groups of illness: the spotted fevers (including Rocky Mountain spotted fever), the typhus group (including classic typhus and murine typhus), and Q fever. Rash is a characteristic feature of all except Q fever. The following discussion focuses on the rickettsial diseases causing rash that are commonest in the United States.

DIAGNOSIS

Differential Diagnosis

The suspicion of Rocky Mountain spotted fever (RMSF) should be raised for a patient with fever, prostration, headache, and a history of tick bite or tick exposure while engaged in work or recreation in a rural or wooded area of known endemicity. Early in the febrile illness before the rash has appeared, differentiation from other acute infections is confusing. The rickettsial rash is initially pink macular, fades on pressure, and becomes petechial or ecchymotic more slowly over several days. This exanthem is not sensitive to palpation. Meningococcemia and measles are common mistaken diagnoses.

The rash of meningococcemia simulates RMSF and epidemic typhus in certain features since it may be macular, maculopapular, or petechial in acute or subacute forms and either petechial, confluent, or ecchymotic in more acute types. Usually the hemorrhagic, purplish, necrotic exanthem develops rapidly in fulminant meningococcemia and is tender to palpation. Significant leukocytosis favors meningococcal infection. The features of gonococcemia resemble those of meningococcemia.

Measles, more often an autumn- and winter-occurring illness, is associated with coryza, cough, conjunctival injection and photophbia, and a characteristic cephalocaudal progression of the rash. It appears about 3 days after onset—first in the face and neck as pink macules—soon becomes maculopapular and extends within a day or two to the trunk and extremities. Petechiae or ecchymoses may occur; Koplick's spots are distinctive. In rubella (German measles), the rash is frequently a flush, not unlike scarlet fever, which soon spreads from the face and neck to the trunk and extremities. It is less extensive and of shorter duration than measles with mild constitutional manifestations. Postauricular adenopathy and absence of Koplick's spots suggest rubella.

The initial lesions of varicella or variola are first exanthematous and later become vesicular. Rose spots in the typhoid fevers are usually on the upper abdomen and lower chest and remain delicate, without hemorrhagic characteristics. The macular lesions in RMSF, in contrast to typhoid, begin on the periphery of the body and later become petechial. The rash of infectious mononucleosis (uncommon except when associated with sensitivity to drugs) is usually morbilliform on the trunk and rarely becomes petechial. In pharyngitis, the presence of a whitish membrane, lymphadenopathy, and atypical lymphocytes in the blood are differentiating features.

Drug rashes, including that of erythema multiforme, often cause fever. Yet such patients are less toxic in their appearance than are those with RMSF, and the rash is frequently diffusely erythematous; the individual lesions are larger, raised, and vesicular.

Epidemic typhus frequently causes all of the pronounced clinical, physiologic, and anatomic alterations noted in cases of RMSF: hypotension, peripheral vascular failure, cyanosis, skin necrosis and gangrene of digits, renal failure with azotemia, and neurologic manifestations. However, the rash of classic typhus occurs initially in the axilla and on the trunk and later extends peripherally, rarely involving the palms, soles, and face. Classic or epidemic typhus occurs in the United States as Brill-Zinsser disease (recurrent epidemic typhus fever) and an endemic type associated with contact with flying squirrels. Each is usually milder than cases of classic typhus.

Murine typhus is a milder disease than RMSF and epidemic typhus, the rash is less extensive, nonpurpuric, and nonconfluent, and renal and vascular abnormalities are uncommon. Differentiation between these three major rickettsial disease must often await the results of specific serologic tests.

An illness that simulates RMSF is caused by *Rickettsia canada*, a member of the typhus group. Rickettsialpox, caused by a member of the spotted fever group of organisms, is easily differentiated from RMSF by the initial lesion, the relative mildness of the illness, and early vesiculation of the maculopapular rash.

Q fever is the one rickettsial infection unassociated with a rash. Usually the illness is mild to moderate. It is manifested by fever for about a week to 10 days, severe headache, and pneumonitis in about 50 percent of cases. The roentgenographic findings are nonspecific and may resemble those of influenza or the atypical pneumonias. Occasionally, a dense infiltrate may suggest a neoplasm. An acute form of hepatitis, with or without jaundice, may progress to chronic granulomatous hepatitis. A chronic form of Q fever endocarditis is becoming clinically significant. In chronic hepatitis or endocarditis, antibodies to phase I antigens are present, which confirm the clinical diagnosis. The Weil-Felix reaction is negative.

Confirmatory Laboratory Diagnosis

In ordinary practice, the available serologic tests are adequate for laboratory confirmation of the rickettsioses provided two and preferably three serum samples are examined during the first, second, and fourth to sixth weeks of illness. This allows demonstration of a rise in titer of specific antibody during convalescence.

Weil-Felix Test

The Weil-Felix test, using *Proteus* strains of OX19, gives positive results in many patients with RMSF and epidemic and murine typhus and negative or nonspecific results in those with rickettsialpox, Q fever, and scrub typhus. In Brill-Zinsser disease (recurrent typhus), *Proteus* OX19 titers are usually negative or low. Proteus OXK agglutinins appear in more than 50 percent of patients with scrub typhus. Although the *Proteus* reaction is a dependable screening test for the presence of certain rickettsioses, it does not distinguish between the spotted fever and typhus groups. A single convalescent serum titer of 160 to 320 is usually diagnostic, but demonstration of a rise in titer is of greater value. Approximately 10 percent of patients with either RMSF or typhus may fail to show *Proteus* OX19 agglutinins, and when specifically acting antibiotics are given early in the first week of illness, the titers may be delayed, but usually reach diagnostic levels. False-positive reactions may occur in urinary tract infections or bacteremia caused by *Proteus* organisms and in enteric, relapsing, and rat-bite fevers, leptospirosis, brucellosis, and tularemia.

Complement-fixation Reaction

Group specific rickettsial antigens clearly differentiate the rickettsial disease group (the typhus fevers, spotted fevers, and Q fever). Using nonspecific, washed rickettsial antigens, it is possible to distinguish between the various member diseases of the spotted fever group (RMSF, rickettsialpox, fièvre boutonneuse, North Asian tick-borne rickettsioses, and Queensland tick typhus).

Complement-fixing antibodies appear during the second or third week in patients who receive no specific therapy and may be delayed when illness is shortened by vigorous antibiotic treatment initiated within several days after onset of fever.

Antibodies present after response to a primary infection of RMSF and typhus are usually 19S globulins (IgM). In Brill-Zinsser disease, antibodies appear rapidly, several days after onset, and are of the 7S (IgG) type. Q fever antigens are usually diagnostic. In acute Q fever infections, such as with pneumonitis, antibodies to phase II antigen appear.

Coxiella burnetii undergoes antigenic phase changes similar to the rough-smooth variation of bacteria. In nature, *C. burnetii* is found only in the smooth phase I. It possesses a cell wall-associated surface antigen. Phase I antigen is antiphagocytic and appears to be related to virulence. Phase II antigen develops after adaptation to growth in chick embryos; the organism lacks a surface phase I antigen and is of lesser virulence than the parent strain. The phase phenomenon is reversible; phase II organisms revert to phase I by passage in animals. High phase I complement-fixing titers are considered pathognomonic of chronic Q fever, such as hepatitis or endocarditis.

Other Specific Serologic Tests

The following serologic tests are becoming standard procedures and are more reliable than the Weil-Felix or complement-fixation tests. Specific diagnoses of RMSF, other tick-borne rickettsioses, and the typhus fevers may be achieved by the rickettsial microagglutination and the indirect fluorescent antibody (or hemoagglutination) reactions.

Early Diagnosis by Identification of Rickettsiae in Tissues

Rickettsia rickettsii are identified by the indirect fluorescent antibody reaction in pink macular skin lesions obtained by biopsy as early as the third day or in ecchymotic lesions as late as the tenth day. The organisms show an identifiable morphology and staining properties. This technique may be used with formalized tissue. Organisms can be demonstrated on heart valves of patients with Q fever endocarditis caused by *Coxiella burnetii.* Undoubtedly, such techniques would apply for epidemic and murine typhus as well as others.

THERAPY

There are important physiochemical changes that merit understanding in planning a therapeutic regimen for patients seriously ill with the spotted fever-typhus group of rickettsioses. Often there is circulatory collapse, oliguria, anuria, azotemia, anemia, hyponatremia, hypochloremia, hypoalbuminemia, edema, and coma. Management is much less complicated in mildly and moderately ill patients when these alterations are absent. The principles of treatment of all rickettsioses are specific chemotherapy and supportive care.

Specific Treatment

Chloramphenicol and the tetracyclines are specifically effective; they are rickettsiostatic and not rickettsicidal. When therapy is initiated during the early stages coincident with appearance of the rash, there is prompt alleviation of clinical signs. Response is less dramatic when therapy is delayed until the rash becomes hemorrhagic and diffuse.

Optimal antibiotic regimens are: chloramphenicol, an initial oral dose of 50 mg per kilogram body weight, or tetracycline, 25 mg per kilogram body weight. Either is acceptable. Subsequent daily doses are calculated as the initial oral dose divided equally and given at 6- to 8-hour intervals. Antibiotic treatment is given until the patient improves and has been afebrile for about 24 hours. In patients too ill to take oral medication, intravenous preparations are employed for the loading and subsequent doses. All patients with rickettsioses respond promptly to antibi-

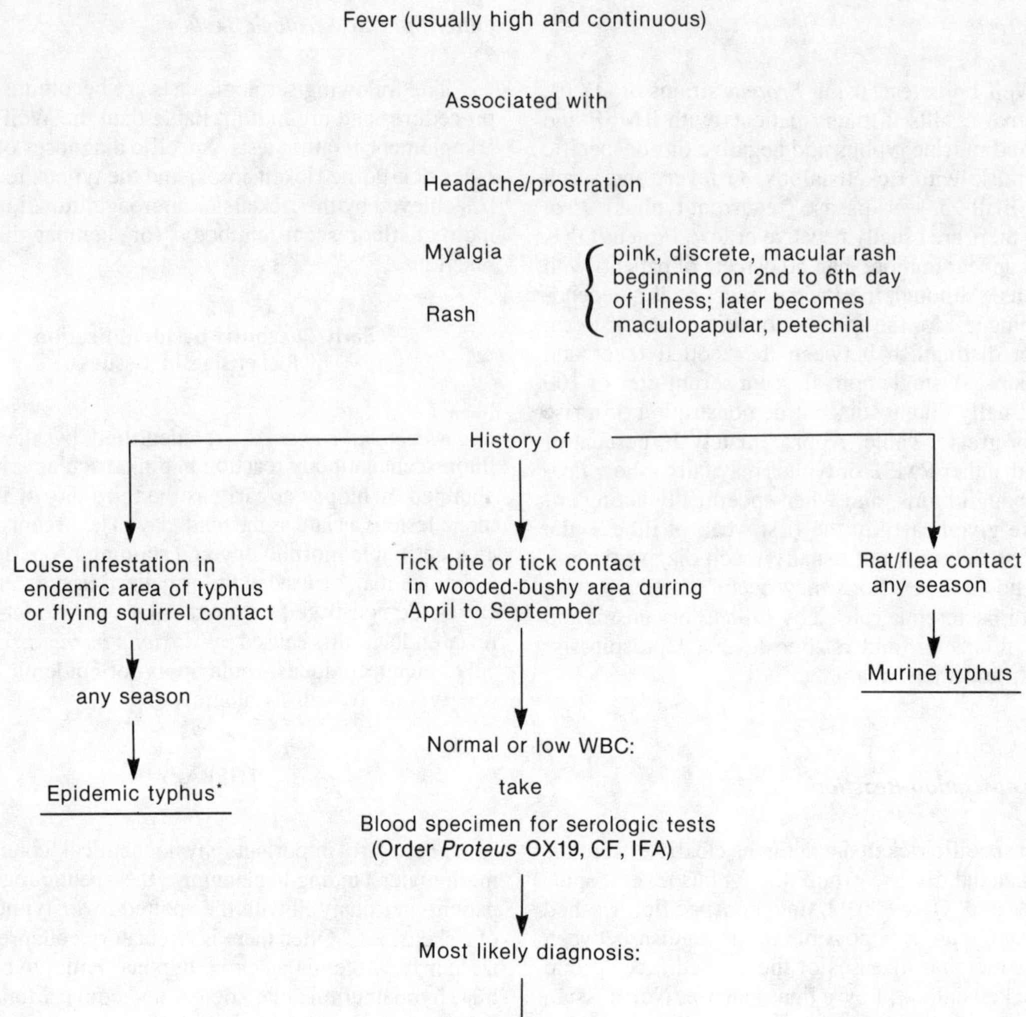

Figure 1 Salient epidemiologic, clinical, diagnostic, and therapeutic features of the major rickettsial diseases. * Serology as for Rocky Mountain spotted fever.

otic treatment when it is initiated early in illness, before serious tissue changes have occurred. Clinical improvement is obvious in 36 to 48 hours, with defervescence in 2 to 3 days. In scrub typhus, the response is even more dramatic.

Clinical improvement is slower and fever extends over longer periods in those patients first treated during the latter stages of illness. Large, single oral doses of chloramphenicol (50 mg per kilogram) have been effective in patients with RMSF and scrub typhus, although this regimen is not recommended. A single oral dose of 200 mg of doxycycline (a lipotropic tetracycline derivative that produces sustained high blood and tissue levels) has been shown in field trials to be practically effective for treatment of louse-borne typhus fever.

Tetracycline and chloramphenicol are quite effective for treatment of patients with the acute manifestations of Q fever. Recovery is usually prompt. Endocarditis is difficult to treat since the vegetations are rather large and the broad spectrum antibiotics are rickettsiostatic and not rickettsicidal. Long-term treatment is necessary; this favors tetracycline as the antibiotic of choice. As a general rule, surgical intervention with valve replacement is necessary for cure. A few patients have recovered following extended antibiotic treatment.

Steroid Treatment

Large doses of adrenal cortical steroids (e.g., prednisone 1.0 mg/kg or solucortef 5.0 mg/kg) given for about 3 days in combination with specific antibiotics are recommended in patients critically ill with spotted fever or with typhus that is first observed late in the course of severe illness. Temperature abates more rapidly than usual, as do the toxic manifestations. Steroids are not recommended for mild or moderately ill patients.

Supportive Treatment

Mouth care—swabbing of the oral cavity and use of mouth washes—may help prevent gingivitis and parotitis. Frequent turning of the patient will help prevent aspiration pneumonia and avert pressure sores over bony prominences. A generous intake of protein supplements with frequent feedings is useful. Protein intake of up to 2.0 g per kilogram normal body weight, with adequate carbohydrate and fat sufficient to make the diet palatable, is usually well tolerated. In uncooperative patients, when there is no abdominal distention, hourly liquid protein feedings by gastric tube are helpful, but such measures are usually obviated by proper intravenous alimentation. Attention is given to parenteral alimentation with glucose and amino acid supplements in critically ill patients with enhanced capillary permeability, edema, and vascular decompensation. Dialysis is indicated if there is clear-cut evidence of acute tubular necrosis.

NONSUPPURATIVE SEQUELAE OF GROUP A STREPTOCOCCAL INFECTION

ALAN L. BISNO, M.D.

Group A *Streptococcus* is the cause of a wide variety of acute infections in humans, including tonsillopharyngitis, otitis media, sinusitis, scarlet fever, erysipelas, pyoderma, cellulitis, lymphangitis, endometritis, pneumonia, septicemia and localized abscesses. This organism is distinguished from other pyogenic bacteria, however, by the occurrence of delayed nonsuppurative sequelae during convalescence from the acute infectious process. The two major nonsuppurative sequelae of group A streptococcal infection are acute rheumatic fever (ARF), which follows streptococcal upper respiratory tract infection, and poststreptococcal acute glomerulonephritis (AGN), which may be a consequence of either upper respiratory or cutaneous infection. Other nonsuppurative disorders, such as Schönlein-Henoch purpura and erythema nodosum, have beeen attributed to group A *Streptococcus*, but an exclusive and specific relationship between Schönlein-Henoch disease and group A *Streptococcus* has not been established, and erythema nodosum is associated with a wide variety of infectious and noninfectious disorders.

ACUTE RHEUMATIC FEVER

Diagnosis

The incidence of ARF has declined dramatically in the last three decades. The diagnosis of ARF can at times be difficult because the clinical presentation is quite variable and there is no diagnostic laboratory test. Certain manifestations, however, are so highly characteristic of the disease that they have been designated as "major manifestations" in the set of diagnostic criteria developed many years ago by T. Duckett Jones. The five major manifestations are migratory arthritis, carditis, erythema marginatum, subcutaneous nodules, and Sydenham's chorea. Certain other clinical and laboratory findings occur frequently in ARF but are too nonspecific to be utilized except as supporting evidence for the diagnosis. These "minor manifestations" include fever, arthralgia, previous rheumatic fever or rheumatic heart disease, prolonged P–R interval on the electrocardiogram, leukocytosis, and the presence of acute-phase reactants in the blood (elevated C-reactive protein level, accelerated erythrocyte sedimentation rate).

The presence of two major—or one major and two minor—criteria make the diagnosis of ARF highly probable provided that there is supporting evidence of recent group A streptococcal infection. Such evidence may consist of a throat culture positive for group A streptococci or a documented recent bout of scarlet fever. In most instances, however, the evidence is provided by an elevated serum titer of one or more antibodies to group A streptococcal extracellular products. Tests currently available include antistreptolysin O, antideoxyribonulease B, and antihyaluronidase. The serum titer of antistreptolysin O is elevated in only approximately 80 percent of ARF patients. However, failure to demonstrate an elevated titer of antistreptococcal antibodies or a significant titer rise by a battery of the above tests makes the diagnosis of ARF most unlikely.

Streptozyme (Carter-Wallace Laboratories) is a rapid and sensitive slide agglutination test that is widely used to screen for streptococcal antibodies. The antigens responsible for the Streptozyme hemagglutination reaction, however, are poorly characterized, and some investigators have reported considerable lot-to-lot variation in the titers obtained. If used, the exact Streptozyme titer of the patient's serum should be determined (titers of 1:200 or less are equivocal in our hands), and local sera of known titer are best included in each run.

The Jones criteria, even when accompanied by evidence of recent streptococcal infection, are not infallible. The criteria are particularly subject to error when satisfied by polyarthritis as a single major manifestation accompanied by minor criteria indicative of acute inflammation. Now that the incidence of ARF in North America has declined to an extremely low level, a variety of other infectious and vasculitic disorders are undoubtedly more frequent causes of acute polyarthritis than is ARF. Thus, diseases such as gonococcal arthritis and Still's disease, to name only two, must be ruled out by therapeutic maneuvers or by careful follow-up before the diagnosis of ARF can be established with confidence.

Therapy: General Measures

The management of patients with ARF depends to a significant extent upon the predominant clinical manifestations. Some patients experience polyathritis, some carditis, some chorea, and some various combinations of the three. Chorea tends to appear after a latent period that is variable but, in general, longer than that of the other major manifestations. It may occur as an isolated disoder (''pure'' chorea), but, mercifully, rarely occurs simultaneously with arthritis. Polyarthritis is usually accompanied by considerable fever and toxicity; patients with pure chorea may present no evidence of acute inflammation; carditis may be fulminant or indolent.

Patients should be placed at bed rest during the acute febrile portion of the illness or while experiencing active carditis. The pulse rate should be carefully monitored; a tachycardia that persists during sleep after fever has abated strongly suggests carditis. Routine base-line laboratory studies should include a complete blood count, erythrocyte sedimentation rate, C-reactive protein determination, throat culture, urinalysis, streptococcal antibody assays, chest roentgenogram, and electrocardiogram. An echocardiogram is useful in detecting subtle pericardial effusions or valvular abnormalities and in establishing a base line for further evaluation. A synovial fluid analysis may be indicated, particularly in problem cases in which other rheumatologic or infectious causes of arthritis are strongly suggested.

In cases in which gonococcal or other forms of septic arthritis are major considerations, the response to a brief (3-day) trial of appropriate antibiotic therapy should, in most instances, precede institution of anti-inflammatory agents. Indeed, in early cases wherein the diagnosis is not clear-cut, it is best to withhold anti-inflammatory agents (treating pain only with codeine) until the disease process has had an opportunity to declare itself. Such management does not influence the long-term prognosis of the rheumatic process. It is important that the diagnosis of ARF be as secure as possible because it has major implications for the patient's long-term management.

Antistreptococcal and Anti-Inflammatory Therapy

Once the diagnosis of ARF has been established, the patient should be given an adequate course of antistreptococcal therapy. In the absence of penicillin allergy, the treatment of choice is a single intramuscular injection of benzathine penicillin G, 600,000 units for children weighing 27 kg (60 lbs) or less and 1.2 million units for heavier individuals. The penicillin-allergic patient should receive erythromycin. Prescribing information for various formulations should be consulted for the precise dosage. For most preparations, the dosage is 40 mg per kilogram per day, not to exceed a total of 1 g. The antibiotic is administered orally in two to four equally divided doses. Throats of family contacts should be cultured; contacts harboring group A streptococci in the pharynx should receive a course of antistreptococcal therapy.

The two time-honored anti-inflammatory agents for use in ARF are salicylates and corticosteroids. Both drugs quiet the acute inflammation when given in adequate doses, but corticosteroids are more potent. The choice of agents depends upon the nature of the rheumatic process and the patient's tolerance of high doses of salicylates. There are inadequate data on the use of the newer nonsteroidal anti-inflammatory agents to allow formulation of firm recommendations regarding their use.

Patients whose only manifestation is mild arthritis may be managed with analgesics such as codeine. Avoiding use of anti-inflammatory agents allows a better assessment of when the attack has actually terminated and avoids posttherapeutic rebounds. For patients with moderate to severe arthritis without carditis, aspirin is the drug of choice. The initial dose of 100 mg per kilogram (not to exceed 6 to 7 g per day) is designed to produce serum levels in the range of approximately 25 mg per deciliter. Aspirin should be given every 4 hours around the clock for the first 1 to 2 days and then in four doses equally spaced through the waking hours. Small amounts of milk given with the aspirin will reduce gastric irritation. Large doses of sodium bicarbonate should be avoided, as they result in decreased blood levels of acetylsalicylic acid. Data are lacking as to the efficacy of enteric-coated aspirin preparations in ARF, but these formulations have been of value in management of patients with inflammatory arthritides of other types. Absorption of the enteric-coated products may be less predictable than that of regular aspirin, but this problem can be circumvented by careful monitoring of serum salicylate levels.

Once the acute signs and symptoms of arthritis have abated and the temperature has returned to normal, the aspirin dose may be reduced to two-thirds of the original dose and maintained at this level until laboratory manifestations of acute inflammation are normal. (The C-reactive protein is a particularly useful measure in this regard.) Thereafter, the dose may be reduced to one-half of that used initially. The total duration of therapy should be at least 6 weeks. Patients with rheumatic carditis who do not exhibit significant cardiomegaly and who do not have congestive heart failure may also be treated with salicylates, but the duration of therapy should be at least 8 weeks.

The above treatment schedules represent general guidelines that must be individualized from patient to patient. The aspirin dose must be titrated against clinical response and patient tolerance. If the patient exhibits severe gastrointestinal intolerance or signs of salicylism (e.g., hyperpnea, tinnitus) at required dosage levels or if the clinical response is inadequate, it is advisable to switch to corticosteroids.

Patients with carditis associated with high fever, prominent systemic toxicity, or congestive heart failure should receive corticosteroids. In very ill patients with carditis, the profound anti-inflammatory effects of corticosteroids may be critical in controlling congestive failure. Authorities differ as to the advisability of using corticosteroids in patients with carditis manifested by cardiomegaly but without overt congestive heart failure; I favor the use of steroids in this situation. An initial starting dose of 40 to 60 mg prednisone may be varied according to the patient's response. In particularly severe cases intravenous methyl prednisolone may be instituted. Methyl prednisolone is approximately 25 percent more potent than prednisolone. Steroids are continued in full dosage for 2 to 3 weeks, at which time salicylates are added while steroids are gradually tapered over an additional 1 to 3 weeks. Aspirin, in a dosage sufficient to suppress clinical and laboratory manifestations of inflammation, is continued for at least 1 month after termination of the steroids to minimize the chances of a rebound.

Treatment of Heart Failure

The usual measures of bed rest, sodium restriction, oxygen as necessary, sedation, and diuretics are indicated in management of congestive heart failure associated with acute rheumatic carditis. As indicated above, corticosteroids, by quieting inflammation and damping fever, decrease the demand on the heart. Although there has been some debate in the past as to the risk-to-benefit ratio of digitalis in acute rheumatic carditis, this drug should be used if the modalities listed above fail to bring congestive heart failure under control.

Rebound of Rheumatic Activity

As anti-inflammatory therapy is reduced or terminated, a flare of rheumatic activity may occur. These exacerbations usually appear within the first 2 weeks, and virtually always within 5 weeks, after cessation of therapy. At times rebounds may be detectable only by monitoring of acute-phase reactants in the blood. Clinically overt rebounds may be mild, consisting of fever, arthralgia, or mild arthritis, or they may be even more severe than the initial attack. A rebound of rheumatic carditis may be manifested by cardiomegaly, appearance of new murmurs, pericarditis, and congestive heart failure. The severity of the rebound seems related to the profundity of suppression of the rheumatic process. Thus, rebounds are thought to occur more frequently and to be more severe in steroid-treated than in salicylate-treated patients. Mild rebounds usually require no specific treatment. In more severe rebounds, reinstitution of anti-inflammatory therapy is indicated, and this should be with aspirin if possible to avoid further rebounds. In patients treated initially with steroids, the occurrence of severe rebounds may be minimized by instituting aspirin therapy while corticosteroids are being tapered.

Sydenham's Chorea

Patients with this disorder should be placed in a quiet, supportive environment and protected from inadvertent physical injury caused by their involuntary movements. Often sedation with phenobarbital or tranquilizaton with drugs such as diazepam, chlorpromazine, or haloperidol is required. The choice must be individualized, depending on the severity of the chorea and the patient's clinical response to the various agents.

Prevention of Rheumatic Fever

Prevention of the first attack of ARF is accomplished by accurate diagnosis and appropriate therapy of group A streptococcal upper respiratory infections (so-called primary prevention). Because the signs and symptoms of group A streptococcal and viral pharyngitis overlap, it is advisable to obtain throat cultures for patients with acute tonsillopharyngitis. Although the throat culture does not distinguish reliably between true streptococcal pharyngitis and asymptomatic streptococcal carriage, it does prevent unnecessary treatment of the majority of patients with sore throat who will have negative throat cultures. Recent technical advances in identification of group A streptococcal carbohydrate antigen directly from throat swabs may make it possible to obtain a positive or negative result shortly after taking the swab. Patients with positive throat cultures should be treated with penicillin if they are not allergic. The most effective therapy is a single intramuscular injection of benzathine penicllin G, 600,000 units for children weighing 60 lbs (27 kg) or less and 1.2 million units for heavier individuals. In epidemiologic settings where the risk of ARF is quite low, for example, in most nonindigent populations of North American and western Europe, a full 10-day course of penicillin V by mouth is sufficient. The standard dosage regimen is 125 to 250 mg three to four times a day. For convenience, penicillin V, 250 mg to 500 mg, may be administered twice daily with equivalent results. The efficacy of these oral regimens, of course, depends upon patient fidelity, which is a considerable factor because the signs and symptoms ordinarily abate long before the 10 days are over. Penicillin-allergic individuals should receive oral erythromycin in the dosage indicated above in the section, Antistreptococcal and Anti-Inflammatory Therapy. Oral cephalosporins are also acceptable alternatives in the penicillin-allergic patient, especially if the patient is known to be able to tolerate these drugs. Oral cephalosporins should not be used in the patient with immediate hypersensitivity to penicillin.

Individuals who have experienced an attack of ARF are inordinately susceptible to repeated attacks following group A streptococcal infections, and such recurrences may lead to progressive cardiac damage. Thus, they should be protected from intercurrent streptococcal infections by continuous antimicrobial prophylaxis (secondary prevention). The most effective form of prophylaxis is benzathin penicillin G, 1.2 million units intramuscularly every 4 weeks. Oral prophylaxis is less reliable, and fidelity is difficult to assure. Oral regimens include sulfadiazine, 0.5 g once a day for children weighing less than 60 lbs and 1 g once a day for heavier patients, or penicillin G or V, 200,000 to 250,000 units twice a day. For the rare patient who is allergic to both penicillin and sulfa, erythromycin, 250 mg twice a day, may be prescribed.

In general, benzathine penicillin G should be used for prophylaxis of patients at greatest risk of recurrence of ARF and of development of progressive cardiac damage. Risk factors include presence of rheumatic heart disease, previous recurrences, less than 5 years since the most recent attack, and intensive exposure to school-aged children at home or at work. Moreover, the rate of ARF recurrence declines with age. Thus, as age and changing epidemiologic circumstances lower the risk, it is permissible to switch from parenteral to oral prophylaxis. Although few patients maintain rheumatic fever prophylaxis for life (especially in the absence of significant rheumatic heart disease), there are no firm guidelines as to when prophylaxis may be discontinued. This decision should be taken only after careful appraisal of the risks and in consultation with the patient.

From a personal viewpoint, I strongly consider discontinuing prophylaxis in patients who have reached their mid-twenties, have had only a single ARF attack that occurred at least 5 years previously, have no evidence of residual rheumatic heart disease, and are not intimately exposed to primary schoolchildren at home or by the nature of their occupation. As stated above, the decision to discontinue prophylaxis in less optimal circumstances must be individualized.

In certain epidemiologic settings, severe and widespread outbreaks of streptococcal pharyngitis may be associated with multiple cases of ARF. Such outbreaks, which are quite rare in the United States today, have in the past occurred primarily in military installations or similar civilian institutional settings. Under such circumstances, mass prophylaxis with benzathine penicillin G may be required to terminate the epidemic.

ACUTE GLOMERULONEPHRITIS

Poststreptococcal acute glomerulonephritis is an inflammatory disease of the renal glomerulus that follows upper respiratory tract or cutaneous infection with certain nephritogenic group A streptococcal strains belonging to a limited number of M-protein serotypes. (Rare common-source outbreaks of group C streptococcal infection have also been reported to be associated with AGN.) The pathology of AGN is characterized by diffuse proliferative glomerular lesions and clinically by edema, hypertension, hematuria, and proteinuria.

The clinical spectrum of AGN ranges from asymptomatic hematuria and hypocomplementemia to severe clinical disease with volume overload and hypertensive encephalopathy. In cases severe enough to require hospitalization, the most immediate problem is usually that of circulatory overload. The patient is placed at bed rest; salt and fluids are restricted, and, if required, a diuretic is administered. Digitalis is usually not indicated for management of the circulatory problems associated with AGN because myocardial function is normal. In most instances specific antihypertensive therapy other than diuretics is unnecessary. Antihypertensives should be used, however, if the clinical situation dictates. If severe hypertension and hypertensive encephalopathy ensues, potent parenteral agents may be required. Acute pulmonary edema or severe and prolonged oliguria occur in a small percentage of patients with AGN and are managed by the measures conventionally employed in these conditions.

The occurrence of a case of AGN signals the presence of a nephritogenic streptococcus in the patient, and often, in his family contacts. Thus, the patient should receive antistreptococcal therapy, preferably with a single intramuscular injection of benzathine penicillin G, or if the patient is penicillin-allergic, with erythromycin. Dosages to be employed are the same as those indicated above for primary prevention of ARF. Family contacts should be screened for asymptomatic nephritis with urinalysis and serum C3 complement determinations. In addition, the contacts should have cultures of the pharynx and any pyoderma lesions. Individuals harboring group A streptococci should receive appropriate therapy in order to eradicate the nephritogenic strain. Although this is an important measure from the epidemiologic standpoint, such treatment will not modify the course of preexistent AGN, nor is it likely to abort the disease in a patient who is within the latent period.

Most patients with AGN are children, and for them the prognosis appears quite good. Death during the acute attack is fortunately rare, but a small percentage of AGN patients never resolve the acute attack. In them, the disease enters a subacute phase, resulting in virtually complete loss of renal function within a few months to two years. For the vast majority of pediatric patients, however, the disease appears to resolve completely and does not lead either to chronic glomerulonephritis or hypertension in later life. The data on adult patients are more limited. It does appear, however, that the prognosis for adults may be poorer.

Unlike ARF patients, those with AGN are not at increased risk of repeated attacks, and continuous antistreptococcal prophylaxis is not indicated.

DIPHTHERIA

CARLOS H. RAMIREZ-RONDA, M.D.

Diphtheria is an acute, infectious, preventable, and potentially fatal disease caused by *Corynebacterium diphtheriae*. The infection is usually localized to the upper part of the respiratory tract and the skin; the infection gives rise to local and systemic signs. These signs are the result of a toxin elaborated by the microorganisms multiplying at the site of infection. The systemic complications particularly affect the heart and the peripheral nerves.

ETIOLOGY

Corynebacterium diphtheriae is a gram-positive rod that grows best under aerobic conditions and is not a gas former. Gram stains of the diphtheria bacilli show a club-shaped rod, arranged in palisade formation or a "Chinese-letter" configuration. A toxin is responsible for most of the clinical manifestations. The toxin is produced by the bacterial cells infected with a lysogenic bacteriophage, beta-prophage. Avirulent diphtheria strains do not have the bacteriophage and fail to produce toxins. Disease can be caused by toxigenic and nontoxigenic strains; however, the disease seen with nontoxigenic strains is mild and behaves like localized disease caused by toxigenic strains. The severity of the illness seen with strains that produce certain colony types—gravis and mitis—seem to be more severe, but all types can produce the same clinical picture. The view that epidemic diphtheria is more frequently associated with gravis strains is no longer tenable.

EPIDEMIOLOGY

Diphtheria is distributed worldwide, with a higher incidence in temperate climates. The disease occurs predominantly under poor socioeconomic conditions where crowding is common and where many persons are either not immunized or inadequately immunized.

The only significant reservoir of *Corynebacterium diphtheriae* is the human host. The organism is transmitted directly from one person to another, and intimate contact is required. The usual habitat for the microorganism is the respiratory tract. There are extrarespiratory locations of diphtheria infection that include skin, wounds, buccal mucosa, vagina, and conjunctiva. Disease spreads from asymptomatic or convalescent carriers, who constitute a reservoir. The organism can multiply in the mucous membranes of the respiratory tract of the immunized host without causing clinical disease. Transmission is usually by way of infected droplets of nasopharyngeal secretions. Infective skin exudate is also involved in human-to-human transmission. Transmission may also be by animals, fomites, or milk.

Morbidity and mortality are highest in children less than 14 years of age. In the United States, attack rates are highest in blacks and Mexican-Americans between 5 and 14 years old and are higher for unimmunized household members and contacts of an index case.

Immunity against the disease depends upon the presence of antitoxin in the host's blood. Antitoxin is formed by immunization or by clinical or subclinical infection, including skin infections. The Schick test consists of an intradermal injection of 0.1 ml of purified diphtheria toxin dissolved in buffered human serum albumin. This is injected into the volar surface of one arm, and 0.1 ml of purified diphtheria toxoid is used as a control in the other arm. The test can be used to assess the immune status of the subject. A positive reaction (reaction to toxin but not to toxoid) is interpreted to mean that the patient is susceptible to diphtheria; a negative reaction (no reaction at site of toxin or toxoid injection) indicates that the patient is immune and that levels of antitoxin exceed 0.03 units per milliliter. The test provides only an estimate of immunity. The lack of ability to perform it should not delay the treatment of asymptomatic contacts of diphtheria.

PATHOGENESIS

The organisms multiply on epithelial cells of the pharynx or other infected site. There they secrete the specific toxin that is responsible for the local signs and that is absorbed into the blood, resulting in systemic illness. The first local changes are necrosis; as a consequence, an exudate is formed that tends to coalesce. The fibrinous exudate contains leukocytes, necrotic epithelial cells, red blood cells, and the diphtheria bacillus. This exudate forms a pseudomembrane with a white center and a gray or brownish periphery; removal of this membrane leads to bleeding. The membrane can extend in the pharynx to the larynx and to the bronchial tree, forming a cast. The edema associated with the inflammation may lead to laryngeal and/or tracheal obstruction.

The soluble toxin is disseminated via blood and lymphatics and can produce effects on the heart, nervous system and kidneys. The toxin gains access to the cytoplasmic portion of the cell by bypassing normal cellular digestive mechanisms. After crossing the cell membrane, toxin inactivates elongation factor, a protein needed in the translocation step of protein synthesis. This results in abrupt arrest of protein synthesis, presumably bringing about degeneration and death of the cell. Although antitoxin may neutralize even absorbed toxin, it does not prevent this chain of events once the toxin penetrates the cell.

CLINICAL FEATURES

Diphtheria may be a symptomless state or a rapidly fatal disease. The incubation period varies from 1 to 7 days, but is most commonly from 2 to 4 days.

Anterior Nares Diphtheria

The infection is localized to the anterior nasal area and is manifested by unilateral or bilateral serous or serosanguinous discharge that erodes the adjacent skin resulting in small crusted lesions. The membrane may be seen in the nose.

Tonsillar (Faucial) Diphtheria

This is the commonest presentation and includes the most toxic forms. The onset is usually sudden, with minimal fever (rarely exceeding 38 °C), malaise, and mild sore throat. The pharynx is moderately injected, and a thick whitish gray tonsillar exudate is frequently seen. There is enlargement of the tonsillar and cervical lymph nodes. The exudate may extend to other areas and result in nasopharyngeal diphtheria and massive cervical lymphadenopathy (''bullneck'' appearance). The commonest complaints reported are sore throat (in 85%), pain on swallowing (23%), nausea and vomiting (25%), and headache (18%).

Pharyngeal Diphtheria

This form is diagnosed when the membrane extends from the tonsillar area to the pharynx.

Laryngeal and Bronchial Diphtheria

This type involves the larynx. The voice becomes hoarse, and inspiratory and expiratory stridor may appear, dyspnea and cyanosis occur, and the accessory muscles of respiration are used. Tracheostomy or intubation is needed.

Cutaneous Diphtheria

Classically described as diphtheria in tropical areas, this form now is seen in nontropical areas. It takes the form of a chronic, nonhealing ulcer, sometimes covered with a grayish membranous exudate. Another form is secondary infection of a preexisting wound. Finally, superinfection with *C. diphtheriae* may occur in a variety of preexisting skin lesions such as impetigo, insect bites, ectyma, or eczema.

COMPLICATIONS OF DIPHTHERIA

Myocarditis

Although electrocardiographic changes have been described in up to 25 percent of cases, overt clinical myocarditis is less common. The onset is insidious, occurring in the second or third week of the infection. The patient exhibits a weak, rising pulse, distant heart sounds, and a profound weakness and lethargy. More overt signs of heart failure can occur. The most common ECG changes are T-wave flattening or inversion, bundle branch block or intraventricular block, and several disorders of rhythm. Serial determination of SGOT levels indentifies most patients with myocarditis. The prognosis is poor, especially when heart block supervenes.

Peripheral Neuritis

The commonest form of cranial nerve palsy is paralysis of the soft palate. There may be nasal regurgitation and/or nasal speech. The condition is usually mild and recovery occurs within 2 weeks. Ciliary paralysis and oculomotor paralysis are the next commonest forms. Peripheral neuritis affecting the limbs may appear during the fourth to the eighth week. It is usually manifest by weakness of the dorsiflexors and decreased or absent deep-tendon reflexes. Diphtheritic polyneuritis has been described after cutaneous diphtheria.

DIAGNOSIS

Diagnosis is made on clinical grounds and can be confirmed by laboratory tests. The clinical features of a fully developed diphtheritic membrane, especially in the pharynx, are sufficiently characteristic to suggest the possibility of the disease and for treatment to start immediately.

A definitive diagnosis of diphtheria requires culture of the microorganism and the demonstration of toxin production.

Specific diagnosis of diphtheria depends completely on demonstration of the organism in stained smears and their recovery by culture. Methylene blue-stained preparations are positive in experienced hands in 75 to 85 percent of cases. The presence of deeply stained granules with methylene blue (metachromatic granules) is suggestive of *C. diphtheriae*. The bacilli can be recovered by culture in Löeffler's medium within 8 to 12 hours if patients have not been receiving antimicrobial agents. The lesion or a piece of membrane should be cultured on Löeffler's medium plus a tellurite plate and a blood agar plate before antibiotics are given. The presence of beta-hemolytic streptococci does not rule out the diagnosis of diphtheria, since such streptococci are recovered in 20 to 30 percent of patients with diphtheria.

Since a patient may have nontoxigenic bacilli, efforts should be made in the laboratory to determine toxigenicity of cultured diphtheria-like organisms. Tests that can be used are the Elek-plate method, guinea pig inoculation, and others.

The differential diagnosis of tonsillar-pharyngeal diphtheria should include streptococcal pharyngitis, adenoviral exudative pharyngitis, infectious mononucleosis, and Vincent's angina, among others (see Table 1).

TABLE 1 Differential Diagnosis of Diphtheria

Localization	*Other Condition*
Nasal	Sinusitis, foreign body, "snuffles" of congenital syphilis, rhinitis
Faucial and pharyngeal	Streptococcal or adenoviral exudative pharyngitis, ulcerative pharyngitis (herpetic, coxsackieviral) infectious mononucleosis, oral thrush, peritonsillar abscess, retropharyngeal abscess, Vincent's angina, lesions associated with agranulocytosis or leukemia
Laryngeal	Laryngotracheobronchitis, epiglottitis
Skin	Impetigo, pyogenic ulcers, herpes simplex infection

TREATMENT

The best and most effective treatment of diphtheria is prevention by immunization with diphtheria toxoid, since this is a preventable disease. The most important aspect of treatment is to administer antitoxin as soon as diphtheria is suspected clinically, without awaiting laboratory confirmation. The patient should be hospitalized and isolated at bed rest for 10 to 14 days.

Use of Antitoxin

Antitoxin is of equine origin, and the minimal effective dose remains undefined; therefore, dosage is based on empiric judgments. It is usually accepted that for patients with mild or moderate cases, including those with tonsillar and pharyngeal membrane, 50,000 units, injected intramuscularly, is enough (for a child, 30,000 units). In severe cases, such as with a more extensive membrane and/or thrombocytopenia, 60,000 to 120,000 units, is the recommended dose, depending on severity, at least half of it being given by slow intravenous infusion in critically ill patients.

Before administration of antitoxin, any history of allergy or reactions to horse serum or horse dander must be determined. All patients must be tested for antitoxin sensitivity. The test is carried out by diluting horse antitoxin in saline and performing an eye test with a 1:10 dilution. This is followed by a scratch test with a 1:100 dilution; if negative in one-half hour, the scratch test is followed by an intradermal test, 1:100 dilution. If all tests are negative, antitoxin can be given. The intravenous route recommended, giving first a slow intravenous infusion of 0.5 ml of antitoxin in 10 ml of saline, followed in one-half hour by the balance of the antitoxin dose in a dilution of 1:20, with saline infused at a rate not to exceed 1 ml per minute. Others give the antitoxin dose intramuscularly in mild to moderate cases only.

If the patient is sensitive to horse serum, desensitization should be carried out with care, preferably in an intensive care unit. Epinephrine should be available as well as intubation equipment and respiratory assistance. The following doses of horse serum antitoxin should be injected at 15-minute intervals, if no reaction occurs:

1. 0.05 ml of 1:20 dilution subcutaneously;
2. 0.10 ml of 1:10 dilution subcutaneously;
3. 0.3 ml of 1:10 dilution subcutanoeously;
4. 0.1 ml of undiluted antitoxin subcutaneously;
5. 0.2 ml of undiluted antitoxin subcutaneously;
6. 0.5 ml of undiluted antitoxin subcutaneously;
7. remaining estimated therapeutic dose intramuscularly.

During all tests and injections of antitoxin, a syringe containing epinephrine, 1:1,000 dilution in saline, should be at hand to be used immediately in a dose of 0.01 ml per kilogram subcutaneously or intramuscularly at any sign of anaphylaxis. A good precaution is to have a venous access open with normal saline prior to the test. If needed, a similar amount of epinephrine diluted to a final concentration of 1:10,000 in saline may be given slowly intravenously and repeated in 5 to 15 minutes. Other information and instructions in the package insert accompanying the antitoxin should be observed.

Antibiotic Therapy

Corynebacterium diphtheriae is susceptible to several antimicrobial agents. After cultures have been performed, antibiotics should be administered to prevent multiplication of the microorganisms at the site of infection and to eliminate the carrier state. Penicillin G is the drug of choice and is usually given as procaine penicillin, 600,000 units intramuscularly every 12 hours for a period of 10 to 14 days. Erythromycin is also very active against the diphtheria bacillus and is given in a dose of 2.0 g per day divided in four doses for the same period. Antimicrobial therapy may be discontinued after the antibiotic course and when three successive daily cultures from both nose and throat are negative.

Supportive Measures

Bed rest is essential during the acute phase of the disease. Return to physical activity must be carefully guided by the physician and will depend on the degree of toxicity and the presence of cardiac involvement.

Complications such as dehydration, malnutrition, and congestive heart failure should be promptly diagnosed and properly treated. The pulse and blood pressure should be measured frequently. The use of digitalis in heart failure associated with diphtheria myocarditis has been questioned and should be individualized on a case-by-case basis (e.g., for an elderly patient with rapidly progressing myocarditis).

In cases of severe laryngeal involvement, marked toxicity, and/or shock, corticosteroids (prednisone, 3 to 5 mg per kilogram per day), have been advocated, but there are no hard data on its effectiveness; I would use corticosteroids in this situation.

In cases of laryngeal obstruction with respiratory stridor, a tracheostomy is necessary and should be performed promptly.

Before the patient is discharged, specimens from throat and nose or local lesion should be cultured; at least two, and preferably three, consecutive negative cultures should be obtained.

After recovery, toxoid administration against tetanus and diphtheria (Td) should be administered to complete a primary series if the patient has not been immunized.

Treatment of Carriers

The chronic carrier state may occur despite immunity derived either from clinical disease or from immunization. The carrier state occasionally occurs and persists in the absence of antecedent disease. Erythromycin (in adults, 0.5 g orally four times a day for 7 days) is the drug of choice for treatment of the carrier state and probably also the acute disease. Alternative antibiotics are procaine penicillin G, 600,000 units intramuscularly daily for 14 days; clindamyin, 150 mg orally four times a day for 7 days; or rifampin, 600 mg by mouth daily for 7 days.

PREVENTION

Prevention of diphtheria has been achieved mainly by active immunization of all children in the population. Primary immunization of children 6 years of age and younger should be carried out with a mixture of diphtheria and tetanus toxoids and pertussis vaccine (DPT), according to the following schedule: 2 months, DPT; 4 months; DPT; 6 months, DPT; 18 months, DPT; 4 to 6 years, DPT; 14 to 16 years, Td (adult type). For primary immunization of children older than 6 years of age, adult type tetanus and diphtheria toxoids (Td) should be used. This combination contains no more than 2 flocculation units (Lf) of diphtheria toxoid per dose, in contrast to 7 to 25 Lf in DPT and is less likely to produce reactions in older recipients. Complete immunization is accomplished with two doses at least 8 weeks apart followed by a third dose a year later.

Children who have had a complete course of primary immunization with diphtheria toxoid (DPT) may be given a booster injection on exposure to diphtheria.

Household and other close contacts of a patient with diphtheria should be observed attentively for 7 days. They should receive either an intramuscular injection of 1.2 million units of benzathine penicillin or a 7-day course of erythromycin by the oral route. Cultures should be performed before and after treatment. An injection of toxoid appropriate for age and immunization status can also be given. Susceptible close contacts who have had no (or only one) prior injections of toxoid should promptly be given 3,000 to 10,000 (depending on body size) units of antitoxin following the usual precautions. When indicated, active immunization with toxoid should be continued to completion.

MANAGEMENT IN EPIDEMICS

1. Identify all primary cases, hospitalize, and treat.
2. Use toxoid in all the population at risk.
3. Culture all contacts for diphtheria, and treat all persons with *C. diphtheriae* in throat, nose, or skin lesions with erythromycin for 7 days to eliminate carrier state (see Prevention, above).
4. Watch primary contacts closely during the first week of exposure and treat at first signs or symptoms. Alternatively, all susceptible primary contacts can be given 1,500 to 3,000 units of diphtheria antitoxin intramuscularly, using the same precautions for antitoxin administration as previously stated in addition to toxoid. This low-level dose will boost them while they are forming their own antibody.

PERTUSSIS

MARGARET H. D. SMITH, M.D.

Pertussis (whooping cough) is an infectious tracheobronchitis characterized by severe, protracted, repeated spasmodic coughing. The etiologic agent is *Bordetella pertussis*, rarely *Bordetella parapertussis*, and very rarely, *Bordetella bronchiseptica*; these organisms multiply only in association with the ciliated epithelium of the tracheobronchial tree, producing marked mucus secretion, desquamation, and necrosis, with resulting bronchial and bronchiolar obstruction of varying degrees. Adenoviruses and parainfluenza viruses, sometimes alone, sometimes in addition to *Bordetella*, have been isolated from children with spasmodic coughs, but their presence in patients with true pertussis is probably coincidental rather than causal. Commonest in the spring and early summer months, and more frequent among females than males, pertussis affects particularly young children and small infants, for whom it is highly infectious and very dangerous.

The incubation period of 7 to 10 days is followed by the invasion or catarrhal stage, which is characterized by cough, lacrimation, and dry, persistent cough—sometimes hoarseness. Within a week or two the cough becomes more severe, especially at night; the older child starts to vomit after coughing, and the coughing attacks occur at rather regular intervals. In the second or paroxysmal stage, paroxysms usually occur at the rate of 10 to 15, rarely up to 30, per day. Each paroxysm consists of many coughs in quick succession—like a machine gun—and is productive of long ropes of thick mucus; the child's face becomes purplish blue and swollen, with bulging eyes. Air is finally inspired with great effort through tense vocal cords, producing the characteristic crowing sound or whoop that gives the disease its name; the whoop is in turn followed by vomiting and sometimes immediately by another attack of coughing. Apnea or "black-out" spells occasionally interrupt the paroxysm in severe cases. The child often senses an oncoming paroxysm, becomes very apprehensive, and runs to an adult, even a strange one, for support; also, the child tries to avoid any stimulus, such as eating, that is likely to precipitate a paroxysm. Finally, after 2 to 6 weeks, the third or convalescent stage gradually sets in, characterized by slow disappearance of the paroxysms, although some children continue to whoop typically, usually without vomiting, for up to a year. Fever is not part of the picture of uncomplicated whooping cough, except possibly at the start of the catarrhal stage.

Infants less than 1 year of age often display a protracted, exhausting, staccato cough, accompanied by listlessness and lack of appetite, sometimes by apneic spells, but usually without whoop or vomiting.

Adolescents and adults probably develop whooping cough more often than is recognized. Although they are rarely so severely affected as children, the "chronic bronchitis," sometimes associated with violent cough, whooping, and vomiting, can be debilitating as well as highly infectious for contacts. Tradition has it that whooping cough in old people tends to be very severe.

Acute complications include those due to:

1. The strain of coughing (edema of the eyelids, face, and tongue; hemorrhages into the conjunctivae and skin; nose bleeds; meningeal and cerebral hemorrhages, often followed by permanent focal neurologic impairment; ulceration of the frenulum of the tongue; temporary loss of sphincter control; umbilical or inguinal hernia; prolapse of the rectum,
2. Respiratory involvement (atelectasis; areas of hyperaeration; pneumothorax, pneumomediastinum, subcutaneous emphysema; pneumonia due to secondary bacterial invaders; activation of a previous tuberculous infection).
3. "Toxic" central nervous system involvement (apnea; convulsions, focal or generalized).
4. Gastrointestinal difficulties (dehydration; unwillingness to eat with resultant loss of weight, avitaminosis, electrolyte disturbances, tetany).

Sequelae, rare nowadays in the United States, can include bronchiectasis and central nervous system damage.

DIAGNOSIS

Lymphocytosis of up to 80 percent of a total white blood cell count of 30,000 or more is characteristic of older children with pertussis, but is often absent in infants, in adults, and in individuals with a previous history of immunization.

Chest roentgenogram often shows heavy peribronchial streaking with patchy atelectasis and hyperaeration, and, in some cases, enlargement of hilar lymph nodes.

Fluorescent antibody identification of *B. pertussis* in nasopharyngeal smears is a quick, reliable diagnostic procedure carried out by many state health departments as well as private laboratories.

Isolation of *Bordetella* by culture from nasopharyngeal swabs is ideal, but, except in times of epidemic, skilled personnel and fresh culture media are rarely available. In competent hands the isolation rate is high.

Differential diagnosis includes viral infection, particularly with adenoviruses, parainfluenza, or even influenza viruses; foreign body; mycoplasma and legionella pneumonia (particularly in adolescents and adults); and, especially in young infants, chlamydial pneumonia.

TREATMENT

Erythromycin estolate (50 mg per kilogram per day divided into four oral doses) is by far the most effective antimicrobial drug yet found for eliminating *B. pertussis* from the nasopharynx, thereby suppressing communicability. If started during the catarrhal stage, it may also shorten the illness. It probably also diminishes the likelihood of secondary bacterial infection. It should be given for 14 days, since relapses have been observed with shorter courses.

Steroids (hydrocortisone sodium succinate 30 mg per kilogram intramuscularly in gradually decreasing doses for 1 week) were found beneficial in one controlled study.

Theophylline (0.3 to 0.5 mg per kilogram per day orally divided into three doses) appeared to reduce whooping in one study but not in another.

Immune globulin has been found ineffectual for both prophylaxis and treatment.

Cough-suppressive medications should not be used since the patient must cough up the large amounts of mucopus from the respiratory tract.

General care is of the utmost importance for the young child with whooping cough. The child older than 2 or 3 years without fever benefits from being up and around and out-of-doors, as long as there is an adult nearby to whom the child can run for comfort and support as a paroxysm comes on. The child should be encouraged to sleep on the abdomen, even in the knee-chest position, with the foot of the bed elevated to promote drainage of the thick mucus. Fluids by mouth should be offered often to prevent dehydration and to liquify secretions; the child should be coaxed frequently with favorite foods to avoid weight loss.

Infants less than 1 year should usually be hospitalized and cared for by a special nurse, since most of the deaths from whooping cough occur in this age group. Discriminating use of antimicrobial drugs, suctioning, monitoring of pO_2 and pCO_2, oxygen therapy, parenteral fluids and nutrition, and even artificial respiration and totally assisted ventilation can be necessary to prevent atelectasis, treat pneumonia, and assure gas exchange, thereby avoiding cerebral anoxia and subsequent bronchiectasis and central nervous system damage. Strict isolation is mandatory for hospitalized patients.

PREVENTION

The high mortality of pertussis in infants—the potential occurrence of serious sequelae; the protracted course in older children and adults, necessitating weeks of absence from day care center, school, and workplace for one or more family members—make complete immunization essential for all but children with a personal history of convulsions. All patients with pertussis should receive erythromycin estolate (50 mg per kilogram per day) for 14 days to minimize dissemination of disease.

The efficacy of prophylactic erythromycin administration to healthy contacts is supported by only very limited data. However, since those data are encouraging and because the drug has very low toxicity and the disease can be serious, I recommend that all close (i.e., household, day care center, school) contacts should likewise receive erythromycin if they have not completed immunization. This applies particularly to very young infants, since neonatal immunity is nonexistent in pertussis. Whether adolescent and adult contacts, whose immunization or exposure occurred many years previously, should also receive prophylactic erythromycin is a matter of opinion. Recent reports of epidemics involving hospital personnel, as well as the serious nature of pertussis in old people, suggest that it is wise to recommend erythromycin prophylaxis at least for these groups, as well as for people of any age who live or work in close contact with neonates, unimmunized infants, or immunosuppressed individuals.

For individuals who are known to have completed their initial course of pertussis vaccine, further booster doses of vaccine are rarely recommended because of the high incidence of adverse effects. Only in the circumstances of an institutional epidemic has it been found necessary to administer booster doses.

ANTHRAX

BORIS VELIMIROVIC, M.D., D.T.P.H.

Anthrax is an acute disease caused by the aerobic, spore-forming, gram-positive, toxin-producing organism *Bacillus anthracis*. It is the oldest known zoonosis with worldwide distribution: infrequent and sporadic in the U.S., moderately frequent in southern, to rare in central and northern Europe, and common in the USSR, tropical and subtropical Africa and Asia.

EPIDEMIOLOGY

The ability to form spores permits the organism to survive environmental and disinfective measures that destroy most other bacteria. Public health problems largely arise from its long persistence in the soil (90 years proved). Infection of the skin comes about by contact with contaminated goat hair, wool, hides, and other similar products or by direct contact with infected tissues. Inhalation anthrax results from aspiration of spores via small aerosol particles; the spores germinate in the alveoli and multiply. Gastrointestinal anthrax results from ingestion of contaminated meat and occurs in explosive outbreaks. There is no evidence that milk from infected animals transmits the disease. Biting flies and other insects may serve as mechanical vectors.

For epidemiologic purposes, the disease is divided into agricultural and industrial anthrax (occupational history is important). Particularly exposed or at potential risk are veterinarians, veterinary assistants, sheep herders, agricultural and ranch workers, slaughterhouse employees, tannery and textile industry workers, home craftsmen using imported yarn from endemic areas, and people handling bonemeal fertilizer.

PATHOGENESIS

The virulence of the organism is determined by at least two factors: an extracellular toxin and the capsular polypeptide. The toxin causes vascular permeability, edema and fluid loss, and oligemic shock, which is the mechanism of death. The toxin consists of at least three components that are each nontoxic but that act synergistically.

CLINICAL PICTURE

There are four major forms of anthrax.

Cutaneous

The commonest form accounts for up to 98 percent of all cases. At the entry point on the skin, a cut or abrasion—usually of the upper extremities, face, or neck, (but also other parts: feet, breast, penis, scrotum)—a small red papule develops after an incubation period of 2 to 5 days (range 1 to 7 days). This papule progresses within 12 to 48 hours to a fluid-filled blister. The fluid in the vesicle is initially clear, but soon becomes dark and bluish black. The blister is surrounded by inflammation, extensive hard induration and edema in the adjacent deeper tissues, lymphadenitis, lymphadenopathy. Fever is mild. The lesion is not painful. Double lesions do occur. Satellite vesicles can develop near the initial lesion. The vesicle ruptures and develops into a pustule (pustula maligna), the tissue necrotizes and progresses to a carbuncle that is relatively painless, and then becomes a dark-colored black eschar (*anthrax* is Greek for "black") of about 1 cm diameter or larger. This heals and the scale falls off, leaving a scar.

In untreated (or unrecognized) cases, there may be hematogenous spread via regional lymph nodes, bacteriemia (fever) and toxemia, which may lead to death in 5 to 20 percent of cases (localization on the head or neck has more serious prognosis). Eighty percent of cutaneous anthrax can heal without treatment.

Pulmonary

The pulmonary form is initially manifested by a mild upper respiratory tract infection, nonproductive cough suggestive of atypical pneumonia, influenza, or mild bronchopneumonia. Roentgenograms may show mediastinal widening. After several days and often after a temporary improvement from the primary phase (at which there is a surprising discrepancy between subjective and objective findings: patient is well-oriented, alert, not agitated), there is a sudden onset of acute dyspnea, cyanosis, stridor, signs of pleural effusion, and an elevated temperature. The patient usually dies within 24 hours of onset of this second stage. Postmortem findings are hemorrhagic mediastinitis.

The first stage may not be clearly observed and the disease is noted in the second stage, which is also called the septicemic form.

Intestinal

The intestinal form appears 2 to 5 days after ingestion of meat contaminated with spores of *B. anthracis* and the penetration of the intestinal mucosa. The lesions in the gut are similar to those of the cutaneous form and are accompanied by nonspecific symptoms such as nausea, vomiting, dizziness, anorexia, fever, abdominal pain, splenomegaly or bloody diarrhea, hemorrhagic ascites (even several liters). There is progression to generalized septicemia, toxemia, shock, and death in about 25 to 50 percent of cases. Postmortem, local lesion, hemorrhagic spots in the serosa and a typical septic, soft, necrotic spleen are characteristic.

Meningeal

The meningeal form occurs mostly following a cutaneous initial disease in up to 3 to 5 percent of cases, rarely as a primary infection, or may result from inhalation. Clinically typical symptoms of bacterial meningitis are present and lead almost invariably to death in 2 to 4 days.

Milder or subclinical cases in cutaneous and pulmonary forms and chronic cases in intestinal form can occur but their incidence is unknown.

Any differential diagnosis of anthrax must consider: staphylococcal contagious pustular dermatitis; in the tropics, cutaneous diphtheria and plague in cutaneous form; any pneumonia in respiratory form, and various enteric infections and sepsis in intestinal form. Recently a renal form has been described.

LABORATORY DIAGNOSIS

Diagnosis is by confirmation of *B. anthracis* in films made from pus, exudates from lesions, cerebrospinal fluid, discharges, or by direct microscopic examination. Bacilli are usually not present in the bloodstream in large numbers until just before death, but a blood specimen must be cultured.

The bacillus can be identified by fluorescent antibody techniques in tissue sections. Examination of paired sera by indirect microhemagglutination or ELISA may be helpful. (*Bacillus subtilis* group may resemble *B. anthracis* and *Bacillus cereus*; it has been found to produce a clinical picture similar to cutaneous anthrax.) The use of radioactively labeled antibodies for rapid detection (indirect immunoradiometric assay) has been reported.

TREATMENT

Procaine penicillin remains the drug of choice: 300,000 to 1.2 million units daily, divided into two intramuscular injections initially and continued as single daily doses thereafter for 7 days. However, in the cutaneous form, a shorter course may be equally effective. If penicillin G is used, doses should be increased. In pulmonary and septicemic forms, which have an unfavorable prognosis, 30 to 40 million units penicillin in infusion have been recommended. Also other broad-spectrum antibiotics, such as tetracyclines, chlortetracycline, erythromycin, aureomycin, achromycin, 3 g per day for 6 to 7 days, and streptomycin (30 mg per kilogram per day divided in two intramuscular injections), cephalosporins, and also trimethoprim-sulphamethoxazole, are fully effective. In plague endemic areas, streptomycin or tetracycline are recommended if diagnostic doubts exist. There is only limited experience with the newer aminoglycoside antibiotics. With antibiotic treatment, there should be no fatal cases with cutaneous anthrax. However, antibiotics have no effect on the toxin already produced. Antiserum is no longer used. Antibiotic ointments have no influence on the healing process. Skin transplantation after extensive cutaneous lesion may be necessary.

PREVENTION

Prevention of cutaneous, and probably inhalation, anthrax by immunization of high-risk persons with a cell-free vaccine prepared from a culture filtrate of a nonvirulent, nonencapsulated strain, containing the protective antigen, is possible. The best control measure is immunization of animals in endemic areas.

LEPROSY

WARD E. BULLOCK, M.D.

Leprosy continues to be one of the major unconquered infectious diseases of mankind. It is estimated that there are 12 to 15 million cases worldwide and that 25 percent of these individuals have incurred physical deformity as a consequence of the disease. The prevalence of leprosy is highest in geographic areas of greatest poverty (regardless of climate), where personal and public health control measures are limited.

The etiologic agent, *Mycobacterium leprae*, is an acid-alcohol-fast bacillus that has not yet been cultured successfully in a synthetic medium or in tissue culture. It does undergo limited multiplication in the footpads of mice. This model is used to determine the antibiotic susceptibility of *M. leprae*—the level of an antibiotic that must be maintained in blood to inhibit growth of the organism in the mouse footpad. *M. leprae* produces disseminated disease in the armadillo and in certain species of monkeys.

EPIDEMIOLOGY

The precise mechanism by which leprosy is spread remains elusive. Patients with lepromatous forms of disease, who carry large numbers of organisms, are believed to be the major source of spread. Nasal secretions of persons with untreated lepromatous leprosy contain up to 10^8 lepra bacilli per milliliter. Thus, others in close and repeated contact with an index case may be infected via the respiratory tract. Firm evidence to support this hypothesis, however, is lacking. Other possible means of transmission include human milk and biting insects in which *M. leprae* can survive for days to weeks. Large numbers of *M. leprae* are not shed from the intact skin surface even in the most advanced cases. Children appear to be more susceptible than adults.

Although a few cases of leprosy indigenous to the United States are detected each year, the vast majority of the 1,835 cases reported between 1971 and 1981 in the United States occurred in persons who were foreign. The most frequent countries of origin were Mexico, the Philippines, Puerto Rico, Vietnam, China, India, and American Somoa. The refugee resettlement programs for large numbers of Southeast Asians have distributed individuals from regions with fairly high prevalences of leprosy throughout the United States. Therefore, it behooves all practicing physicians caring for these individuals to be alert to the possibility of leprosy.

DIAGNOSIS

The *sine qua non* for diagnosis of leprosy is a meticulous examination of the entire skin surface under optimal lighting, preferably daylight. Any patches of depigmentation, plaques, macules, or nodules should bring leprosy to the forefront of diagnostic considerations, as should the presence of multiple burn scars over the hands, forearms, or lower extremities. If careful testing of the involved skin areas for perception of light touch, pain, and temperature indicates anesthesia or hypoesthesia and other causes are excluded, a presumptive diagnosis of leprosy can be made. Additional diagnostic support is provided by visualizing or palpating enlarged nerves that typically have a firm, rope-like consistency. Nerves that should be examined routinely are the lesser occipital, the greater auricular, the ulnar, and the peroneal.

Individuals with leprosy frequently manifest clinical findings secondary to nerve damage that always should raise the possibility of this disease. Commonest among these are (*1*) flexion deformities of the hands that produce claw-like appearance; (*2*) loss of ability to oppose the thumb; (*3*) footdrop; (*4*) shortening of the digits; (*5*) ulceration of weight-bearing areas of the foot; (*6*) corneal ulceration secondary to anesthesia of the ophthalmic division of the Vth cranial nerve; and (*7*) lagophthalmos secondary to involvement of the VIIth cranial nerve.

Leprosy is not an easily defined disease entity, but, rather, a broad spectrum of disease activities. Thus, an accurate assessment of individual cases with respect to a spectral classification of leprosy is important for prognosis and treatment. At one pole of the spectrum are people with tuberculoid forms of leprosy who generally are capable of mounting a cell-mediated immune (CMI) response to the leprosy bacillus. In fact, some of those with very limited disease are capable of self-cure without therapeutic intervention. Because the host CMI response in tuberculoid leprosy is relatively vigorous, motor and sensory deficits tend to be greater as a result of the damage produced by granulomatous inflammation within the nerve trunks. At the opposite pole of the leprosy spectrum is lepromatous leprosy, a severe form of the disease. Persons with diffuse lepromatous leprosy may be deceptively normal in their appearance except for a diffuse sheen or thickened appearance to the skin. Since they are unable to mount an effective CMI response to the enormous numbers of acid-fast bacilli that infiltrate their tissues, they generally suffer less extensive nerve damage. Likewise, the skin lesions, except for certain allergic reactions, generally are less active or inflammatory in appearance. Loss of eyebrows, epistaxis, thickened facies, and testicular atrophy are all late signs of lepromatous leprosy.

Definitive diagnosis requires performance of a generous skin biopsy of sufficient depth to obtain subcutaneous tissue. The pathology of tuberculoid forms of leprosy is characterized by well-formed, mature granulomas within the dermis that resemble those observed in sarcoidosis. Organisms are difficult to detect within these granulomas even with special techniques, such as the Wade-Fite stain, to preserve the acid-fastness of the lepra bacilli. The finding of granulomatous inflammation within nerve twigs of the dermis is strongly suggestive of leprosy since no other bacterial disease of humans attacks nerves directly. In lepromatous leprosy, the inflammatory response within the dermis is poorly organized, consisting of sheets of macrophages, many of which are vacuolated. Large clumps of acid-staining bacilli are present within these vacuoles.

DIFFERENTIAL DIAGNOSIS

In the United States, leprosy frequently is mistaken for a variety of other conditions including nonspecific dermatitis, ringworm, arthritis, and allergic reactions, including arteritis. Failure to recognize that erythema nodosum-like lesions are a frequent manifestation of lepromatous leprosy is a common cause of diagnostic error. Of note is that erythema nodosum leprosum (ENL) is typically distributed over the entire body, including the face, torso, and upper extremities. In other conditions associated with classic erythema nodosum, the nodular rash is usually confined to the lower extremities.

TREATMENT

All forms of leprosy should be treated with a multiple antibiotic regimen. The necessity for use of such a regimen stems from the fact that the prevalence of acquired resistance to dapsone by *M. leprae* is increasing throughout the world. Moreover, resistant organisms are being transmitted, as evidenced by the appearance of primary dapsone resistance among patients with lepromatous leprosy.

In patients with tuberculoid forms (pauci-bacillary) of leprosy, the load of lepra bacilli is relatively small. Thus, a relatively short course of chemotherapy is feasible. As a minimum, the World Health Organization (WHO) recommends treatment with rifampin, 600 mg by mouth once a month for 6 months, plus dapsone, 100 mg (1 to 2 mg per kilogram body weight [1 mg per kilogram for a large person, 2 mg per kilogram for a small person] by mouth daily for 6 months. The rifampin administration should be supervised. If the treatment regimen is interrupted, it should be restarted at the point where it was stopped to complete a full course. The long-term efficacy of intermittent rifampin administration for treatment of pauci-bacillary leprosy has not been established fully. Therefore, it is the author's practice to treat these cases with rifampin, 450 mg (small person) or 600 mg (large) by mouth daily for 6 months, and to continue dapsone as recommended above for a period of 2 or more years (for more severe forms of leprosy, treatment is longer; see below). Patients should be checked on a regular basis for satisfactory progress, for evidence of neuritis or reactional activity, and for possible adverse effects of drugs. After completion of therapy, they should be examined annually for 4 years. Retreatment is on the basis of failure of symptoms to resolve.

Lepromatous forms (multibacillary) of leprosy present a serious therapeutic challenge and should be treated with a triple-drug regimen according to the following minimum WHO recommendations: (*1*) rifampin, 600 mg by mouth once a month under supervision; (*2*) dapsone, 100 mg by mouth daily, self-administered; (*3*) clofazimine (Lamprene), 300 mg by mouth once a month under supervision and 50 mg daily by mouth, self-administered. Clofazimine currently is an investigational drug for treatment of leprosy in the United States. However, it is recognized worldwide as a principal antileprosy drug by virtue of its potent inhibitory effect on the growth of *M. leprae*. Clofazimine is available on an individual basis from the National Hansen's Disease Center, Carville, Louisiana (telephone 504-642-7771). The drug is very lipophilic and is deposited mostly in the fatty tissues and cells of the reticuloendothelial system. The compound is a red dye and, therefore, produces a dose-related pigmentation of the skin that ranges in color from pink to purplish black. Pigmentaion is most noticeable over exposed areas of the skin and is slowly reversible after cessation of therapy. In patients who refuse clofazimine for reasons of pigmentation, substitution of ethionamide should be considered in a self-administered dosage of 250 to 375 mg by mouth daily (on the basis of body size).

Combined therapy should be given for at least 2 years and, if possible, until all skin smears become negative for the presence of acid-fast bacilli. Smears of skin scrapings are a valuable means by which to follow the course of treatment. They are performed at intervals of approximately 6 months, always in the same skin sites, e.g., the ears, elbows, and knees. By means of these smears the clinician can determine the morphologic index (MI), a crude estimate of the viability of organisms, as well as the numbers of bacilli (the bacteriologic index, BI). Generally, 3 to 5 years of antibiotic therapy are required for the BI to become negative in lepromatous leprosy.

Since the WHO recommendation for intermittent rifampin therapy is based on data that are still incomplete, the author prefers to administer the drug in a dosage of 450 to 600 mg by mouth (on the basis of body size) for 2 years to patients with lepromatous leprosy, if possible. During treatment, patients with multibacillary disease should be checked monthly to ensure satisfactory progress, to check for drug toxicity, and to monitor for onset of neuritis and other reactions outlined below. Those failing to demonstrate clear improvement in skin lesions after documented combined therapy for a period of 6 months should be considered for referral to a leprosy treatment center to be evaluated for the possibility of drug resistance. After the therapy of lepromatous patients has been completed, they should be examined for recurrence annually for a period of 8 years.

ADVERSE REACTONS TO ANTILEPROSY DRUGS

Dapsone

Dapsone is a relatively nontoxic drug that also appears to be safe to administer during pregnancy. The side effect observed most frequently is a mild hemolytic anemia. Dapsone is more hemolytic to erythrocytes deficient in glucose-6-phosphate dehydrogenase (G6PD). Therefore, patients should be screened for this deficiency, and, if it is present, dapsone treatment must be instituted with considerable caution. Other reactions to dapsone that occur uncommonly are agranulocytosis, hepatitis, exfoliative dermatitis, and, rarely, severe hypoalbuminemia.

Rifampin

Rifampin as intermittent therapy for tuberculosis on a weekly or biweekly basis has been associated with adverse reactions. However, with the once monthly regimen of rifampin for treatment of leprosy, the prevalence of serious reactions such as thrombocytopenic purpura, shock, renal failure, or the less severe influenza-like syndrome has been very low. Rifampin may cause hepatitis with diffuse hepatic cell damage, most commonly during early phases of administration. Preliminary screening of hepatic function, therefore, is advisable, especially in immigrants from Southeast Asia, who may manifest chronic active hepatitis more frequently in association with a high prevalence of chronic hepatitis virus B surface antigenemia (approximately 10% to 12%). Rifampin is a potent inducer of drug metabolism by the liver and is known to diminish the pharmacologic effects of oral contraceptives, warfarin, glucocorticoids, digitoxin, quinidine, hypoglycemic agents, and others. Consequently, increased dosages of these drugs may be required during rifampin therapy.

Clofazimine

Aside from its troublesome staining of the skin, side effects caused by this drug are uncommon when it is given in dosages of 100 mg per day or less. If higher dosages of 300 to 400 mg per day are required to treat persistent reactional states in leprosy (see below), gastrointestinal adverse reactions may be encountered. These include nausea, vomiting, and anorexia. Clofazimine crystals are deposited in the submucosa of the small intestine and, rarely, can produce colicky abdominal pain and symptoms of obstruction secondary to edema of the bowel wall. With very high dosages of clofazimine over prolonged periods, linear brownish streaks on the cornea of the eye have been observed. These streaks appear to produce no functional disturbance and the changes are reversible.

Ethionamide

Gastrointestinal adverse effects are the commonest. These include a metallic taste, anorexia, nausea, and vomiting. Mental disturbances such as depression, asthenia, and anxiety may be encountered. The drug may cause hepatitis with cellular necrosis, and concomitant administration of rifampin increases the risk of hepatotoxicity.

TREATMENT OF REACTIONS IN LEPROSY

Two major classes of reactions may be encountered during the treatment of leprosy. The first of these is erythema nodosum leprosum (ENL) that is observed only in those with lepromatous forms of disease. It occurs in up to 50 percent of cases, usually during the first year of two of therapy. ENL is an Arthus-like reaction believed to be precipitated by release of *M. leprae* antigens in tissues, with local antigen-antibody-complex formation that triggers a panniculitis. Although ENL tends to be transient, frequently it is recurrent, and in severe cases it may be life threatening. In association with ENL, patients may experience one or more of the following: neuritis, polyarthritis, orchitis, iridocyclitis, and glomerulonephritis.

Steroids are effective as acute therapy for severe ENL. Initially, the author uses prednisone, 80 mg per day, with cautious tapering over a 3- to 4-week period to lessen the chance of flare-up. Thalidomide also is very effective in treating severe ENL at an initial dosage of 200 mg by mouth twice daily. Usually the drug can be tapered over several weeks to maintain levels of 50 to 100 mg per day in individuals prone to recurrent ENL. In severe cases, the combination of a steroid and thalidomide is quite effective and allows the steroid to be tapered with less chance of rebound. Thalidomide is an investigational drug for the treatment of ENL in the United States. It can be obtained by special arrangement with the National Hansen's Disease Center after approval by the Committee on Human Research of a local hospital. Because of its teratogenicity, thalidomide is not recommended for treatment of women who are of childbearing age. It is absolutely contraindicated in pregnancy. The adverse effect most commonly reported is drowsiness; ankle edema, blood eosinophilia, and peripheral neuropathy also have been associated with thalidomide administration.

High-dosage clofazimine therapy (300 to 400 mg per day; 400 mg to start, decrease if not tolerated) also is useful in the management of ENL, although 4 to 6 weeks may be required to achieve an effect. It has been employed in lieu of thalidomide for control of ENL during pregnancy.

A second type of inflammatory response experienced by leprosy patients is the so-called reversal reaction. Such reactions occur predominantly among patients whose disease classification falls within the middle of the leprosy spectrum, namely, those with more extensive tuberculoid leprosy and those with less severe forms of lepromatous leprosy. In contrast to ENL, reversal reactions are slow to develop and last for weeks to months. These reactions appear as indurated, erythematous areas within the skin. Usually, they indicate improvement in the patient's CMI response to *M. leprae*. Frequently however, the inflammatory response of reversal reaction also takes place in peripheral nerves, thereby producing severe neuritis and further loss of nerve function if untreated.

Steroids in high dosage are the therapy of choice. However, these reactions are more persistent than ENL and generally require prolonged anti-inflammatory treatment. Thalidomide is ineffective in reversal reactions. Clofazimine (300 to 400 mg per day; as above) has been reported by some to exert an anti-inflammatory effect upon these reactions. Concomitant administration of clofazimine and steroids may permit the latter to be discontinued after careful tapering or to be employed at a lower dosage than otherwise would be the case.

TREATMENT OF OTHER COMPLICATIONS

Plantar ulceration secondary to sensory loss responds well to medical and surgical management that prohibits bearing weight on the involved area. Once ulcers have healed, the patient must be provided with custom-designed footwear to distribute pressure more evenly over the weight-bearing surface. Excellent surgical procedures are available for correction of hand deformities, for correction of footdrop, and for repair of facial damage, including the replacement of eyebrows. The eye is especially prone to damage in leprosy. In lepromatous patients, iridocyclitis is an insidious and painless complication that requires treatment with mydriatics and steroids to prevent destruction of the ciliary body. Trichiasis (inverted eyelashes) and lagophthalmos are complications that require correction to prevent blindness. Treatment is critical in individuals with corneal anesthesia secondary to leprotic damage of the ophthalmic division of the Vth cranial nerve.

PREVENTION

A multidrug regimen for treatment of patients with multibacillary disease rapidly decreases the number of viable organisms in secretions and tissues. This is determined by the physical appearance of bacilli and their failure to multiply when injected into the footpads of mice. Hence, lepromatous patients can be considered to be noninfectious after receiving therapy for only a few weeks. Even in the untreated patient with lepromatous leprosy, the risk of contagion is so low that isolation procedures are not required for those who may require initial hospitalization.

Individuals who are household contacts of leprosy cases, especially children, should be examined for signs of leprosy and biopsy specimens obtained for any suspicious skin lesions. Dapsone prophylaxis is not recommended for adult household contacts. Previously, dapsone administration has been shown to be of prophylactic value in children under the age of 16 years who have had household exposure to multibacillary disease. Although it may be advisable to administer dapsone prophylaxis to children under these conditions at the present time, recently developed techniques for quantitation of serum antibodies to *M. leprae*-specific antigens may make it possible to render prophylaxis more selectively in the relatively near future. This author makes the decision to use or not use prophylaxis on a case by case basis. When dapsone prophylaxis is used, the dosage is according to the following: older than 12 years, 50 mg daily; 6 to 12 years, 25 mg daily; 2 to 5 years, 25 mg three times per week; 6 to 23 months, 12 mg three times per week; younger than 6 months, 6 mg three times per week. Dapsone is available as 50- and 25-mg tablets; for pediatric use these can be crushed and dissolved in syrup. Although the degree of protection against clinical leprosy afforded by BCG vaccination is variable, it is the author's practice to vaccinate tuberculin-negative children who are household contacts of multibacillary cases.

NOCARDIAL INFECTION

EDWARD J. SEPTIMUS, M.D.
RICHARD J. WALLACE, Jr., M.D.

EPIDEMIOLOGY

Nocardia is an environmental organism that is an infrequent serious pathogen except in patients with specific underlying diseases or who have received immunosuppressive drugs. Clinical disease is produced by any of three *Nocardia* species: *N. asteroides, N. brasiliensis*, or *N. caviae*.

Four clinical syndromes due to *Nocardia* are recognized: primary cutaneous disease, pulmonary infections, disseminated disease, and central nervous system disease. Although several of these disease states can coexist, this separation is useful for both prognostic and therapeutic reasons.

Primary cutaneous disease is usually due to *N. brasiliensis* and occurs as a consequence of local inoculation into the skin. A suppurative, pyodermatous lesion, often with surrounding cellulitis, is the commonest type of infection. Ascending subcutaneous nodules can occur, a finding referred to as sporotrichoid nocardia. The patients usually have no underlying disease, dissemination of the infection is rare, and recovery without specific therapy is not uncommon.

Pulmonary disease, usually due to *N. asteroides*, is the commonest type of nocardial disease. The use of corticosteroids is the predisposing factor in the majority of patients. Cancer, alcoholism, chronic lung disease, and pulmonary alveolar proteinosis can be associated with nocardiosis in the absence of corticosteroids. The majority of patients will have one or more of these predisposing factors. Fever followed by productive cough is the usual disease presentation.

Disseminated disease and CNS disease almost always occur in the setting of pulmonary *Nocardia*, although infrequent cases of CNS disease have no detectable pulmonary infiltrate. The commonest sites of dissemination with pulmonary disease are skin and brain, and these occur in approximately 10 to 20 percent of patients. Patients with nocardial brain abscess will present with headache, fever, nausea, and vomiting, as with brain abscess due to other organisms.

DIAGNOSIS

Nocardia elicits an intense pyogenic response, so draining material is usually available from skin or sputum. The organism appears as beaded, branched gram-positive filaments that occur in small clumps in a background of many white blood cells. It is weakly acid-fast, and its acid fastness can be demonstrated in samples with 1 percent-acid decolorization or in tissue by the use of the Fite's stain. The organism grows best on blood or chocolate agar as fuzzy white colonies in 2 to 5 days. It will also grow well on Lowenstein-Jensen medium, but Sabaroud's medium should be avoided, since many strains grow poorly or not at all on it. If suspected, the organism can almost always be detected after 48 hours growth with a dissecting microscope (40×), appearing as white, fungal-like colonies.

For patients with pulmonary disease, the chest roentgenogram is often helpful. The majority of patients show nodular alveolar infiltrates that may undergo cavitation, frequently with an air-fluid level. The presence of one or more nodular infiltrates with air-fluid levels in patients on high-dose steroids is highly suggestive, almost diagnostic, of nocardiosis. In some patients, however, the disease can look like a regular bacterial pneumonia.

The majority of patients with pulmonary nocardiosis can be diagnosed on the basis of expectorated sputa. Because of the pyogenic nature of the disease, purulent sputum is produced by almost all patients, and the organism is usually easily demonstrated by gram stain when examined by an experienced observer. Occasionally, bronchoscopy with sterile brushings may be necessary. Invasive techniques such as needle aspiration or lung biopsy are rarely necessary with adequate laboratory facilities and use of the Gram stain.

THERAPY

Before the discovery of sulfonamides, pulmonary nocardiosis was almost invariably fatal. More recent studies show a dramatic improvement with a mortality rate now of less than 25 percent. Primary cutaneous and pulmonary nocardiosis usually respond well to therapy, while central nervous system nocardiosis is a more serious disease and less responsive to antimicrobial agents. Sulfonamides remain the treatment of choice for all types of nocardiosis. There is no good evidence that one sulfonamide preparation is clinically superior to another. Despite their historical importance, sulfadiazine and triple-sulfa should be avoided, since they are highly insoluble, and urinary complications are common with high doses. Despite the demonstration of in vitro synergy of trimethoprim and sulfamethoxazole, there are no comparative clinical data to prove the superiority of the combination over that of sulfisoxazole or sulfamethoxazole alone. The potential increased toxicity of the combination must be weighed against the theoretical advantage of the in vitro synergy. The daily doses of these agents are shown in Table 1. Necessary serum levels of sulfonamide have not been established, despite the traditional reference to the need for 150 to 200 μg per ml (15 to 20 mg per 100 ml). We think that serum levels between 75 and 150 μg per ml (7.5 to 15 mg per 100 ml) are clearly adequate.

Ampicillin in vitro inhibits approximately 40 percent of strains. Ampicillin has been effective, either alone or in combination with erythromycin in a limited number of patients. The combination of amoxicillin/clavulanic acid is also active against many strains of *N. asteroides* and

TABLE 1 Therapy for Nocardiosis

Regimen	Daily Adult Dose	Method of Administration
Drugs of choice		
Sulfamethoxazole	3.0 g (50 mg/kg)	PO
or		
Sulfisoxazole*	6–8 g (100 mg/kg)	PO
Alternative drugs†		
Trimethoprim-sulfamethoxazole	480/2,400 mg (50 mg/kg of SMZ)	PO
Ampicillin-amoxicillin	2.0 g	PO
Erythromycin	2.0 g	PO
Minocycline	300 mg	PO
Doxycycline	300 mg	PO
Amikacin	15 mg/kg	IV
Cefotaxime	175 mg/kg	IV

* These are therapeutically equivalent.
† Should be based on in vitro susceptibilities except for TMP/SMZ.

TABLE 2 Duration of Therapy

Type of Nocardiosis	Preferred	Minimum
Primary cutaneous disease	12 weeks	6 weeks
Pulmonary, disseminated disease without CNS involvement	6 months	4 months
CNS disease	12 months	6 months

all strains of *N. brasiliensis* in vitro. Although it offers a greater therapeutic potential than ampicillin alone, there has been only one report of its use clinically.

Amikacin is the most active agent other than the sulfonamides, inhibiting more than 90 percent of strains at 1 μg per ml or less; however, clinical experience is very limited, and, therefore, it cannot be recommended as single-drug therapy.

Of the tetracyclines, minocycline has consistently demonstrated that best in vitro activity, inhibiting approximately 90 percent of strains by 3.1 μg per ml. A dose of 300 mg per day is generally recommended for treatment. Limited clinical experience suggests that this drug may be useful for the patient allergic to sulfonamides.

Some of the new beta-lactam antibiotics (cefotaxime, cefuroxime, and imipenem, but not moxalactam) appear to be active in vitro. Minimal clinical experience has been favorable with cefotaxime, which has the added advantage of having good penetration into the CNS. The major disadvantage of these beta-lactams, as well as of amikacin, is that they are parenteral agents for a disease in which long-term therapy is usually necessary. For patients who are unable to tolerate sulfonamides, susceptibility testing is essential to choose optimal alternative agents. This can be performed by disk diffusion on Mueller-Hinton agar, or by an MIC dilution method. Cefotaxime and amikacin are the best agents to use empirically while awaiting results of susceptibility testing.

The duration of treatment will vary with the type of disease (Table 2). Six to 12 weeks are usually sufficient to treat primary cutaneous nocardiosis, while 4 to 6 months are required for isolated pulmonary and most forms of disseminated nocardiosis that do not involve the CNS. CNS disease remains the most challenging and difficult to treat. Therapy should probably be continued for 6 to 12 months. Aspiration and/or surgical drainage of isolated brain abscesses is an important, often essential, adjunct to antimicrobial therapy. Decrease or discontinuation of immunosuppressive drugs is probably important, but not essential, in successful therapy.

The mortality in patients with nocardiosis varies with the type and extent of disease. Approximately 90 percent of patients with pulmonary disease will survive, with death usually a result of overwhelming pneumonia with respiratory failure or medical complications. The mortality in patients with CNS nocardia is 50 percent, a figure that results from the frequent poor response of this disease to sulfonamides alone and problems with drainage.

ACTINOMYCOSIS

ROBERT L. PERKINS, M.D.

Actinomycosis in humans is a chronic suppurative infection, most often caused by *Actinomyces israelii*. Rare causative species include *A. naeslundii*, *A. viscosus*, *A. odontolyticus*, and a related but serologically distinct organism, *Arachnia propionica*. Occasional cases initially present with acute or subacute cellulitis or organ involvement. Sources for infection are endogenous, primarily from mucosal or paramucosal structures including surfaces of teeth, tonsils, the gastrointestinal tract and the cervicovaginal vault. The presence of dental plaque or caries, dentogingival disease, foreign bodies in the gastrointestinal tract, intrauterine devices, and coincidental trauma or surgical manipulation of colonized areas may presage the development of local actinomycotic invasion. Aspiration of upper airway mucosal secretions and debris containing actinomycetes may lead to pulmonary-thoracic infection. Any disease of mucosal structures or related organ systems resulting in chronic anatomical or functional changes may predispose to this infection. Opportunism by actinomycetes in patients with chronic illnesses, malignancies, or immunosuppression due to other causes has been observed.

SITES OF INFECTION

Cervicofacial

The initial lesion, usually submandibular in location, may be asymptomatic or mildly painful and may enlarge slowly or more acutely in occasional cases. Although lymph node involvement is unusual, adenopathy and submandibular or parotid gland adenitis may be simulated. Untreated, the pyogenic process extends across tissue and fascial planes, evolving into an abscess. Contiguous involvement of the thyroid gland, larynx, lacrimal gland, orbit and contents, and bones, and eruption through the skin aptly demonstrate the capacity for local spread and sinus formation.

Thoracic

Recognition of pulmonary infection is often delayed. Irregular and chronic dense infiltrates occur in the presence of relatively nonspecific symptoms suggestive of chronic illness. The lesions are commonly suspected to represent tuberculous or fungal infection or malignancy. Hemoptysis or radiographic evidence of parenchymal cavitation may become prominent. Late extension to the pleural space, chest wall, ribs or vertebrae, and muscles—with sinus formation—are typical in a small percentage of cases. Hematogenous dissemination from thoracopulmonary sites may lead to infection of distant organs including the central nervous system.

Abdominal

Ileocecal infection is characteristic of most cases, although secondary spread to contiguous adjacent bowel, abdominal wall, or solid organs results in a variety of clinical presentations. Prior abdominal surgery for acute or chronic inflammatory bowel diseases is typical. The relationship of the antecedent disorder or procedure to the actinomycosis is frequently unknown. Chronic abdominal pain, evidence of partial bowel obstruction, or a mass lesion simulating tumor commonly leads to surgical intervention. Anorectal infection with perianal extension and sinuses may occur alone or may accompany ileocecal actinomycosis. Infection of other gastrointestinal locations is significantly less common except that involvement of the liver by contiguity or via the portal-venous route must be excluded in each case.

Pelvic

Association of localized or extensive pelvic infection with intrauterine contraceptive devices (IUDs) or pessaries has been recognized relatively recently. Endometrial tissue injury due to the IUDs may provide conditions suitable for actinomycete proliferation after introduction from the vagina or perineal surfaces. Involvement of adnexa, ovaries, tubes, and bowel may cause pain, fever, mass effect, or bowel obstruction. Sinuses and fistulae may occur.

Central Nervous System

Infection of brain after hematogenous dissemination commonly presents as a single hemispheric abscess that may be multiloculated. Extension from primary cervicofacial lesions across cranial bones and meninges to cerebral tissue has occurred in chronic cases. Microbiologic evaluation of cultured material from brain lesions must carefully exclude the presence of accompanying organisms.

DIAGNOSIS

The anatomic locations and physical characteristics of evolving lesions noted at the bedside or radiographically should stimulate the alert clinician to pursue the possibility of actinomycosis. Notably, suppuration, sinuses, and scarring ("the three S's") along with microscopic evidence of abscess formation, granulation tissue, and fibrosis should trigger the search. Lesions may exude typical macroscopic sulfur granules, individual ray fungi, or thin gram-positive filaments. Beaded gram-stained filaments may also resemble diphtheroids or *Nocardia* and less often may be confused with *Lactobacillus* or *Listeria*. Further differentiation of *Actinomyces* and *Nocardia* on the basis of partial acid-fast staining of the latter is useful. In occasional patients, the etiologic diagnosis of actinomycosis may in retrospect rest solely on the results of stained materials, since inadequate or improperly handled patient samples and cultures can yield false-negative results. The fastidious anaerobic or facultative anaerobic requirements of *Actinomyces*, especially if accompanied by inadvertent antibiotic therapy that may suppress in vitro growth, also contribute to problems in laboratory confirmation. Specific fluorescent antibody staining of patient samples is feasible, but currently serves as a laboratory serotyping method. Thus, recovery of the infecting organism in anaerobic cultures may require repeated careful sampling of exteriorized lesions or even biopsies while withholding antibiotic therapy. These circumstances underscore the importance of planning and of initial processing of material from sites not amenable to repeated sampling, such as visceral abscesses, intraperitoneal pus, or major organ sections. Successful recovery of an actinomycete from an appropriate sample, with species identification by appropriate biochemical tests and chromatographic patterns, confirms the clinical diagnosis.

Visualization of microscopic forms consistent with *Actinomyces* in stained oropharyngeal samples or even bronchopulmonary secretions may be considered uncertain evidence unless they are clearly associated with a pyogenic response and consistent clinical findings. Similarly, positive cultures of such secretions may indicate normal residence or colonization of those mucosal surfaces. The meaning of positive biopsy cultures from such anatomic sites is usually clarified by the histopathology revealed in microsections.

TREATMENT

The essentials of initial therapy include prolonged, high-dosage penicillin G and carefully selected surgical procedures. It should be emphasized that zealous surgical intervention, especially for cervicofacial infection, may be unnecessary and may yield unsatisfactory cosmetic results. Initial incision for diagnostic sampling and drainage usually is essential for closed lesions. Similarly, large collections of pus in any location require drainage, and life-threatening lesions must be dealt with surgically as necessary. Excision of fibrosed granulation tissue should be discouraged. Decisions regarding elective extensive debridement, resections of visceral abscesses, or removal of infected organs should be reasonably delayed to allow maximal response to antibiotic therapy. Sound judgment on the timing of elective major surgical interventions usually involves an expectant attitude based on past observations in other patients of slow but favorable responses to nonsurgical therapy.

Intravenous penicillin G should be administered to adults for 6 weeks. Modest-to-moderately severe cervicofacial infections usually respond to 5 g (8 million units) per day in four divided doses. Extensive infections of soft tissues, the lungs, or intra-abdominal sites will require 10 g (16 million units) per day in four divided doses. Specialized problems such as intracerebral abscesses, acute cerebritis, ophthalmitis, or extensive involvement of other relatively inaccessible sites may require 15 g (24 million units) per day given in divided doses as frequently as every 2 hours.

Favorable responses to parenteral penicillin with obvious resolution of masses and closure of sinuses should be followed by oral phenoxymethyl penicillin 2 to 4 g (3.2 to 6.4 million units) per day, depending upon tolerance, for 6 to 12 months. Patient intolerance may occasionally limit the size of individual oral doses to 0.5 g. Compliance by patients over a long treatment period may be improved by an every 8 hour rather than an every 6 hour schedule. The higher more frequent dosage is recommended (1 g every 6 hours).

Alternate agents may be required because of penicillin allergy or discovery of the actinomycosis may occur after an already-favorable response to one or more such drugs. In that regard, in vitro susceptibility data indicate high activity of a variety of beta-lactams, tetracyclines, macrolides, lincomycins, sulfonamides, and chloramphenicol. Although agreement is incomplete among investigators as to all the methodologic aspects of *Actinomyces* susceptibility testing, the collective data derived is generally agreed to indicate little variation in responses among various first-line antimicrobials. Innumerable reports of treatment cures using all of the mentioned penicillin alternates attest to the clinical relevance of the in vitro results. However, the utility and effectiveness of clindamycin, and tetracycline to a lesser extent, dictate their use as the two alternate agents of choice. Intravenous clindamycin, 1,200 to 4,200 mg per day (17 to 34 mg per kilogram per day) divided in doses every 6 to 8 hours may be given to adults (average, 70 kg) during the initial acute phase, followed by oral administration of 900 to 1,800 mg per day (13 to 25 mg per kilogram per day) divided every 6 to 8 hours. The higher dosage ranges are recommended only for life-threatening or disseminated forms of the disease. Intravenous tetracycline hydrochloride, 1 to 2 g per day divided every 6 or 12 hours, may be given initially to adults for 1 or more weeks, but local venous intolerance or other adverse effects may limit use of the high dose intravenous route. Oral tetracycline, 1.5 to 2 g per day, in divided doses every 6 to 8 hours may be tolerated for an extended period. However, gastrointestinal intolerance may require use of the lowest oral dosage ranges for either tetracycline or clindamycin. Neither clindamycin or tetracycline should be used for central nervous system involvement or other highly inaccessible sites. Actinomycete meningitis in the penicillin-allergic patient may require use of a third-generation parenteral cephalosporin, such as cefotaxime or ceftriaxone, known to enter the cerebrospinal fluid. If a cross-reaction with a cephalosporin is anticipated, consideration of chloramphenicol may be appropriate. Metronidazole may be applicable in the rare instances of ventriculitis because of known high penetration. Awareness of the potential for development of antibiotic-induced colitis and superinfections is important, especially with high-dose long-term treatment with any of the agents for actinomycosis.

Antibiotic treatment failures should cause consideration of possibilities such as (*1*) undrained pus; (*2*) unrecognized foreign body, sinus tract, fistula, bony sequestrium, or coexistent malignancy; (*3*) poor oral absorption of antimicrobic agent or poor patient compliance; and (4) unrecognized concomitant infection. Acquisition of antibiotic resistance by *Actinomyces* during treatment has not been adequately documented as a cause of therapeutic failure.

TULAREMIA

TOM MADHAVAN, M.D., F.A.C.P.

Tularemia, also known as rabbit fever, deerfly fever, and Ohara's disease, is an acute infectious disease caused by *Francisella tularensis*, a very small coccoid, aerobic gram-negative bacillus. This organism is predominately infectious for wild mammals and blood sucking anthropods. In humans, this disease is characterized by high fever and severe constitutional symptoms that may persist for weeks to several months. Initially, this disease was discovered in Tulare, California, and is endemic in the central and southwestern United States. Since 1975, 30 people have died in the United States. In 1983, 40 patients contacted the disease.

The organism is widely distributed in nature, predominately in wild mammals—for example, rabbits, hares, squirrels, muskrats—occasionally in domestic animals, and in many anthropods such as ticks, deerflies, and mosquitoes. The most important reservoir hosts are the cottontail white rabbits and ticks. The rabbit-associated infection (type A) tends to be more virulent than rodent-associated illness (type B).

Tularemia is transmitted to humans by direct contact with infected animals or by the insect vectors—wood ticks (*Dermacentor andersoni*) or fleas. Humans are highly susceptible to the disease, and it is frequently seen in hunters, butchers, and housewives.

The incubation period is 3 to 7 days, followed by the sudden onset of flu-like symptoms. A primary lesion may be present. If so, regional lymphadenopathy will be present and may become tender, fluctuant, erythematous, and suppurative. Rarely, a generalized maculopapular rash is seen.

The clinical manifestations of tularemia are highly variable. There are several forms of the disease. The ulceroglandular form is the commonest, occurring in 80 percent of all reported cases. This form presents with a slow healing ulcer at the site of entry and painful regional lymphadenopathy. The ulcers usually occur in the hands or lower extremities with localized lymphadenopathy. This form of infection is often caused by handling infected animal carcasses or from the bite of an infected tick or flea.

Oculoglandular tularemia is manifested by conjunctivitis, with edema, congestion, photophobia, pain, and lacrimation. Regional lymphadenopathy is present with suppuration. This results from direct contamination of the eyes with infected material.

Gastroenteritis may also occur following ingestion of contaminated meat. Typhoidal tularemia is a severe form of the disease and difficult to diagnose. It occurs following ingestion of the organism. Lymphadenopathy is usually not seen, but severe constitutional symptoms are present. Pneumonia can be a complication of all forms of tularemia. It is usually hematogenous, but can occur from inhaling an infectious aerosol or dust. Severe tularemia accompanied by pneumonia or pleuritis has a poor prognosis. Rarely, other forms such as endocarditis, meningitis, osteomyelitis, and pericarditis are seen.

Diagnosis is based primarily on clinical suspicion. Both Gram stain and routine culturing are often difficult in a hospital microbiology laboratory. Hence, repeated negative cultures do not rule out the disease. Positive diagnosis is made retrospectively by serologic identification. A fourfold rise in the tularemia agglutination titer is diagnostic of infection. A single convalescent titer of greater than or equal to 1:160 by currently available serologic methods is diagnostic of past or current infection. More often the serologic tests are negative during the acute phase of illness and are positive after 2 weeks of illness. The titers may also remain elevated at diagnostic levels for many years after the acute episode. Even though a skin test may be of some help, it is not commercially available. Tularemia agglutinins may cross-react with *Brucella* antigens, but may not be positive until the end of the second week.

Prevention of tularemia involves avoiding skinning or eviscerating rabbits and other wild mammals, especially if they appear ill. Wearing gloves while performing such tasks reduces the risk of infection. Avoidance of tick bites and immediate removal of the tick from the body will help prevent infection. Insect repellents such as diethyltoluamide or dimethylphthalate may be of value for persons whose occupation or vocation results in repeated tick exposures. The inactivated tularemia vaccine administered intradermally by multiple puncture technique is effective, but does not provide complete protection.

For infected patients, streptomycin hydrochloride is the drug of choice for all forms of tularemia. Streptomycin, 15 to 20 mg per kilogram per day intramuscularly in two divided doses for 7 to 10 days, is effective. For severe infections, larger doses (30 to 50 mg per kilogram) may be given for 2 to 3 days, followed by 15 to 20 mg per kilogram per day. Streptomycin is primarily ototoxic in elderly patients, so this must be monitored carefully. Gentamicin (5 mg per kilogram per day) is an acceptable alternative to streptomycin. Tetracyclines or chloramphenicol may also be given, but clinical relapses occur more frequently with these compounds, particularly when administered for less than 2 weeks. A loading dose of tetracyclines or chloramphenicol, 30 mg per kilogram orally, is given followed by 30 mg per kilogram per day orally in four divided doses for 14 days. Tetracycline is preferably avoided in pregnant women in the last trimester, in patients with azotemia, and also in children prior to permanent dentition. Chloramphenicol carries the risk of dose-related bone marrow depression and occasional aplastic anemia.

LEPTOSPIROSIS

CARLOS E. LOPEZ, M.D.

Leptospirosis is an acute febrile illness caused by pathogenic members of the genus *Leptospira*. Although it exists primarily as an endemic zoonosis, infection in humans occurs and may at times be severe. Since clinical manifestations may vary greatly, diagnosis rests on a high index of suspicion based on epidemiologic history. Confirmatory testing is possible, but requires attention to the inherent microbial characteristics of the leptospire and proper timing of clinical specimens. Although the antimicrobial therapy of leptospirosis has for a long time been a subject of controversy, recent work has shown conclusive evidence of benefit in human infection. Figure 1 summarizes the approach to diagnosis and management of the patient with suspected leptospirosis.

EPIDEMIOLOGY

Leptospirosis exists primarily as a zoonotic infection, affecting a wide range of wild and domesticated animals. Infection in humans occurs accidentally, usually as a result of either occupational or recreational exposure. Infected animals are known to excrete viable leptospires in the urine in large numbers and may continue to do so for a long time after an acute infection. Under favorable conditions of humidity, warmth (about 25 °C), and a neutral or alkaline pH, leptospires may survive in urine-infected surface waters for several weeks and in infected soil for about 15 days. Although urine probably serves as the main vehicle maintaining the zoonotic reservoir of infection with leptospires in nature, venereal transmission through infected semen is known to occur among some animal species and may play a role in disease transmission among these.

Leptospira belong to the Spirochaetaceae and pathogenic strains are grouped under the species complex *L. interrogans* which consists of about 160 different serovariants (serovars). Based on antigenic relationships and for epidemiologic and diagnostic purposes, serovars are grouped together into serogroups. During a 6-year period (1973–1978), 733 cases of leptospirosis were reported to the United States Centers for Disease Control, and of these, the infecting serogroup was known for 575 cases. The commonest serogroups implicated were *icterohemorrhagiae* (150 cases), *canicola* (67), *autumnalis* (50), *grippotyphosa* (32), *hebdomadis* (30), *australis* (23), *pomona* (20), and *ballum* (16). Although some serogroups have in the past been associated with specific clinical syndromes (e.g., Weil's disease or icterohemorrhagic fever with *L. icterohemorrhagiae* and "Fort Bragg" or "pretibial fever" with *L. autumnalis*), it is now apparent that there is no clinical syndrome that can be linked exclusively to a specific serotype. For example, severe icteric leptospirosis (Weil's disease) can be caused by various leptospiral serotypes, and mild, even asymptomatic, leptospirosis may be seen with infection with *L. icterohemorrhagiae*, as well as with other leptospiral serotypes.

Although leptospirosis occurs through the year in the United States, a peak incidence is seen during a 4-month period from July to October. Two-thirds of all cases reported from 1973 to 1978 were from 11 states (in descending order of frequency): Florida, Hawaii, Texas, Louisiana, California, Georgia, Alabama, Missouri, Ohio, New York, and Oregon. However, the disease occurs in practically all states with the possible exceptions of Alaska and North Dakota. Most cases (78%) are in males, and nearly 70 percent are in those younger than 40 years of age. In about one-half of civilian cases of leptospirosis, infection results from occupational exposure (i.e., farmers, slaughter-house and meat packing-house workers, loggers, fresh-water prawn raisers, trappers, miners, veterinarians, biologists, rice-field workers, sewer workers, and waste collectors). Soldiers in jungle-survival training are also known to be at high risk of infection.

With the exception of some laboratory-acquired infections, humans acquire leptospirosis through either direct or indirect contact with the urine of infected animals. In the Unites States, implicated sources of infection have more recently been, in descending order of frequency, pets (dogs or cats) or farm animals (cattle or swine), water or sewage, rodents, and wild animals. That water is an important vehicle of infection is testified by the fact that the largest common-source outbreaks of leptospirosis have in the past been associated with swimming in contaminated pools that are accessible to farm, pets, and wild animals. History of exposure to contaminated water or mud by means other than swimming (wading in shallow pools of water, riding recreational vehicles through muddy farm fields) have been implicated in other outbreaks of leptospirosis. Leptospira may gain entry into humans by penetration through interrupted skin or through mucosal surfaces.

CLINICAL MANIFESTATIONS

In leptospirosis illness may vary from a self-limited, mildly symptomatic or asymptomatic infection to a severe illness with icterus, renal failure, and hemorrhagic manifestations. Most persons (90% to 95%), however, will experience an acute illness without jaundice that may easily escape detection by the clinician. The incubation period is usually from 7 to 12 days, but it may be as few as 2 days or as many as 3 weeks before the first clinical manifestations appear.

The initial manifestations are usually of sudden onset and coincide with the appearance of leptospires in the blood and the cerebrospinal fluid. This is termed the first or septicemic phase and usually lasts from 3 to 7 days. The majority of patients (more than 80%) will experience headache, fever, and myalgias (usually of calves, abdomen, and lumbosacral musculature). Conjunctival injection is an important physical finding and is seen in up to

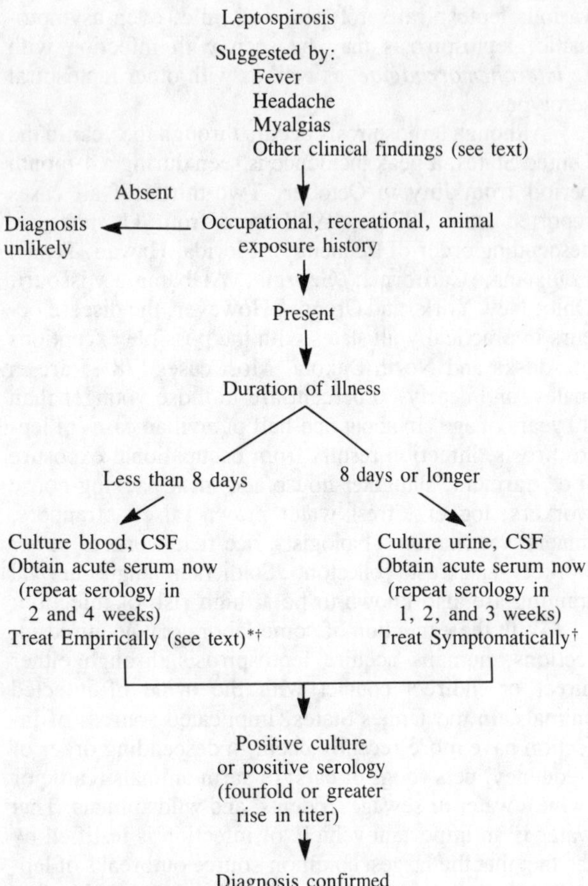

Figure 1 Diagnosis and management of leptospirosis. *First choice: doxycycline or, when cost considerations are of importance, tetracycline; second choice: penicillin plus streptomycin. Antibiotic treatment initiated beyond the fourth day of illness is of doubtful benefit in leptospirosis. †Tetracycline should be given in appropriate dosage as for Rocky Mountain spotted fever and regardless of duration of illness, if the latter is also suspected on clinical or epidemiologic grounds.

two-thirds of the patients during the leptospiremic phase, but it may not be obvious in the markedly icteric patient. Gastrointestinal symptoms (nausea, vomiting, and diarrhea) occur in 30 percent to 40 percent of cases. Other symptoms or signs occur less frequently and include, in descending order of frequency, cough, arthralgias, hepatosplenomegaly, lymphadenopathy, pharyngitis, neck rigidity, and rash. Since fever may be the only manifestation of infection in some patients, the diagnosis may easily escape detection without due regard to occupational or other exposure risk factors.

In anicteric leptospirosis, a symptom-free period of 1 to 3 days will typically follow the first phase of illness, coinciding with the disappearance of leptospires from the blood and the spinal fluid. The appearance of circulating antileptospiral antibodies and the excretion of leptospires in the urine typically start during the second week of illness, which also marks the onset of meningeal inflammation. This is termed the second or immune phase of leptospirosis, and it is symptomatic in about two-thirds of cases, primarily with fever, headache, and vomiting. However, symptoms tend to be less severe and of shorter duration than during the first or leptospiremic phase. Cerebrospinal fluid pleocytosis is seen in 80 percent to 90 percent of cases of anicteric leptospirosis during this second week of illness and is most likely the result of an antigen-antibody reaction. Only one-half of these patients will have detectable clinical signs of meningeal irritation.

WEIL'S DISEASE

Weil's disease (leptospirosis with icterus) represents the most severe end of the spectrum of leptospiral infection. Virtually any leptospiral serovariant may produce this syndrome, although it was originally described as a manifestation of infection with *L. icterohemorrhagiae*. Aside from the symptoms and signs present in anicteric leptospirosis, jaundice is the hallmark of infection in the patient with Weil's disease, and in its most severe form includes renal dysfunction, mucosal and cutaneous hemorrhages, and vascular collapse. The pathogenesis of Weil's disease is most likely a diffuse vasculitis, probably as a result of direct endothelial damage by the leptospires, but the exact mechanism of injury remains unclear. Hepatic injury occurs most likely at a subcellular level, since only modest elevation of serum transaminases and only slight hepatocellular necrosis are evident even in markedly icteric patients. Renal function abnormalities occur characteristically as a result of tubular damage, but interstitial nephritis may also play a role later in the course of the disease.

The biphasic illness seen in the anicteric form of leptospirosis may be absent in a patient with Weil's disease, with no defervescence between the leptospiremic and the immune stages of infection. Fever tends to be higher and last longer than in cases of anicteric leptospirosis. The patient may present primarily with either hepatic, renal, or vascular dysfunction or with an incomplete syndrome (e.g., jaundice without azotemia). Jaundice and azotemia may appear as early as the third day, but may be delayed until the second week of illness. There seems to be a direct correlation between the magnitude of icterus and the severity of illness in Weil's disease, with severe renal, hemorrhagic, and cardiovascular complications occurring most commonly in those patients with marked icterus. Death occurs in 5 percent to 10 percent of patients with Weil's disease, usually as a result of profound anuric renal failure, hemorrhagic diathesis, or refractory vascular collapse.

MISCELLANEOUS CLINICAL MANIFESTATIONS

An acute acalculous dilatation of the gallbladder has been observed in children with leptospirosis, and it may require surgical intervention. Lungs may be affected in up to 40 percent of patients, and symptoms may range from only cough in mild cases to respiratory distress and, at times, profuse hemoptysis due to a hemorrhagic pneumonitis in others. Skin lesions occur in about one-fourth of the patients, and the eruption may be macular, maculopapular, urticarial, or hemorrhagic. Pretibial eruptions were originally described with *L. autumnalis* infections (Fort Bragg fever), but other serotypes have also caused illness with pretibial eruptions. Erythema nodosum may be seen. A desquamative eruption with stomatitis, acral edema, and lymphadenopathy mimicking Kawasaki syndrome has been described. Neurologic manifestations other than aseptic meningitis are not commonly seen in leptospirosis, but, when present, usually occur during the second or immune phase of illness. Manifestations may include peripheral and cranial neuritis, transverse myelitis, encephalitis, and the Guillain-Barré syndrome. Cardiac abnormalities may occur even in mild leptospirosis, more commonly being a subclinical event with electrocardiographic abnormalities only (T-wave changes, arrhythmias, conduction abnormalities). In Weil's disease, a severe myocarditis may lead to severe left ventricular failure and cardiogenic shock. Pericarditis and endocarditis have been reported sporadically.

LABORATORY FINDINGS

Neutrophilia, commonly with a normal or slightly increased total leukocyte count, is frequently seen in leptospirosis. Serum transaminase (SGOT, SGPT) levels are elevated in about 40 percent of patients with anicteric leptospirosis and almost universally in icteric cases. These enzyme levels, however, are only moderately elevated even in the presence of marked hyperbilirubinemia, a feature of leptospirosis that serves to distinguish it from viral (A or B) hepatitis. The serum bilirubin level, mostly of the conjugated type, is usually less than 20 mg percent, but levels as high as 80 mg percent may be seen in the most severe cases of Weil's disease. Elevation of the creatine phosphokinase (CPK) may be seen, reflecting an underlying myolysis. Severe acute rhabdomyolysis has been observed and may lead to acute renal failure. An abnormal urinalysis is very common during the initial (septicemic) phase and includes albuminuria, cylindruria, pyuria, and microhematuria, changes that may persist beyond the first stage in those with Weil's disease. Azotemia is seen in up to one-fourth of anicteric cases of leptospirosis, but marked azotemia is seen only in icteric leptospirosis (Weil's disease). Cerebrospinal fluid abnormalities are very common during the second (or immune) phase of leptospirosis. Elevation of the CSF cell count (initially polymorphonuclear white cells, then predominantly mononuclears) is seen with counts being generally less than 600 per cubic millimeter although, rarely, counts may be in the thousands. The CSF protein may be elevated, but the CSF glucose concentration is generally normal.

LABORATORY DIAGNOSIS

Only culture and serology can reliably establish the diagnosis of leptospirosis. With attention to proper timing and handling of clinical specimens—and with the use of appropriate growth media—cultural confirmation of infection can be expected in the majority of patients. Since leptospires are killed quickly in acid urine, alkalization is suggested before attempting specimen collection for either culture or direct microscopy. Sodium bicarbonate or chewable calcium carbonate tables (e.g., Tums) taken the day before, can effectively render the urine alkaline.

Direct examination by darkfield microscopy will occasionally reveal leptospires when blood or spinal fluid specimens are screened during the first week of illness or urine specimens, thereafter. However, since leptospires will only occasionally be seen in direct examination of clinical specimens and since artifacts (pseudoleptospira) occur commonly (which may confuse even the experienced observer), darkfield microscopy is considered an unreliable method of diagnosis for leptospirosis. Double centrifugation of cerebrospinal fluid and oxalated or heparinized blood or urine may potentially increase the yield of direct microscopy by removing other cellular elements at slow speed (1,500 rpm for 15 minutes) followed by higher speed (5,000 to 10,000 rpm) centrifugation of the supernatant for 20 minutes, to sediment the leptospires. Only when live, active forms showing the characteristic morphology and motility are observed can a presumptive diagnosis of leptospirosis be made by darkfield microscopy of clinical specimens.

The length of leptospires varies from 6 to 20 μm, and they are considerably thinner than treponemes, (that cause syphilis and other diseases) with a width of only 0.1 to 0.2 μm. In wet suspensions they are visible by darkfield microscopy, and they are characterized by a large number of spiral coils of narrow width and short amplitude, giving the appearance of a thread of tightly packed beads. The characteristic motion consists of (1) rapid spinning along their long axis, (2) slower, boring or serpentine movements, (3) bending angular movements at the midsection, and (4) active hooking movements at both ends; only these active forms can be differentiated from the artifacts (pseudoleptospirae) seen frequently, particularly in blood specimens. In contrast to the active movements displayed along their axis, as described above, they are otherwise rather stationary, showing only a very slow linear movement through the field. They may be seen at times in smears of blood stained by the Giemsa method and in tissues stained by silver-impregnation techniques. They can be cultured in artificial media (see below).

On culture leptospires can be recovered from blood or spinal fluid obtained during the first week or septicemic phase of leptospirosis. During the immune or second phase of infection, only urine, and occasionally cerebrospinal fluid, will reveal leptospires on cultures. Incubation is carried out at about 30°C, and darkness is not essential. A selective, agar-containing, semisolid medium (Fletcher's) to which pooled rabbit sera is added is considered the standard for isolation for leptospires, but an albumin-enriched medium (E.M.J.H. medium) is preferred by others. Pre-prepared, ready-to-use culture media are commonly available from state health department laboratories upon request. Since bedside inoculation of cultures is preferred, the physician who suspects leptospirosis ought to obtain these pre-prepared isolation media for *Leptospira* from the local state health department laboratory in anticipation of specimen collection, preferably before the institution of antibiotic therapy. Blood should be cultured several times during the acute phase of illness by use of at least 3 separate culture media tubes to which 1, 2, and 3 drops of blood are added, respectively, and mixed well with the media. Spinal fluid is inoculated more liberally (0.5 ml per culture tube). Urine is frequently inhibitory to the growth of leptospires. Since urinary bacteria may inhibit the growth of leptospires, the addition of either 5-fluorouracil to a final concentration of 200 μg per milliliter or a 30-μg neomycin disk to the medium is suggested. Urine should be drawn into a tuberculin syringe through an 18-gauge needle and a drop of undiluted urine mixed with the medium in the first culture tube (e.g., 5 ml of Fletcher's medium). Serial dilutions of urine in phosphate-buffered saline (pH 7.4) are then made in the syringe from 1:10 to 1:1,000 (i.e., 0.1 ml of urine plus 0.9 ml of buffered saline, and so on), and a drop from each of these dilutions is inoculated into 3 separate culture tubes. Cultures are then examined weekly by darkfield microscopy for 6 weeks before being discarded as negative. Species identification of positive cultures is then carried out by a reference laboratory, usually by the microagglutination method, using specific antisera. Necropsy material (preferrably renal cortex, liver, lung, and brain) should be secured as soon as possible after death, ground (1 g of tissue to 9 parts of buffered saline) and cultured as in the method for urine. If a delay is anticipated before culture of organ specimens, these should be rapidly frozen at −60 °C or transported on dry ice. Inoculation of clinical specimens into hamsters or weanling guinea pigs, where practical, is a very efficient and rapid method of isolation of leptospires.

Serology is probably the method most widely used by the clinician in the diagnosis in leptospirosis. The microagglutination (MA) method employs live organisms and is the standard performed at the Centers for Disease Control in Atlanta, Georgia (U.S.A.). A slide macroagglutination method uses killed or formalinized antigens and, although titers are considerably lower than with the MA method, it remains a useful screening procedure. Antibodies are detectable by the end of the first week of illness, reach maximal levels by the third or fourth week, and low levels of antibodies may remain detectable for years. A single serum specimen is seldom useful in diagnosing acute illness, but a titer of equal to or greater than 1:1,600 by MA may be considered strong presumptive evidence of recent infection. An acute serum should be obtained as soon as the diagnosis is suspected, followed by two convalescent specimens obtained 2 and 4 weeks later. A fourfold or greater change in titer between the acute and convalescent sera is evidence of active leptospirosis. On occasion, and particularly when the acute specimen is obtained late during the course of illness, antibody titers may not change appreciably. A few patients will fail to show a demonstrable antileptospiral antibody titer even in culture-proven infection. Antibiotic therapy may also be responsible for suppressing or delaying the appearance of antileptospiral antibodies. The identification of the infecting leptospiral serotype is most accurately done through typing of culture isolates. Serologic titers will frequently show nonspecific cross-reactions between several different leptospiral serotypes, particularly in the first few weeks of illness. These cross-reactions tend to disappear after the first month of illness.

DIFFERENTIAL DIAGNOSIS

In severely ill patients, the hepatic, renal, hemorrhagic, and circulatory manifestations of leptospirosis may mimic rickettsial infection (e.g., Rocky Mountain spotted fever) and overwhelming bacterial sepsis, including meningococcemia. Other causes of aseptic meningitis must be considered including enteroviral, Epstein-Barr viral, and mycoplasmal infections, Rocky Mountain spotted fever, tuberculosis, cryptococcosis, syphilis, and partially treated bacterial meningitis. The multisystem form of secondary syphilis with hepatitis, lymphadenopathy, and cutaneous eruption duplicate some of the manifestations of leptospiral illness. Other acute infections that share some of the clinical manifestations of leptospirosis include systemic salmonellosis, tularemia, Q fever, psittacosis, severe toxoplasmosis, trichinosis, rubeola, and viral hepatitis. Other diagnostic considerations may include the acute form of sarcoidosis and collagen vascular diseases (particularly systemic lupus erythematosus and Wegener's granulomatosis). Leptospirosis may deserve consideration when pancreatitis, prostatitis, or epididymo-orchitis occur in the context of an acute, febrile, multisystem disease.

TREATMENT

The benefit of antimicrobial therapy in leptospirosis has been a matter of controversy in the past. A recent randomized, placebo-controlled study among U.S. troops attending jungle training in Panama showed convincing evidence of benefit of doxycycline (100 mg twice a day) in reducing the duration of fever, headache, and myalgias and in preventing leptospiruria. It is widely accepted that if it is to be of benefit, treatment must be started before the fourth or, preferrably, by the second day after onset of illness. Since in vitro sensitivity of leptospires varies widely, it remains to be seen whether the favorable experience with doxycycline in the study noted above will be reproduced in infection due to other serovars of *Leptospira*. Only penicillin and tetracycline derivatives are considered to be of any benefit in this infection. In adults, doxycycline, 100 mg twice a day, or tetracycline, 500 mg four times a day, are the regimens of choice in leptospirosis and are generally given for 1 week. Doxycycline is preferred, but tetracycline is a good alternative when cost considerations or patient compliance become paramount. Penicillin (2.4 to 4 million units) intravenously every 24 hours) has also been found effective when treatment is started by or before the fourth day of illness. Since penicillin does not prevent leptospiruria, the addition of intramuscular streptomycin (1.0 g per day) to the treatment is recommended. A Jarisch-Herxheimer reaction has been observed in those treated with penicillin, but the reaction has not been of sufficient severity to prevent penicillin use. Doxycycline is also effective prophylaxis in those at high risk of infection; 200 mg are administerd on a weekly basis during exposure. Neither chloramphenicol nor sulfonamides have been found effective in leptospirosis.

General supportive measures are of critical importance in the management of the severely ill patient with leptospirosis. Bed rest is advised for all febrile patients and while myalgias persist. Decreased intravascular volume may occur as a result of gastrointestinal fluid losses and hemorrhage or extravascular fluid shift because of wide-spread endothelial damage; this situation demands meticulous attention to fluid and electrolyte replacement. Although shock is most often due to a decrease in intravascular volume, cardiovascular collapse may be caused by either severe myocarditis or myopericarditis or by acute adrenal insufficiency secondary to intra-adrenal hemorrhage. Plasmapheresis or exchange transfusions have been advocated by some as an adjunct in the management of the patient with marked hyperbilirubinemia and renal failure. The role of steroids in the treatment of leptospirosis is not clear, but an occasional patient with marked thrombocytopenia has benefited from short-term steroid therapy.

PLAGUE

PHILIP J. SPAGNUOLO, M.D.

Plague—the Black Death of earlier centuries—although no longer a significant cause of epidemic or pandemic disease, remains a significant problem. Recent surveillance estimates confirm the continued presence of sylvatic, enzootic plague in the western United States as well as an increase in the number of documented human cases. The clinical presentation is sufficiently nonspecific to make diagnosis difficult for physicians in nonendemic areas. In view of the potential for widespread transmission of the pneumonic form of the disease and the high mortality if untreated, the public health implications of undiagnosed plague are significant.

EPIDEMIOLOGY

The first North American cases of plague occurred on the West Coast in the first few years of the twentieth century, having been imported from the Orient and eastern Europe. Although plague was originally an urban disease in the United States, since 1927 all cases have been associated with the sylvatic environment of the American West, where it has remained enzootic in wild rodents and their fleas. From 1974 through 1983, 177 cases were reported from 11 western states. In 1983 alone, 40 human cases were documented, the largest number reported since 1920. Plague also has been reported from areas of Africa, South America, and Southeast Asia. The vast majority of cases have occurred in residents of plague-endemic areas; however, approximately 4 to 5 percent of cases occurred in travelers within 1 week of visiting endemic areas.

An epidemiologic history of exposure to wild rodents is helpful in suspecting the diagnosis, but is only documented in a minority of patients. In the United States, the major enzootic reservoirs for the plague bacillus include prairie dogs, squirrels, chipmunks, rats, field mice, coyotes, bobcats and rabbits. Recent studies have demonstrated that domestic animals such as cats and dogs also may develop plague and transmit disease to humans through infected secretions or carriage of infected fleas acquired in the wild. The groups at highest risk of acquiring infection are males (4:1 incidence versus females); children (55% of cases reported from 1950 to 1979 occurred in the pediatric age group); and western American Indians, particularly the Navajo, who have an attack rate of 1.4 per 100,000 population compared to 0.1 per 100,000 for non-Indians. The majority of cases of plague have occurred during late spring and summer (May to September), although cases occurring during the winter hunting season are not unheard of.

CLINICAL PRESENTATION

The commonest clinical syndrome, bubonic plague, accounts for more than 90 percent of reported cases. Following a flea bite or other skin exposure, the plague bacilli migrate to regional lymphatics where they induce an intense inflammatory response, lymphatic obstruction and, ultimately necrosis. Fever, malaise, and headache may precede the development of painful lymphadenitis; more frequently, however, the bubo and systemic symptoms appear simultaneously and may progress rapidly. Classically, the bubo is unilateral and localized to one group of nodes, most commonly the inguinal/femoral area, but any nodal region may be involved including axillary, cervical, epitrochlear, and popliteal nodes. Typically, the bubo is firm, erythematous, and exquisitely tender to palpation.

Primary septicemic plague may occur in the absence of a bubo in a minority of patients. Recent reports from New Mexico suggest that primary septicemic plague may account for an increasingly larger percentage of cases, especially in patients over the age of 60 years. Plague pneumonia may result from secondary seeding of the lung during transient bacteremia or direct inoculation of lung by aerosolized secretions from infected animals or humans. Pneumonic disease is a rapidly progressive illness characterized by hemoptysis, diffuse alveolar infiltrates, hypoxemia, and, ultimately, death due to septic shock and disseminated intravascular coagulation. Uncommon forms of plague include meningitis, ophthalmic involvement, renal tubular necrosis, and hepatic disease.

Laboratory evaluation of plague cases demonstrates a peripheral leukocytosis with a shift to band forms in most cases. In general, the laboratory work-up is otherwise noncontributory.

DIAGNOSIS

The diagnosis of plague should be seriously considered in any patient with the clinical triad of fever, malaise, and painful lymphadenitis who resides in or has traveled through rural western United States or other plague-enzootic areas of the world within 1 week of onset of illness. The diagnosis may be readily confirmed by smear and culture of *Yersinia pestis* from the bubo aspirate. Aspiration should be performed with a large-bore needle (19- or 20-gauge) and a 10 to 30 ml syringe. When no liquid is aspirated, injection of sterile non-bacteriostatic saline into the bubo and reaspiration may facilitate culture and smear. The aspirate should be plated on sheep's blood agar, MacConkey's agar, and inoculated into broth culture. Smears of the aspirate should be stained with Gram stain, Wayson stain and fluorescent antibody directed against *Y. pestis*, which is available through the Centers for Disease Control (CDC, Atlanta, Georgia) and many state health department laboratories. The organism appears as gram-negative, bipolar-staining coccobacilli or as light blue bacilli with darker polar bodies by Wayson stain. In some patients with high-grade bacteremia, smears of blood or buffy coat may be positive by these techniques, thus establishing the diagnosis more rapidly.

Microbiologic confirmation of the diagnosis from bubo aspirate, blood, or sputum requires the demonstration of nonhemolytic, nonmotile organisms that fail to hydrolyze urea and indole or utilize citrate. In the decade 1970 to 1979, *Y. pestis* was recovered from 98 of 105 reported cases. Thus, given the appropriate suspicion of the disease, the microbiology laboratory can substantiate the diagnosis in nearly every case. Definitive identification should be undertaken by the CDC. Serologies play no role in the prospective diagnosis of acutely infected patients, but serve only a confirmatory purpose.

THERAPY

If left untreated, bubonic plague has a mortality rate of 40 to 80 percent; primary septicemic and pneumonic plague are uniformly fatal untreated. Thus, accurate diagnosis and rapid institution of antibiotic therapy are critical. Recent mortality figures of 5 to 18 percent attest to the increased awareness of the disease, especially in endemic areas. Selection of antimicrobials should be based on the type and severity of the illness. Streptomycin is the drug of choice in this disease and should be used in all cases of pneumonic and primary septicemic plague as well as for severely ill patients with bubonic disease. The dosage in adults is 30 mg per kilogram intramuscularly daily in two or three divided doses. Children should receive 25 mg per kilogram daily in two divided doses. In adults and children older than 8 years of age with uncomplicated bubonic plague, oral tetracycline may be used (loading dose of 15 mg per kilogram followed by 30 mg per kilogram in four divided doses). The total duration of therapy with either regimen should be 10 days. Oral tetracycline (2.0 g per day in four divided doses for 7 days) has been used successfully for prophylaxis of plague-exposed individuals.

All patients with evidence of meningitis should receive parenteral chloramphenicol in a dosage of 75 mg per kilogram in four divided doses. With clinical improvement, oral therapy may be substituted to complete a 10-day course. Although other drugs may be suggested as a result of sensitivity testing of *Y. pestis* isolates, the disparity between in vitro testing and efficacy prohibits the use of penicillins or cephalosporins.

All patients with suspected plague must be placed in strict isolation until the disease is excluded or there is no evidence of development of pneumonic disease. All specimens from patients (bubo aspirate, blood, and sputum) should be handled with gloves and attention to the prevention of aerosolization. After 48 to 96 hours of appropriate antimicrobial therapy, patients should be considered noninfectious. Buboes may require incision and drainage during the first week of therapy for suppuration. Appropriately treated patients rarely relapse. The most important complications of the disease include endotoxic shock, disseminated intravascular coagulation, and metastatic infection.

The potential transmissibility of plague mandates that local and state health departments be made aware of all suspected and confirmed cases immediately. The microbiologic and clinical expertise provided by these departments as well as by the CDC may prove invaluable in managing individual patients, especially in nonendemic areas.

BABESIOSIS

MURRAY WITTNER, M.D., Ph.D.
HERBERT B. TANOWITZ, M.D.

Babesiosis is a common hemolytic disease of wild and domestic animals which occasionally occurs in a similar form in man. Infection ordinarily is transmitted through the bite of hard (Ixodid) ticks, although recently there have been several human cases acquired through blood transfusion. Human babesiosis may present with mild to severe intermittent fever, splenomegaly, hemolysis, and jaundice.

During the past 20 years cases of human infection with *Babesia* species have been reported with increasing frequency in Europe and the United States. In this country the primary endemic area is the northeastern coastal region, especially Nantucket Island, Massachusetts, and eastern Long Island, New York, although infection has been reported as far away as California. It appears that all human cases of babesiosis occurring in the eastern United States are caused by the murine species, *B. microti*, which is transmitted by the bite of the small deer tick, *Ixodes dammini*. In Europe the bovine species, *B. divergens* and *B. bovis*, have been implicated.

Babesia species are intraerythrocytic protozoan parasites of mammals and birds, presently classified in the subphylum Apicomplexa, together with those organisms that cause malaria (*Plasmodium* species) and toxoplasmosis (*Toxoplasma gondii*). The 71 species of *Babesia* are frequently distinguished as the ''small'' (1.0–2.5 μm) and ''large'' (2.5–5.0 μm) species. Until now, however, only the ''small'' species have been found causing disease in humans.

As in wild animals, human resistance to *Babesia* infection seems to depend upon the functional integrity of the spleen. Fatal and near-fatal cases have occurred almost exclusively in patients who were splenectomized for a variety of reasons, including trauma, thrombocytopenic purpura, or Hodgkin's disease. Studies in calves and hamsters have demonstrated that splenectomy performed after apparent recovery from experimental infection may result in parasitic relapse. In experimental infection in athymic nude mice and mice immunized with BCG, immunity to *Babesia* was shown to be, in part, T-cell dependent. The protective role of immune serum in babesiosis remains unclear. Asymptomatic infections seem to be common, as suggested by seroepidemiologic studies on Nantucket Island, Massachusetts, Shelter Island, New York, and Mexico. Some of these asymptomatic individuals may have a low number of circulating parasites for many weeks or months and thus have been the source of transfusion babesiosis. Despite the prevalence of asymptomatic infection, clinical disease has not been reported from immunocompromised patients during the course of corticosteroid and/or cyclophosphamide therapy. It should be emphasized, however, that *B. microti* often causes symptomatic infection in otherwise immunocompetent individuals.

DIAGNOSIS

The diagnosis of babesiosis should be considered in anyone with fever who has been in an endemic area, regardless of a history of tick bite, or who has received a blood transfusion. It is not unusual for the laboratory technician to report the presence on a blood smear of ring forms of malaria. The morphologic resemblance in man between *B. microti* and trophozoites of *Plasmodium falciparum*, especially when they assume a peripheral position in the erythrocytes, should be emphasized. However, *Babesia* species do not produce residual hemazoin pigment, a by-product of hemoglobin digestion, as is usual with malarial parasites. In some instances cruciate, maltese cross, or tetrad forms lacking pigment can be found on blood films. These are diagnostic. An indirect immunofluorescence test performed by the Centers for Disease Control can be helpful, but low-titer, cross reactions between *Babesia* and *P. falciparum* and *P. vivax* occur. High *Babesia* antibody titers $\geq$1:1024) are present during acute disease and decline over the ensuing year to 1:256–1:32 or less. Moreover, if 1.0 ml of the suspected patient's blood is inoculated intraperitoneally into a golden hamster, parasitemia will be evident within 12 to 14 days and should help to confirm the diagnosis.

When fever, chills, marked fatigue, weakness, and myalgias are present, babesiosis may be confused with malaria, especially when the unwary examine a blood smear and discover intraerythrocytic ring-shaped parasites.

Babesiosis can also be confused with rickettsial illness, especially when patients present with a history of tick bite, fever, myalgias, headache, hemolysis, and thrombocytopenia. However, a blood smear will usually reveal the true etiologic agent. In several of the fatal cases of babesiosis hemolysis was rapid and serum bilirubin was markedly elevated; Weil's disease and viral hepatitis were seriously considered until the intraerythrocytic parasites were discovered.

THERAPY

Treatment for human babesiosis until recently has had limited success. Most patients have received chloroquine, primarily because of the morphologic similarities of *B. microti* to *P. falciparum*. While a limited slow response has been reported to a prolonged (14 days or more) course of chloroquine at doses similar to those used to treat malaria, there is little evidence to support its efficacy. Hamsters experimentally infected with *B. microti* were shown to be unaffected by chloroquine, sulfadiazine, primaquine, or metronidazole in combination with pyrimethamine. Minocycline and tetracycline, when employed in extraordinarily high and toxic doses, had some effect in reducing parasitemia; at usual therapeutic levels, however, tetracycline had no antiparasitic activity. Pentamidine isethionate (Lomidine, Specia [Société Parisienne d'Expansion Chemique], Paris, France) used to treat hu-

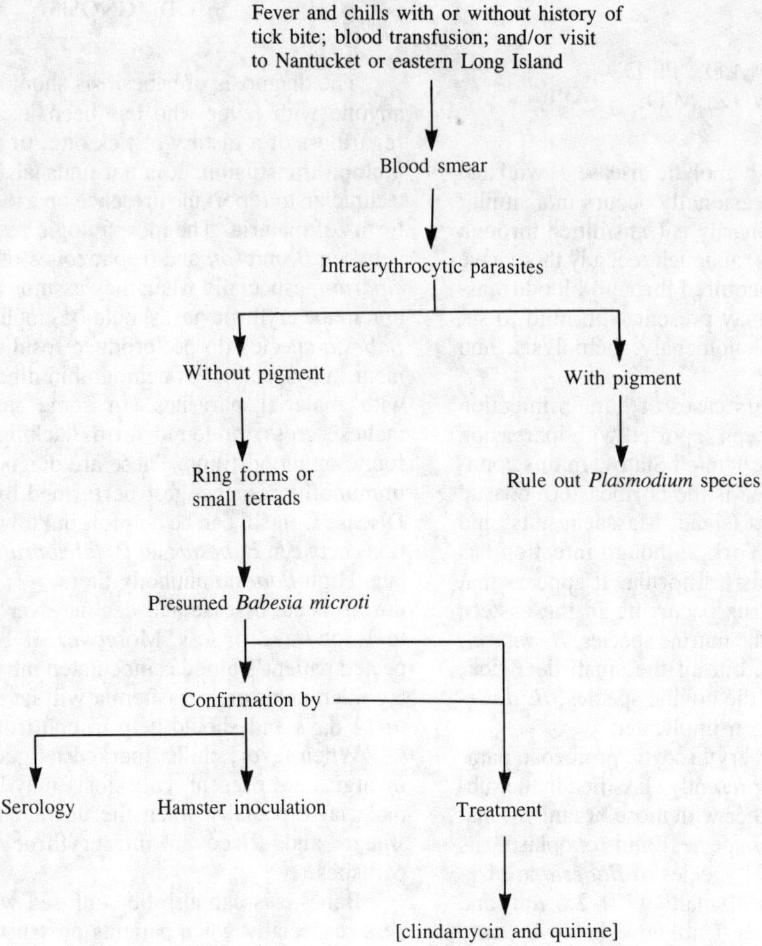

Figure 1 Diagnosis and treatment of *Babesia microti* infection

man *B. microti* infection (4 mg per kilogram per day for 14 days by deep intramuscular injection) has had limited success in lowering but not eliminating the parasitemia in human babesiosis. Moreover, relapse has been reported after completion of therapy. In hamsters similar results were obtained and the parasitemia increased significantly once drug therapy was discontinued. Significant side effects have been reported with pentamidine, including evidence of renal insufficiency, pain at the injection site, and formation of sterile abscesses. Diminazene aceturate (Berenil, Hoechst-Roussel Pharamaceuticals, Inc., Somerville, New Jersey), an aromatic diamidine that is highly effective against *Babesia* infection in animals, has been tried in human *B. microti* infection. A 50-mg test dose was given, followed by a 3-day course of 2 mg per kilogram per day. Upon completion of the course of therapy the patient became afebrile and no parasites could be detected after 48 hours. However, the patient developed severe, life-threatening acute polyneuritis. During treatment electrocardiographic changes, including atrial premature beats, and nonspecific STT wave changes in the precordial leads were noted. Subsequently these reverted to normal. Severe pain at the injection site also occurred. In hamsters experimentally infected with *B. microti*, diminazene (6 mg per kilogram) reduced the parasitemia but parasitic relapse occurred once therapy was discontinued. Diminazine was used unsuccessfully to treat a fatal human case of *B. divergens*.

Several reports have underscored the therapeutic efficacy of either red cell or whole-blood exchange. The latter procedure was chosen to provide free haptoglobin, to decrease extracellular and intracellular parasitemia, and to eliminate serum factors that have been described as possibly responsible for the pathogenesis of the renal complications of babesiosis.

Clindamycin (20 mg per kilogram per day intramuscularly for 7 to 10 days), together with quinine (25 mg per kilogram per day orally for 7 to 10 days), was used successfully to treat severe transfusion-induced *B. microti* infection in a premature baby. Experimental hamster studies have confirmed the efficacy of this regimen. While clindamycin alone consistently cleared the infection, when oral quinine was added the infection cleared more rapidly. A febrile splenectomized adult treated for *B. microti* infection with clindamycin (600 mg intramuscularly four times per day for 7 days) and quinine (650 mg orally three times a day for 7 days) had rapid lysis of fever (within 24 hours) and the parasitemia declined.

Currently it appears that clindamycin alone or together with quinine may represent the safe, effective treatment of choice for babesiosis caused by *B. microti*. Figure 1 outlines recommendations for diagnosis and treatment of babesiosis.

PROPHYLAXIS

Specific chemoprophylaxis is not available. Those who are immunocompromised, especially postsplenectomized individuals, should avoid tick-infected areas. However, since normal or immunocompetent individuals may acquire symptomatic and sometimes severe disease, they too should be wary when entering these areas. Moreover, since *Ixodes dammini* is small and often is not obvious, individuals should carefully inspect themselves for ticks daily and remove them completely. Gentle traction with forceps applied close to the capitulum usually will suffice to remove the entire tick. If the ticks are deeply entrenched, mineral oil or even a hot needle should be applied and the arthropod will usually relax its hold. In tick-infested areas clothes should be coated with repellent, and especially the lower parts of trousers should receive such treatment. It is advisable to wear long-sleeved garments, and shirts should be tucked under the belt.

Individuals from known endemic areas should be screened for asymptomatic infection before they are accepted as blood donors.

HUMAN BRUCELLOSIS

EDWARD J. YOUNG, M.D.

Brucellosis, a disease of animals transmissible to humans (zoonosis), remains an important human health problem, especially in countries where brucellosis in domestic animals has not been controlled or eradicated. Epidemiologic studies have shown that man's risk of contracting brucellosis is closely linked to his methods of animal husbandry, standards of hygiene, and food habits. Since human infection usually occurs from direct contact with infected animals, certain occupations present an increased risk of exposure; these include farmers, veterinarians, abattoir workers, and laboratory personnel. Although a history of animal contact should always be sought, clinicians must also be aware that brucellosis can be transmitted by ingestion of unpasteurized milk or other dairy products, such as cheese that is prepared from "raw" milk. Human-to-human transmission of brucellosis is rare, associated with blood or bone marrow transfusions from infected donors.

PATHOGENESIS

Among the six recognized species in the genus *Brucella*, four are known to cause human disease: *B. abortus* (cattle), *B. melitensis* (goats and sheep) *B. suis* (swine), and *B. canis* (dogs). Animal studies suggest that *B. melitensis* and *B. suis* are the most virulent, but specific virulence factors are poorly understood. The *Brucella* are facultative intracellular bacteria that have the capacity to survive and even multiply within phagocytic cells of the host. Normal human serum and polymorphonuclear leukocytes have a limited ability to kill *Brucella*; macrophages of the reticuloendothelial system (RES) "activated" by specifically sensitized thymus-derived lymphocytes appear to be the principal defense against *Brucella* and other facultative intracellular pathogens. It has even been suggested that intracellular survival may aid in the spread of *Brucella* throughout the body and may protect the bacteria against antimicrobial agents.

CLINICAL MANIFESTATIONS AND COMPLICATIONS

The spectrum of human brucellosis ranges from subclinical (detected by specific antibodies or skin test reactivity in the absence of a known overt infection) to chronic infection characterized by recurrent symptoms over many years. The incubation period varies from weeks to months, and the onset of symptoms is insidious in approximately one-half of cases and acute in the remainder. Patients often have multiple nonspecific complaints, notably, lethargy, body aches, fever, sweats, anorexia, fatigue, and depression. Because there is often a paucity of physical findings, these symptoms may be considered psychosomatic. If empiric antibiotic treatment is given with a penicillin or oral cephalosporin, symptoms may abate, only to recur, since these drugs have little clinical efficacy.

Since *Brucella* localize in tissues rich in elements of the RES, involvement of lymph nodes, spleen, liver, bones, and the genitourinary system is common. Mild lymphadenopathy may be the only physical abnormality in many cases; the spleen may also be enlarged, perhaps more commonly in cases due to *B. abortus*. The liver is probably involved initially in all cases, although icteric hepatitis is rare. Often patients have only mild or no abnormalities demonstrable by hepatic cell function tests, despite the demonstration of lesions on hepatic biopsy. Noncaseating hepatic granulomas, indistinguishable from sarcoid, are characteristic of infection due to *B. abortus*, and diffuse hepatic inflammation with focal microabscesses is often found in infection caused by *B. melitensis*;

however, disease caused by the two species is difficult to distinguish clinically.

Skeletal involvement—most often in the spine (60% in the lumbosacral regions)—is frequent in brucellosis. Brucellar spondylitis begins in the intervertebral disk and spreads to contiguous vertebral bodies producing osteomyelitis occasionally with paravertebral abscesses. Inflammation results in narrowing of the intervertebral foramen, causing irritation to dorsal nerve roots. Sacroiliitis is reported to be the commonest joint involvement, occurring alone or in combination with other joints in some 15 percent of cases.

Genitourinary complications occur in up to 20 percent of men infected with *Brucella*, notably, involvement of the testes and epididymis. Pyelonephritis and prostatitis have been reported infrequently. Although abortion is common in animals infected with *Brucella* (due to massive growth of bacteria in placental tissues rich in the growth stimulant erythritol), there is little evidence that *Brucella* causes reproductive failures in humans. Abortion can occur in pregnant women in the course of acute bacteremic brucellosis, but this is not unique to *Brucella*.

DIAGNOSIS

Routine laboratory studies, like physical findings, are few and nonspecific. The white blood count is generally normal or low, and granulocytopenia is commoner than lymphopenia. Blood coagulation abnormalities have been attributed to disseminated intravascular coagulation (DIC), and, rarely, erythrophagocytosis is present in the bone marrow. The diagnosis of human brucellosis rests with isolation of the organism from the blood, bone marrow, or other tissues. One caveat relative to blood cultures in brucellosis is the slow growth of the bacteria in artificial media. If brucellosis is suspected, the laboratory should be instructed to observe routine blood cultures for a minimum of 4 weeks before assuming that they are negative.

In the absence of a positive culture, the diagnosis rests with the demonstration of a rise in specific antibodies. A variety of serologic tests have been employed to diagnose human brucellosis; however, the standard tube agglutination (STA), 2-mercaptoethanol (2-ME) agglutination, and complement fixation (CF) tests are the most useful. The STA test measures total agglutinating immunoglobulins (IgM plus IgG), whereas the 2-ME test measures only IgG (2-ME-resistant) agglutinins. Both IgM and IgG antibodies rise in acute brucellosis, but titers of IgG agglutinins disappear or decrease with treatment and recovery, and low levels of IgM antibodies may persist for many years. This observation is useful in distinguishing chronic brucellosis, relapse, or reinfection, in which IgG antibodies are often elevated and are resistant to treatment with 2-mercaptoethanol. Antigen prepared from *B. abortus* is routinely used in these tests, since cross-reactions between the three major species is sufficient to detect infection due to all but *B. canis*. Caution is advised in interpreting low levels of *Brucella* agglutinins (less than 1:160), especially in patients previously immunized or infected with cholera, tularemia, or *Yersinia enterocolitica* serotype 9. A variety of impure and nonstandardized antigens have been employed in the past to test type IV immune responses to *Brucella*; however, skin tests are not useful in the clinical diagnosis of human brucellosis.

TREATMENT

The evidence for subclinical brucellosis suggests that the body may be capable of recovery from infection without specific chemotherapy; however, the practice of prescribing empiric antibiotics for a variety of nonspecific symptoms precludes the assumption that all such cases were untreated. In fact, the literature is replete with reports of spontaneous, often sudden, recovery from brucellosis without specific treatment. Nevertheless, most authorities agree that antibiotics shorten the course of infection as well as reduce the incidence of complications, some of which may be life threatening.

Sulfadiazine and streptomycin were the first antibiotics used to treat human brucellosis, but the toxicity associated with this combination soon led to the discovery that tetracycline provided an effective and less toxic alternative. In vitro the majority of *Brucella* strains are inhibited by concentrations of tetracycline from 0.1 to 0.5 μg per millimeter, but the drug is not bactericidal. Oral tetracycline (250 mg four times daily) for a minimum of 21 days is adequate theray for uncomplicated cases of brucellosis. Oral doxycycline or minocycline (100 mg twice daily) produces comparable results and may be tolerated better, but is more expensive. Although some studies have reported in vitro synergy between tetracycline and streptomycin, conflicting results have been obtained in clinical studies regarding the incidence of relapses between single versus combination drug therapy. Regardless, most authorities recommend treating seriously ill patients or cases complicated by deep tissue involvement (arthritis, osteomyelitis, among others) with a combination of oral tetracycline for 6 weeks plus intramuscular or intravenous streptomycin (1 to 2 g daily) for the first 1 or 2 weeks. Gentamicin is more active in vitro than streptomycin, but no controlled comparative study using different aminoglycosides in human brucellosis has been reported. The ability of trimethoprim-sulfamethoxazole (TMP/SMZ) to penetrate into cells suggests that this drug combination might be useful for the treatment of human brucellosis. The in vitro sensitivity of TMP/SMZ against *Brucella* ranges from 0.39 to 6.25 μg per millileter (some strains may be higher), and several uncontrolled studies have indicated that it is a reasonable alternative therapy. Since the tetracyclines may cause irreversible staining of deciduous teeth, TMP/SMZ is particularly useful for treating brucellosis in children, and the relapse rate is reportedly less than 5 percent. The usual dose of TMP/SMZ (combination containing 80 mg trimethoprim and 400 mg sulfamethoxazole) is four tablets daily in adults or two tablets daily in children administered for 6 to 12 weeks, depending on response.

Rifampin is another drug with promise in the treatment of human brucellosis. *Brucella* are inhibited in vitro at concentrations of rifampin between 0.15 and 2.5 μg per millileter, and the drug is bactericidal at concentrations approximately four times the MIC. Unfortunately, rifampin-resistant variants are produced in vitro which suggests that it should not be used as single-drug therapy. Several uncontrolled studies using rifampin have reported encouraging results, but it is still too soon to know what role this agent has in the treatment of human brucellosis.

Other drugs such as erythromycin and chloramphenicol have been used to treat brucellosis, but they are less active in vitro than tetracycline, show variable effects against different strains of *Brucella*, and are not recommended alternatives. The penicillins, including ureidopenicillins, and first- or second-generation cephalosporins have little activity against *Brucella* and appear to be ineffective clinically. Some new beta-lactam antibiotics such as thienamycin and moxalactam are effective in vitro against some strains of *Brucella* but are unproved clinically.

Complications of brucellosis, such as meningitis and endocarditis, that require a bactericidal antibiotic remain a difficult problem. Tetracycline penetrates the blood-brain barrier but is only bacteriostatic; aminoglycosides do not penetrate the blood-brain barrier well when given intravenously. Moxalactam and some other new beta-lactam antibiotics achieve adequate CSF levels after intravenous injection, and are useful in treating some gram-negative meningitis without the need for intrathechal or intraventricular administration. Rifampin also enters the CSF in adequate concentrations, and we have successfully treated one case of meningoencephalitis caused by *B. suis* with moxalactam and rifampin after treatment with tetracycline plus streptomycin failed to sterilize the CSF. Additional experience will be required with these agents before a definitive recommendation can be made.

Endocarditis is another rare, but usually fatal, complication of human brucellosis. Most authorities recommend surgical replacement of the infected valve in addition to antibiotics in order to achieve a cure of *Brucella* endocarditis. In order to determine the optimal antibiotic treatment of specific complications, in vitro studies using newer antibiotics may be useful.

CHRONIC BRUCELLOSIS

Perhaps no aspect of human brucellosis is more controversial or difficult to treat than so called chronic brucellosis. This is, in part, due to the disagreement over what constitutes chronicity in a disease that has an insidious onset, extending over many months in half of the cases. If one defines chronic brucellosis as that of patients complaining of ill health for more than a year after the initial diagnosis, then some proportion will represent treatment failures with relapsing infection, and another portion will be patients with an identifiable focus of infection, such as an abscess in the liver, spleen, or other tissue. The majority, however, appear to be patients with no evidence of active disease, but who, after prolonged illness, ascribe all nonspecific symptoms (lethargy, depression, headache, body aches) to the persistence of brucellosis. These patients may have low levels of 2-ME-sensitive (IgM) aggutinins in their serum, which tempts clinicians to retreat with antibiotics. However, residual antibodies are not unusual in the course of adequately treated infection because polysaccharide antigens are very slowly metabolized by the body. Such patients may benefit from assurance, but are more often refractory to all attempted therapy.

ORNITHOSIS

VERNON KNIGHT, M.D.

Ornithosis is a febrile respiratory and systemic illness caused by *Chlamydia psittaci* that ranges in severity from a mild influenza-like syndrome to severe pneumonia. Infrequent extrapulmonary complications are endocarditis, meningoencephalitis, and vasculitic skin lesions.

THE CHLAMYDIAE

The chlamydiae are obligate intracellular parasites. The other chlamydial species pathogenic for humans is *Chlamydia trachomatis*, the several antigenic variants of which are the cause of trachoma, other eye infections, and genital infections in men and women. *C. trachomatis* tends to cause localized infections in contrast to the systemic involvement caused by *C. psittaci*. *C. trachomatis* is distinguished from *C. psittaci* by its synthesis of folic acid and consequent susceptibility to sulfonamides and by the production of glycogen-containing inclusions in the cytoplasm of infected cells.

EPIDEMIOLOGY

C. psittaci infection is primarily a disease of birds. It was first called psittacosis because of the recognition that infection in psittacine birds was the source of infections of humans, but the name is now generalized to ornithosis with the discovery that more than 130 species of birds may be host to the infection. In addition, it is found in sheep, cattle, felines, and some other animals. In recent years in the United States, somewhat more than 100 cases of ornithosis have been reported annually. The cases have largely occurred in owners of pet birds (psittacines and pigeons) and pet shop operators, but one-fifth or more of patients have had no history of exposure to birds. The disease is uncommon in children and is about equally distributed between men and women. Human-to-human transmission is considered likely since the organism is shed in sputum. Some recovered patients have prolonged respiratory tract shedding. In 1974, 1976, and 1981, outbreaks of orinthosis occurred in turkey processing plants in the United States, with the highest incidence among persons who killed, picked, or eviscerated the birds; this suggests aerosol transmission of the infection by dried particles of feces or droplets from infected tissues. In Europe and Great Britian, well-defined cases of infection have been associated with exposure to infected sheep; other reports implicate infected cattle and felines as sources. Birds may be latently infected and become symptomatic under stress. When the infection is either latent or active, fecal shedding occurs and can be the source of infection. Sick birds have diarrhea, anorexia, and lethargy. Conjunctivitis also occurs. The mortality in sick birds ranges from 5 to 30 percent. Chlortetracycline, 0.44 percent in feed for 45 days or longer, has been used to control infection in pet caged birds.

COMMON CLINICAL MANIFESTATIONS

After an incubation period of 1 to 2 weeks, an abrupt onset of high fever and chills, headache, sore throat, malaise, and dry cough is most characteristic of ornithosis. A relative bradycardia may occur. Up to one-third of patients have developed pneumonia in some outbreaks. The pneumonia is about equally divided between single- and multi-lobe involvement. Pleural effusion and pulmonary collapse occur in a minority of patients, and cavitation may be rarely encountered. Physical signs of pneumonia are less than radiographic changes, similar to the situation with *Mycoplasma pneumoniae* pneumonia. Clearing of radiographic changes during recovery occurs at about the same rate as in patients with mycoplasmal pneumonia, a period of 4 to 6 weeks, but is more rapid than in patients with severe pneumococcal pneumonia or pneumonia of legionnaires disease. A rash resembling rose spots of typhoid is sometimes seen. Gastrointetinal symptoms of nausea, vomiting, and diarrhea may accompany the initial stages of infection of all types. Blood counts are usually within a normal range and the red cell sedimentation rate is greatly increased. Arterial oxygen pressures may be reduced when pneumonia is extensive. Other laboratory findings are nonspecific.

UNCOMMON CLINICAL MANIFESTATIONS

Endocarditis

This unusual but serious complication of *C. psittaci* infection is usually detected weeks to months after onset of illness and is suspected when other causes of endocarditis are not demonstrable. The history is usually one of developing dyspnea, fever, night sweats, and weight loss. Aortic and mitral valves may be involved. The disease often occurs on bicuspid aortic valves or valves damaged by rheumatic fever. Other manifestations of endocarditis—petechiae, clubbing of fingers, and glomerulonephritis—may occur. Vegetations vary from warty to friable, and valve replacement has been successfully accomplished. Two patients with probable endocarditis presented with brachial artery emboli requiring surgical removal. Patients with endocarditis due to *C. psittaci* infection exhibit the highest titers of complement fixing antibody detectable with this infection (1:128 to 1:1,024). A history of exposure to pet psittacine birds or pigeons is often obtained. Treatment with tetracycline, erythromycin, or rifampin has been successful in a few cases, but four of seven reported patients died, primarily because of congestive failure, possibly resulting from the advanced state of illness before treatment was begun.

Other Complications

Disseminated intravascular coagulation may complicate ornithosis with increases in prothrombin and partial thromboplastin times and increase in fibrin degradation products. Superficial venous thrombosis may accompany this complication. Delerium, stupor and hepatitis have occurred in severely ill patients. Pericarditis and myocarditis are also reported.

PATHOGENESIS AND PATHOLOGY

The disease primarily involves the respiratory tract and spreads hematogenously to other organs. The pulmonary lesion is an inflammatory process, with infiltration of mononuclear cells principally confined to interstitial tissue and alveolar septa. As the infection progresses, proteinaceous exudate and mononuclear cells accumulate in alveoli in involved portions of the lung. *C. psittaci* elementary bodies can be visualized as inclusions, 300 to 400 nm in diameter in infected mononuclear cells by Macchiavello or Castaneda technique. Focal necrosis or frank abscess of alveolar septa may occur in severe cases. Diffuse mononuclear cell infiltration and focal necrosis of liver, spleen, brain, and other organs are evidence of dissemination of infection.

DIAGNOSIS

A complement fixation test employing fluids from infected cells as antigens is most commonly used for diagnosis. The antigen preparation contains reticulate bodies that possess the group antigen that detects both *C. psittaci* and *C. trachomatis* (2-keto-3-deoxyoctanoic acid). For this reason, the test does not discriminate between the two species of *Chlamydia*. Among serotypes of *C. trachomatis*, lymphogranuloma venereum exhibits the closest relationship to *C. psittaci*. Two to 3 percent of normal adults may have complement-fixation titers to chlamydiae of more than 1:16. Individual titers of 1:32 or greater or a fourfold or greater rise in paired specimens are considered diagnostic of chlamydial infection. Differentiation between infections caused by the two species of *Chlamydia* is based on clinical grounds. Early treatment with tetracycline and probably other antimicrobial drugs can delay the appearance of antibody. The agent of legionnaires disease may stimulate low titers of chlamydial antibody. *C. psittaci* is readily isolated in embryonated eggs or in cell culture, but is hazardous to laboratory workers, and the procedure is not generally available.

TREATMENT

Tetracycline is the usual treatment. Two grams daily in four divided doses orally in adults are given for 3 weeks. Clinical response may not be detectable for 2 or 3 days after start of treatment. Relapse may occur if treatment is shortened. Children 8 years of age and younger should be given erythromycin stearate, based on severity of infection, 30 to 50 mg per kilogram per day orally in four divided doses fasting or before meals, for a similar period. Larger doses of erythromycin may be given to severely ill children. Erythromycin, 2 g daily in four divided doses for 2 to 3 weeks should be used to treat women in the last half of pregnancy.

Patients with endocarditis are given tetracycline for 4 to 6 weeks or longer. Rifampin was used successfully in treatment of one patient with endocarditis; until experience is greater, this treatment should be reserved for cases unresponsive to other regimens.

Since tetracycline is the preferred treatment for ornithosis and erythromycin is preferred for legionnaires disease, there may be difficulty in selection of treatment for cases in which these etiologies cannot be differentiated. Strategies for treatment of such patients will have to be individualized.

LYME DISEASE

LAURI E. MARKOWITZ, M.D.
ALLEN C. STEERE, M.D.

Lyme disease is a systemic, tick-borne spirochetal disease with protean manifestations, including rheumatic, neurologic, cardiac, and dermatologic abnormalities. The best clinical marker for the disease is the initial skin lesion, erythema chronicum migrans (ECM), that occurs at the site of the tick bite. ECM was first reported in Europe in 1910, and the first case of ECM acquired in the United States was reported in 1970. However, it was not until 1975 that investigation of a cluster of cases of arthritis in Lyme, Connecticut, led to the description of the full clinical spectrum of what is now known as Lyme disease. Through subsequent studies, *Ixodes dammini* and *Ixodes pacificus* were identified as the principal vectors of Lyme disease in the United States. In 1981, the etiologic agent of the disease was identified, a previously unrecognized spirochete. This spirochete has been referred to as the Lyme disease spirochete or the *Ixodes dammini* spirochete, but has now been classified taxonomically as a *Borrelia* and named *Borrelia burgdorferi*.

EPIDEMIOLOGY

Lyme disease has been recognized in three major areas in the United States: the coastal areas of the Northeast (Connecticut, Delaware, Maryland, Massachusetts, New Jersey, New York, Rhode Island, and Pennsylvania); the Midwest, (Minnesota and Wisconsin); and the West (California, Oregon, Utah, and Nevada). These areas correspond to the range of *I. dammini* in the Northeast and Midwest and of *I. pacificus* in the West. However, sporadic cases have been reported from states outside the known range of these ticks, including Arkansas, Florida, Georgia, Indiana, Kentucky, Montana, North Carolina, Tennessee, Texas, and Virginia. The occurrence of these cases suggests that there are vectors other than *I. dammini* and *I. pacificus* and/or that these ticks may be spreading to new areas. Recently, *B. burgdorferi* has also been recovered from *Amblyomma americanum* and *Dermacentor variabilis*, suggesting that these ticks may be vectors for Lyme disease. In Europe, where *I. ricinus* is the vector, Lyme disease is known to occur in almost all countries on the continent. The illness has also been reported in Australia, but the vector there is unknown.

The peak incidence of Lyme disease is during the summer months. In more than 80 percent of cases, the patients have onsets in May through August. All age groups have been affected. In 1980, 226 cases were reported to the Centers for Disease Control and in 1982, 487 cases were reported. It is unclear to what extent the increase in reported cases is a result of increased awareness of the disease rather than a true increase in incidence.

CLINICAL MANIFESTATIONS

The manifestations of Lyme disease have been divided into three stages that may overlap or occur alone. During the first stage of Lyme disease, most patients have ECM and constitutional symptoms. ECM occurs at the site of a tick bite after an incubation period of 3 to 32 days (median, 7 days). The skin lesion begins as a red macule or papule that expands to form an annular erythema as large as 70 cm in diameter (median, 15 cm). As it expands, the center of the lesion often clears. Lesions may appear on any part of the body, and multiple lesions occur in about 50 percent of patients (Fig. 1). The lesions are usually not painful, but some patients describe them as burning or pruritic. Atypical ECM may lack central clearing or have a vesicular center. Other cutaneous manifestations have also been reported including localized or generalized urticaria, diffuse erythema, and malar rash. The dermatologic manifestations last for a median of 3 weeks (range, 1 day to 14 months). In untreated patients, skin involvement may recur.

A wide range of symptoms may accompany the skin lesions, including fatigue, headache, stiff neck, chills, sore throat, arthralgia, myalgia, abdominal pain, nausea, and vomiting. On physical examination, fever and regional lymphadenopathy are the commonest findings. Some patients have generalized lymphadenopathy or splenomegaly. These signs and symptoms are typically intermittent and changing. During early Lyme disease, laboratory findings include an elevated sedimentation rate (50% of patients), elevated white blood cell counts (10% of patients), elevated total serum IgM (33% of patients), and abnormal hepatic function tests (20% of patients). Complement levels are usually normal, and tests for both antinuclear antibody and rheumatoid factor are almost always negative.

Several weeks to months later, approximately 15 percent of untreated patients develop frank neurologic abnormalitis (stage 2) including aseptic meningitis, encephalitis, cranial neuritis, motor and sensory radiculoneuritis, mononeuritis multiplex, or myelitis. The most frequent neurologic presentations are aseptic meningitis, Bell's palsy (which may be bilateral), or radiculoneuritis. While the cerebrospinal fluid may be normal during the first 1 to 2 weeks of illness, most of these patients develop a predominately lymphocytic pleocytosis (40 to 450 cells per cubic millimeter), sometimes accompanied by an elevated protein or a slightly decreased glucose. Multiple neurologic abnormalities can be present simultaneously or, as with all manifestations of Lyme disease, the manifestations may be intermittent and fluctuating. They typically last for months and then resolve, but chronic neurologic involvement may occur later.

Also during stage 2, approximately 8 percent of patients develop cardiac complications, which include conduction abnormalities, myopericarditis, cardiomegaly, and left ventricular dysfunction. Electrocardiographic abnormalities include varying degrees of atrioventricular block, and diffuse T-wave and ST-T segment changes. In patients with atrioventricular block, progression from first to third degree may be rapid. Radionucleotide angiography reveals depressed left ventricular ejection fractions in some patients. Cardiac abnormalities last from 3 days to 6 weeks; they may recur.

Weeks to years after the tick bite or ECM about 60 percent of untreated patients develop arthritis (stage 3), which typically occurs in brief, intermittent attacks for several years. The arthritis can be mono-, oligo-, or polyarticular and typically affects large joints, particularly the knee. However, any joint in the body may be involved. The synovial fluid typically shows evidence of moderate inflammation (2,000 to 100,000 cells per cubic millimeter) with a predominance of neutrophils. Synovial fluid complement levels are normal or slightly reduced. In approximately 10 percent of patients, the arthritis becomes chronic, with pannus formation and cartilage erosion, resembling the process seen in rheumatoid arthritis.

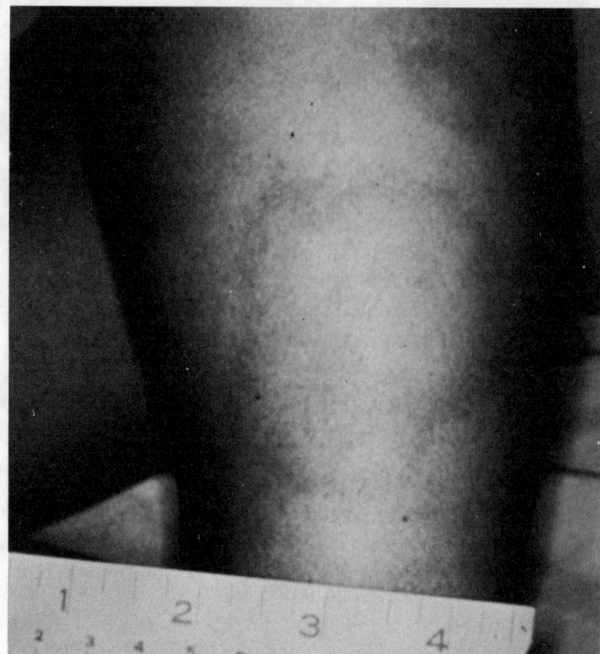

Figure 1 Secondary annular skin lesions of Lyme disease showing the cleared center of the expanded lesions.

Although the three stages of Lyme disease usually occur separately, it is important to emphasize that they may overlap or occur together. Incomplete pictures are also common. Some patients have only ECM. Others lack this lesion, and in such cases, neurologic, cardiac, or arthritic manifestations may be the presenting features of the illness.

PATHOGENESIS

After inoculation by the tick, *B. burgdorferi* may migrate outward in the skin and produce the enlarging ECM lesion. The organism may also disseminate in the blood to almost any site early in the disease. Spirochetes have been isolated from blood as well as from ECM lesions. Most of the manifestations of stages 2 and 3 Lyme disease, initially thought to be immune mediated, are now thought to be due to tissue invasion by the spirochete. *B. burgdorferi* has been isolated from cerebrospinal fluid several months after disease onset and has been seen in the synovium. The efficacy of antibiotic therapy in patients with these manifestations also suggests spirochetes are alive late in the illness.

DIAGNOSIS

In endemic areas the diagnosis of stage 1 Lyme disease can usually be made on clinical grounds if the charac-

TABLE 1 Suggested Antibiotic Therapy for Lyme Disease

Stage of Disease	*Treatment* — *Adults*	*Children*
ECM (stage 1)	Tetracycline 250 mg PO qid for 10–20 days	Penicillin V 50 mg/kg/d in divided doses for 10–20 days
	Alternatives	
	Penicillin V 500 mg PO qid for 10–20 days Erythromycin 250 mg PO qid for 10–20 days	Erythromycin 30 mg/kg/d in divided doses for 10–20 days
Neurologic (stage 2)	Penicillin G 20 million units/d IV for 10 days	Penicillin G, 300,000 units/kg/d IV for 10 days
Arthritic (stage 3)	Penicillin G 20 million units/d IV for at least 10 days *or* Benzathine penicillin 2.4 million units/week IM × 3	Penicillin G 300,000 units/kg/d IV for at least 10 days

teristic ECM lesion is present. Because the tick vector is tiny, most patients do not give a history of a tick bite. Later in the illness, a history of preceding ECM may be helpful, but some patients lack such a history. If confusion exists in diagnosis, laboratory tests can be used to confirm the clinical suspicion of Lyme disease. Examination and culture of blood, skin, and CSF, if positive for spirochetes, are definitive; at present, these are low-yield procedures. Serologic tests (immunofluoresence assay or enzyme-linked immunosorbent assay) are the most practical diagnostic aid. In stage 1 Lyme disease, these tests have low sensitivity. Only 50 percent of patients with only ECM have elevated antibody titers. However, almost all patients with later manifestations of Lyme disease have elevated titers. Antibody to *B. burgdorferi* cross reacts with other spirochetes, and patients with syphilis may have false-positive Lyme serologic tests. Similarly, patients with Lyme disease may rarely have a false-positive RPR. However, patients with Lyme disease can be distinguished from those with syphilis by the VDRL and MHA-TP tests, which are negative in patients with Lyme disease.

TREATMENT

The treatment of Lyme disease has evolved over the past several years as understanding of the illness has advanced. Before identification of the etiologic agent, studies suggested that antimicrobial treatment was effective for stage 1 Lyme disease. Trials of antimicrobial therapy were then undertaken for both late neurologic and arthritic complications. Antimicrobials are now recommended for treatment of all manifestations of Lyme disease (Table 1).

For patients with stage 1 Lyme disease, tetracycline 250 mg four times per day for 10 to 20 days is the treatment of choice. Penicillin V 500 mg four times per day and erythromycin 250 mg four times per day for 10 to 20 days are alternative treatments. For children less than 8 years of age, penicillin V, 50 mg per kilogram per day (not less than 1 g and not more than 2 g) in divided doses for 10 to 20 days is recommended. All three antimicrobials effectively treat ECM and usually prevent the late complications of the disease. About 15 percent of patients develop an intensification of symptoms (Jarisch-Herxheimer-like reaction) within 24 hours of antimicrobial therapy. A second course of antimicrobials should be given to patients who do not respond to the initial course or for those with recurrent symptoms.

For patients with neurologic complications or who develop them after treatment of early Lyme disease, intravenous penicillin G, 20 million units per day in six divided doses (penicillin G, 300,000 units per kilogram per day in children) is effective therapy. Although meningitic and sensory symptoms often improve quickly, 6 to 8 weeks are often required for the resolution of motor deficits. For patients with arthritis, this intravenous regimen, as well as intramuscular benzathine penicillin, 2.4 million units per week for 3 weeks, are sometimes effective. Although systematic trials have not been undertaken for patients with cardiac complications, antimicrobials should be used for these manifestations as well. Patients with a PR interval greater than 0.30 seconds should be admitted to the hospital for observation because of the risk of progression to higher grade AV block. If high-grade block develops, temporary pacing may be necessary.

The role of corticosteroids in the treatment of any stage or manifestation of Lyme disease appears limited. It is possible that corticosteroids may have some role in patients with Bell's palsy if they are seen within 24 hours of onset and in patients with complete heart block or congestive heart failure if they do not improve on antimicrobial therapy alone within 24 hours.

Prevention

Protective clothing and/or insect repellents may offer some protection against tick bites for those engaged in outdoor activities in endemic areas.

HERPES SIMPLEX VIRUS INFECTION

RICHARD J. WHITLEY, M.D.
DAVID W. BARNES, M.D.

Of the recent advances in antiviral therapy, the treatment of herpes simplex virus (HSV) infections has provided the most gratifying results. In the early 1960s, effective topical antiviral therapy for the management of herpes simplex keratoconjunctivitis was introduced. A decade later significant advances were achieved in the treatment of life-threatening herpes simplex encephalitis and neonatal herpes. More recently, with the development of acyclovir, mucocutaneous HSV infections have become treatable. HSV infections of the skin are among the most common diseases of humans. The successful treatment of cutaneous herpex simplex virus infections has been predicated, in large part, upon the physician's ability to diagnose these infections rapidly because of clinically apparent and characteristic skin lesions. A broad spectrum of infection with HSV exists, ranging from totally asymptomatic or benign nuisance infections, such as recurrent labial or genital herpes, to those that are life-threatening, such as herpes simplex encephalitis or neonatal herpes simplex virus infections. With most clinical therapeutics, successful therapy is facilitated by prompt and accurate diagnosis. Treatment of viral infections is no exception. A delay in diagnosis, particularly when organs such as the brain are involved, only leads to progressive disease and poor therapeutic outcome. Similarly, successful therapy of primary genital infections is most beneficial when drug is administered within a few days of the onset of clinical symptoms and signs.

The propensity for HSV infections to be more severe during symptomatic primary disease or when occurring in the immuncompromised host provides a broader therapeutic window for evaluation of antiviral efficacy than with recurrent infection. As with other antimicrobials, the definition of a therapeutic index or ratio of efficacy to toxicity must balance recommendations for application of antivirals to human disease. In defining the numerator of the therapeutic index, efficacy must equate with an enhanced clinical effect beyond that of simply promoting cessation of viral excretion. Similarly, assessment of toxicity must consider both acute laboratory and clinical aberrations associated with the administration of the medication and the long-term consequences of the administration of these drugs. For example, nucleoside analogues must be assessed for potential mutagenicity and teratogenicity, particularly if therapy is to be administered for long periods. Furthermore, the potential for the development of viral resistance must be included in the risk-to-benefit ratio for any treatment modality.

This chapter focuses on the current application of antiviral therapies in the treatment of HSV infections. Each disease state is considered separately; the importance of prompt and accurate diagnosis is emphasized. Although a number of unproven or investigational antiviral agents have potential uses in therapy for herpesvirus infections, they will not be addressed in this summary.

HERPES SIMPLEX ENCEPHALITIS

Herpes simplex encephalitis (HSE) is the commonest cause of sporadic, fatal encephalitis in the United States, with an estimated annual incidence of approximately one in 500,000 individuals. Patients with HSE have clinical evidence of an acute febrile encephalopathy, signs of temporal lobe involvement with disordered mentation, seizures, evidence of localized central nervous system disease by diagnostic studies (brain scan, computerized tomography, and/or electroencephalography), and cerebrospinal fluid findings compatible with viral encephalitis. Even in the presence of these clinical findings, establishment of a diagnosis of HSE is particularly problematic. The only unequivocal method by which the diagnosis of HSE can be confirmed is by brain biopsy. As shown in Figure 1, a logical approach to the evaluation of individuals who present with evidence of localization by neurodiagnostic assessment is the performance of brain biopsy with detailed tissue examination. Such an approach will lead to confirmation of HSV infection of the brain by rapid diagnostic tests and isolation of virus in culture and, of equal importance, to the prompt and expeditious diagnosis of diseases that may mimic herpes simplex encephalitis (Table 1). Complications from the biopsy procedure itself and the likelihood of obtaining a false-negative result for virus are exceedingly small. It should be emphasized that if the patient does not have evidence of a focal encephalitic process, the probability of HSE is very low.

Historically, double-blinded, placebo-controlled studies of vidarabine therapy have demonstrated a reduced mortality in treatment of HSE. Mortality in placebo recipients is 70 percent, with 11 percent of survivors, or 2.5 percent of patients overall, returning to normal function. Vidarabine therapy decreases mortality to 40 percent 6 months after onset of disease. Twenty percent of patients overall return to normal function. These data led to the licensure of vidarabine for the treatment of HSE at a dosage of 15 mg per kilogram per day given intravenously over 12 hours for 10 to 14 days. However, recent data indicate that acyclovir is superior to vidarabine for the treatment of HSE. A further reduction in mortality rate—to 20 percent 6 months after the onset of treatment—has been demonstrated. Normalcy is achieved in 30 to 56 percent of patients six months after treatment. Thus, acyclovir is now the treatment of choice for HSE. As shown in Table 2, the dosage of acyclovir is 10 mg per kilogram administered every 8 hours for a period of 10 days. It should be noted that in adults simple menin-

These studies were supported in part by contract No. 1-AI-12667 from the Development and Applications Branch of the National Institute of Allergy and Infectious Diseases, grant NCI-13148 from the National Cancer Institute, and grant RR-032 from the Division of Research Resources.

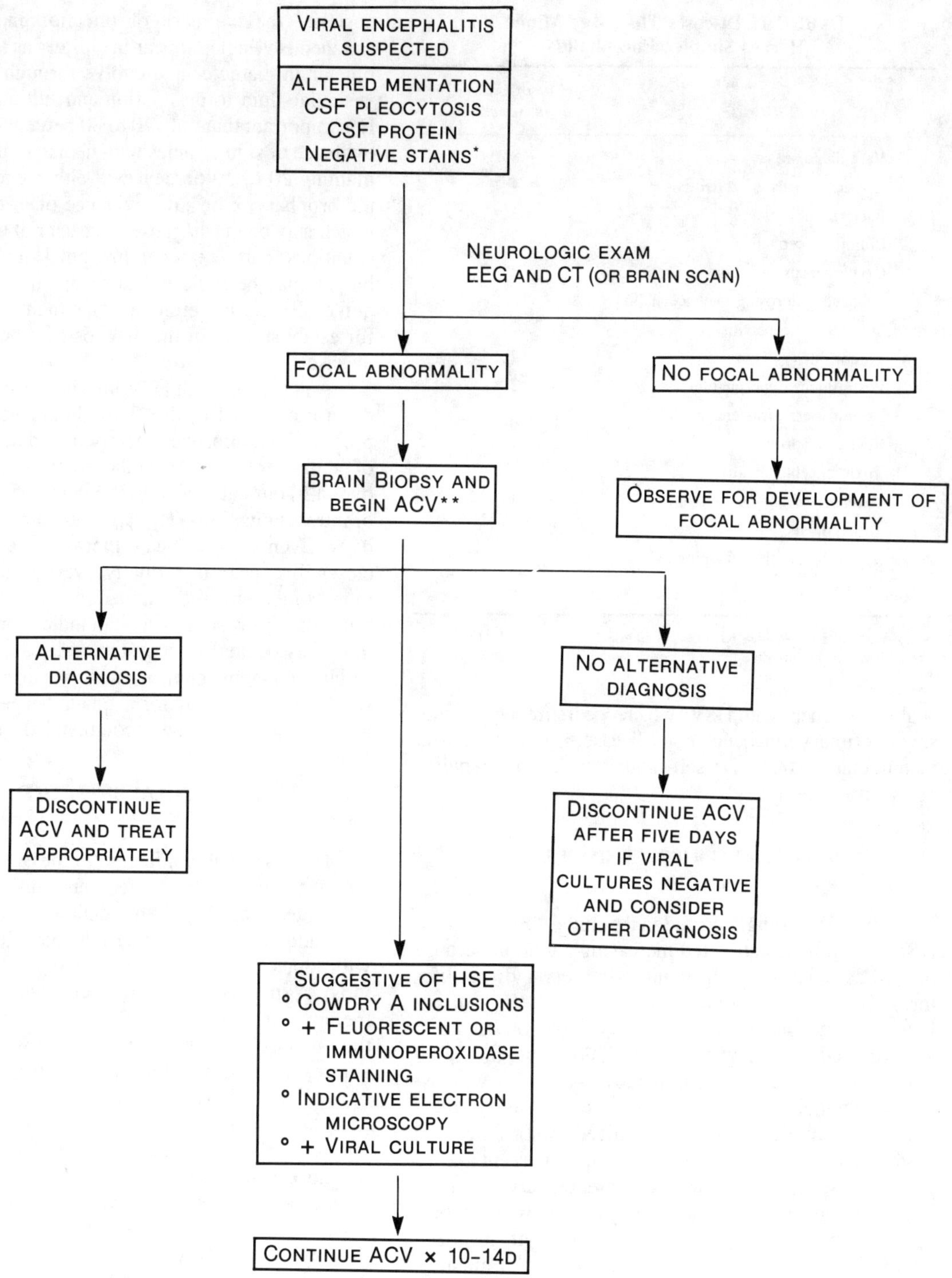

Figure 1 Suggested evaluation and therapy for herpes simplex encephalitis. * = gram, AFB, and India ink stains; ** = 10 mg per kilogram IV every 8 hours.

TABLE 1 Diseases That May Mimic Herpes Simplex Encephalitis

Disease	*No. of Cases in Series*
Vascular disease	8
Coxsackievirus encephalitis	4
Bacterial abscess	3
Mumps encephalitis	3
Cryptococcus infection	2
Subacute sclerosing panencephalitis	2
St. Louis encephalitis	2
Tumor	2
Postinfluenza encephalitis	2
Epstein-Barr virus encephalitis	2
Reye's syndrome	1
Toxic encephalopathy	1
Toxoplasma gondii infection	1
Tuberculosis	1
Lymphocytic choriomeningitis	1
Total	32

Note: Adapted from Whitley RJ, et al. N Engl J Med 1981; 304:313–8. Used with permission.

geal involvement with HSV, which occurs frequently with severe primary mucocutaneous disease, is like other viral meningitides in that it is a self-limited process and requires no specific therapy.

NEONATAL HERPES SIMPLEX

After first being reported in the mid-1930s, neonatal HSV infection has attracted increasing attention because of its association with genital herpes and its life-threatening nature with a known propensity for causing long-term morbidity. Neonatal HSV infection occurs at an estimated frequency of one in 3,000 to one in 15,000 live births per year. Without therapy, the disease will disseminate widely in more than 80 percent of cases. Multiple organ involvement and localized central nervous system disease have mortality rates of 80 percent and 50 percent, respectively. With severe disease, survivors rarely escape significant neurologic impairment without therapy. As many as 30 percent of babies with localized neonatal HSV infection of the skin, eye, and/or mouth—although not at risk for mortality—can have evidence of neurologic impairment on follow-up.

Important observations which suggest a diagnosis of neonatal HSV infection are viral excretion from the maternal genital tract, a maternal history or a sexual partner with genital herpes, the inability to grow bacteria from cerebrospinal fluid or blood cultures of an infant with suspected meningitis or encephalitis, characteristic findings on electroencephalogram or CT scan, and progressively increasing levels of cerebrospinal fluid protein in the presence of clinical deterioration. Confirmation of the diagnosis remains dependent upon the isolation of HSV from vesicles, the hallmark of infection in these children. Cutaneous vesicles appear in clusters as small as one millimeter in diameter and evolve through phases of clear vesicular fluid to pustulation and, ultimately, scabbing. It is important that only 70 to 80 percent of children have evidence of skin vesicles with neonatal infection. The remaining 20 to 30 percent will either excrete virus from the oropharynx or have evidence of brain involvement, which may be misdiagnosed as bacterial infection. In such situations, cultures of cerebrospinal fluid and even brain biopsy may be indicated to establish the diagnosis unequivocally. Serial serologic assessment is of limited value for establishment of the diagnosis in the early phases of disease.

Any neonate with HSV infection, including those with disease confined to the skin, should be treated. At the present time, approved therapy is vidarabine at a dosage of 30 mg per kilogram per day administered intravenously over 12 hours at a concentration of 0.5 mg per milliliter of intravenous fluid. Therapy should be continued for 10 days. Even with adequate therapy, recurrent skin vesicles will appear in virtually every child within 2 to 3 months following the completion of treatment. The recurrence of skin vesicles is not an indication for retreatment unless associated with systemic disease. Eventually the results of ongoing clinical trials comparing vidarabine versus acyclovir therapy for neonatal herpes infections may lead to changes in the recommended therapy.

OCULAR INFECTION

Herpes simplex infection of the eye is recognized as one of the commonest infectious causes of blindness in the United States. Of all modalities of herpesviral therapy available to date, the earliest benefits were achieved with topical therapy of herpes simplex keratoconjunctivitis. A persistent problem encountered with topical therapy—as well as for other modalities of therapy—is the propensity for recurrences even with successful initial treatment. Idoxuridine, trifluorothymidine, and vidarabine all can abort individual attacks with varying but acceptable degrees of toxicity. The most pronounced toxicity is local allergic reaction to idoxuridine. For optimal diagnosis and therapy, care of HSV infections of the eye should be provided by a qualified ophthalmologist. The concomitant prescribing of corticosteroids with antiviral therapy should only be undertaken by physicians experienced in the management of herpes simplex keratoconjunctivitis. The drug of choice at the present time for the treatment of this disease appears to be trifluorothymidine.

MUCOCUTANEOUS HERPES SIMPLEX

Herpes simplex labial and genital infections have been a major focus of antiviral research in the United States. Significant advances in the treatment of human HSV infections from a therapeutic and suppressive standpoint have been achieved in this area. At the present time, the management of these infections is dependent in large part upon host immune status (normal or immunocompromised) and the nature of the infection (primary or recurrent). Aside from the classic clinical presentation of vesicular/ulcerative lesions, the standard of diagnosis is the isolation of virus in tissue culture. Evidence of cytopathic effect in tissue culture usually occurs within 48 to 72 hours. More rapid diagnostic techniques have included lesion scrapings followed by staining with monoclonal antibodies, although these techniques may lack sensitivity and specificity. Humoral antibodies to HSV, types 1 and 2 are common, even in persons without clinical disease, and are of limited diagnostic usefulness.

As shown in Figure 2, there is no established or approved therapy for primary herpes simplex gingivostomatitis or recurrent herpes simplex labialis in the normal host. By contrast, in the immunocompromised host who suffers from recurrent orolabial HSV infections, three preparations of acyclovir—topical, oral, and intravenous—have all been shown to be useful. At the present time the topical and intravenous formulations of acyclovir are approved by the U.S. Food and Drug Administration for treatment of labial lesions, progressive stomatitis, and cutaneous disease in the immunocompromised patients. The appropriate dosage regimens for utilization of these compounds in each circumstance appear in Table 2. The recent licensure of the oral formulation of acyclovir should provide an effective therapy for HSV infections in immunocompromised patients who are not systemically ill. Intravenous vidarabine appears to be of limited utility in the treatment of mucocutaneous HSV infections in immunocompromised patients and is not recommended.

The management of genital HSV infections has undergone even more striking advances. Following the demonstration that topical acyclovir accelerated viral clearance and decreased clinical symptomatology in primary genital HSV infections by 24 to 48 hours, further therapeutic advances were achieved with both the intravenous and oral formulations of acyclovir. Although intravenous acyclovir has demonstrated efficacy in the treatment of primary genital herpes infections, its cost as well as the requirement for hospitalization for drug administration restrict this form of therapy to particularly severe cases. The recent licensure of the oral formulation of acyclovir may offer a more efficacious and cost effective treatment for primary genital HSV infections. Significant reductions in the duration of viral shedding, the time to healing, and the duration and severity of the clinical symptoms comparable to those seen with intravenous acyclovir can be achieved with oral therapy. The drug can be administered to the patient in an ambulatory setting, avoiding the expense of hospitalization and the hazards of intravenous therapy.

The effect of acyclovir in the treatment of recurrent episodes of genital HSV infection is less marked. Topical acyclovir, when applied very early in the course of a recurrence, may be of some benefit in decreasing the duration of viral shedding. The effect of topical therapy on the events of healing is minor, but greater benefit may be achieved by beginning application of the ointment during the prodromal phase of a recurrence rather than waiting for lesions to appear. Such an approach has not been proved efficacious. Oral acyclovir has been shown to be effective in shortening the clinical course of recurrent genital herpes simplex infections, but has no significant effect on the frequency of recurrences when taken intermittently. Recent trials have shown that continuous administration of oral acyclovir is effective in suppressing attacks in patients with frequent recurrences. However, discontinuation of suppressive therapy results in the recurrence of disease, with an attack frequency no different from that prior to therapy. The adverse effects of long-term acyclovir administration are not yet known, and caution should be used in prescribing this drug on a continuous-use basis. The use of systemic (oral or intravenous) acyclovir should be avoided in pregnancy because of the potential for adverse effects on the fetus. If therapy is indicated in this setting, topical acyclovir should be used. In addition, acyclovir-resistant herpes simplex viruses have been found in clinical isolates even without prior exposure to drug. Several studies have demonstrated the emergence of acyclovir-resistant herpes simplex virus during acyclovir therapy, but the clinical significance of this observation is unknown. With cessation of acyclovir therapy, there is reversion to acyclovir sensitivity in most cases, perhaps because of reduced pathogenicity of the resistant strain. Thus, intermittent therapy may be perferrable to chronic continuous therapy in the management of recurrent genital herpes.

Acyclovir has also been shown to be effective in the suppression and treatment of recurrent HSV infections in immuncompromised patients. These infections can be particularly troublesome in those patients with hematologic malignancies as well as those on high doses of immunosuppressive agents or with defects in cellular immunity. Oral prophylactic therapy may offer such patients with persistent or recurrent mucocutaneous herpes simplex infections effective outpatient therapy. Intravenous and oral acyclovir prophylaxis have been used successfully in patients undergoing bone marrow transplantation while awaiting marrow recovery.

VISCERAL INVOLVEMENT

Visceral disease associated with HSV infection is generally encountered in two circumstances: newborns with disseminated involvement and immunocompromised hosts, particularly organ transplant recipients. In these individuals, the most common visceral HSV complications include esophagitis, hepatitis, and pneumonitis. Although no controlled data exist to substantiate the clinical utility of therapy in these situations, a reasonable choice for severe or life-threatening disease is the administration of acyclovir, at the dosages indicated in Table 1.

Diagnosis of visceral complications can be difficult and is achieved by isolation of virus from biopsy material (lung, liver, or esophagus). Confirmation of HSV infection can be made in culture either by monoclonal stain-

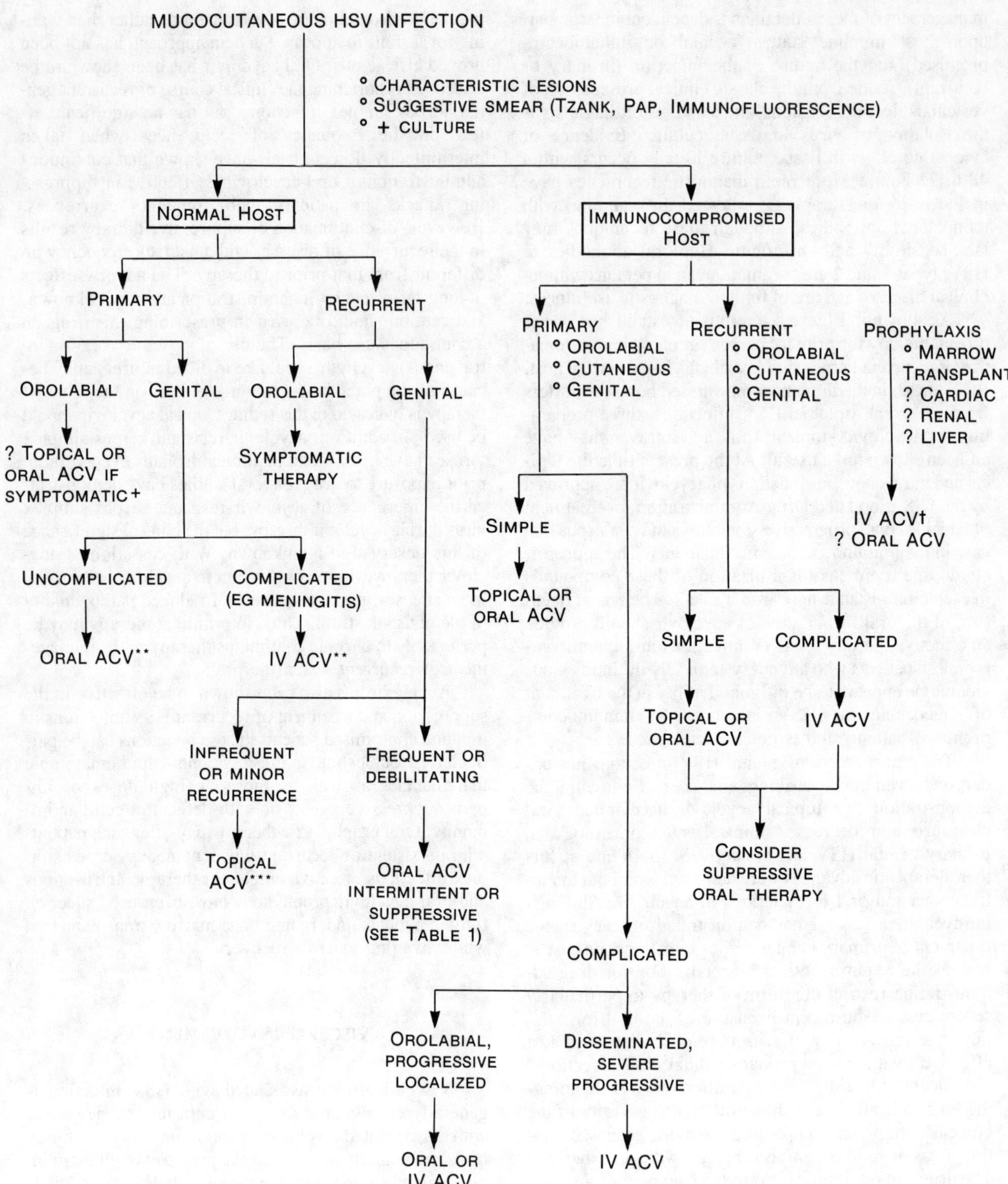

Figure 2 Therapeutic approaches to mucocutaneous herpes simplex virus infections. * = 200 mg PO five times per day for 10 days; ** = 5 mg per kilogram IV every 8 hours for 10 days; *** = 5 percent ointment applied every 3 to 4 hours (initiated during prodrome if recurrent); + = not of proven efficacy; † = 5 mg per kilogram IV every 8 to 12 hours while susceptible.

TABLE 2 U.S. Food and Drug Administration Approved Antiviral Modalities for Herpes Simplex Virus (HSV) Infections

Antiviral	*Formulation*	*Indication*	*Dosage Administration*	*Some Reported Side Effects*
5-iodo-2′-deoxyuridine (Idoxuridine, IDU, Stoxil)	Topical ophthalmic 0.1% solution or 0.5% ointment	HSV keratitis	Solution: 1 gtt q1h while awake and q4h at night; ointment: q4h while awake	Contact dermatitis, pruritis, tearing, viral resistance
9-β-D-arabinofuranosyladenine (vidarabine, adenine arabinoside, ara-A, Vira-A)	Topical ophthalmic 3% ointment	HSV keratitis	q4h while awake and qhs	Contact dermatitis, pruritis, tearing, viral resistance
	Intravenous	HSV encephalitis	15 mg/kg/day IV; dilute to 0.5 mg/ml and administer over 12h × 14 days	Nausea and vomiting, diarrhea, megaloblastosis, tremors, myoclonus, seizures
	Intravenous	Neonatal herpes	30 mg/kg/day IV; dilute to 0.5 mg/ml and administer over 12h × 14 days	Elevated SGOT; allopurinol is a relative contraindication-accumulation of toxic metabolites; viral resistance (decreased dose necessary in renal impairment)
2′-deoxy-5-(trifluoromethyl) uridine (TFT, Viroptic)	Topical ophthalmic 1% solution	HSV keratitis	1 gtt q2h × 7 days 1 gtt q4h × 7 days (do not exceed 21 days therapy)	Contact dermatitis, pruritis, tearing, viral resistance
9-[(2-hydroxyethoxy) methyl] guanine (Acyclovir, ACV, Zovirax)	Topical ointment 5%	Primary genital or mucocutaneous HSV	Cover lesions q3h while awake and qhs × 7 days	Drug sensitization, viral resistance
	Oral capsule 200 mg	Primary genital HSV	1 cap PO q4h while awake × 10 days	Vomiting, nausea, headache, ? decreased spermiogenesis, viral resistance
		Suppressive therapy with recurrences >6 times/year	1 cap PO q8h for <6 months*	
	Intravenous	Primary genital HSV and immunocompromised patients with primary or recurrent disease†	Adults: 5 mg/kg IV over 1h q8h × 7 days; children (<12 yrs), 750 mg/m²/day as above	Elevated BUN, nausea, viral resistance, headache, thrombophlebitis (with IV formulation) (decreased dose necessary in renal impairment)
	Intravenous	HSV encephalitis	Adults: 10 mg/kg IV over 1h q8h × 10 days; children (<12 yrs), 1,200 mg/m²/day as above	

* Another option is intermittent therapy initiated by the patient while in the prodromal stage of a recurrent episode and continued for 5 days. Dose is the same as primary infection.

† Oral therapy may be appropriate in some instances.

ing of cellular debris or the cell sheet, immunoperoxidase staining, or antigen detection using a variety of procedures. It does not appear that vidarabine is useful in the management of these infections.

CONCLUSIONS

Antiviral therapy has been shown to be effective for many herpes simplex virus infections, particularly those of the genital tract, in the immunocompromised host, and neonatal and encephalitic diseases. However, recurrences cannot be prevented with existing modalities of therapy, even when therapy is administered shortly after the onset of primary infection. This observation is true for all antiviral medicines presently in use. As with other forms of antimicrobial therapy, continual monitoring for potential toxicity is imperative, particularly in the setting of chronic therapy. The evolution of antiviral therapy over the last decade has allowed us to successfully manage severe and life-threatening HSV infections and has allowed for control, albeit not yet optimal, of less severe yet psychologically debilitating mucocutaneous infections. Such advances will provide a foundation for developments in antiviral therapy that will lead to the discovery of more effective drugs and the prevention of recurrent disease.

VIRAL HEMORRHAGIC FEVER

C. J. PETERS, M.D.
ALEXIS SHELOKOV, M.D.

Several RNA viruses transmitted to humans from animals or arthropods may cause a syndrome referred to as viral hemorrhagic fever or VHF (Table 1). The target organ for the VHF syndrome is the vascular bed; correspondingly, the dominant clinical features are usually related to microvascular damage and changes in vascular permeability. Common presenting complaints are fever, myalgia, and prostration; clinical examination may reveal only conjunctivitis, mild hypotension, flushing, and petechial hemorrhages. Full-blown VHF typically proceeds to shock and generalized mucous membrane hemorrhage and is often accompanied by evidence of neurologic, hematopoietic, or pulmonary system involvement. Hepatic involvement is common, but a clinical picture dominated by jaundice and other evidence of hepatic failure is only seen in some cases of Rift Valley fever, Congo-Crimean HF, Marburg HF, Ebola HF, and yellow fever. Renal failure is proportional to cardiovascular compromise, except in hemorrhagic fever with renal syndrome (HFRS), where it is an integral part of the syndrome. Mortality is substantial, ranging from 5 to 20 percent or higher in recognized cases.

EPIDEMIOLOGY

Since these viruses are all zoonotic agents, the major determinant of human infection is rural exposure to the appropriate reservoir (Table 1). Several exceptions exist: (*1*) Dengue is typically an urban disease, although a sylvatic cycle exists. (*2*) Yellow fever may develop an urban transmission cycle by involving *Aedes aegypti* mosquitoes; the last time this occurred in coastal U.S. cities was in 1905 (New Orleans), but in recent years urban outbreaks have been recognized in Africa. (*3*) Viruses causing HFRS may infect rats; rats in turn have transmitted disease to urban dwellers in Asia and to laboratory personnel working with rat colonies in Europe and Asia. It should be noted that distinction between ''urban'' and ''rural'' can be ambiguous if meat products or ectoparasite-laden domestic animals are present within large cities.

All the viruses in Table 1 (exception: dengue virus) are infectious by aerosol or fomites. Since most patients are viremic, there is a potential for transmission to patients, medical staff, and particularly laboratory personnel (exception: Hantaan virus infection).

The age and sex distributions of each disease generally reflect the opportunities for zoonotic exposure. The exception is DHF/DSS which has typically been a childhood disease in its major focus in Southeast Asia. (DHF/DSS will be used to refer to hemorrhagic fever and shock syndrome, the life-threatening complications of dengue fever). DHF/DSS is also unique since it is thought to result most often from infections with a second dengue virus serotype. Although this is the general epidemiologic pattern, dengue virus may, rarely, cause hemorrhagic fever in adults and in primary infections.

DIFFERENTIAL DIAGNOSIS

Because of the ecologic determinants of virus circulation, a detailed travel history is essential in making the diagnosis of VHF. VHF should be suspected in any pa-

TABLE 1 Recognized Viral Hemorrhagic Fevers of Humans

Viral Group	*Disease (virus)*	*Natural Geographic Distribution*	*Source of Human Infection**	*Incubation Period (days)*
Arenavirus	Lassa	Africa	Rodent (nosocomial)	5–16
	Argentine HF (Junin)	South America	Rodent (nosocomial)	7–14
	Bolivian HF (Machupo)	South America	Rodent (nosocomial)	7–14
Bunyaviridae				
Phlebovirus	Rift Valley fever	Africa	Mosquito (slaughter of domestic animal)	2–5
Nairovirus	Congo-Crimean HF	Europe, Asia, Africa	Tick (slaughter of domestic animal; nosocomial)	3–12
Hantavirus	Hemorrhagic fever with renal syndrome (Hantaan and related viruses)	Asia, Europe; possibly worldwide	Rodent	9–35
Filovirus	Marburg and Ebola HF	Africa	Unknown (nosocomial)	3–16
Flavivirus (mosquito-borne)	Yellow fever	Tropical Africa, South America	Mosquito	3–6
	Dengue HF	Asia, Americas, Africa	Mosquito	†
Flavivirus (tick-borne)	Kyasanur Forest disease	India	Tick	3–8
	Omsk HF	Soviet Union	Tick (muskrat-contaminated water)	3–8

* Usual source in nature (other routes in parentheses).
† Unknown for DHF, but 3–15 days for uncomplicated dengue.

tient presenting with a severe febrile illness and evidence of vascular involvement (lower than normal blood pressure, postural hypotension, petechiae, easy bleeding, flushing of face and chest, edema) who has traveled to an area where the virus is known to occur (Table 1). Signs and symptoms suggesting additional organ system involvement are common, but rarely dominate the picture (headache, photophobia, pharyngitis, cough, nausea or vomiting, diarrhea, constipation, abdominal pain, hyperesthesia, dizziness, confusion, tremor). The macular eruption present in most Marburg-Ebola cases should be sought because of its diagnostic importance.

For much of the world, the major differential diagnosis is malaria. It must be borne in mind that parasitemia in patients partially immune to malaria does not prove that symptoms are due to malaria. Typhoid fever and rickettsial and leptospiral diseases are major confounding infections, with nontyphoidal salmonellosis, shigellosis, relapsing fever, fulminant hepatitis, and meningococcemia being some of the other important diagnoses to exclude. Any condition leading to disseminated intravascular coagulation could present in a confusing fashion, as well as diseases such as acute leukemia, lupus erythematosus, thrombotic thrombocytopenic purpura, idiopathic thrombocytopenic purpura, among others.

Because of recent recognition of their worldwide occurrence, additional consideration should be given to infections with Hantaan-related viruses. The classic HFRS, including Korean hemorrhagic fever syndrome, progressing from fever through hemorrhage, shock, renal failure, and polyuria, has a well-described and severe course. However, the Scandinavian and some European virus strains usually produce a much milder disease (referred to as nephropathia epidemica) with prominent fever, myalgia, and abdominal pain and only a brief period of oliguria. The full spectrum of Hantaan-like virus infections in humans is still being defined and may include mild influenza-like illness, aseptic meningitis, and hemorrhagic pneumonitis.

The clinical laboratory can be very helpful. Thrombocytopenia (exception: Lassa) and leukopenia (exceptions: Lassa and Hantaan) are the rule. Proteinuria and/or hematuria are common, being the rule in Argentine HF, Bolivian HF, and Hantaan-related viral infections. A positive tourniquet test has been particularly useful in DSS/DHF, but should be sought in other HF as well.

Definitive diagnosis in an individual case rests on specific virologic diagnosis. Most patients are viremic at presentation (exception: Hantaan-related viral infections). These viruses (exceptions: dengue and Hantaan) require specialized microbiologic containment for safe handling, so the virus laboratory should be consulted before submission of samples for isolation or serology. Both the Centers for Disease Control (CDC; Atlanta, Georgia) and the U.S. Army Medical Research Institute of Infectious Diseases (USAMRIID; Frederick, Maryland) have diagnostic laboratories functioning at the highest (P4) containment level (see end for addresses).

Rapid diagnostic tests for Rift Valley fever or Lassa viral antigens can be performed on inactivated samples. Lassa- and Hantaan-specific IgM are often detectable during the acute illness. Otherwise, diagnosis by virus cultivation and identification will require 3 to 10 days.

THERAPY

Specific antiviral therapy of proven value (Table 2) is available for Lassa virus (the antiviral drug ribavirin) and the Argentine HF (2 units of convalescent plasma before the first 8 days of illness). The lifesaving value of appropriate supportive management of DHF/DSS is emphasized by its inclusion in this table, even though the treatment is syndrome specific and not virus specific.

Because they often come from malarious areas, patients should either be evaluated by an experienced laboratory to exclude malaria or should be empirically treated for falciparum malaria with a regimen known to be effective for the geographic parasite strain. Conversely, the presence of malarial parasites, particularly in the immunes, should not preclude the management of a patient for VHF, if clinically indicated. Several nonspecific measures apply to all the VHF: additional capillary damage and hemostatic impairment should be minimized by prompt hospitalization, gentle handling, avoidance of acetylsalicylic acid, and other antiplatelet-anticlotting-factor drugs. Restlessness, confusion, myalgia, and hyperesthesia frequently are problems and should be managed by reassurance and other supportive measures. Judicious use of oral opiates, diazepam, or chloral hydrate may be indicated at times. Secondary infections are common and should be monitored and vigorously treated. Intravenous lines, catheters, and other invasive procedures must be avoided unless clearly indicated in management. Attention should be given to pulmonary toilet, the usual measures to prevent superinfection, and supplemental oxygen. Immunosuppression with steroids or other agents has no empiric or theoretical basis, except possibly in HFRS. In this disease the onset of the immune response coincides with the onset of disease, and uncontrolled observations have suggested that cyclophosphamide therapy may be useful. However, these observations require confirmation before such therapy can be recommended.

The management of bleeding is controversial. Uncontrolled clinical observations support vigorous administration of clotting factor concentrates and platelets, as well as early use of heparin, for expectant management of disseminated intravascular coagulation. In the absence of definitive evidence, it is recommended that mild bleeding manifestations not be treated at all. More severe hemorrhagic defects should receive appropriate replacement therapy. When definite laboratory evidence of disseminated intravascular coagulation develops, heparin therapy should be employed if appropriate laboratory control is available. Plasma levels of coagulation factors may decrease from lack of synthesis and/or vascular leakage, and viral involvement of bone marrow and liver can complicate interpretation of the usually employed coagulation parameters.

TABLE 2 Therapy and Prophylaxis of Viral Hemorrhagic Fevers

	Therapy		
Disease	*Indicated*	*Speculative**	*Prophylaxis*
Lassa fever	Ribavirin;† convalescent plasma‡	----	Ribavirin; convalescent plasma
Argentine HF	Convalescent plasma†	Ribavirin	Convalescent plasma; vaccine in phase I testing
Bolivian HF	Convalescent plasma‡	Ribavirin	Convalescent plasma
Rift Valley fever	Ribavirin;‡ convalescent plasma‡	----	Vaccine (investigational); interferon;* convalescent plasma;† ribavirin‡
Congo-Crimean HF	----	Convalescent plasma‡; ribavirin; heparin	----
Hemorrhagic fever with renal syndrome	----	Ribavirin	Convalescent plasma‡
Marburg and Ebola HF	----	Convalescent plasma plus interferon; heparin	----
Yellow fever	----	Convalescent plasma	Vaccine (licensed)
Dengue HF	Vigorous fluid therapy†	----	Vaccine (investigational for DEN-2)
Kyasanur Forest disease	----	----	Vaccine (investigational)
Omsk HF	----	----	----

Note: Before proceeding with therapy of a suspected case, physician should contact a laboratory with an ongoing program in VHF, such as those listed at the end of the chapter.
* Some clinical or laboratory data suggest possibility of limited applicability in specific circumstances.
† Shown to decrease human morbidity and mortality in controlled study or by strong clinical evidence.
‡ Laboratory data in non-human primates and/or anecdotal human data suggest that potential benefits outweigh risks.

Management of hypotension and shock is difficult. Patients are often modestly dehydrated from heat, fever, anorexia, vomiting, and/or diarrhea. There are covert losses of intravascular volume through hemorrhage and increased vascular permeability. Nevertheless, these patients often respond poorly to fluid infusion and readily develop pulmonary edema, possibly due to myocardial impairment or increased pulmonary vascular permeability. Fluid should be given cautiously and colloid should be used. Dopamine would seem to be the agent of choice for shock, but has never been properly evaluated. Alpha-adrenergic agents have not been clinically helpful except when there is need to temporize; vasodilators have never been systematically evaluated. Cardiac stimulants, such as digitalis glycosides, could reasonably be applied. Pharmacologic doses of corticosteroids (30 mg methylprednisolone per kilogram) provide another reasonable but untested therapeutic modality in treating shock.

Two hemorrhagic fevers should be clearly separated from the other diseases. Severe consequences of dengue infection are largely due to systemic capillary leakage syndrome and should be managed initially by brisk infusion of crystalloid, followed by albumin or other colloid if there is no response. Severe Hantaan-like virus infections present many of the management problems of the other hemorrhagic fevers, but will culminate in acute renal failure with a subsequent polyuria during recovery. Careful fluid and electrolyte management, and, often, renal dialysis, are necessary for optimal treatment of these cases.

ISOLATION AND CONTAINMENT

With the exceptions of dengue (no secondary infection hazard) and Hantaan-like viruses (not present in excreta or blood at the time of hospitalization), HF patients have significant quantities of virus in blood and, perhaps, in other secretions. Experience in field situations suggests that the mask-gown-glove precautions and other barrier nursing procedures commonly employed will halt transmission in most cases. Careful attention to needle disposal and other sources of parenteral exposure is mandatory. Rarely, these infections may disseminate by the aerosol route, in which case secondary infections among contacts and medical personnel should be expected, unless maximal containment precautions have been observed. It should also be borne in mind that most experience wtih various VHF has been gained in situations where respirators, arterial lines, routine blood sampling, and extensive laboratory analysis of contaminated samples were not available. No carrier state has ever been observed with any VHF, but excretion of virus in urine or semen may occur in convalescence; also, late-onset complications such as uveitis may be associated with the local presence of infectious virus.

Laboratories experienced in dealing with P4 level pathogens include: *United States of America*—United States Army Medical Research Institute of Infectious Diseases, Disease Assessment Division, Ft. Detrick, Frederick, Maryland, 21701-5011 (telephone

301-663-7193 or evenings 301-663-7655); Centers for Disease Control, Special Pathogens Branch, Atlanta, Georgia 30333 (telephone 404-329-3308); *United Kingdom*—Center for Applied Microbiology and Research, Special Pathogens Unit, Salisbury, Porton Down, Wiltshire, SP4 0JG, England; *South Africa*—National Institute for Virology, Private Bag X4, Sandringham, Johannesburg (telephone 27-11-6405031).

The views of the authors do not purport to reflect the positions of the U.S. Department of the Army or the U.S. Department of Defense.

INFECTIONS AFFECTING MORE THAN ONE SYSTEM CAUSED BY PARASITES OR FUNGI

MALARIA

JOEL G. BREMAN, M.D.

Human malaria is a protozoal infection with any of four species of the genus *Plasmodium (P. falciparum, P. vivax, P. malariae, P. ovale*). An acute infection typically manifests fever, chills, shivering, sweats, and malaise; severe attacks, usually caused by *P. falciparum*, may lead to convulsions, loss of consciousness, and death if the illness is not diagnosed and treated promptly.

The disease is endemic throughout the tropical developing countries in Central and South America, Haiti, the Dominican Republic, Africa, the Middle East, the Indian subcontinent, Asia and Oceania. Although about 7 to 11 million cases are reported to the World Health Organization (WHO) each year, the actual number is at least 20 times greater, because of incomplete reporting. In the United States, where the disease was eradicated in the 1950s, 1,013 cases of malaria were reported in 1984. As in previous years, about one-third of these cases were in U.S. citizens who were infected during travel abroad. From 1966 to 1984, 70 deaths due to malaria were reported in the United States, and 92 percent of these were due to *P. falciparum*.

LIFE CYCLE OF *PLASMODIUM*

A description of the natural cycle of malaria is important to understand the basis of diagnosis, treatment, and prevention. The infected female mosquito injects malaria sporozoites as it feeds, and within 30 minutes these enter hepatocytes (exoerythrocytic stage). After parasitic maturation (primary tissue schizogony), that takes 7 to 15 days, the merozoites rupture from an hepatic cell containing a mature schizontand enter red blood cells (RBCs) beginning the erythrocytic schizogonic cycle. The parasites again mature in the RBCs, become schizonts, containing daughter blood-stage merozoites. The infected RBCs rupture, and the blood stage cycle is continued, with the invasion of other RBCs by merozoites. Most of the blood-stage parasites are asexual, but some parasites differentiate into gametocytes. These sexual forms, when ingested by the feeding mosquito, develop into oocysts in the gut of the mosquito, then into sporozoites, allowing the transmission cycle to begin once again when the mosquito takes another blood meal.

P. vivax and *P. ovale* are relapsing species, meaning that some of the sporozoites may become hypnozoites, or dormant forms in the liver, with the potential to complete development and initiate renewed cycles of RBC infection months or even years later. Parasite density in RBCs may be at very low levels for prolonged periods due to partial immunity of the host, use of incompletely effective drugs or both. Recrudescences are renewed manifestations of an infection due to survival of the erythrocytic forms of the parasite; infectin with *P. falciparum* and *P. malariae* is the commonest cause of recrudescences.

DIAGNOSIS

The individual with malaria almost always reports fever lasting for one or more days; other symptoms are those resembling influenza—chills, sweating, headache, muscle pain, and malaise. In infants the classic signs and symptoms may not be present; there may only be irritability, lethargy, and decreased appetite. Cerebral malaria is the most severe complication. Malaria can cause adult respiratory distress syndrome (ARDS), renal failure, hemolytic anemia, and hypoglycemia in addition to central nervous system complications. A positive blood smear is necessary to confirm the diagnosis.

Patients with malaria have almost always been to malarious areas recently or have had the disease before. This information should be actively sought by the clinician. In nonendemic areas the clinician should ask the patient's residence and travel history and determine which antimalarial drugs, if any, have been taken for prevention. In endemic areas any patient with a febrile illness should be suspected of having malaria. The areas of the world with endemic malaria have not changed greatly over the past 25 years (Fig. 1).

Malaria can also be transmitted by RBC-containing products, either via blood transfusions or from shared needles and syringes of drug abusers; transfusion malaria occurs fewer than nine times per year in the United States. Congenital malaria, also a rare event, occurs when the newborn is inoculated with RBC-containing parasites from the infected mother during delivery. In general, the incubation period for transfusion malaria is about 10 days

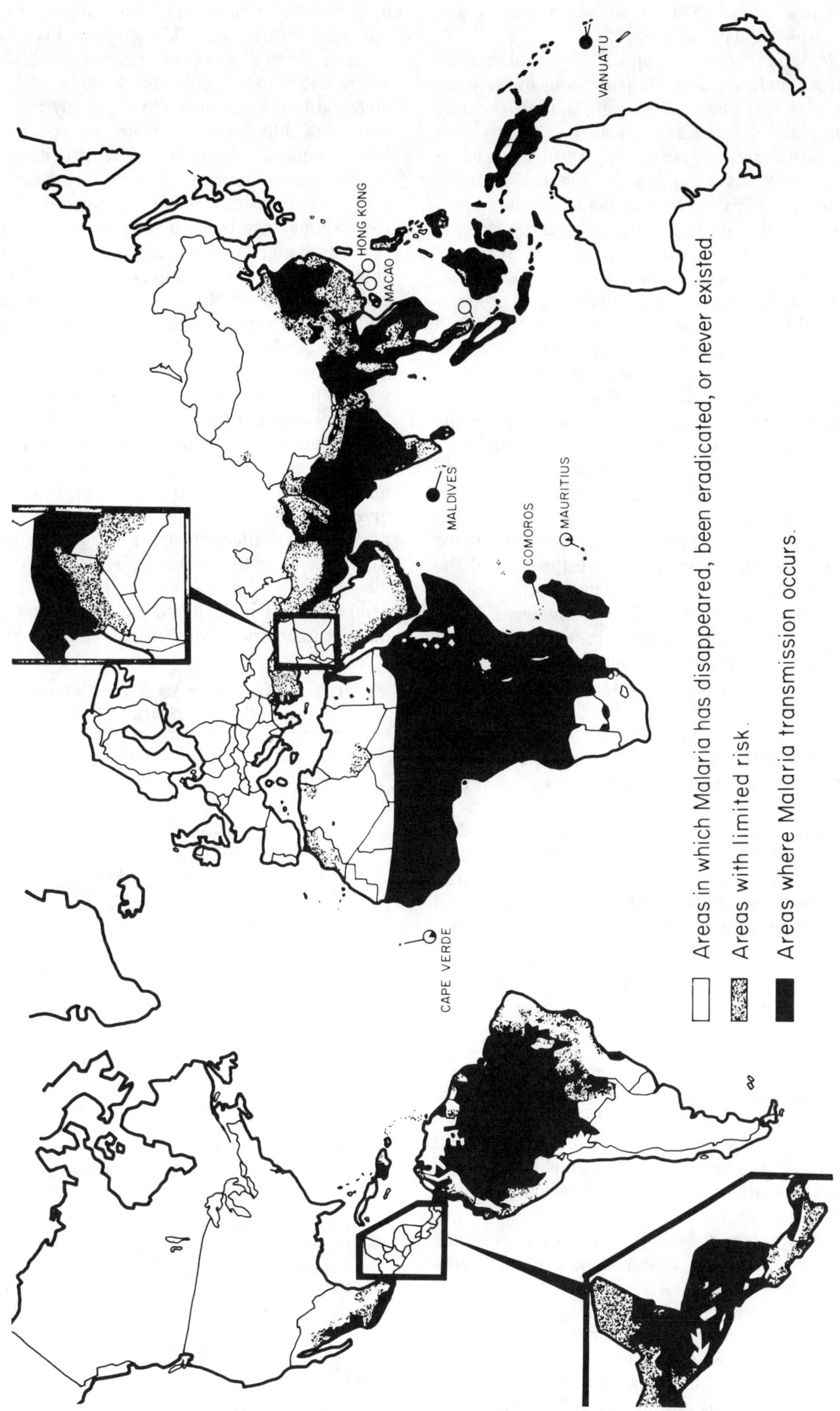

Figure 1 Areas of the world with endemic malaria.

for *P. falciparum*, for *P. vivax* usually about 16 days, and for *P. malariae* 40 days or longer.

P. falciparum, *P. vivax*, and *P. ovale* have been called tertian malarias because the paroxysms of fever and chills were first described as occurring at approximately 48-hour intervals; *P. malariae* is a quartan (72-hour) parasite. The intervals reflect the asexual parasite cycle in the blood, and symptoms occur when the merozoite-laden RBCs rupture. Cyclical fevers may not be common, particularly in patients with *P. falciparum* malaria, because parasite development may be asynchronous.

The definitive diagnosis of malaria is made by detecting malaria parasites in a blood smear that is properly taken, stained and examined. A thick and thin blood film should be taken at the time the disease is suspected, and Giemsa stain should be used. The thick film should be examined first, since low-density infections will be more easily detected here; on a thick film, about 40 times the blood volume is represented per microscopic field than on a thin blood smear. The thin smear is used to identify the species of parasite. The distinction between *P. falciparum* and other *Plasmodium* species is important because special treatment may be required, particularly for drug-resistant strains. A quantitative estimation of the parasitemia should be done to follow the clearance of the infection after treatment begins. The percentage of RBCs parasitized can be made by estimating the number of RBCs with parasites in a representative thin blood film. If malaria is highly suspected, and the initial blood smear is negative, several repeat blood smears should be taken at 12 hour intervals and examined carefully. Gametocytes of *P. falciparum* can be observed in the blood for weeks after treatment begins, and their presence does not reflect treatment failure.

Serologic testing for immunofluorescent antibodies is useful in diagnosing a prior malaria infection in donors of blood products given to patients with transfusion-induced malaria. Serologic methods are not very useful in diagnosing an acute attack of malaria.

TREATMENT

Prompt diagnosis and effective treatment are key to a rapid recovery from malaria. Objectives of treatment are rapid elimination of parasitemia and prevention of complications due to malaria. The critical factors in determining treatment are the clinical status of the patient, species of parasite present, and the geographic origin and the potential for drug-resistance if the infecting species is *P. falciparum*. Strains of chloroquine-resistant *P. falciparum* (CRPF) are now found in Africa, Asia, and South America (Table 1). They appear to be extending geographically, particularly in Africa where the phenomenon was first reported there in 1978.

Drugs used clinically are directed toward the asexual parasite within RBCs. These include the 4-aminoquinolines (i.e., chloroquine and amodiaquine), the cinchona alkaloids (i.e., quinine and quinidine), the combination of pyrimethamine and sulfadoxine (Fansidar), and the tetracyclines. Antimalarial drugs and dose schedules for treating mild and severe malaria are shown in Table 2. For *P. falciparum* infections acquired in areas where CRPF exists, patients should be treated with quinine and either Fansidar (25 mg of pyrimethamine and 500 mg of sulfadoxine per tablet) or tetracycline. Parenteral quinine should be given if a patient has had vomiting or manifestations of cerebral malaria, such as obtundation or convulsions. In general, the parenteral route should also be used for nonimmune patients (persons living outside of endemic areas) having greater than about 5 percent parasitemia (about 250,000 parasites per cubic millimeter of blood). Nonimmune and comatose individuals with greater than 10 percent of RBCs parasitized are candidates for exchange blood transfusions. Very rapid recovery has occurred in some critically ill patients with high parasite levels where exchange transfusion was initiated soon after diagnosis was made.

Quinine, given by intravenous infusion to a severely ill (often unconscious) patient over 4 hours, is recommended to assure close regulation of the amount of drug given and absorbed. In the United States, parenteral quinine is only available from the Malaria Branch, Centers for Disease Control, Atlanta, Georgia 30333; telephone 404–452–4046 (nights, weekends: 404–329-2888). Recently, studies in Thailand has shown that quinidine, a diastereoisomer of quinine, may be more effective than

TABLE 1 Areas with Reported Chloroquine-Resistant *Plasmodium falciparum*, November 1985

Africa	*Asia*
Angola	Burma
Burundi	China (Hainan Island and southern provinces)
Cameroons	Indonesia
Central African Republic	Kampuchea
Comoros	Laos
Congo	Malaysia
Gabon	Philippines (Luzon, Basilan, Mindoro, Palawan Mindanao Islands, and Sulu Archipelago)
Kenya	Thailand
Madagascar	Vietnam
Malawi	
Mozambique	*Indian Subcontinent*
Namibia	Bangladesh (north and east)
Rwanda	India (Orissa, Assam, Uttar Pradesh, Andhra Pradesh, Madhya Pradesh)
Sudan (northern provinces)	Pakistan (Rawalpindi, Punjab)
Tanzania	Sri Lanka
Uganda	
Zaire	*Oceania*
Zambia (northeastern)	Papua New Guinea
Zimbabwe	Solomon Islands
South America	Vanuatu
Bolivia	
Brazil	
Colombia	
Ecuador	
French Guyana	
Guyana	
Panama (east of the Canal Zone including the San Blas Islands)	
Peru (northern provinces)	
Surinam	
Venezuela	

Note: In some countries relatively few sites have been sampled.

TABLE 2 Drugs of Choice for the Treatment of Active Malaria Infections

Clinical Setting	*Drug(s) of Choice**	*Dosage†*
Uncomplicated attacks of all species of malaria EXCEPT *P. falciparum* acquired in areas of chloroquine resistance	Chloroquine phosphate (Aralen)	10 mg base/kg (up to maximum of 600 mg base), then 5 mg base/kg (maximum of 300 mg base for follow-up doses) 6 hr later, then 5 mg base/kg per day for 2 days
Uncomplicated attacks of *P. falciparum* acquired in areas of chloroquine resistance	Quinine sulfate	25 mg/kg per day in 3 divided doses for 3 days (maximum of 650 mg/dose)
	plus	
	Pyrimethamine/sulfadoxine (Fansidar)‡	2–11 months; ¼ tablet 1–3 years: ½ tablet 4–8 years: 1 tablet 9–14 years: 2 tablets >14 years: 3 tablets Above as a single dose
	or	
	Quinine sulfate	Same as above
	plus	
	Tetracycline§	5 mg/kg qid for 7 days (maximum of 250 mg/dose)
Severe illness, due to *P. falciparum*; oral therapy cannot be administered for any reason	Quinine dihydrochloride‖	25 mg/kg per day: administer half of dose in a 4-hr IV infusion of 500 ml of 5% glucose and 1 N saline solution, plasma, or dextran; then give the other half 6–8 hr later in the same volume over the same time if oral therapy still cannot be started (maximum dosage: 1,800 mg per day); continue q8h for 3 days of treatment; adjust volume of fluids for pediatric patients.
	plus	
	Pyrimethamine/sulfadoxine or tetracycline, as above, after IV quinine completed	
After treatment of acute attack of *P. vivax* or *P. ovale* to prevent further relapses ("radical cure")	Primaquine phosphate#	0.3 mg base/kg per day for 14 days (maximum dose: 15 mg base/day)

* Consult experts, including the Malaria Branch of the Centers for Diseases Control, Atlanta, Georgia 30333, (404–452–4046; nights, weekends, 404–329–2888), for information regarding alternative regimens.

† Dosages are oral unless otherwise stated.

‡ Fansidar should not be given to persons with known allergy to sulfonamides or pyrimethamine.

§ For the treatment of malaria, the U.S. Food and Drug Administration (FDA) considers tetracycline an investigational drug. Tetracycline has been shown to be effective in the treatment of *F. falciparum* strains resistant to Fansidar and acquired in Southeast Asia. Physicians must weigh the benefit of tetracycline therapy against the possibility of known adverse effects in children under 8 years of age.

‖ In the United States, quinine for parenteral use is available from the Malaria Branch of the Centers for Disease Control. Intravenous administration of quinine can produce arrhythmias and hypotension, and should be given slowly. Constant monitoring of the pulse and blood pressure is recommended. Oral quinine sulfate should be substituted as soon as possible, accompanied by the other drugs recommended for an uncomplicated attack.

\# As primaquine may cause severe hemolysis in persons with a G6PD deficiency, this trait should be tested for before this drug is given. Congenital malaria and transfusion malaria do not require treatment with primaquine.

quinine when administered intravenously to patients with *P. falciparum* malaria.

Patients with cerebral malaria must have airway maintenance, tracheal suction, and other care to assure that aspiration and bacterial pneumonia do not occur. Convulsions may be due to high fever or to hypoglycemia; depending on the cause, an anticonvulsant or glucose infusion is given. Dexamethasone is not advised for patients with cerebral malaria, because controlled trials have indicated that the drug was associated with prolonged unconsciousness, increased gastrointestinal bleeding, and sepsis. Since cerebral edema is not usually part of the pathologic process in cerebral malaria, tissue diuretics such as urea and mannitol are not advised.

Salt and water loss—associated with high temperature, sweating, and decreased fluid intake—leads to oliguria. In general, fluid and electrolyte replacement will be sufficient to restore hypovolemia and renal function. Diuretics, such as furosemide, should be considered when a rise in blood urea nitrogen and creatinine occurs. Renal dialysis may be required if the patient does not respond.

Red blood cells or whole blood may be given slowly (to limit the danger of pulmonary edema) when severe anemia develops. Platelet transfusions are generally not needed, since the platelet count returns to normal rapidly with treatment.

Pulmonary edema may develop in severely ill patients who have very high parasite counts or who are pregnant, as well as in those who are given excess fluids, blood transfusions, or who have oliguria. Treatment includes sitting the patient up, giving oxygen, diuretics, venesection, and positive end expiratory ventilation.

Hypoglycemia is a recently recognized complication of severe malaria, particularly cerebral malaria. Persons receiving quinine may develop severe hypoglycemia from the hyperinsulinemia effect of this drug; these effects may

TABLE 3 Drugs Used in the Prophylaxis and Presumptive Treatment of Malaria Acquired in Areas with CRPF

	Routine Prophylaxis		Presumptive Treatment§	
Drug	*Adult Dose*	*Pediatric Dose*	*Adult Dose*	*Pediatric Dose*
Chloroquine phosphate (Aralen)	300 mg base (500 mg salt) orally once a week	5 mg/kg base (8.3 mg/kg salt) orally once a week, up to maximum adult dose of 300 mg base	Chloroquine is not recommended for the presumptive treatment of malaria acquired in areas of known chloroquine resistance	
Amodiaquine (Camoquin, Flavoquine)*	400 mg base (520 mg salt) orally once a week	7 mg/kg base (9 mg/kg salt) orally once a week, up to maximum adult dose of 400 mg base	Amodiaquine is not recommended for the presumptive treatment of malaria acquired in areas of known chloroquine resistance	
Pyrimethamine-sulfadoxine (Fansidar)†	1 tablet (25 mg pyrimethamine and 500 mg sulfadoxine) orally once a week	2–11 months: ⅛ tab/wk 1–3 years: ¼ tab/wk 4–8 years: ½ tab/wk 9–14 years: ¾ tab/wk >14 years: 1 tab/wk	3 tablets (75 mg pyrimethamine and 1,500 mg sulfadoxine) orally as a single dose	2–11 months: ¼ tab 1–3 years: ½ tab 4–8 years: 1 tab 9–14 years: 2 tabs >14 years: 3 tabs As a single dose
Doxycycline‡	100 mg orally once a day	>8 years of age: 2 mg/kg per day orally, up to adult dose of 100 mg/day	Tetracyclines are not recommended for the presumptive treatment of malaria	

* Unavailable in the United States, but widely available overseas.
† The use of Fansidar is contraindicated in persons with histories of sulfonamide or pyrimethamine intolerance, in pregnancy at term, and in infants under 2 months of age. Physicians who prescribe the drug to be used as presumptive treatment in the event of a febrile illness when professional medical care is not readily available should ensure that such prescriptions are clearly labeled with instructions to be followed in the event of a febrile illness. If used as weekly prophylaxis, travelers should be advised to discontinue the use of the drug immediately in the event of a possible adverse effect, especially if any mucocutaneous signs or symptoms develop.
‡ The use of doxycycline is contraindicated in pregnancy and children under 8 years of age. The FDA considers the use of tetracyclines as antimalarials to be investigational. Physicians who prescribe doxycycline as malaria chemoprophylaxis should advise their patients to limit direct exposure to the sun to minimize the possibility of a photosensitivity reaction.
§ Not confirmed by blood slide.

occur even with continuous infusions of glucose. Patients with malaria and deepening coma or seizures should be assessed for hypoglycemia and treated for this condition until laboratory studies indicate otherwise.

As with many infections during pregnancy, *P. falciparum* malaria can be life threatening to the mother and the fetus; abortion, stillbirth, and an infant with low birth weight can result from malaria. The effect on the fetuses of primagravidae are more severe than on those of multigravidae. The potential risks of using quinine in pregnant women with severe malaria are far outweighed by the need for prompt treatment of these patients. Hypoglycemia and anemia need to be assessed carefully in pregnant women with malaria.

PREVENTION OF MALARIA

The major dilemma in the prevention of malaria is the continuing spread of drug-resistant strains of *P. falciparum*. While most persons can be protected with available drugs, 100 percent assurance of prevention is not possible. Hence, travelers must understand these issues before departure.

Travelers going to malarious areas are strongly advised to take preventive drugs, even if their visit is as brief as an airport stopover. Factors to consider before advising or taking antimalarial drugs include the area to be visited, the predominance of *P. vivax* or *P. falciparum*, the presence of chloroquine-resistant strains of *P. falciparum*, the length and intensity of exposure to infected *Anopheles* mosquitoes, the traveler's history of drug allergy or intolerance, and the pregnancy status of women.

In most areas of the world, malaria transmission in urban areas is much less intense than in rural zones; in some cities, particularly in malarious Asian and South American countries, malaria transmission is limited or nonexistent. *P. vivax* is the most prominent species in most malarious Asian and Central and South American countries, and all *P. vivax* strains are sensitive to chloroquine. The major risk areas for getting severe CRPF malaria are in East and Central Africa, although CRPF strains do exist in South America and Asia.

Table 3 lists the drugs used in the prophylaxis and presumptive treatment of malaria acquired in areas with CRPF. Those travelers spending 3 weeks or less in areas with CRPF are advised to take chloroquine weekly. In addition, they should take along a treatment dose of Fansidar (Table 3) to use in case they develop symptoms and cannot get medical assistance and a slide-confirmed diagnosis. Those with a history of sulfonamide or pyrimethamine allergy should not take this drug.

Fansidar can be considered for persons with prolonged or intense exposure to malaria in areas of CRPF transmission. Physicians who advise these travelers and expatriate residents must assess individual living conditions, availability of local medical care, and the local malarial transmission pattern. Fansidar has recently been associated with erythema multiforma, Stevens-Johnson syndrome, and toxic epidermal necrolysis in persons taking the drug to prevent malaria. Several deaths have occurred, presumably as a result of sulfonamide allergy. Fansidar should be stopped immediately if a reaction occurs; mucocutaneous signs or symptoms such as pruritus, erythema, rash, orogenital lesions, or pharyngitis are indicative of such a reaction. In case of febrile illness during or after the trip , professional care should be sought promptly and a blood smear taken. If such care is not available, the treatment dose of Fansidar should be taken and follow-up care obtained as soon as possible. Alternates to chloroquine and Fansidar are amodiaquine (like chloroquine, a 4-aminoquinoline compound), which is currently not available in the United States but appears to be more effective than chloroquine in areas with CRPF, and tetracycline, for which limited therapeutic studies indicated effectiveness against CRPF. Tetracyclines should not be used in pregnant women or in children younger than 8 years of age. Some persons taking tetracyclines may develop a sunburn-like rash due to photosensitivity. A sun screen should be used when tetracyclines are taken. Other drugs are available throughout the world as preventives against malaria. However, they cannot be recommended because their efficacy is not proved or they are not yet licensed or available in the United States.

Primaquine, an 8-aminoquinoline, is effective against the hepatic phase of the parasite. Some populations of Africa, Mediterranean, Middle Eastern or southeast Asian origin have glucose-6-phosphate dehydrogenase (G6PD) deficiency and may develop hemolysis after taking primaquine; therefore a test for this trait should be done before the drug is given. Primaquine is used for radical cure of patients with a relapsing form of malaria (*P. vivax* or *P. ovale*) and is used as terminal prophylaxis in areas where prolonged exposure to these parasites may have occurred (Table 2). Peace Corps volunteers, missionaries, or others living in areas with relapsing forms are at higher risk. In general, most individuals taking short trips to malarious areas are not candidates for primaquine unless they develop a relapsing form of malaria after returning home.

Travelers should make strong efforts to reduce exposure with mosquitoes. These measures include screening of windows and doors, use of mosquito nets, application of insect repellants containing high concentrations of N,N-diethylmetatoluamide and wearing clothes that cover most of the body, particularly at dawn and dusk. It is also useful to carry a spray for flying insects to use in living and sleeping quarters during night hours.

AMEBIASIS AND GIARDIASIS

ROGER I. GLASS, M.D.
PETER SPEELMAN, M.D.

AMEBIASIS

Amebiasis is an infection with the protozoan parasite *Entamoeba histolytica*. The organism is most commonly found as a commensal in asymptomatic individuals, but it can invade the colon to produce disease ranging from mild bloating gas or nonspecific diarrhea to severe bloody dysentery. Following tissue invasion, spread to the liver can result in abscesses that may rupture into the peritoneum, pleura, lung, or pericardium. The disease is caused by the vegetative forms—trophozoites. These live in the gut and produce cysts that are passed, can remain infective in the environment for months, and develop into trophozoites after ingestion by a new host.

Epidemiology

E. histolytica is found in approximately 10 percent of the world's population and is more prevalent in tropical areas with poor water and sanitation than in the developed countries. Infection occurs in 2 to 5 percent of Americans, most of whom are asymptomatic cyst passers. Man is the prime reservoir for the organism and, once infected, may excrete cysts for years. In a moist environment these cysts can survive and remain infective for months. Infection is spread by the fecal-oral route, primarily through exposure to contaminated food or water, although both venereal and person-to-person spread have been documented. High-risk groups for infection in developed countries include travelers to tropical areas, homosexuals, prisoners, residents in homes for the mentally retarded, and patients who are immunocompromised or are taking immunosuppressive drugs such as corticosteroids. Untreated water in endemic areas, foods prepared by carriers, and uncooked vegetables that may be contaminated with human excreta are to be avoided.

Pathophysiology

After *E. histolytica* cysts are ingested, they survive passage through the gastric acid of the stomach, mature by cell division, and release motile vegetative trophozoites in the small intestine. These trophozoites migrate to the large intestine where they most commonly survive without producing disease. The host suffers no symptoms although he may periodically pass cysts. It is still unclear why some individuals have an asymptomatic infection or suffer only mild symptoms, whereas others develop severe dysentery.

Trophozoites near the mucosa release cytolytic enzymes that prepare the way for tissue invasion and ulcer formation, especially in the cecum and rectosigmoid areas. These ulcers may be small at the mucosal surface and larger in the submucosa, giving a flask-like appearance. The mucosa between ulcers is usually normal. Progression of this process is associated with larger ulcers capped with dense yellow sloughs and sometimes with hematophagous trophozoites in the depths of these ulcers. Deep ulcers through the muscular layers may lead to hemorrhage, perforation, and peritonitis. The process is essentially one of necrosis with lysis of cells.

Most of the cellular reaction in the ulcers is lymphocytic. Polymorphonuclear white blood cells are found only with secondary bacterial invasion. In some cases a large granulomatous reaction can occur leading to a tumorlike lesion called an ameboma that can constrict the bowel wall. Hematogenous spread to the liver can occur following tissue invasion, and this results in abscess formation. Many patients with amebic liver abscess show no symptoms prior to or at the time of the intestinal invasion.

Clinical Presentation and Differential Diagnosis

The most common illness associated with infection with *E. histolytica* is a mild, chronic gastrointestinal illness with cramps, loose stools, flatulence, and malaise which may continue for weeks to months. As bowel wall invasion becomes more extensive, symptoms of colicky pains, particularly in the right iliac fossa, diarrhea with or without blood and mucus and vomiting become more prominent. In severe dysentery, the patient may have low-grade fever, bloody stool, tenesmus, liver tenderness, and abdominal distention. The development of the full dysentery picture is more gradual, less toxic, and less commonly associated with dehydration than in patients with shigellosis. Other infectious agents, including *Salmonella, enterotoxigenic* and enteroinvasive *Escherichia coli, Campylobacter jejuni*, giardiasis, and schistosomiasis (in endemic areas), should be considered in the differential diagnosis as well as ulcerative colitis, Crohn's disease, and diverticulitis. The presence of a discrete palpable abdominal mass in the right of left iliac fossa may suggest an ameboma, which must be distinguished from a colonic carcinoma and Crohn's disease.

Perforation with peritonitis occurs in about 3 percent of patients with severe amebic dysentery. Amebiasis should be included in the differential diagnosis of acute abdominal pain, particularly when preceded by dysentery.

Hematogenous spread of *E. histolytica* from the right colon most commonly seeds the right posterior lobe of the liver, which can lead to the formation of an abscess. Half of the patients presenting with this complication give no previous recent history of dysentery. These patients may have often suffered weight loss from an insidious illness associated with fever, sweats, and tender hepatosplenomegaly. Cholecystitis, pancreatitis and ulcer disease must be ruled out. In 10 to 20 percent of patients with liver abscesses, extension into the pleura, lungs, pericardium, or peritoneum will occur. Lesions or ulcers in the perianal area and the abdominal wall are uncommon but can occur by direct extension from the colon.

Diagnosis

The diagnosis of amebiasis requires identification of the organism in stool or in tissue. Microscopic examination should be performed on fresh stools, because trophozoites survive only a few hours at room temperature. Stool examination should include direct, flotation, and staining methods. The finding of motile *E. histolytica* trophozoites with ingested red blood cells is indicative of invasive amebiasis in some cases of amebic dysentery, but not all trophozoites will have ingested red blood cells.

If the stool examination is negative, material scraped from the mucosa during proctoscopy may show hematophagous trophozoites. Cysts and trophozoites are shed intermittently from the colon. Therefore, additional stool samples should be retested on each of 3 separate days. Many laboratory technicians are unfamiliar with the morphology of *E. histolytica* cysts and trophozoites and may have difficulty differentiating the pathogenic large form of *E. histolytica* (up to 50 μm) from the small forms (10 to 20 μm) whose pathogenicity is unclear as well as from other amebae such as *Entamoeba coli* and *E. hartmanni* whose pathogenicity is also unclear. Microscopic examination should be performed on fresh stool since trophozoites remain active for a short period. Alternatively, specimens can be preserved in a 1:3 dilution of 10 percent formalin and examined with PVA fixative.

In the presence of amebic liver abscesses, patients will often show liver tenderness, elevation of the right hemidiaphragm with blunting of the costophrenic angle, and basilar atelectasis. Radionuclide, sonographic, and CT scans are helpful in confirming the presence of an abscess, its size, and monitoring response to therapy. Serologic tests are extremely helpful in making a diagnosis of amebic abscess, especially when the stool examination is negative for *E. histolytica*. The expected rapid response to treatment makes a therapeutic trial both diagnostic and potentially curative. Surgery should only be considered when hepatic abscesses are in danger of perforation or are not responding to treatment.

Treatment

The objectives of therapy are to control symptoms, to destroy amebae in the lumen (luminal amebicides), to eradicate invasive amebae (tissue amebicides), and to prevent the spread of amebae to other tissues. Metronidazole, 750 mg orally three times per day for 10 days, is the most effective drug for the treatment of symptomatic amebiasis. It has been shown to produce mutations in bacteria and cancer in rats and mice. This drug should not be given to pregnant or lactating women or to patients who are at increased risk of developing cancer. It can be given orally and parenterally. Side effects of metronidazole include nausea, abdominal pain, and development of a metallic taste and brown urine. Because of an antabuse reaction, use of alcohol during treatment should be avoided. For cases of amebic abscess or in severe advanced cases that do not respond to intravenous metronidazole, the drug of choice is dihydroemetine (1.0 to 1.5 mg per kilogram daily IM or SC for 10 days). This synthetic drug is excreted rapidly but may produce cardiac toxicity, although less so than emetine, which was previously recommended.

The asymptomatic cyst passer should be treated with a luminal amebecide. Of the available drugs, diloxanide furoate, 500 mg orally three times per day for 10 days, is the drug of choice and is available in the United States from the Centers for Disease Control (the Parasitic Diseases Division, Center for Infectious Diseases, Centers for Disease Control, Atlanta, GA 30333). An alternative luminal amebacide is iodoquinol (formerly known as diiodohydroxyquin), 650 mg three times per day for 20 days. Use of iodoquinol has been associated rarely with optic atrophy and blindness. Accordingly the recommended dosage should not be exceeded and it should be used only when other drugs are not available. Paromomycin has also been utilized, 25 mg per kilogram per day, given as three doses per day for 7 days. Corticosteroids are contraindicated in patients with amebiasis.

Prevention of *E. histolytica* infection is a great challenge. Endemic amebiasis can be controlled by improvements in general levels of sanitation and personal hygiene. Travelers to endemic areas should be warned not to eat fresh vegetables and not to drink unfiltered water. Chlorination is ineffective in destroying amebic cysts.

GIARDIASIS

Giardia lamblia is a flagellate protozoan that infects the upper small bowel. The patient may be asymptomatic or the parasite may cause disease ranging in severity from mild abdominal discomfort, to acute diarrhea, to chronic diarrhea with severe malabsorption and weight loss.

Epidemiology

Giardia lamblia is one of the most common intestinal protozoa and is found worldwide; it is particularly prevalent in areas with poor sanitation. However, it is also endemic in parts of the United States (Rocky Mountain areas, New York, New England, Washington state), the USSR (particularly Leningrad), and Europe. The major source appears to be water that becomes contaminated from human waste or from animals such as beavers or muskrats. Transmission occurs by the fecal-oral route, either from drinking contaminated water or occasionally by person-to-person contact. There are many asymptomatic carriers; in the United States alone these may comprise from 3 to 7 percent of the population. Diarrheal outbreaks due to *Giardia* have occurred in areas with contaminated water supplies, in residential and custodial institutions, day care centers, and in travelers, homosexuals, and hikers and backpackers. Cysts can survive for weeks in water and are killed by bringing water to a boil. Iodine treatment and routine chlorination are not always effective.

Pathophysiology

Ingestion of as few as 10 to 100 *Giardia* cysts can lead to infection. Cysts must survive passage through stomach acid and bile to reach the small intestine where each cyst divides into two trophozoites. Trophozoites have a sucking disk that promotes attachment to the mucosa. Attachment can damage the microvilli and lead to focal areas of acute inflammation in the lamina propria. The lesions are scattered so there is no good correlation between density of infection and severity of symptoms. Once the infection has occurred, intestinal function can be impaired, deficiency of disaccharidases (particularly lactase), defects in vitamin B_{12} absorption, a mild deficiency of intestinal immunoglobulin, and overgrowth of bacteria have been noted. These conditions can lead either to acute diarrhea or to chronic diarrhea with malabsorption. Circulating IgG antibodies develop in response to infection and have been employed in serologic tests with some success. Conditions that predispose to clinical giardiasis are hypochlorhydria, gastric resection, and hypogammaglobulinemia.

Clinical Presentation

Most patients infected with *G. lamblia* have no symptoms or suffer only vague abdominal pains which persist until a diagnosis is finally made. Some individuals will present with acute self-limited diarrhea with anorexia, nausea, and occasional fevers, while others go on to chronic diarrhea with cramping and malabsorption marked by weight loss, flatulence, and foul-smelling, frothy stools.

Diagnosis requires identification of cysts and trophozoites by microscopic examination of stool specimens, but because *Giardia* are not shed continuously, multiple stool examinations may be necessary in a patient with typical symptoms who is stool-negative. Concentration techniques can be used to increase sensitivity. When stool examination is negative but the index of suspicion is high, examination of duodenal or jejunal aspirates obtained by string capsule or endoscopy can be helpful. Also, mucosal imprint smears have been employed when duodenal biopsy is done.

Treatment

Quinacrine hydrochloride (100 mg three times per day after meals for 5 days in adults or 2 mg per kilogram three times per day after meals for 5 days but not exceeding 300 mg per day) is the drug of choice, although metronidazole (250 mg three times per day for 5 days for adults and 5 mg per kilogram three times per day for 5 days in children) is commonly used and better tolerated. Metronidazole has been given effectively in both 1-day and 3-day courses (for example, 2 g daily for 3 days) with only a slight loss of efficacy. Furazolidone (6 mg per kilogram per day for 5 days) is also recommended for children. While *Giardia* infection is often self-limited, treatment is recommended, since symptoms can recur and diagnosis is often difficult to establish.

TOXOPLASMOSIS

JACOB K. FRENKEL, M.D.

Toxoplasma infection occurs worldwide in animals and humans. Asymptomatic acute infection is common, and persistent, chronic latent infection usually follows. The disease, toxoplasmosis, may occur during the acute, subacute, or chronic phase of infection, including congenital infection and recrudescence of a chronic latent infection.

THE ORGANISM

Toxoplasma gondii is a tissue protozoan that occurs in three forms. Tachyzoites are actively multiplying in tissues and lead to most cell and tissue destruction during acute infection. Bradyzoites are slowly multiplying or resting forms causing chronic infection. They are present in cysts in many tissues such as brain, muscle, and retina. Usually bradyzoites give rise to few lesions except when cysts rupture in the retina. Cysts maintain the chronic infection in animals and are important sources of infection for cats—the final host and source of all toxoplasmosis. The sporozoites within oocysts are the resistant infectious stage; they are eliminated in the feces by cats that have eaten bradyzoites.

TRANSMISSION

Humans are infected mainly from oocysts or tissue cysts (Fig. 1). Oocysts come from soil contaminated with cat feces. Most cats get infected from meat, birds, or mice. In the United States, transmission occurs mainly during adulthood and is probably related to meat ingestion. Tissue cysts infect people who eat undercooked meat, mainly pork and mutton. Infection, documented by seroconversion, occurs at a rate of 0.5 to 1 percent per year in the United States. In many developing countries, close to 50 percent of children become infected from oocysts. If a pregnant woman contracts infections, her fetus may be infected in utero, and congenital toxoplasmosis may result. This devastating disease entity should be considered preventable.

CLINICAL ILLNESS

The clinical spectrum of toxoplasmosis includes acute acquired, congenital, ocular, and recrudescent toxoplasmosis.

Acute Acquired Toxoplasmosis

Following an incubation period of 1 to 3 weeks, a febrile illness develops in an estimated 10 to 20 percent of primary infections, irrespective of infecting stage. Signs and symptoms may include headache, myalgia, stiff neck, anorexia, maculopapular rash (sparing palms and soles), arthralgia, signs of hepatitis, and, sometimes, hepatomegaly. Lymphadenopathy is common and appears simultaneously with other signs and symptoms, or it may be the first sign, persisting for weeks or months. Atypical lymphocytes are commonly present in the peripheral blood. Signs of myocarditis, hepatitis, pneumonitis, pericarditis, polymyositis, or meningoencephalitis occur occasionally, singly, or in combination. Retinochoroiditis may follow.

Toxoplasmosis in Pregnant Women

Toxoplasmosis acquired during pregnancy is symptomatic in only 10 to 20 percent of pregnant women. However, the fetus is at risk whether or not symptoms are present. Congenital infections are rare but severe when transmitted in the first and second trimesters and more frequent but less severe in the third trimester.

Congenital Toxoplasmosis

Four patterns of congenital toxoplasmosis can be distinguished. 1. The asymptomatic infection is commonest and usually follows transmission in the third trimester. 2. A mild form, characterized by gestational prematurity, intrauterine growth retardation, abnormal spinal fluid, and failure to thrive. 3. Severe generalized toxoplasmosis, accompanied by one or several of the following: splenomegaly, jaundice, fever, anemia, thrombocytopenia, hepatomegaly, splenomegaly, lymphadenopathy, pneumonia, myocarditis, and a petechial rash. 4. Severe neurologic toxoplasmosis, characterized by convulsions, nystagmus, fever or hypothermia, retinochoroiditis, anemia, intracerebral calcifications, internal hydrocephalus, microencephaly, strabismus, trophic cataracts, glaucoma, optic atrophy, deafness, psychomotor retardation, abnormal spinal fluid findings (including xanthochromia), elevated protein levels (grams percent in the ventricular fluid), and mononuclear pleocytosis.

Transitional forms occur; retinochoroiditis especially may also be present in the third pattern, and it may follow many years after the first and second patterns.

Ocular Toxoplasmosis

Ocular toxoplasmosis is usually an isolated manifestation of chronic latent toxoplasmosis in children or adults. Retinochoroiditis may occur as a single episode or recurrently in the same eye, without generalized symptoms, local pain, or changes in the blood levels of antibody. The acute lesions consist of a focus of retinal necrosis with fuzzy borders accompanied by a cellular exudate in the vitreous that often obscures the lesions and vision in general. The lesion and the vitreous exudate usually start

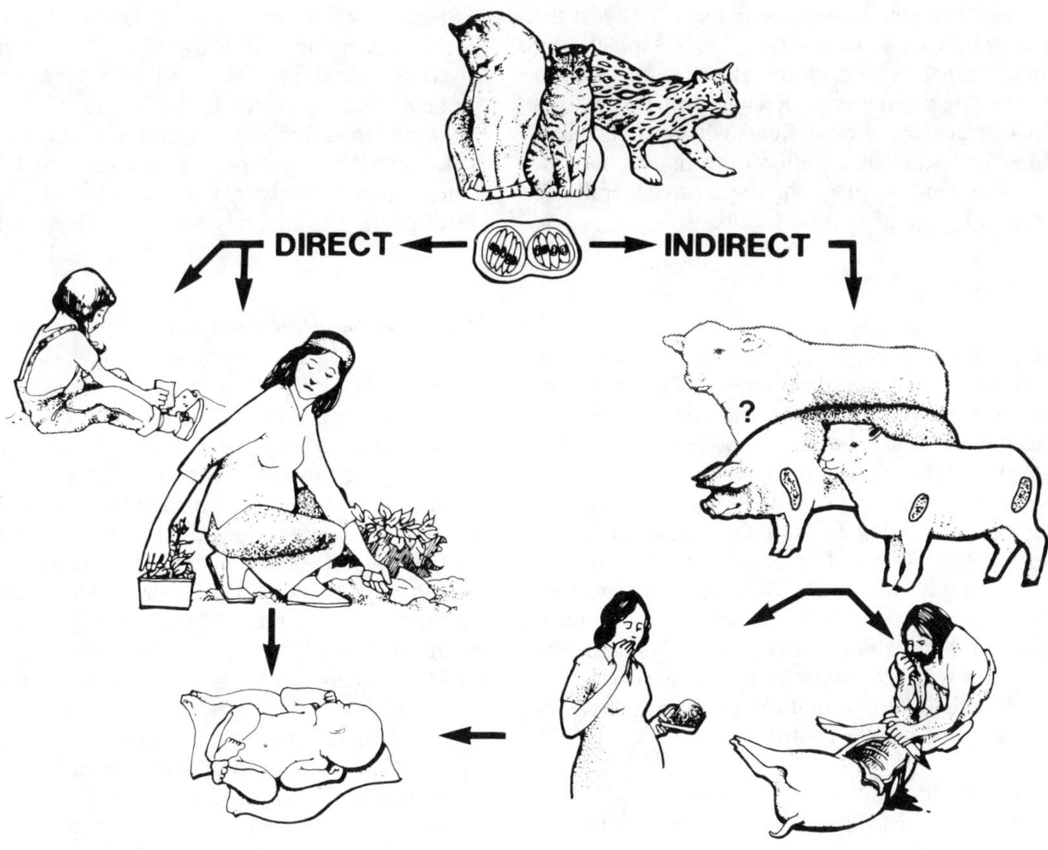

Figure 1 Transmission of *Toxoplasma* to humans.

to clear after 2 to 3 weeks. Visual acuity may return to normal if the lesion was distant from the macula. The retinal lesion becomes hyperpigmented. Smoldering lesions with exacerbations have been described. Progressive lesions may result in blindness and glaucoma.

Toxoplasmosis in the Immunocompromised Patient

Two patterns are seen: recrudescent chronic infection and severe primary infection.

Relapsing chronic infection is most commonly manifested as encephalitis; this is characteristically focal and stimulates an abscess or tumor, but can also be multicentric. CT scans may show one or more ring-shaped lesions. Retinochoroiditis, myocarditis, and pneumonia occur less commonly. Most of these patients receive immunosuppressive drugs for a lymphoreticular or other neoplasm or to support an organ transplant; others are immunosuppressed by HTLV-3 that destroys T lymphocytes, resulting in acquired immunodeficiency syndrome.

A severe primary infection may have been acquired from a transplanted heart or kidney, or it may have been contracted accidentally. Because of the impaired immunity, the primary infection may last longer, and may be more severe.

DIAGNOSIS

Identification of the Organism

Histologic Examination

Biopsy diagnosis may be useful when one or several enlarged lymph nodes are present, preceded or accompanied by fever. Toxoplasmic lymphadenopathy can be differentiated from a lymphoma by the presence of normal architecture, reticular cell hyperplasia, prominent histiocytic infiltration of germinal centers, and by slight periadenitis; however necrosis or Reed-Sternberg cells are absent. Very few Toxoplasma organisms, usually in cysts, may be found in serial sections.

Brain biopsy—used to differentiate a variety of infections, tumors, and vascular phenomena—may demonstrate large numbers of tachyzoites or a few cysts with much necrosis and inflammation. To differentiate between tachzyoites and nuclear debris, an immunoperoxidase stain can be used.

Isolation of Toxoplasma

Inoculation of mice, hamsters, or cell cultures can be attempted with biopsy, placental, or autopsy material in order to enhance the sensitivity and specificity of the histologic examination. In addition, blood, spinal, and ventricular fluids can be used in patients with generalized or neurologic symptoms. Recovery of toxoplasma from blood, placenta, or body fluids generally indicates active infection, whereas isolation from tissues may indicate active or chronic infection. These can generally be differentiated by the histologic picture.

Serologic Diagnosis

Rising antibody titers in the acute infection have been traditionally used to support the diagnosis of clinical toxoplasmosis. However, in immunosuppressed patients, antibody responses cannot be relied upon: it is here that demonstration of the organisms with tissue destruction or demonstration of antigen in the blood is most helpful.

Five types of serologic tests are available for the diagnosis of toxoplasmosis. Usefulness depends on both availability and reliability of the tests. Often kits are used that embody unrealistic assumptions of useful titers and size of test run. Most laboratories will run only occasional specimens and will need more control material than is generally supplied. The laboratory performing the tests must use adequate quality controls.

1. The Sabin-Feldman dye test (DT) is based on antibody-complement-mediated lysis of *Toxoplasma*. Although this is the standard test, it is performed by only a few laboratories in the United States because it requires living *Toxoplasma* and complement from normal human plasma. It measures total antibody.
2. The indirect fluorescent antibody test (IFAT) is the next most useful test, giving results similar to those obtained with the DT. Its drawback is the need for appropriate antisera (separate for humans and mice) and a fluorescent microscope. If antihuman globulin is used, it measures the total antibody. With antihuman IgG, the IgG fraction can be categorized.
3. The indirect hemagglutination test (IHA) is available in kit form and is attractive because of its simplicity. Its drawback is the lack of sensitivity of the antigen usually used, so that it is not dependable for diagnosis of early acute infection nor for congenital toxoplasmosis.
4. The IgM fluorescent antibody test (IgM-IFA), like IFAT, measures, by means of antihuman IgM serum, the binding of IgM antibody in the patient's serum to killed *Toxoplasma* organisms on a slide. This test was designed to distinguish active infection in babies from passively transferred maternal IgG antibody. The large IgM molecule is not transferred past the intact placenta, and in case of a leak, IgM quickly disappears, since it has a half-life of only 3 to 5 days. This test, however, gives false-positive results in the presence of antinuclear antibody and rheumatoid factor and false-negative results when a large quantity of IgG is present in the baby's serum and competes with IgM.
5. IgM capture tests are designed to capture the IgM in the patient's serum and to determine whether this IgM contains antibody to toxoplasma. These capture tests avoid the false-positive and false-negative reactions mentioned above for IgM-IFA. These tests are performed in several laboratories, and at least one kit by Litton has reached the U.S. market. The IgM capture tests give higher titers than the conventional IgM-IFA tests, and the antibody persists longer—perhaps 2 to 3 years.

Strategy of Serologic Diagnosis

When seeking to link an acute illness to *Toxoplasma*, it is important to distinguish preexisting antibody due to a remote infection or passively transferred antibody (acquired by transfusion or in utero, which decays 10-fold every 3 months) from antibody related to the illness. In the United States, DT, IFA, or IHA titers of 1:1,000 suggest acute infection. In areas where such titers are common in a normal population, stable high titers can not be interpreted, but IgM titers correlate with acute or recent infection. The algorithms, Figures 2 to 6, illustrate the sequence of steps and the considerations applied to acute infection (Fig. 2), encephalitis (Fig. 3), retinochoroiditis (Fig. 4), neonatal illness (Fig. 5), suspicion of infection in a pregnant woman (Fig. 6), and the use of IgM antibody titers to analyze the meaning of antibody present in the IgG fraction (Fig. 7).

Serologic diagnosis is generally based on the demonstration of a 4-fold rise in IgG antibody titers between two specimens compared in the same test run. Elevated IgM titers are presumptive evidence of recent infection; conventional IgM-IFA titers persist 6 to 10 months, but with the capture techniques, 2 years or longer.

In immunosuppressed patients, IgG antibody, if present, is interpreted as usual; however, negative titers do not exclude toxoplasmosis. Histologic diagnosis is useful. A test for antigenemia has been developed that appears promising for the rapid diagnosis of acute infection. However, it is not generally available.

Differential Diagnosis

The signs and symptoms of toxoplasmosis are usually so nonspecific that the etiology is not suspected. Most illnesses are mild and they are often not recorded. In a small outbreak in Atlanta, days absent from work or from school were not ascertained, and none of the five students in the New York "hamburger epidemic" became ill enough to be incapacitated. However, patients have been seen with fevers of up to 39.5 °C and malaise lasting for 2 months, sometimes with sore throat and myalgia suggesting infectious mononucleosis or cytomegaloviral infection, which must be excluded. The persistent lymphadenopathy, sometimes with splenomegaly and a Coombs' test–negative hemolytic anemia may suggest a lymphoma; lymph node biopsy is diagnositic. The algorithms (Figs. 2 to 6) outline diagnostic steps and con-

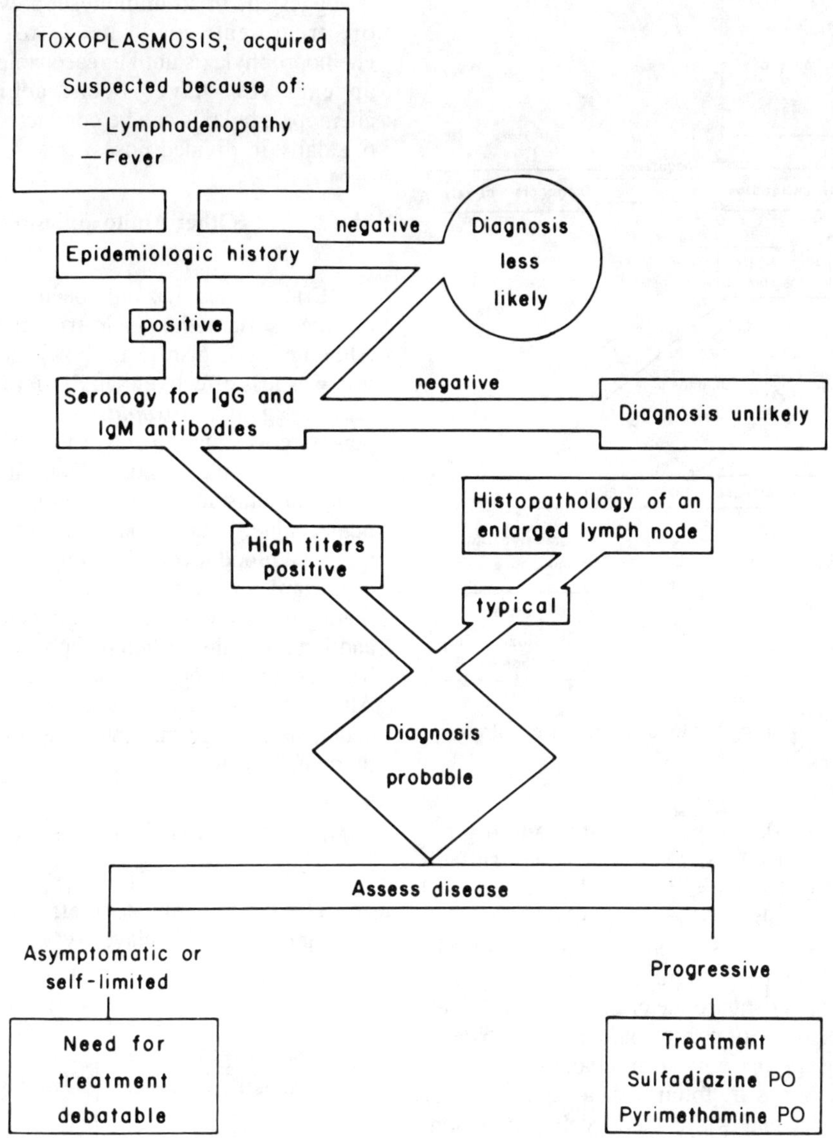

Figure 2 Evaluation of suspected acute toxoplasmosis and lymphadenopathy. (Modified from Mahmond AAF and Warren KS. Toxoplasmosis. J Inf Dis 1977; 135:493)

siderations to follow with several presenting symptoms.

Isolated anterior segment inflammation in the eye is not likely to be due to toxoplasmosis. The differential diagnosis includes cytomegaloviral infection, syphilis, brucellosis, leptospirosis, tuberculosis, visceral larva migrans, and retinoblastoma; all of these entities should also be considered in the presence of retinochoroiditis.

TREATMENT

Indications for treatment are: diagnosed clinical illness (Figs. 2 and 3), active lesions in the eye (Fig. 4), congenital infection, whether the infant is symptomatic or not (Fig. 5), and signs and symptoms compatible with toxoplasmosis in immunosuppressed patients (Fig. 3). Treatment of a pregnant woman infected during pregnancy is controversial (Fig. 6). The presence of a high antibody titer is not an indication for treatment.

Therapeutic Agents

The most effective treatment for toxoplasmosis employs sulfadiazine together with pyrimethamine (Daraprim, Chloridin, Malocide) because the individual inhibitory effects of each drug become synergistic when used together.

Sulfadiazine (SD, or sulfamerazine, sulfamethazine, sulfapyrazine, sulfalene, sulfadoxine, trisulfapyrimidine)

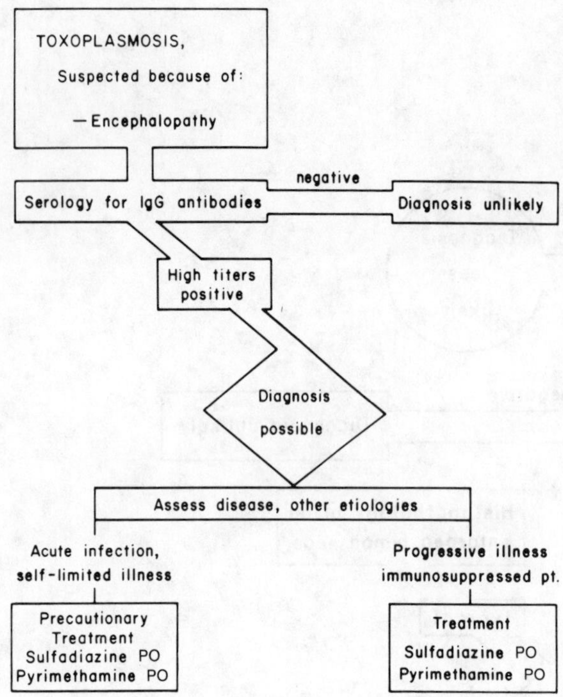

Figure 3 Evaluation of suspected toxoplasmic encephalopathy.

is given in doses of 100 mg per kilogram up to 4 g per day in two to four divided doses. The half-life of sulfadiazine is about 10 to 12 hours. Tablets, liquid oral, and parenteral forms of sulfadiazine are available.

Pyrimethamine (PYR) is given in doses of 40 mg per square meter or 1 mg per kilogram for the first 3 days, followed by 15 mg per square meter or 0.3 mg per kilogram daily. The half-life of pyrimethamine is 4 to 5 days. Tablets of 25 mg are the only form available.

Because these drugs are folinic acid antagonists, they may impair platelet and white blood cell production. Counts of platelets and leukocytes should be performed twice weekly. If platelets decline below 100,000 per cubic millimeter, folinic acid (calcium leucovorin), 3 to 10 mg daily, is given either orally or subcutaneously; it is available as 5 and 25 mg tablets and in 3 and 5 mg ampules and 50 mg vials. When folinic acid is not available, 5 to 10 g of fresh yeast (such as Fleischman's, Red Star) daily can be substituted (100 mg for children). It is mixed with food or tomato juice to disguise the taste. These antagonists do not impair the chemotherapeutic effect of the drugs. When platelet counts are not feasible, 5 g of yeast should be given daily.

Toxicity effects of sulfonamides include rashes, the Stevens-Johnson syndrome, crystalluria, hematuria, vasculitis, and hemolytic anemia with deficiency of glucose-6-phosphate dehydrogenase.

Duration of treatment depends on subsidence of signs and symptoms, and immunity can be assumed to have been acquired. If the patient appears to be immunologically competent, treatment for approximately twice the time necessary for disappearance of signs and symptoms is suggested. In an immunosuppressed patient, a period of treatment may need to be followed by chemoprophylaxis until a reasonable immunocompetence appears to have been achieved. Long-term chemoprophylaxis can be conducted with SD alone, 4 to 6 g daily in divided doses.

Other Antitoxoplasmic Agents

Effectiveness has only been shown for the first drug of the sulfamethoxazole-trimethoprim combination. Although synergism was shown in vitro, this combination was less effective than SD-PYR. Clindamycin is effective against *Toxoplasma*. However, it does not penetrate well into the central nervous system, and with its potential enteric side effects, it should be used only under circumstances where SD-PYR toxicity appears unmanageable. Fetal blood levels were about 50 percent of maternal blood levels. Spiramycin, chemically related to erythromycin, is not generally available in the United States; however, it can be obtained from the U.S. Food and Drug Administration (telephone 301-443-4310). It has been used in Europe to treat pregnant women and babies. Although it reaches sufficient concentrations in the placenta, its passage into the fetus appears insufficient for therapeutic effects.

Anti-Inflammatory Treatments with Corticosteroids

The anti-inflammatory effects are useful to moderate manifestation of delayed type hypersensitivity with fo-

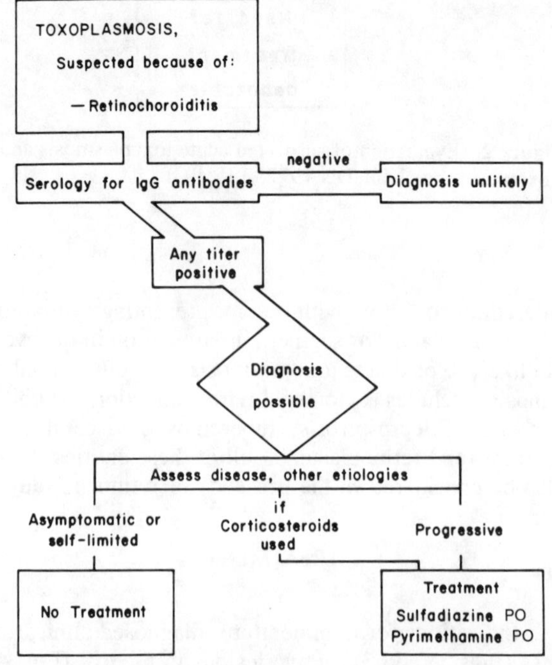

Figure 4 Evaluation of suspected toxoplasmic retinochoroiditis.

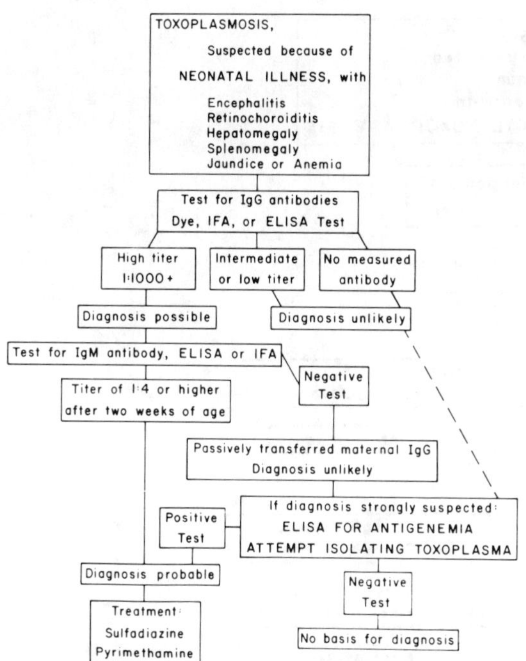

Figure 5 Evaluation of suspected neonatal toxoplasmosis.

cal retinochoroiditis in or adjacent to the macula or the optic nerve. Because anti-inflammatory doses are also immunosuppressive, corticosteroids should be used together with the sulfadiazine-pyrimethamine combination. Prednisone, 50 to 100 mg per day (1 to 1.5 mg per kilogram or 10 to 20 replacement doses) are given orally in two divided doses daily until the acute inflammation begins to subside, which usually takes 5 to 10 days, and it is then tapered to zero while the SD-PYR is continued. The corticosteroids should not be injected periocularly.

Therapy of Specific Clinical Illness

Generalized Acute Toxoplasmosis

Diagnosis and treatment is outlined in Figure 2. Defervescence and improvement of signs, symptoms, and abnormal laboratory tests usually occur promptly, and treatment for an additional week appears sufficient. If manifestations recur, treatment can be resumed.

Immunosuppressed Patients

Diagnosis and treatment are as outlined in Figure 3. Because multiple infections may be present, therapeutic response should be measured by regression of toxoplasmic lesions; e.g., in the brain. Sulfadiazine-pyrimethamine treatments should extend approximately a month beyond clinical improvement. Because treatment does not usually eradicate the infection and immunity may not be sufficient to contain it, sulfadiazine prophylaxis should be continued indefinitely until the immune status has improved, as after remission of the underlying neoplasm or stabilization of the graft. The sulfadiazine or combined treatment with pyrimethamine would be also effective prophylaxis against pneumocystosis.

The sulfadoxine-pyrimethamine combination (Fansidar) should be more effective against both toxoplasmosis and pneumocystis infections than sulfamethoxazole-trimethoprim.

Toxoplasmosis in the Pregnant Woman

Diagnostic and management considerations are outlined in Figure 6. If an infection was presumably acquired in first trimester, the chances of severe lesions of the fetus are great, and therapeutic abortion should be considered. The possibility of a severely damaged baby will often extend this consideration into the second trimester. Because pyrimethamine can be teratogenic, it should not be given in the first or second trimester. However, treatment with SD alone, which passes into the fetus, is a reasonable alternative in the second trimester. In the third trimester, when the risk of lesions is less, the possibility of toxic effects of SD-PYR can be controlled with folinic acid and yeast. Once diagnosed, treatment should extend throughout pregnancy until the status of the baby can be evaluated after birth. No controlled studies have been published concerning this treatment.

Clindamycin passes the placenta and fetal blood levels are about half the maternal levels. It could reasonably be used if SD–PYR are not tolerated, keeping in mind its poor penetration into brain end eye and its side effects.

Spiramycin, by concentrating in the placenta, can be expected to diminish the chance of fetal infection; however, it is not effective once infection has passed into the fetus.

Congenital Toxoplasmosis

Figure 5 outlines the diagnostic considerations. Diagnosis depends on finding *Toxoplasma* antibody in the IgM fraction, which, because of its size, is not passively acquired. Because antibody in the IgG fraction is quantitatively transferred from mother to fetus it does not aid in the diagnosis or exclusion of fetal infection. IgM antibody can be measured at birth. However, occasionally a placental leak and mixing of maternal and fetal blood occurs, in which case maternal IgM decays, with a half-life of 4 to 5 days; hence the need to check a positive finding after 2 weeks. The conventional IgM antibody tests may be negative because of competition with IgG for the antigen sites; therefore, a test based on the IgM capture technique is preferred.

Treatment for congenital toxoplasmosis should be started, at least with SD alone, when suspicion is strong, if serologic testing takes more than 24 hours. Once the diagnosis is confirmed, treatment with SD–PYR should

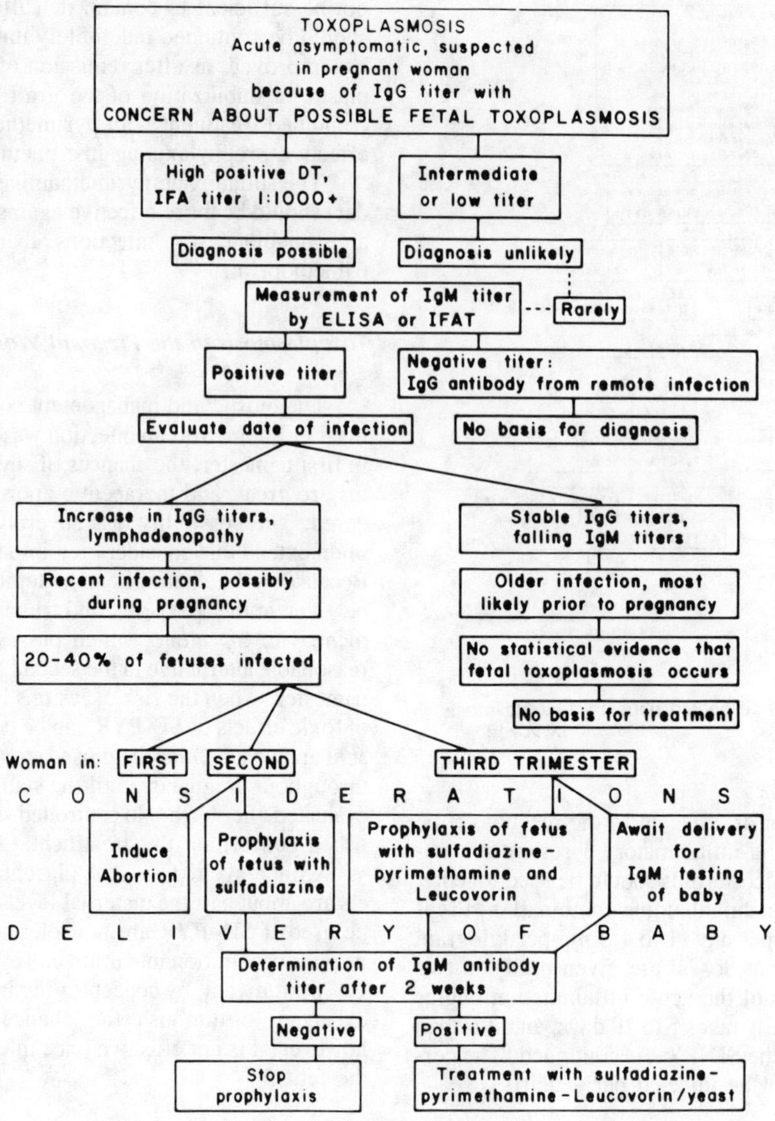

Figure 6 Evaluation of suspected toxoplasmosis in a pregnant woman.

be initiated and extended for at least 4 to 8 weeks beyond resolution of manifestation of illness. This diminishes the number of organisms and provides time for the immune potential of the newborn baby to mature. After 3 to 6 months, treatment can be given intermittently for 1 month followed by no treatment for another month, or prophylaxis can be maintained with SD alone. Duration of treatment is controversial. Some treat arbitrarily for 1 year. However, the decisive criterion is the ability to mount a sufficient cellular immunity to contain the chronic infection, and this may be reached earlier. The objective is to prevent all possible cell destruction of nonregenerating brain and retinal tissues while avoiding unnecessary and costly treatment. Treatment with SD–PYR—alternating with SD only or nontreatment—for periods of 1 month appears preferable to monthly treatments with SD–PYR alternating with spiramycin, as is practiced sometimes in Europe.

Ocular Toxoplasmosis

Diagnostic and treatment considerations are outlined in Figure 4. The mere presence of *Toxoplasma* antibody in the IgG fraction indicates that *Toxoplasma* may be the etiology of a retinal lesion. Until CMV, herpes, and other causes of retinitis can be diagnosed and treated, it does not seem imperative to confirm a specific diagnosis. (This could be accomplished by simultaneous measurement of antibody in the aqueous of the anterior chamber and the serum and comparing the antibody ratios for each of the several agents.) Treatment with SD–PYR should be started as soon as possible in patients with periodic relapses without waiting for an appointment with the physician because of the risk of irreparable retinal damage. Oral anti-inflammatory corticosteroid treatment may be added for lesions involving or adjacent to the macula or optic nerve, but they should not be given without drugs

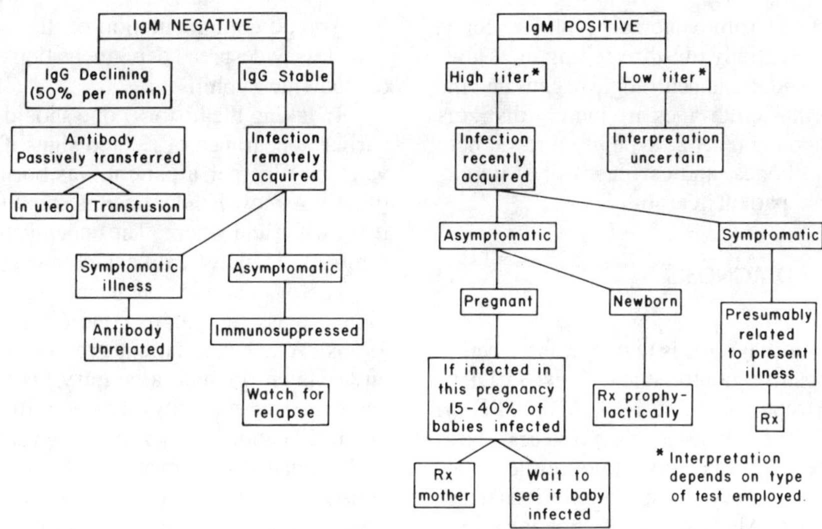

Figure 7 Analyzing IgG antibody to *Toxoplasma* with the IgM technique.

that inhibit *Toxoplasma*. The anti-inflammatory corticosteroids should be tapered as soon as the vitreous inflammation begins to subside and should be stopped while the SD–PYR medication is continued for a total of approximately 4 to 8 weeks.

Clindamycin has been used orally or by periocular injection for retinochoroiditis refractory to SD–PYR. If this treatment is successful, it would suggest another etiology rather than drug-resistant *Toxoplasma*. No control studies employing either regimen have been published.

PREVENTION

Toxoplasma oocysts remain viable in moist and shaded soil for a year or longer. Oocysts are ingested by geophagia, whether compulsive (pica) or inadvertent. Hands should be washed after contact with soil potentially contaminated with cat feces. Oocysts are destroyed by exposure to heat over 60 °C, but chemical disinfectants are not effective.

Tissue cysts that have persisted for months or years in the animal remain viable in pork, mutton, and other meats for days at room or refrigerator temperatures. Most of the organisms are destroyed when meat is frozen and thawed, but they are destroyed more effectively by heating to 60 °C, as indicated by a change in color of the meat. Hands should be washed after contact with raw meat. Soap and water, alcohol, and chemical disinfectants inactivate bradyzoites from tissues cysts on the skin. Prevention of toxoplasma infection is most important during pregancy and early childhood, and in immunosuppressed patients, when the consequences of infection tend to be more serious. The admonition to wash hands after contact with cats, soil, and raw meat, and before eating or touching the face and to cook meat thoroughly should be incorporated into the general instructions for pregnant women. Work gloves should be used when handling soil potentially contaminated by cat feces. Because infection of older children, especially young girls, is of value for immunization and the risk of appreciable illness is small, prevention becomes less important in this group. The possibility of a vaccine to protect women during pregnancy is under investigation.

Because toxoplasma cysts are often present in the heart, transplant recipients should be serologically screened and, if negative, the donor should also be screened. If a donor is positive and the recipient negative, toxoplasma infection should be expected and managed by treatment. Once a vaccine is available, negative recipients could be immunized 2 to 4 weeks prior to transplantation.

NONVENEREAL TREPONEMATOSES

DONALD R. HOPKINS, M.D.

The nonvenereal treponematoses include yaws, endemic syphilis (bejel), and pinta. Pinta is restricted to tropical parts of the Americas, where it is diminishing in incidence and prevalence. Endemic syphilis still occurs in parts of the Middle East and is highly endemic in the Sahel region of West Africa. Yaws is resurgent in West Africa and also still occurs sporadically elsewhere in tropical Africa, Latin America, and Asia.

In diagnosing and treating these infections, one must remember that the nonvenereal treponematoses cannot be distinguished from each other absolutely, nor can they always be distinguished from venereal syphilis. Since venereal syphilis is potentially life-threatening in its ability to attack cardiovascular and neurologic organs and the nonvenereal treponemal syndromes are merely disfiguring (pinta) and/or crippling (enemic syphilis or yaws, both of which attack skin, bones, and cartilage), it is important to evaluate these patients carefully.

DIAGNOSIS

The main basis for diagnosis is to determine whether the patient has a positive nontreponemal test (VDRL, RPR) and a positive treponemal test (FTA-ABS, TPHA). In early stages of the infection (less than 5 years' duration), it should be possible to demonstrate motile treponemes in exudate from primary or secondary lesions under a darkfield microscope. Alternatively, treponemes may be demonstrated in fixed smears of exudate from early lesions by fluorescein-labeled antitreponemal antibody. The most secure diagnosis is based on a positive serologic test (high-titer nontreponemal test and/or reactive treponemal test) plus demonstration of treponemes in exudate from a lesion. In latent stages, and in infections more than 5 years old, the latter will obviously not be possible.

The combination of positive serologic and microscopic tests in the same patient can only confirm that the patient has a treponemal infection, since the venereal and nonvenereal treponemes are physically and antigenically identical (by all current tests), and the serologic reactions in humans also do not differ in any reliable way. In order to determine which of the four syndromes the patient most likely has, one must consider other clues from physical examination and history (Fig. 1)

Typically, yaws manifests first with a large primary lesion on one of the extremities, followed after a few weeks or months by multiple, raised, raspberry-like papillomata. Early lesions of endemic syphilis most commonly appear as patches in and around the mouth, and these are also sometimes followed by a generalized secondary rash, the lesions of which tend to be less exuberant than in yaws. Early yaws and endemic syphilis tend to occur among children younger than 15 years. Early pinta is characterized by slightly elevated, red or bluish circular plaques on the skin. In late stages, both yaws and endemic syphilis may leave a legacy of atrophic superficial scars on the extremities or deep mutilating lesions of the nose or bones. Untreated pinta characteristically results in widespread depigmentation of the skin, although somewhat less widespread depigmentation can also follow yaws or endemic syphilis.

In taking the history, one should seek clues as to the earlier appearance of related signs if the infection is advanced. Whether a patient was born, grew up, or later lived in a known endemic area should be determined and, if so, when and where. The endemic treponematoses were rampant in many tropical countries in the 1940s and 1950s, for example, but were much less prevalent following mass campaigns conducted in many areas in the 1960s. Whether a patient grew up in an urban or rural environment in such a country (as well as the patient's age or sexual maturity) makes a difference in establishing the likelihood of exposure to a venereal or nonvenereal treponematoses. In men, a history of homosexuality increases the likelihood that one is faced with venereal syphilis rather than one of the other treponematoses.

TREATMENT

For patients with an established diagnosis of nonvenereal treponematoses—whether pinta, yaws, or endemic syphilis—an injection of long-acting penicillin G, such as benzathine penicillin G (BPG) is the treatment of choice. Children younger than 10 years old should be given 0.6 million units of BPG. Persons 10 years old and older should be given a total of 1.2 million units of BPG intramuscularly.

Because of the potential confusion with venereal syphilis and the fact that the latter may be life threatening, it is recommended that if, after a careful history and physical examination, there is still some doubt as to whether the treponemal infection in question is venereal or nonvenereal in origin, it may be wisest to treat such patients (pharmacologically, at least) as if they had venereal syphilis. Due to the high transmissibility of yaws and endemic syphilis and the frequency of latent infections, family and other close contacts of confirmed cases should also be treated, prophylactically, at the same time as the index patient.

Little is known about the treatment of endemic treponematoses with antibiotics other than penicillin. A course of oral tetracycline or erythromycin, 0.5 g four times a day for 5 days, is probably adequate therapy in penicillin-allergic adults; children younger than 7 years should not be treated with tetracycline.

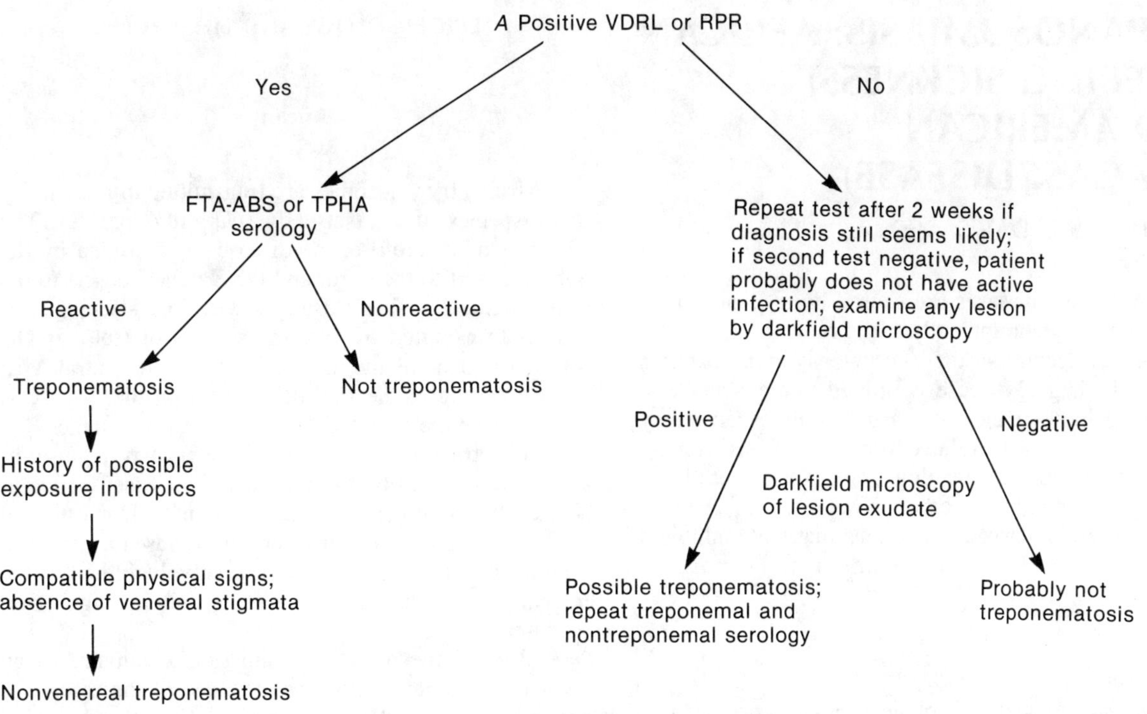

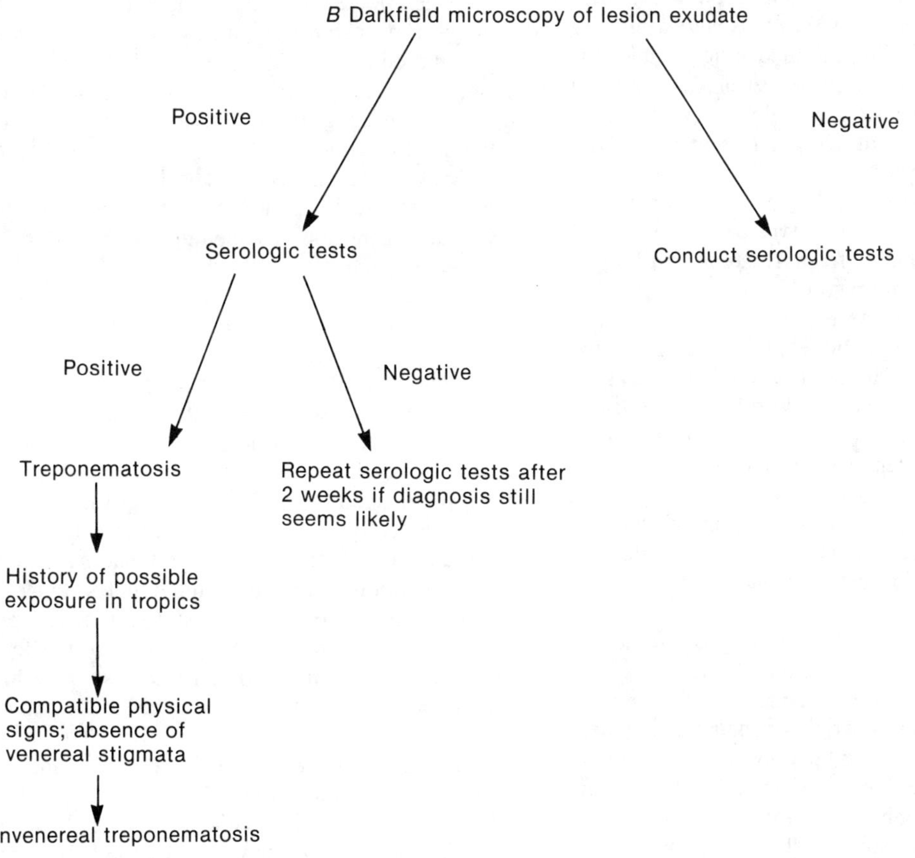

Figure 1 Diagnosis of nonvenereal treponematoses, beginning with serologic (*A*) or darkfield examination (*B*)

TRYPANOSOMIASIS: AFRICAN (SLEEPING SICKNESS) AND AMERICAN (CHAGAS' DISEASE)

CHARLES E. DAVIS, M.D.

Two distinct diseases are caused by trypanosomes. Each is limited geographically to the range of its vector, so that Africa sleeping sickness occurs only in sub-Saharan Africa and Chagas' disease is limited to the Americas. They are included in the same chapter only because they are caused by closely related protozoa. Their clinical manifestations, pathophysiology, and treatment differ markedly. Considered together, however, they are surpassed only by malaria as infections that have inhibited the development of tropical countries.

ETIOLOGY

Trypanosomes are flagellated parasitic protozoa of the family Trypanosomatidae, which also includes *Leishmania*. Chagas' disease is caused by *Trypanosoma cruzi*, which also infects wild and domestic animals. Two species of African trypanosomes infect human beings: *Trypanosoma rhodesiense* and *Trypanosoma gambiense*. These species are morphologically indistinguishable from one another and from *Trypanosoma brucei*, which cannot infect humans because it is killed by high-density lipoproteins of human serum. Domestic animals and wildlife are commonly infected by *T. rhodesiense, T. brucei*, and two other species that cannot infect human beings, *Trypanosoma congolense* and *Trypanosoma vivax*. *T. gambiense* has been isolated from livestock, but humans are probably its major reservoir.

Divergent behavior of American and African trypanosomes in the mammal probably explains the differences in the diseases caused by these closely related parasites. African trypanosomes circulate and reproduce extracellularly in the bloodstream of infected mammals. *T. cruzi* circulates, but does not replicate in the mammalian bloodstream. Instead, it invades cells and multiplies as amastigotes. Thus, *T. cruzi* is basically an intracellular parasite that tends to cause chronic disease, while African trypanosomes multiply extracellularly and often cause acute systemic disease.

The bloodstream forms of African trypanosomes and *T. cruzi* are morphologically similar. Both are spindle-shaped, motile protozoans with a nucleus and a separate kinetoplast that serves as the origin of an undulating membrane that terminates in a long, anterior flagellum. *T. cruzi*, however, tends to assume the shape of the letter *C* and is 15 to 20 mm long, unlike the straighter, longer (23 to 30 mm) African trypanosomes. The amastigote form of *T. cruzi* resembles *Leishmania*; it is a round, 3- to 5-mm body with a separate kinetoplast and nucleus.

EPIDEMIOLOGY AND LIFE CYCLE

Afican

African trypanosomes are transmitted to humans by many species of the tsetse fly (*Glossina* species). The vector—and, therefore, the disease—is confined by the Sahara desert to the north and the Kalahari desert to the south. Generally, West African or Gambian sleeping sickness is transmitted by riverine species of tsetse in the forests surrounding the streams of West and Central Africa. Accordingly, the risk of contracting the disease is greater near the forested water sources of villages.

In contrast, East African or Rhodesian trypanosomiasis is transmitted by the bite of infected tsetse flies of species that favor the dry savannah country. Domestic and wild animals are the major reservoir because they are easily infected and many species are relatively tolerant to the infection, which usually causes acute, fulminating disease of human beings.

Although mechanical transmission of human African trypanosomes can occur, maintenance of the disease is dependent upon a developmental cycle in the fly. Near the peak of parasitemia in the mammal, the long, slender African trypanosome undergoes morphologic differentiation into a form called the short stumpy trypanosome. When the infected mammal is bitten by a tsetse fly, short stumpy trypanosomes ingested with the blood meal transform in the insect midgut to procyclics, which resemble longer, beaked stumpy forms. After 3 to 4 weeks, the procyclics migrate to the salivary gland where they develop into infective metacyclics, which resemble the long, slender bloodstream form. The life cycle is completed when the infected tsetse inoculates the skin of another mammal during its next feeding.

American

Chagas' disease affects millions of people in South and Central America and extends northward through Mexico into the southern United States. Although only a handful of clinically apparent infections of people have been recognized in the United States, serologic studies and a relatively high prevalence of infections in opossums and other vertebrates suggest that inapparent infections may not be rare in the United States. In Central and South America, however, transmission occurs primarily in rural areas, where true bugs of the family Reduviidae (kissing or assassin bugs) can find a suitable habitat in animal burrows or the cracked walls and thatch of adobe huts.

The bugs defecate when they feed and infective trypomastigotes are deposited with the feces into the bite or rubbed into the bite by the host. After local multiplication, motile trypanosomes reach the bloodstream and invade cells, where they transform into amastigotes and multiply by binary fission until the cells rupture. After leaving cells, amastigotes transform into trypomatigotes again and are infective to reduviid bugs. In the midgut of the bug, trypomastigotes transform into epimastigotes, which multiply in the midgut and invade the hindgut and rectum, where they again transform into infective trypomastigotes that are deposited with the feces during the next blood meal.

Chagas' disease is a true zoonosis since large numbers of cats, dogs, oppossums, and armadillos are infected in and around villages in the endemic area.

PATHOLOGY AND PATHOGENESIS

African

When an infected fly inoculates metacyclics into the skin, the trypanosomes multiply subcutaneously and establish a focus of infection that invades the lymphatics and enters the bloodstream in 7 to 10 days. Tissue damage at the site of inoculation and multiplication of trypanosomes result in the formation of a typical chancre at the site of inoculation. Continued release of trypanosomes causes proliferative lymphadenopathy near the lesion. After trypanosomes reach the bloodstream, they multiply rapidly for several days, producing high levels of parasitemia that remit after a few days because of differentiation into the nonreplicating, short stumpy forms and because of the action of lytic antibody. Parasitemia recurs within a week or 10 days, however, with antigenically distinct trypanosomes. This phenomenon, antigenic variation, occurs because the parasite sheds one outer variant surface-glycoprotein coat (VSG) and replaces it with another. Each VSG is immunogenic, but contains different epitopes from preceding VSGs and shields the trypanosome from attack by antibodies directed against common, internal antigens. Antigenic variation can go on almost indefinitely because each parasite can code for more than 100 different VSGs. One gene is expressed at a time, and variation occurs when one gene is shut off and another turned on by genetic mechanisms that are still under study.

Recognition of each new surface coat by the immune system induces antibody that kills most of the trypanosomes, although a few escape by antigenic variation. This process continues, and the net result is recurring waves of parasitemia with localization of parasites in the heart, central nervous system, and many other organs. Multiple antigenic stimuli induce the production of very high concentrations of IgM, including specific lytic antibodies, heterophile antibodies, and rheumatoid factor. Destruction of trypanosomes releases internal trypanosomal antigens that eventually induce the production of immune complexes and inflammatory mediators. In association with these multiple antigenic challenges, lymphadenopathy, splenomegaly, and vasculitis are common. Small lymphocytes in germinal centers become replaced by plasma cells and macrophages, the patient finally becomes immunosuppressed, and the lymph nodes become atrophic and fibrotic. Myocarditis, pericarditis, glomerulonephritis, anemia, and thrombocytopenia have also been attributed to immune complex disease. Interstitial hemorrhage and perivascular mononuclear infiltration are characteristic of the myocardial lesions.

Changes in the central nervous system include diffuse meningoencephalitis, edema, lymphocytic infiltration, and "felting" of the dura-arachnoid onto the surface of the brain. The most dramatic lesion is perivascular cuffing, which may be 20- to 30-cells thick and completely separate the vessels from the brain parenchyma. Morula or Mott cells that resemble lymphocytes with a large eosinophilic, mulberry-like inclusion are prominent in the perivascular cuffs and are thought to be IgM-producing plasma cells.

Not all patients who die of Rhodesian trypanosomiasis exhibit such marked pathology. In fact, East African trypanosomiasis often resembles acute bacterial septicemia with disseminated intravascular coagulation and a fulminating course. This presentation has led some investigators to postulate a role for putative trypanosomal toxins in this syndrome, and there is experimental evidence supporting such a possibility. It seems likely that trypanosomal products are responsible for many of the clinical manifestations of acute disease and that immune-complex vasculitis accounts for many of the pathologic findings of long-standing disease.

American

Within a week or two after the bite of the reduviid bug, a chagoma develops around the parasites, which are mulitplying rapidly at the site of inoculation. Infiltration of polymorphonuclear cells and lymphocytes is accompanied by interstitial edema and lymphangitis. About the time that the chagoma is formed, *T. cruzi* begins to invade the blood and can be found in almost any organ or tissue. At this time the parasite begins to invade cells, especially those of mesenchymal origin (skeletal and cardiac muscle), reticuloendothelial cells, and neuroglia. There is a predilection for macrophages and fat cells in the chagoma. As cellular penetration occurs, *T. cruzi* loses its flagellum and undulating membrane, rounds up, and assumes the leishmanial (amastigote) form. Parasites multiply intracellularly by binary fission until the cytoplasm is full, the cellular membrane is distended, and the infected cell becomes a pseudocyst. When pseudocysts rupture, some amastigotes transform into trypomastigotes, which cannot multiply in the mammal and must either invade new cells, infect a new reduviid bug, or die.

There is little reaction to intracellular *T. cruzi*, but rupture of cells with release of amastigotes and their products produces a severe inflammatory reaction. In the acute stage of disease, the reaction consists primarly of polymorphonuclear leukocytes followed by lymphocytes, plasma cells, and histiocytes. As immunity develops, the inflammatory response becomes more localized and granulomatous, with the formation of pseudotubercles and giant cells. Healing is often accompanied by fibrosis.

Lesions in the CNS include lymphocytic perivascular cuffing, endarteritis, leptomeningitis, and neuronal degeneration. Because the CNS involvement is usually focal, scattered glial nodules are a common presentation. Myocardial manifestations in the acute stage are often due to infection of muscle cells in the conduction system. Chronic disease can cause myocardial fibrosis. Megaesophagus and megacolon are severe complications that are probably caused by invasion and destruction of the autonomic nervous plexuses that control peristalsis. Autoimmune processes may contribute to continuing damage in the chronic phase of illness when the number of parasites is low.

CLINICAL MANIFESTATIONS

African

The manifestations of African trypanosomiasis can conveniently be divided into first and second (CNS involvement) stages. The first sign of disease is the development of a chancre within 1 to 3 weeks of the tsetse bite. It is an indurated, inflamed lesion at least 10 to 12 cm in diameter that resolves into an area of shiny desquamation. The other hallmarks of early disease are fever and chills, headache, tachycardia (often out of proportion to the fever), shiny edema (especially of the face and extremities), an erythematous, circinate rash, aimless pruritis, and myalgia. Fever usually persists for about 1 week, corresponding to waves of parasitemia that are aborted by antibody, only to recur a week later with the appearance of a new antigenic variant. After several febrile periods, hepatosplenomegaly develops and lymphadenopathy becomes prominent, especially in the posterior cervical chain (Winterbottom's sign). Deep hyperesthesia, especially over the ulna (Kerandel's sign) may occur during the early stage. Thrombocytopenia, consumption coagulopathy, and frank bleeding diastheses may also occur during this stage.

CNS invasion may occur very early in Rhodesian (East African) trypanosomiasis, or the patient may die of systemic disease before the CNS is involved. The CNS symptoms of West African trypanosomiasis may not become manifest for months or years. Typically, however, the late stage of the disease occurs within a few months and is defined clinically by symptoms of interference with mental function including headache, irritability, insomnia, changes in mood, and frank psychosis. Nuchal rigidity and continuing irregular fever may suggest tuberculosis or pyogenic meningitis. Splenomegaly, lymphadenopathy, and severe facial edema usually persist. As the disease progresses, the patient becomes amenorrheic, or impotent, and emaciated. Tremors of the hands, muscle fasciculations, a shuffling gait, and muscular rigidity progress to somnolence, loss of sphincter control, and coma. Death is usually caused by starvation, bronchopneumonia, or other intercurrent infections.

The entire spectrum of these manifestations may occur in both Gambian and Rhodesian trypanosomiasis, but Rhodesian disease is often acute and may be confused with bacterial septicemia or acute malaria. The acute manifestations of Gambian disease are typically milder, and it may even present in the late stage with no obtainable history of acute disease. Patients usually die of Rhodesian disease within months, whereas patients with Gambian disease often live for 3 to 5 years and may survive for as long as 10 years.

American

The manifestations of Chagas' disease are protean, but can generally be broken down into acute, subacute, and chronic. Acute Chagas' disease occurs mainly in children younger than the age of 2 years. Its cardinal manifestation are fever to 40 °C, vomiting, diarrhea, and anorexia, often accompanied by unilateral edema of the eyelid and conjunctivitis (Romana's sign). Swelling of the lacrimal glands and submaxillary nodes usually accompanies Romana's sign, so that acute Chagas' disease is one of the causes of an oculoglandular complex. The ocular edema may spread to the entire face and the extremities. Severe illness is accompanied by generalized lymphadenopathy, hepatosplenomegaly, myocarditis, and meningoencephalitis. The mortality rate of at least 5 percent is usually due to cardiac arrhythmias, heart failure, or meningoencephalitis.

The acute stage is usually not recognized, however, and when it is, it usually resolves spontaneously with little or no damage. Some patients may eliminate the parasite, but many continue to harbor *T. cruzi* in a latent infection that may either remain asymptomatic or cause the manifestations of subacute or chronic Chagas' disease.

Subacute disease occurs in young adults, who present with massive involvement of the heart, often without other manifestations of the disease. *T. cruzi* is the major cause of severe and fatal myocarditis in Central and South America.

The unknown percentage of patients who pass into the chronic stage present either with cardiac manifestations, megaesophagus, or megacolon. Distention of the stomach, duodenum, urinary bladder, and ureters also occurs, but is less common. Thus, chronic Chagas' disease may present with arrhythmias, cardiomegaly, heart failure, esophageal or abdominal distention, severe constipation, pyelonephritis and hydronephrosis, or any combination of these manifestations.

Since *T. cruzi* can invade the placenta and can also survive in stored blood, neonates or patients who have received contaminated blood may present with the manifestations of acute Chagas' disease without exposure to the reduviid vector.

LABORATORY DIAGNOSIS

African

A flow sheet for the laboratory diagnosis of African sleeping sickness is presented in Figure 1. Establishment

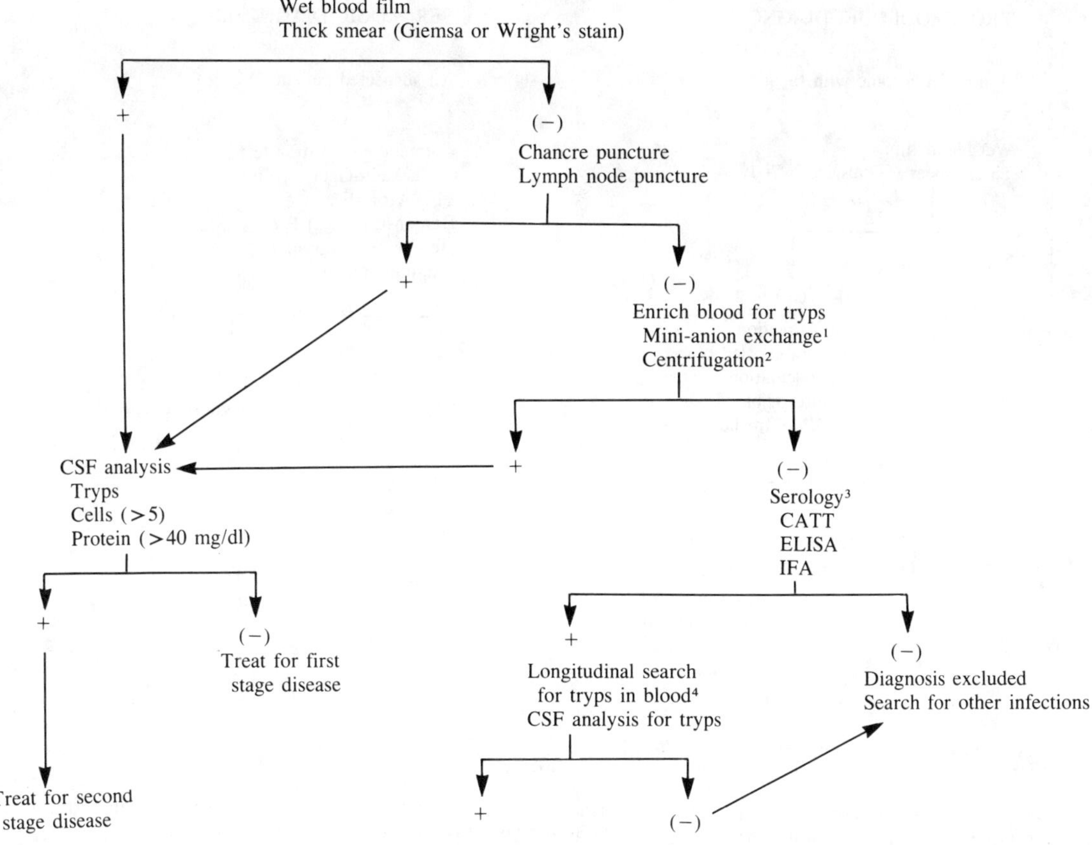

Figure 1 Laboratory diagnosis of African trypanosomiasis. [1]Mini-anion exchange kits are provided to endemic countries by WHO, but anion exchange enrichment can be done easily by mixing citrated blood with phosphate-buffered saline/glucose solution (PSG) (1:3) and eluting trypanosomes from a small column of DEAE with several volumes of PSG (6 parts PBS + 4 parts distilled water + 1.5% glucose, adjusted to pH 8.0). [2]Separate plasma and examine buffy coat for trypanosomes. [3]Available at CDC. Specimens should be forwarded by county health departments. CATT = card agglutination trypanosomal test. [4]Examine daily by direct and, every second to third day, by enrichment procedures during febrile periods. Rats should also be inoculated as described in the text.

of this diagnosis is ultimately dependent upon the demonstration of the trypanosome in a body fluid. During the acute, early stage of disease, the wet film and thick smear are usually positive in febrile patients. If they are negative, aspiration of tissue fluid from enlarged lymph nodes or the chancre will usually establish the diagnosis, but the blood should also be enriched by either passing a few milliliters of citrated or heparinized blood over an anion exchange column or centrifuging 5 to 10 ml of anticoagulated blood. Trypanosomes are less negatively charged than the formed elements of the blood and will elute rapidly from a column of DEAE flushed with phosphate-buffered saline glucose solution (PSG) adjusted to a pH of 8.0. The eluate can be examined directly under the microscope (100× to 400×) or pelleted by centrifugation before examination. The buffy coat from centrifuged blood should be collected and examined in the same way. If trypanosomes are found by any of these techniques, the cerebrospinal fluid must be analyzed. The presence of trypanosomes, a pleocytosis of greater than 5 cells per cubic millimeter, or an elevated protein indicate CNS invasion. If trypanosomes are not detected in the CSF, the fluid should be centrifuged and the pellet examined for trypanosomes.

In endemic areas a serologic test, the CATT (card agglutination trypanosomiasis test), is provided by the World Health Organization. This simple test is based on the agglutination of trypanosomes by the blood of a patient with antibody and is performed with fingerstick blood on reaction cards with trypanosomes provided by WHO. This test is not available to physicians in the United States, but the Centers for Disease Control in Atlanta can perform agglutination tests and may also be able to conduct ELISA or immunofluorescence tests that identify stable, internal antigens. The CATT is used in Africa as a screening test for entire villages, and a positive CATT is, therefore, often the reason for implementing the rest of the diagnostic scheme shown in Figure 1.

If another diagnosis has not been established and trypanosomes have not been demonstrated, the blood should be repeatedly examined for trypanosomes, especially during fever. Inoculation of rats, as described be-

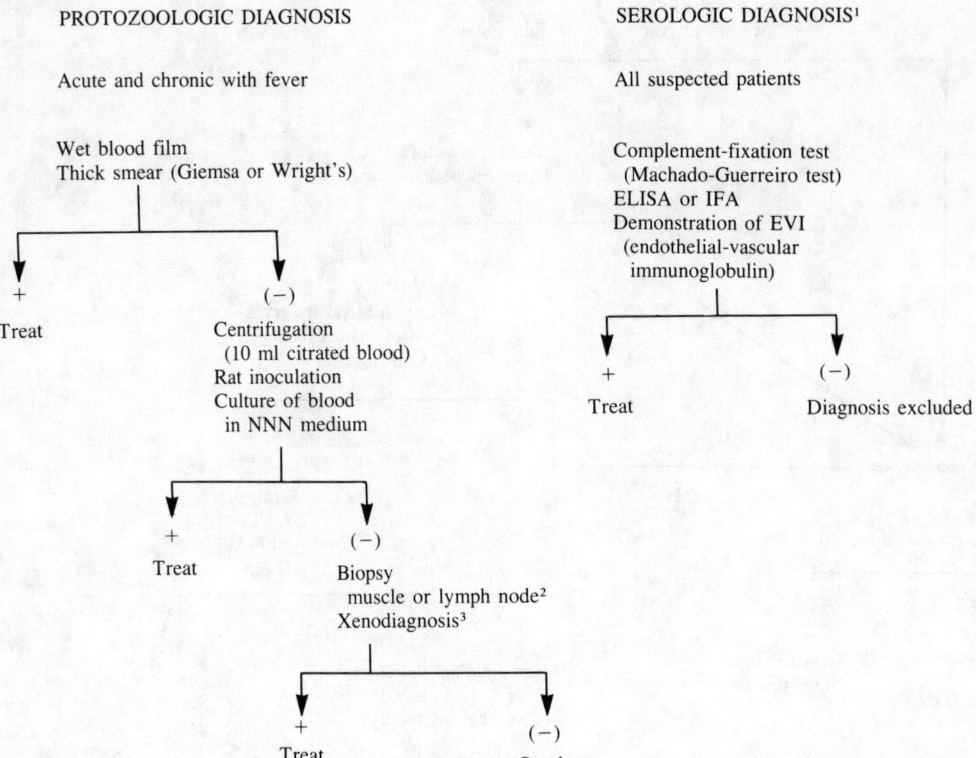

Figure 2 Laboratory diagnosis of American trypanosomiasis. See text and Figure 1 for explanation of centrifugation, inoculation, and culture in NNN medium. [1]Serologic procedures available at CDC. Specimens should be forwarded by county health departments. [2]Skeletal muscle or lymph node sections stained by Giemsa. [3]Uninfected reduviid bugs are fed on patients and examined periodically for *T. cruzi*. This painless and sensitive, but distasteful, procedure is not available in the United States.

low, for American trypanosomiasis is helpful for the diagnosis of East African trypanosomiasis, but *T. gambiense* seldom causes infections in rats.

American

Acute Chagas' disease occurs primarily in young children who are exposed to an environment appropriate for infected reduviid bugs. Chronic or subacute Chagas' should be considered in any patient with idiopathic myocarditis, megacolon, or megaesophagus who has lived in or visited rural areas of the southern United States, Mexico, and Central and South America.

Protozoologic diagnosis of acute Chagas' disease or chronic disease in a febrile patient is approached by the same techniques as African disease except that anion exchange is not of proven value and animal inoculation and culture of *T. cruzi* should be attempted (Fig. 2). Five to 10 rats should be injected intraperitoneally with 0.5 to 1.0 ml each of whole heparinized blood. Beginning 10 days to 2 weeks after rat inoculation, tail blood should be examined every 2 to 3 days for trypanosomes. After 60 days, the rats should be killed, and histopathologic sections of heart, spleen, and liver should be stained with Giemsa and examined for the presence of leishmanial forms. A small amount of patient's blood should be cultured on NNN (Novy, MacNeal, and Nicolle's) medium or on blood-agar slants overlaid with Locke's solution. The medium should be examined daily for 14 to 21 days for *T. cruzi* colonies or free trypanosomes in the liquid overlay.

More commonly, physicians in the United States will attempt to establish the diagnosis of Chagas' disease in a patient with idiopathic myocardopathy. The Machado-Guerreiro complement fixation (CF) test is valuable because it is positive in more than 95 percent of cases. Cross-reactions occur primarily with mucocuataneous leishmaniasis and other diseases with different manifestations than Chagas' disease. ELISA and indirect immunofluorescence tests are promising new developments, but have not replaced the CF test. An immune globulin, EVI (endothelial-vascular immunoglobulin), that seems to be specific for the damaged myocardium of patients with Chagasic myocardopathy has been demonstrated but testing is not yet generally available.

TREATMENT

African

The treatment of African trypanosomiasis varies with the stage of the disease and with the geographic location of the exposure. Before invasion of the CNS, East African

TABLE 1 Treatment of African Trypanosomiasis, First Stage

Day of Rx	*T. rhodesiense* (*East Africa*) *Suramin (IV)*	*T. gambiense* (*West Africa*) *Pentamidine*
1	0.2 g (test dose)	3–4 mg/kg base
2	---	3–4 mg/kg base
3	10 mg/kg	3–4 mg/kg base
4	---	3–4 mg/kg base
5	20 mg/kg (up to 1 g)	3–4 mg/kg base
6	---	3–4 mg/kg base
7	---	3–4 mg/kg base
8–10	---	---
11	20 mg/kg (up to 1 g)	---
17	20 mg/kg (up to 1 g)	---
23	20 mg/kg (up to 1 g)	---
30	20 mg/kg (up to 1 g)	---

Note: Recommendations are modified from those of the World Health Organization and the dedicated physicians working in Trypanosomiasis Network Hospitals throughout Africa. Suramin and pentamidine are available from the Parasitic Disease Drug Service, Centers for Disease Control, Atlanta, Georgia 30333; telephone (404) 329–3670. Suramin (Bayer 205, Germanin, Naganol, Moranyl) is a whitish powder that is freely soluble in water and should be freshly prepared with sterile, pyrogen-free distilled water to a 10% solution. Pentamidine isothionate is supplied as a white powder that is made up in sterile, pyrogen-free distilled water to a 4% solution of base. Lomidine is pentamidine methanesulfonate that is already prepared as a 4% solution. The dose of the base is 3 to 4 mg per kg for either product, but 1.74 mg of pentamidine isothionate and 1.56 mg of lomidine equals 1 mg of base.

trypanosomiasis (*T. rhodesiense*) can be treated successfully with suramin as outlined in Table 1. Suramin clears the blood of trypanosomes within a few hours, and a full course will cure almost 100 percent of people with first-stage disease. About one person in 20,000 has an idiosyncracy to suramin, and this ratio is greatly increased in patients with onchocerciasis. Consequently, a small test dose of 0.2 to 0.25 g is recommended for the first injection. The remainder of the course is presented in Table 1. Suramin is a complex organic chemical that combines with plasma proteins and remains in the circulation for long periods. It is deposited in the renal tubules and can cause albuminuria and granular casts. Rare instances of nephritis and uremia have been reported. Accordingly, a urinalysis and blood urea nitrogen should be performed after each day of treatment and further treatment delayed if significant abnormalities occur.

Pentamidine is as effective as suramin against *T. gambiense* and has fewer adverse effects. Consequently, this aromatic diamidine is the drug of choice against first-stage infections with West African trypanosomes, unless it has already been used as mass prophylaxis in the area where the infection was contracted. Mass prophylaxis is associated with the development of resistance to pentamidine and has generally been discontinued. Suramin is an effective alternative. Side effects of pentamidine are usually minor and can often be avoided by rest after the injection to avoid the hypotensive effect. Severe hypoglycemia and peripheral neuritis have been reported.

All patients who are treated for first-stage infections should have repeat CSF analysis at the end of treatment and 3, 6, and 12 months later to detect CNS disease that was latent at the time of diagnosis.

Neither suramin nor pentamidine cross the blood-brain barrier, and second-stage infections with both East and West African trypanosomes must be treated with Melarsoprol, a combination of the trivalent arsenical, melarsen oxide, and dimercaprol (BAL) (Table 2). A test dose and one full injection of suramin are given first to clear the blood and tissues of trypanosomes rapidly. Melarsoprol is usually begun on the fifth day when the condition of the patient has improved, but can be instituted earlier if the patient's condition is critical. The principal adverse reaction of treatment is reactive arsenical encephalopathy, which usually begins after the third injection or at the onset of the second series (day 14; Table 2). The onset may be sudden or develop more slowly with headache, tremor, high fevers, seizures, and coma. It is sometimes difficult to differentiate from progressive sleeping sickness. The risk of this complication is about 5 percent, and it has a high mortality. Its pathogenesis is thought to be associated with the release of trypanosomal products, but it is unclear whether it is a true Herxheimer reaction or immunologic in nature. Hydrocortisone is given to second-stage patients (Table 2) in the hope of decreasing the incidence of this reaction. Other adverse effects of Melarsoprol include conjunctivitis, severe diarrhea, jaundice, and exfoliative dermatitis.

Reactive encephalopathy should be treated by discontinuing Melarsoprol, administering phenobarbital or valium for convulsions, mannitol for cerebral edema, and oxygen as necessary. French clinicians in West Africa believe that epinephrine administered at the rate of 2 mg subcutaneously every 2 hours until improvement may be life-saving. The patient should be isolated and protected from light and noise.

TABLE 2 Treatment of African Trypanosomiasis, Second Stage (CNS Involved)

Day of Rx	*Anti-Trypanosomal Drug, IV Dose*		*Hydrocortisone*
1	Suramin	0.2 g	50 mg
2	---	---	50 mg
3	Suramin	20 mg/kg (1 g max)	50 mg
4	---	---	50 mg
5	Melarsoprol	1.5 mg/kg	50 mg
6	Melarsoprol	2.0 mg/kg	50 mg
7	Melarsoprol	2.2 mg/kg	50 mg
8	---	---	37.5 mg
9–13	---	---	37.5 mg
14	Melarsoprol	2.5 mg/kg	37.5 mg
15	Melarsoprol	3.0 mg/kg	37.5 mg
16	Melarsoprol	3.6 mg/kg	37.5 mg
17–22	---	---	25 mg
23	Melarsoprol	3.6 mg/kg	---
24	Melarsoprol	3.6 mg/kg	---
25	Melarsoprol	3.6 mg/kg	---

Note: Treatment for either East African or West African trypanosomiasis. See Table 1 and text for source of recommendations and more detail about suramin and melarsoprol. Melarsoprol (Mel B, Arsobol) is supplied as a 3.6% solution in propylene glycol and must be given intravenously because propylene glycol is highly irritating. The maximum daily dose is 3.6 mg per kilogram, which must be reached gradually as indicated in the table in order to minimize the chance of reactive arsenical encephalopathy. Available from CDC (see Table 1).

Nitrofurazone (0.5 g PO four times per day every day for 7 days for two series with an interval of 1 week) and difluoromethyl ornithine (DFMO; appropriate doses and schedule have not been established) have been used for melarsoprol failures, but should not be used primarily.

American

There is as yet no effective proven treatment for chronic Chagas' disease. Acute disease can be treated with nifurtimox (Lampit; Bayer 2502), a nitrofurazone that clears the blood of circulating trypomastigotes. It is not very active against intracellular *T. cruzi*, but proven chronic cases should also be treated. The dose for either acute or chronic disease of adults is 10 mg per kilogram PO daily for 60 days in acute disease and 120 days in chronic. Children have been treated with 25 mg per kilogram for 14 days, followed by 15 mg per kilogram for 100 days with no increased incidence of side effects. Adverse effects (5% to 10% of patients) include rashes, gastrointestinal reactions, leukopenia, and polyneuritis. Side effects are reversible after treatment is discontinued.

Benzonidazole is the only alternative to the nitrofurans. At 5 mg per kilogram PO for 60 days (adults and children), it may be as effective as nifurtimox. Side effects are similar and reversible.

Both drugs are available from the Parasitic Disease Drug Service, Centers for Disease Control, Atlanta, Georgia 30333; telephone (404) 329-3670.

Chlortetracycline and steroids, which have been used in the past, should be avoided because they may exacerbate the disease.

LEISHMANIASIS

DAVID J. WYLER, M.D., F.A.C.P.

Leishmaniasis is caused by infection with any of several pathogenic species of protozoa of the genus *Leishmania. Leishmania* in mammalian hosts are obligate intracellular parasites of mononuclear phagocytes where they exist in the aflagellate amastigote form. The parasites are transmitted by the bites of vector sandfly species (*Phlebotomus, Lutzomyia*, and *Psychodopygus*) in the guts of which they develop as flagellated promastigotes. Generally, leishmaniasis exists as a zoonosis; natural reservoirs and sandfly vectors differ within specific endemic regions. In some regions, such as India, no nonhuman reservoir has been identified, suggesting that transmission via sandfly is directly person to person. Rare cases of transmission by means other than sandfly bite (congenital, transfusion, organ transplantation) have been reported.

Three major forms of clinical disease are recognized: cutaneous, mucocutaneous, and visceral leishmaniasis. Clinical manifestations are largely dependent on the species of infecting parasite, but host factors clearly contribute. Epidemiologic studies suggest that asymptomatic infections also occur and are not rare. Longitudinal studies defining the outcome of asymptomatic infections are lacking, however. Taxonomy of the *Leishmania* is confusing. New taxonomic criteria are being applied using sophisticated technologies that employ monoclonal antibody reagents, and restriction endonuclease- and DNA hybridization-probes. Results of the studies should improve our understanding of the precise relationship between infection with a particular *Leishmania* species and the resulting clinical manifestations. Earlier taxonomic studies relied heavily on the clinical features of patients in defined geographic regions from which parasites were isolated. The classification scheme in Table 1 is clinically useful but represents an intentional over-simplification of present taxonomy.

The geographic location where the infection was acquired and the clinical form of the disease are important in deciding on approaches in diagnosis and therapy. Diagnostic methods available include tissue biopsy for the identification of *Leishmania* histologically or by in-vitro cultivation, serology, and skin test. The mainstays of antileishmanial chemotherapy are the pentavalent antimonial compounds (sodium stibogluconate and *N*-methyl glucamine antimonate). Pentamidine and amphotericin B are considered second-line agents used mainly in cases unresponsive to antimonials. Allopurinol and related pyrazolopyrimidines as well as other compounds are being experimentally assessed for their clinical efficacy.

TABLE 1 General Classification of Leishmaniasis and Etiologic "Species Complex"

	Species Complex in	
Clinical Forms	*Old World*	*New World*
Cutaneous	*L. tropica* complex (also *L. major*)	*L. brasiliensis* complex *L. mexicana* complex
Mucocutaneous	Rarely occurs	*L. brasiliensis* complex (esp. *L.b. brasiliensis* subspecies)
Visceral (Kala-azar)	*L. donovani* complex (also *L. infantum*)	*L. donovani* complex (also *L. chagasi*)

Note: The concept of a species complex as used in this classification implies that different subspecies in the complex (elevated to species level in some classification schemes) may cause patterns of disease that differ in details of clinical manifestations, natural history, or epidemiology. Names in parentheses are species designation used in some other classification system and may be encountered in the medical literature.

Conventional alternative drugs such as metronidazole or rifampin have been used successfully in some cases, but are not presently widely accepted as standard drugs in the antileishmanial armamentarium.

CUTANEOUS LEISHMANIASIS

In the Old World this can be acquired in the Mediterranean littoral, Africa, India, China, and Asia Minor. Lesions begin as erythematous papules or macules that become elevated and may ulcerate. Smaller satellite lesions, generally papules that also can ulcerate, may form adjacent to larger ones. Ulcerated lesions are characteristically well demarcated and have raised edges that contain the highest density of parasites (thus, these are the preferred site for biopsy). Lesions generally are nonpruritic, painless, and nontender unless ulcers become superinfected with bacteria, a complication that occurs frequently. Even in the absence of superinfection, nodule formation can occur along draining lymphatics and lymphadenopathy may develop. Uncomplicated lesions usually progress to heal spontaneously over a period of about 6 months, a process that may be heralded by ulceration. Healing results in scar formation. Because of the tendency for spontaneous resolution, chemotherapy is not generally necessary in Old World cutaneous leishmaniasis. It is indicated when lesions progress in size, fail to heal after 5 to 6 months, or are cosmetically embarrassing.

Diagnosis can be established by identifying *Leishmania* in skin biopsies. Impression smears of the biopsy, stained with Giemsa, frequently prove the most rapid and accurate procedure. Parasites are generally harder to identify in tissue sections. Growth of promastigotes may require maintaining cultures of biopsy material at 22 °C to 26 °C for up to 4 weeks. Special culture media are required. Delayed hypersensitivity responses (Montenegro skin test) to injection of killed promastigote suspensions (leishmanin) often develop in these patients. Skin test antigen is not commercially available. It can be obtained from the World Health Organization Leishmaniasis Reference Center in Jerusalem, Israel. Serologic tests (in the United States obtainable from the Centers for Disease Control, Atlanta, Georgia) are usually negative and therefore of uncertain diagnostic value in cutaneous leishmaniasis.

In the New World, skin lesions caused by *Leishmania* can resemble those characteristic of Old World cutaneous leishmaniasis or they can have distinctive patterns. Clinical features characteristic of disease acquired in a particular geographic region may be encountered. Cutaneous disease can be acquired in Central and South America, in areas from the Yucatan peninsula to northern Argentina. Transmission of cutaneous leishmaniasis has not been identified in Uruguay or Chile. A common entity, resulting from *Leishmania mexicana* infection, is characterized by lesions on the pinna of the ear called chiclero's ulcers, so named after the harvesters of chicle gum prone to this occupational hazard. Lesions generally worsen and infrequently undergo self-healing; they do not cause mucosal destruction. Some patients with other forms of New World cutaneous leishmaniasis can, however, progress to mucocutaneous disease. Accordingly, chemotherapy should generally be instituted in all cases of cutaneous leishmaniasis acquired in the New World. Diagnostic approaches to New World cutaneous are indistinct from those described above for Old World leishmaniasis, although parasites may be harder to retrieve in cultures of biopsies.

Chemotherapy of cutaneous leishmaniasis entails one to three courses of pentavalent antimony (Sb V) in a daily dose of 20 mg per kilogram (maximum, 850 mg Sb V per day) in 50 ml of saline or dextrose-in-water, administered intravenously over 20 minutes. The duration of each course must be individualized. Since the total amount of drug administered does not determine toxicity, earlier recommendations of a 10 day observation period between courses is now being abandoned. Therefore, courses of 30 days duration at the recommended daily dose can be safely administered if necessary. Duration of each course of therapy can vary from 10 to 30 days. An observation period of at least 10 days between each course is recommended. The decision to administer the second or third course depends largely on the clinical response, although parasitologic evidence of cure can be helpful in the decision process. Treatment failures (insufficient clinical response) can be treated with intramuscular pentamidine, (2 to 4 mg per kilogram per day for up to 15 days). Amphotericin B (0.5 mg per kilogram daily or 1 mg per kilogram every other day) for up to 8 weeks has also been successful and is an acceptable second-line drug. Treatment of bacterial superinfection with appropriate antibiotics is important. Intralesional administration of antileishmanials, local application of heat, cryosurgery, and chemotherapy with agents other than those mentioned have been reported to be effective in some cases. The relative efficacy of neither the conventional nor exceptional therapies has been subjected to careful experimental scrutiny.

Because of potentially similar clinical features, cutaneous leishmaniasis must be distinguished from infections due to certain mycobacteria, fungi, and spirochetes, as well as from sarcoidosis and neoplasms. Because of the rarity of importation of leishmaniasis, physicians in nonendemic countries must continue to suspect cutaneous leishmaniasis in patients with an appropriate history of exposure and suggestive lesions.

MUCOCUTANEOUS LEISHMANIASIS

During the course of cutaneous infection with *Leishmania brasiliensis*, or after its resolution, mucosal lesions can develop. These lesions may be recognized as late as 24 years after the cutaneous lesions heal; some patients with mucocutaneous leishmaniasis lack historic and clinical evidence of antecedent cutaneous leishmaniasis altogether. The risk of developing mucocutaneous complications varies geographically. In Brazil, this complicaton rate seems to increase progressively from the north to the south.

Nasal lesions can present with stuffiness, coryza, or epistaxis and progress gradually to septal perforation, destruction of the bridge, and soft tissue erosion. Oral lesions can involve the tongue and lips as well as buccal, pharyngeal, and laryngeal mucosa. Perforation of the soft palate occurs. Biopsies reveal granulomas similar to those seen in cutaneous lesions, but parasites are usually sparse and often difficult to identify and isolate. Patients have reactive Montenegro skin tests and usually also positive leishmanial serology (indirect fluorescent antibody or direct agglutination assay being the tests frequently employed). Therapy is similar to that described for cutaneous leishmaniasis. When, as often is the case, patients fail to respond to pentavalent antimonials, amphotericin B is employed in total doses similar to those used for deep-seated mycoses (1.5 to 2 g for adults). Restorative plastic surgery and use of prostheses are helpful in patients with extensively destructive lesions, but should be undertaken only after successful completion of chemotherapy and a subsequent extended period of observation for relapse (for example, 1 year).

Mucocutaneous leishmaniasis can clinically resemble other infections including syphilis, paracoccidiodomycosis, yaws and histoplasmosis, as well as sarcoidosis, basal cell carcinoma and midline granuloma.

VISCERAL LEISHMANIASIS (kala-azar)

Members of the *Leishmania donovani* complex can disseminate to infect mononuclear phagocytes present in virtually any organ and even circulating monocytes. Spleen, liver, and bone marrow are the favored sites, however. Occasionally, patients will recall having had a skin lesion that represents the initial cutaneous infection, but generally cutaneous lesions are absent by the time the patient manifests features of visceral disease. The incubation period between infection and development of clinical features can be as long as 34 months. Therefore, this diagnosis should be considered even in patients whose exposure in an endemic area was temporally remote from the time of clinical presentation. Kala-azar occurs in South America, Asia, Africa, and the Mediterranean littoral.

Progression of symptoms and signs in visceral leishmaniasis (kala-azar) can vary in tempo from abrupt to insidious, and different features may dominate the clinical presentation in different patients. Additionally, some patients manifest a biphasic pattern of disease with a discrete acute phase followed by a more chronic phase. Typical symptoms include fever, abdominal discomfort, cough, and weight loss. Splenomegaly is present and may be massive, and hepatomegaly and lymphadenopathy are usually present. Kala-azar often is complicated by reactivation of tuberculosis, pneumonia, sepsis, or dysentery. These complications contribute to serious morbidity and mortality. Patients characteristically have pancytopenia that leads to pallor, petichiae, ecchymosis, and epistaxis. Spontaneous internal hemorrhage in these patients can lead to exsanguination. Markedly elevated immunoglobulins, especially IgG, is a characteristic laboratory finding, and rheumatoid factor and circulating immune complexes are also frequently identified in these patients.

The most sensitive (98% positive) and specific diagnostic procedure is splenic aspiration with demonstration of parasites in tissue smears or by culture. The use of small-gauge needles minimizes the likelihood of complications (hemorrhage; splenic rupture), which of course is greatest in patients with coagulation defects. Splenic aspiration should be carried out only by physicians experienced in the procedure. Accordingly, this is not a procedure commonly employed in nonendemic regions. Bone marrow aspiration is the next most sensitive specific procedure (50% to 90% positive). Liver biopsy and lymph node aspiration may also provide the diagnosis, but with lesser accuracy. In some cases, parasites can even be identified in buffy coat cells. The Montenegro skin test is characteristically negative, as patients with kala-azar have suppressed *Leishmania* antigen-specific T-cell responsiveness (anergy). Responsiveness returns within weeks to months after treatment. Antileishmanial antibodies measured by standard serologic tests are present, often at high titers. From a practical point of view, patients with marked splenomegaly, pancytopenia, hyperimmunoglobulinemia (IgG), an appropriate exposure history and positive antileishmanial serology can be considered as having kala-azar. Efforts to identify organisms by bone marrow aspiration are reasonable in view of a low risk of complications involved with this procedure. Liver biopsy should be considered if marrow aspiration fails, but splenic aspiration may be harder to justify in nonendemic areas.

The differential diagnosis of kala-azar includes a large number of infectious and noninfectious diseases that have splenomegaly and pancytopenia as features. For physicians practicing in areas where kala-azar is not endemic, the risk is greater that a diagnosis of kala-azar will be missed than that diseases in the differential diagnosis will not be considered.

The efficacy of treatment with pentavalent antimonials differs in different geographic regions. Patients in India and South America generally have good responses, whereas resistance is encountered more frequently in China and the Mediterranean, and especially East Africa. One approach to dealing with disease acquired in areas where relative drug resistance is encountered is to treat for longer periods. Second and third courses are sometimes required, and the second-line drugs (pentamidine and amphotericin B) may be needed if these fail.

RARER DISEASE FORMS

Other clinical forms of leishmaniasis, some with distinct geographic distribution, are occasionally encountered. These include diffuse cutaneous leishmaniasis, a condition that occurs mainly in Venezuela, Ethiopia, and the Dominican Republic and is associated with anergy to leishmanial antigens. Leishmania recidivans, in contrast, is a recrudescent cutaneous infection associated with exuberant T-cell hypersensitivity. Post kala-azar dermal leishmaniasis is characterized by nodular lesions in some patients who have recovered from kala-azar.

PREVENTION

Patients who recover from leishmaniasis apparently are resistant to reinfection by the homologous species. This observation led to the practice in the Middle East and USSR of inoculating children wth material from infected patients as a form of vaccination against cutaneous leishmaniasis. No widely accepted vaccines are available, however, and no chemoprophylactic regimens are in use. Sandfly bites can be minimized by wearing protective clothing, using insect repellents, and employing fine-mesh netting around beds. Travelers to endemic regions should be alerted to the risk of acquiring the disease, so that they can seek early medical attention when signs and symptoms appear.

SCHISTOSOMIASIS

KENNETH S. WARREN, M.D.

The therapy of schistosomiasis has undergone a remarkable change within the last several years with the advent of an oral, nontoxic drug administered in a single day for the treatment of all species of human schistosomes. Prior to this, treatment required different drugs of varying efficacy and toxicity for each of the different species of schistosomes and even for different geographic strains.

Before going on to details of treatment, it is necessary to point out that schistosomes, like most helminths, do not multiply within the human definitive host. Thus, for each schistosome larva (cercaria) that penetrates the skin while the host is immersed in fresh water, one worm may develop. Furthermore, the distribution of schistosomes in human populations is negative binomial—only a small proportion of those infected (usually less than 10%) bear heavy worm burdens. With rare exceptions, it is only that small proportion of individuals that tends to develop the classic syndromes of hepatosplenic disease in *Schistosoma mansoni* and *Schistomsoma japonicum* infections and urinary tract disease in schistosomiasis haematobia. Thus, most infected individuals will have no signs or symptoms of disease. In the relatively small number of treated patients in whom cure is not achieved, there is at least a 90 percent reduction in worm burdens, bringing even heavily infected individuals to the level where overt disease does not occur. (The major exception to this situation is the rare occurrence of schistosomiasis of the central nervous system, in which a single worm pair putatively causes severe disease.)

Signs and symptoms of schistosomiasis are rarely seen in patients in developed countries and then largely in migrants rather than in travelers. Eosinophilia indicates the presence of the helminth infection; in schistosomiasis mansoni and japonica, the patient may appear with hepatosplenomegaly or, in the most extreme case, have a hematemesis; in *S. haematobium* infection, hematuria and dysuria will suggest the diagnosis. Once schistomsomiasis is suspected, a geographic history must be obtained—*S. mansoni* occurs in Africa, the Middle East, parts of South America and the Caribbean; *S. japonicum* occurs in the Far East, and *S. haemotobium*, in Africa and the Middle East. If the geographic history is positive, the next step is to establish whether there has been significant contact with fresh water within an endemic area. If both the geographic history and the history of water contact are positive, definitive diagnosis can then be made by demonstration of characteristically shaped schistosome eggs in the patient's feces or urine. Simple and quantitative methods for doing this are the Kato thick fecal smear for the diagnosis of schistosomiasis mansoni and japonica and the Nuclepore filtration method for the diagnosis of schistosomiasis haematobia. Immunologic diagnostic techniques, such as serology or skin tests, are not as yet adequate for definitive diagnosis.

The drug of choice is praziquantel (Biltricide). Praziquantel appears to have an effect on the permeability of the cell membrane, inducing rapid contraction of the schistosomes. The schistosome tegument shows vacuolization and disintegration. The drug is rapidly metabolized and is eliminated by the kidneys. The treatment regimen for *S. mansoni* and *S. haematobium* infection is a single dose of 40 mg per kilogram, and for *S. japonicum*, 20 mg per kilogram given three times in one day for a total of 60 mg per kilogram. The pediatric dose is the same. Adverse effects include sedation, abdominal discomfort, fever, sweating, and nausea. Cure rates are approximately 85 percent, and in those not cured, egg counts are reduced by 95 percent.

SUPERFICIAL FUNGAL INFECTION

ERNESTO GONZALEZ, M.D.

Superficial fungal infections, collectively called dermatomycoses, are among the most prevalent of all infectious diseases. According to a national health survey published in 1978, 10 percent of the population of the United States is infected with these fungi. It is estimated that these infections account for 15 to 20 percent of new cases in dermatology clinics in tropical countries.

Three groups of fungal infections are included in the dermatomycoses: tinea versicolor, dermatophytosis, and candidiasis. All of the fungi causing these have the proclivity to grow in keratinized tissues, especially the stratum corneum of the skin, and some will also invade skin apendages such as the hair and nails. Tinea versicolor is caused by a lipophilic yeast, *Pityrosporum orbiculare*, which is part of the normal flora of the skin, but which, under specific circumstances, becomes a pathogen. It causes the most superficial of all the dermatomycoses, producing a chronic, usually asyptomatic infection with a characteristic change in the color of the skin. Tinea versicolor does not affect the hair or nails.

Dermatophytoses are the commonest of the dermatomycoses and are produced by several species of true fungi of three different genera: *Trichophyton, Microsporum*, and *Epidermophyton*. A wide spectrum of clinical presentations is produced by these species on the basis of their characteristic growth patterns, which are dependent on the type of keratin and anatomic location where the colonization occurs as well as the host-parasite interaction that is established. Skin, hair, and nails can be affected, depending on the specific predilection of the genus.

Candidiasis of the skin represents one of the protean clinical manifestations of colonization by *Candida albicans*, an opportunistic yeast that can colonize the skin as well as many other organs. A normal resident of the gut, *C. albicans* can invade not only the skin but the mucosal surfaces. Invasion of the mucosal surfaces and other organs is a distinguishing feature of candidiasis, which is not shared by the other dermatomycoses. Although the majority of cases of candidiasis of the skin remain confined to the integument or mucosal surfaces, this infection should always heighten one's awareness for systemic disease or complications.

PATHOGENESIS

The pathogenesis of tinea versicolor is poorly understood. The metamorphosis of *P. orbiculare* from a saprophytic yeast inhabiting the stratum corneum to a pathogen is influenced by environmental factors such as heat and humidity. Application of lipids to the skin seems to enhance the growth of this lipophilic yeast. The host-parasite interaction is not well understood since the yeasts presumably only colonize the nonviable, very superficial, keratinized layers of skin. Recent studies, however, have shown *P. orbiculare* in the viable epidermal cell layers. Furthermore, an inflammatory response observed in some patients with tinea versicolor suggests that an immunologic response induced by the yeasts on their products might be taking place. The characteristic pigmentary changes of hypo- and hyperpigmentation are also a source of controversy. The hypopigmented changes are postulated to be due to the inhibition of tyrosinase by the dicarboxylic acids produced by *P. orbiculare*; however, the pathogenesis of the hyperpigmented lesions is still a debatable issue. Some observers postulate that there is an increased number of melanocytes and melanosomes in these pigmented lesions, although others have observed no such increase.

The pathogenesis of dermatophytoses has been studied more extensively. It is apparent that although colonization by these fungi is limited to keratinized tissues, the disease produced is a consequence of the host's reaction to the antigenic products of the fungus rather than to the invasion of living tissue by the organism. The inflammatory response is manifested clinically by an eczematous reaction induced by a delayed hypersensitivity response by the host. It is postulated that as the inflammatory reaction breaches the skin barrier, the fungal colony is directly exposed to certain host-defense mechanisms that inhibit its growth. As transferrin diffuses into the stratum corneum and binds to iron, this essential nutrient for fungal growth becomes inaccessible. If a delayed hypersensitivity response is not developed by the host, a chronic parasitic state ensues that is difficult to eradicate even with aggressive therapy. Infections with *Trichophyton rubrum* are characterized by this chronic, indolent colonization with no inflammatory response. Immunodeficient patient or patients with atopic diathesis are also unable to express a cellular immune response and are infected chronically.

Animal studies suggest that the pathogenesis of candidiasis is due to the penetration of the fungal elements into the viable layers of the skin. Complement is fixed through the alternative pathway, and chemotaxis of polymorphonuclear leukocytes occurs, inducing not only the inflammatory reaction, but the development of pustules that are characteristic of this infection. The role of cellular immune response is still not clear, but this mechanism might limit invasion by the yeast.

CLINICAL FEATURES

Tinea Versicolor

The reported prevalence of tinea versicolor varies from 5 to 50 percent of the population, being greater in hot and humid climates. The true prevalence may be higher since the disease produces minimal discomfort and patients usually do not seek medical attention. Apparently, tinea versicolor is unique to humans, and some observers postulate that it is not contagious and the pathogenic potential of the saprophyte causing it depends on endogenous and exogenous factors such as genetic predisposition, hyperhidrosis, heat, humidity, and immunologic events that impair host resistance.

The most characteristic features of tinea versicolor are the pigmentary changes and the superficial scaling. Hypopigmented, small, annular lesions with fine, velvety scales appear early and eventually coalesce to form larger hypopigmented, scaly patches. Hyperpigmented lesions are less common and sometimes can appear adjacent to the hypopigmented ones. Enough inflammatory changes can occasionally develop when the patient is exposed to heat and humidity that the lesions become pruritic and can be confused with urticarial lesions. The upper trunk and neck are the areas of predilection, but extremities can also be affected. Face, palms, and lower legs are usually not involved.

The diagnosis of tinea versicolor can be established by examination of the skin lesions under Wood's lamp and confirmed by direct microscopic examination of the scales with a 10 to 20 percent potassium hydroxide solution. An orange-yellow fluorescence under Wood's lamp is characteristic, but is not a constant finding. The typical short, plumpy hyphae and budding yeasts ("spaghetti and meatball"), however, are invariably present on a potassium hydroxide mount, and this is diagnostic. *P. orbiculare* is a lipophilic yeast that cannot be cultured on readily available media unless natural oil (olive oil) is added.

Dermatophytoses

Dermatophytoses account for approximately 5 percent of the dermatology outpatients in large clinics. It is estimated that about 90 percent of men experience at least transient dermatophytic infection by middle adult life, and about 15 percent of men are chronically infected.

Dermatophytes can be transmitted from human to human (anthropophilic), from animal to human (zoophilic), and from soil to human (geophilic). Depending on the source of the infection, the immunologic response by the host will vary. Zoophilic fungi, for example, will induce an inflammatory reaction, whereas anthropophilic fungi will not. Indolent infections with anthropophilic fungi become chronic and are the most important source for dissemination of these infections.

The invasion of tissue (skin, hair, nails) by dermatophytes varies with the species. Species from the *Microsporum* genus, for example, do not invade nails, and *Epidermophyton floccosum* does not affect hair. These characteristics are helpful in the diagnosis and prognosis of these infections.

Since the therapeutic approach and response of dermatophyte infection is so intricately associated with the clinicoanatomic presentation, their clinical features will be highlighted.

Clinicoanatomic Presentation of Dermatophytoses

Infections of Scalp and Hair. Tinea capitis can be classified into an acute inflammatory type and a chronic indolent type. The acute type, also called kerion, is induced by dermatophytes acquired from animals (*Microsporum canis*) or from the soil (*Microsporum gypseum*). The inflammatory response is characterized by edema, erythema, follicular pustules, and eventual scar formation. The course of the infection is relatively short and self-limited. The chronic type, on the other hand, is more insidious, frequently asymptomatic, and characterized by scales and patchy hair loss. Anthropophilic species (*Microsporum audouini* and *Trichophyton tonsurans*) are the frequent etiologic agents and the infection has a prolonged clinical course.

Infections of the hair are also classified according to the manner in which the fungus invades the hair. Ectothrix defines the location of the spores as being outside of the cuticle, whereas in endothrix infection the spores are within the hair shaft. Endothrix infection is usually produced by anthropophilic species. *T. tonsurans* produces an endothrix infection that will cause the hair to break at the scalp surface, and the hair stubs will appear as black dots (black-dot tinea). Ectothrix infections are produced by *Microsporum* species (*M. audouini, M. canis*) that show a characteristic fluorescence of the hair under Wood's lamp, which can help in the diagnosis of the infection.

Thirty years ago the commonest cause of tinea capitis in the United States was *M. audouini*; the infection was confined to children since a natural host resistance developed during adolescence, and adults were not affected. In the last three decades, however, *T. tonsurans* has become the commonest cause of tinea capitis, and, although commoner among children, adults are also susceptible to the infection. The chronicity and insidiousness of this type of infection as well as the susceptibility of all age groups has created a difficult epidemiologic problem. Early diagnosis and therapy of tinea capitis, therefore, has become of paramount importance, especially in school children.

Dermatophyte infection of the bearded areas, tinea barbae, can also appear in two clinical forms. The commonest form resembles inflammatory tinea capitis with follicular pustules and a kerion-like, suppurative presentation that can eventually scar. *Trichophyton mentagrophytes, Trichophyton verrucosum*, and *M. canis* are the most frequent pathogens, and only the hairy part of the face is involved. The other form can affect any part of the face and resembles dermatophytic infections on nonhairy skin. An advancing papulosquamous border can be identified leaving a trace of pigmentation and dull scaling in the center. *T. rubrum* and *Trichophyton mentagrophytes* are the most frequent causitive agents.

Therapy for all forms of tinea capitis and tinea barbae requires oral antifungal agents; topical therapy is ineffective.

Infections of Nonhairy (Glabrous) Skin (Tinea Corporis). This dermatophytic infection best typifies the term *ringworm* since the lesion starts as a small, expanding, inflammatory ring with a healing center. The border is scaly and erythematous with papules, vesicles, and/or pustules and is pruritic. Depending on the inflammatory reaction elicited by the species, tinea corporis can be self-limited or chronic. Children are more susceptible than adults, although immunosuppressed patients are susceptible to extensive, recalcitrant tinea corporis at any age. All species of dermatophytes are able to produce lesions on glabrous skin, although *T. rubrum* and *T. mentagrophytes* are the commonest offenders. *T. tonsurans* causes tinea capitis in children and is a common agent of tinea corporis in adults who handle children.

Although the inflammatory tinea corporis can resolve spontaneously in a few weeks, treatment is indicated to prevent spreading of the infection to others. The chronic form should be treated early to prevent dissemination. Both forms of tinea corporis require oral antifungal agents (see Tables).

Infection of the Groin (Tinea Cruris). Tinea cruris is characterized by an advancing, serpiginous, papulosquamous border and involves primarily the inner aspects of the thighs. Lesions may extend anteriorly to the pubic region and posteriorly to the perineum and perianal and gluteal regions, but, characteristically, it spares the scrotal sac. Lesions are frequently bilateral and can be associated with intense pruritus.

Tinea cruris occurs predominantly in males probably because of the increased heat and humidity produced by wearing slacks. The infection is established in most cases by contamination from other anatomic regions since most of these patients have concurrent infection of the feet or toenails. *T. rubrum* and *Epidermophyton floccosum* are the commonest dermatophytes affecting this area.

Topical therapy with antifungal agents usually suffices to control tinea cruris, but other infected anatomic areas should be treated concomitantly. In extensive, recalcitrant cases oral antifungal agents might be required (see Tables).

Infections of the Hands and Feet. The feet are infected with dermatophytes more frequently than any other anatomic area. Heat and humidity from occlusive footwear as well as trauma predispose this area to infection, which is probably contracted through contaminated fomites such as floors and shoes. Adults of both sexes are equally susceptible, but tinea pedis is rare among children.

As with other clinicoanatomic forms, tinea pedis may be either acute inflammatory or chronic noninflammatory. The acute inflammatory type is usually produced by *T. mentagrophytes* and is characterized by pruritic vesicles and pustules on the soles and lateral aspects of feet, rarely involving the dorsal aspect. The chronic form elicits no inflammatory response by the host and is characterized by an asymptomatic, scaling of soles in a "sandal" distribution. This type of tinea pedis is usually produced by *T. rubrum* and is frequently associated with involvement of the toenails (onychomycosis). The commonest form of tinea pedis, however, is the one manifested as interdigital maceration, which frequently starts in the fourth interdigital space. Maceration of the space is invariably present. Secondary bacterial infection sometimes complicates the clinical picture, producing a painful, purulent process that can eventuate in cellulitis.

The hands, conversely, are infrequently colonized by dermatophytes. Three clinical forms of hand involvement have been described. The first form is similar to tinea corporis; an expanding, inflammatory, serpiginous border extends along the dorsal aspect of the hand. Frequently unilateral, the infection can involve both hands. The second form affects almost exclusively the palm of one hand as part of a chronic, noninflammatory process that affects both feet with a "moccasin" distribution ("two foot–one hand" syndrome). Nail involvement of both feet and the affected hand is very common. The etiologic agent in this chronic, recalcitrant form of tinea is *T. rubrum*. The third clinical presentation is characterized by pruritic papules and vesicles with desquamation on both palms as a hypersensitivity response to a dermatophytic infection elsewhere, usually on the feet. The lesions on the hands are sterile and disappear once the infection on the feet is eradicated.

Tinea pedis of the toewebs responds to topical antifungal therapy. If secondary bacterial infection is present, appropriate oral antibiotic therapy should also be instituted. Inflammatory tinea pedis can be treated topically, but in severe, symptomatic cases, systemic antifungal agents may be necessary. Chronic tinea pedis with or without palmar involvement requires oral therapy (see Tables).

Infection of the Nails. Tinea unguium and onychomycosis are terms used interchangeably to describe fungal infection of the nails, although tinea unguium refers exclusively to infections by dermatophytes, whereas onychomycosis includes infections by other fungi. Tinea unguium occurs more frequently in the toenails and can be manifested in two forms. The commoner of these is characterized by early yellow discoloration of the distal or lateral part of the nail that eventually produces deformity of the nail by accumulation of subungual keratotic debris. The nail plate becomes opaque and dull and crumbles with minimal trauma. Chronic tinea pedis, usually produced by *T. rubrum*, is a constant companion. The other form of tinea unguium is limited to the nail plate and is referred to as superificial white onychomycosis because a white discoloration is seen in the nail plate with no subungual hyperkeratosis. *T. mentagrophytes* is the causative agent of this form of tinea unguium, and is frequently associated with tinea pedis of the toewebs.

The treatment of tinea unguium requires oral agents, but the success rate is low and recurrences are common. Some success has been reported with topical treatment for the superficial white onychomycosis.

Diagnosis of Dermatophytoses

Diagnosis requires direct microscopic examination of specimens from the affected area. Scales from the skin should be examined with 10 to 20 percent potassium hydroxide after gentle heating to remove debris. Hair and nails must be heated and/or allowed to sit for at least 15 to 20 minutes—or use 40 percent potassium hydroxide for a more complete digestion of keratin. Hairs from scalp or beard should be plucked rather than shaved. Slides should always be reviewed with reduced light and examined under low power to identify hyphae.

Identification of species of dermatophytes cannot be performed by direct microscopic examination and, hence, fungal culture is important to establish the specific etiologic agent. Sabouraud's glucose agar with antibacterial agents are available commercially and allow a colony of dermatophytes to grow in about 3 weeks. The species can be identified by a competent laboratory or mycologist on the basis of morphologic characteristics of the colony. It is important to identify the species since the clinicoanatomical entity, prognosis, and response to therapy will be intimately related to the type of dermatophyte and its relationship to the host.

The use of Wood's lamp is only helpful to identify certain dermatophytes that produce tinea capitis such as *M. audouini* and *M. canis*, which produce a blue-green fluorescence. Dermatophytoses of other anatomic areas will not fluoresce.

Candidiasis

The clinical manifestations of candidiasis are extremely varied, ranging from acute, subacute, and chronic to episodic. Involvement may be localized to mucosal surfaces, mucosae and skin, or skin alone. Except for hair, any part of the integument can be colonized by *C. albicans*. The pathologic processes are also diverse and vary from irritation and infection to chronic and acute suppuration or granulomatous response.

Since *C. albicans* is a normal inhabitant of the gastrointestinal system, the disease represents an opportunistic infection. Some of the factors implicated in establishing this fungus as a pathogen include pregnancy, diabetes mellitus, antibiotic and steroid therapy, cancer, infections, and genetic deficiencies. When candidiasis is localized to the skin, these systemic factors might not be present, and the yeast infection is established secondary to local environmental factors that alter the skin barrier. Heat and humidity, occlusion, and maceration are the most important of these factors.

Clinicoanatomic entities have been established for this infection that assist the practitioner in assessing prognosis and response to therapy. The entities discussed in this chapter will only include those manifestations involving the skin.

Clinicoanatomic Presentation of Candidiasis

Intertriginous Candidiasis. The most common cutaneous manifestation of candidiasis involves the axillae, groin, intermammary folds, intergluteal folds, interdigital spaces, and penis glans. Most of these patients are otherwise healthy. These flexural infections are characterized by bilateral involvement with variable, but symmetrical, extension to the adjacent areas of the skin. The lesions are bright red, with fine desquamation that is rolled at the periphery, and multiple satellite pustules outside the affected area. Candidal balanitis is more commonly seen in uncircumcised men, where the glans is constantly occluded. Interdigital infection can occur between the toes or between the third and fourth fingers (interosio digitalis blastomycetes). In obese patients any extra folds of the skin produced by the panniculus adiposus may also be affected.

Topical therapy with anticandidal or broad-spectrum antifungal agents is effective, but successful treatment requires that the affected areas be dried out.

Chronic Paronychia. *C. albicans* is the commonest cause of chronic paronychia in healthy adults and is associated with frequent immersion of the hands in water. The proximal and lateral folds of the fingernails are readily colonized by *C. albicans*, producing painful, red swelling of the paronychial skin. As a chronic state is established, the nail becomes involved, showing greenish yellow discoloration in the lateral aspects, with striation or waving of the nail plate. Hyperkeratotic debris or crumbling of the nail is not a feature of candidal paronychia as it is of tinea unguium.

Topical therapy is usually effective for paronychia, although relapses are common and treatment is prolonged. Keeping the area dry and avoiding trauma to the nail fold is of paramount importance.

Chronic Mucocutaneous Candidiasis. Chronic mucocutaneous candidiasis (CMC) is the most severe and recalcitrant of all the *C. albicans* infections of the skin because of the inherent immunologic deficiency that allows this fungus to grow unchecked. The same areas of the skin that are involved in the other types of candidiasis are affected, but the lesions are hyperkeratotic, verrucous, and crusted. The nails of the hands and feet are invariably involved, with marked destruction of the nail plate that resembles that of severe tinea unguium or psoriasis. Periorificial skin, such as the oral commissure, is also affected as an extension of the mucosal involvement.

Treatment of CMC is primarily systemic and palliative as long as the cell-mediated immunologic response is impaired. Topical antifungal agents can be used as an adjunctive therapy.

Diagnosis

Direct microscopic examination of scales, pustules, or crusts with potassium hydroxide, 10 to 20 percent concentration, will demonstrate the yeast elements, namely pseudohyphae, budding yeasts, or spores. Culture in Sabouraud's glucose agar should be done to confirm the diagnosis since some of the yeast structures can be confused with the hyphae of dermatophytes and the spores of other yeasts. A mucoid, creamy colony that grows within 10 days is characteristic of *C. albicans*.

GENERAL PRINCIPLES OF ANTIFUNGAL THERAPY

Most superficial fungal infections are treated with topical antifungal agents. Some of these infections, however, are not responsive to topical therapy, and systemic treatment, with or without topical treatment, is indicated. Several factors influence the selection of topical antifungal agents over systemic therapy. The species of fungus, especially in the cases of dermatophytic infections, es-

TABLE 1 Topical Antifungal Agents

	Available Formulations	*OTC**	*Relative Cost†*	*Comments*	*Irritation*
Dermatophytosis					
Benzoic acid–compound ointment (Whitfield's ointment)	Ointment	Yes	0.83	---	Yes
Undecylenic acid	Ointment, powder	Yes	2.51 (0.9 oz)	---	Mild
Tolnaftate	Cream, powder aerosol, solution	Yes	3.05	---	Rare
Candidiasis					
Polyenes:					
Nystatin	Ointment, powder	Yes	6.83	---	No
Amphotericin B	Lotion, ointment	No	8.70	---	No
Tinea versicolor					
Sodium thiosulfate	Lotion	Yes	5.75 (6 oz)	---	Mild
Selenium sulfide 2.5%	Shampoo, lotion	No	4.28 (6 oz)	Adjunctive for tinea capitis	Mild
Dermatophytosis, candidiasis, and tinea versicolor					
Imidazoles					
Miconazole	Cream, lotion	Yes	4.36	---	No
Clotrimazole	Cream, solution	No	4.26	---	No
Econazole	Cream	No	4.05	---	No
Haloprogin	Cream, solution	No	4.91	---	No
Ciclopirox olamine	Cream	No	4.25	---	No

* Cost to pharmacist in U.S. dollars for 15 g of cream unless otherwise noted.
† Over the counter (no prescription required).

tablishes an important host-parasite relationship that can affect the response to therapy. Infections with *T. rubrum*, for example, are more chronic and recalcitrant to therapy. In these cases, prolonged topical therapy and, sometimes, systemic therapy might be required to reduce the incidence of recurrences. On the other hand, species that stimulate an inflammatory response by the host, e.g., *T. mentagrophytes*, will be more responsive to therapy.

The anatomic location of the infection, especially in the case of dermatophytes, is also an important consideration in the choice of topical versus systemic antifungal therapy. Characteristically, fungal infections involving the scalp, body, palms, and face are notoriously resistant to topical therapy alone and almost invariably will require a systemic approach. It should be borne in mind that dermatophytic infections are classified by anatomic areas since one species can produce different infections, depending on the anatomic location, and, conversely, many species can produce similar morphologic changes in the same anatomic area.

The severity and extent of infection is also another factor in the selection of therapy. In tinea versicolor, for example, the amount of skin surface involved will determine the use of a cream versus a lotion. Systemic therapy will be the treatment of choice in severe and extensive cases of dermatophytoses and candidal infections.

Other factors that have a bearing on therapy are age, sex, habitus, occupation, and general health. The two most important environmental variables that optimize fungal growth, however, are heat and humidity.

Table 1 provides a partial list of topical antifungal agents with indications, formulations, and cost for each product.

Tinea Versicolor

The treatment for tinea versicolor should be topical, and, until a safe oral antifungal agent is developed, the use of oral antifungal agents (e.g., ketoconazole) is not recommended. Although most of the old remedies with keratolytic activity and the newer broad-spectrum agents can be used, the present standard treatment is selenium sulfide 2.5% shampoo or lotion or zinc pyrithione shampoo. My preference is selenium sulfide 2.5% because, in my experience, longer remissions are obtained. With the aid of Wood's lamp, the areas of pigmentary changes and/or fluorescence can be identified so that all of the affected areas can be treated. Otherwise, the medication should be applied to the glabrous skin surface, avoiding the face and intertriginous areas, but including the forearms and thighs. Two methods of application have been described: weekly overnight application or 30- to 45-minute daily applications for 2 weeks. I prefer the second method because irritation is reduced. Relapse rates are about 50 percent after one year and, therefore, retreatment at periodic intervals is recommended. The use of imidazole creams is advised for the face and intertriginous areas to prevent irritation.

Dermatophytic Infection

Selection of Therapeutic Agents

The newer, broad-spectrum antifungal agents, such as imidazoles and haloprogin, have replaced some of the traditional remedies, such as benzoic acid-compound ointment (Whitfield's ointment), undecylenic acid ointment, and even tolnaftate. This is due in part to the fact that the broad-spectrum antifungal agents are effective for three types of superficial mycoses, and it is, therefore, not necessary to establish a diagnosis of the specific group before instituting therapy.

The new agents are not irritating and are cosmetically more acceptable than the traditional remedies. Interestingly, however, controlled studies show that some of the established medications, such as undecylenic acid, Whitfield's ointment, and, more recently, tolnaftate, fared very well when compared with the newer broad-spectrum antifungal agents. Even when these new broad-spectrum antifungal agents are compared, there is no evidence that one is more effective than another. The consensus indicates, however, that miconazole or clotrimazole are preferred over haloprogin and tolnaftate. Clotrimazole is my first choice, followed by miconazole, tolnaftate, and haloprogin.

In addition to clotrimazole and miconazole, a new imidazole—econazole—has recently become available in the United States. It appears to be equal in effectiveness and safety to the previous imidazole preparations. I cannot pass clinical judgement on this new product at this time, but since the price is competitive (see Table 1), its use might increase in the future.

Ciclopirox olamine is a hydroxypyridone with in vitro activity against a wide variety of fungi, yeasts, and bacteria. Its effectiveness and safety seem comparable with those of the imidazoles.

The dilemma for the practitioner is not so much what type of topical agent to use, but when and where and for how long. Systemic therapy is required to eradicate certain infections on glabrous skin as well as all dermatophytic infections of the hair and nails. Although no controlled data are available, empiric observations suggest that the duration of therapy is variable and dependent not only on the species of the fungus and anatomic area involved, but on other factors as well.

Relapse or reinfection still remains the most important problem in the therapy of dermatophytic infection. The cause of this phenomenon has not been elucidated, but it is probably dependent on the host-parasite relationship. The emergence of resistant strains of dermatophytes during treatment with imidazoles or other topical antifungal agents has never been reported.

Treatment Based on Clinicoanatomic Infection

Topical therapy alone can eradicate lesions from glabrous skin. Widespread and chronic infections, however, particularly those caused by *T. rubrum* as well as the more severe types of granulomatous lesions produced by *T. verrucosum* and other fungi of animal origin, will require systemic therapy.

Systemic treatment, as mentioned previously, is essential for infections of nails and hair. Chronic, indolent dermatophytic infections tend to be extensive and more difficult to eradicate because of the host immune response to the pathogen. Conversely, intense inflammatory dermatophytic infections are limited to small areas of the skin and can either remit spontaneously or respond to antifungal agents.

The duration of topical antifungal therapy should continue until no clinical evidence of acute or chronic changes is evident; this observation should be confirmed by negative direct examination and/or culture. When laboratory facilities are not available, the treatment should continue

TABLE 2 Recommended Therapy for Dermatophytic Fungal Infections

Clinico-Anatomic Type	*Topical**	*Oral*	*Maintenance†*	*Remarks*
Tinea pedis				
Web space	4 weeks	No	Yes, topical	Topical maintenance therapy; can be irritating
Vesicular	4 weeks	Yes	No	---
Diffuse-scaly	4 weeks	Yes	Yes, topical	Keratolytics might be helpful if scales are thick‡
Tinea cruris	4 weeks	Extensive cases only	Yes, topical	Topical maintenance therapy might irritate scrotal skin
Tinea corporis				
Acute, inflammatory	3 weeks	Extensive cases only	No	---
Extensive, chronic, scaly	No	Yes	Yes, topical	---
Tinea manum	No	Yes	No	Keratolytics might be helpful if scales are too thick‡
Tinea facei	No	Yes	No	---
Tinea capitis	No	Yes	No	Selenium sulfide might reduce infectivity
Tinea barbae	No	Yes	No	---
Onychomycosis	No	Yes	No	---
Majocchi's granuloma	No	Yes	No	---

* Clotrimazole, miconazole, econazole, ciclopirox, or haloprogin (in order of preference).
† Undecylenic acid ointment or powder, tolnaftate cream or powder.
‡ Whitfield's ointment.

for 2 weeks after all clinical evidence of infection has disappeared. In indolent, chronic infection of the feet and recurrent infection of the groin, maintenance therapy with less expensive medications, e.g., undecylenic acid or tolnaftate, is recommended. Table 2 provides guidelines for duration of therapy according to the clinicoanatomic area. Recently, the adjunctive use of selenium sulfide shampoo or lotion 2.5% twice a week has been recommended to reduce the infectivity in children with tinea capitis produced by *T. tonsurans*.

Candidiasis

Selection of Therapeutic Agents

As with dermatophytoses, superficial candidiasis presents a spectrum of clinical entities that require individualized treatment according to anatomic location and host-parasite interaction. Topical therapy specific for candidiasis includes four groups of medications: the polyene antibiotics (including nystatin and amphotericin B), the imidazole group (clotrimazole, miconazole, and econazole), haloprogin, and, more recently, ciclopirox olamine. The polyene group has a narrow spectrum of activity, and both medications seem to be equally effective against *C. albicans*. The other three groups are broad-spectrum antifungal agents that are effective against all superficial mycoses as well as bacteria. Since, not infrequently, gram-negative bacteria act as copathogens in superficial candidiasis, the broad-spectrum agents are preferred to the polyenes. Controlled studies, however, have not shown any advantage of haloprogin and the imidazoles over nystatin in the treatment of candidiasis. It also appears that there is no significant difference in effectiveness among the different imidazoles. I prefer the imidazoles over nystatin to treat candidiasis because they prevent bacterial colonization of macerated areas. Similarly, the imidazoles are less expensive than haloprogin. As with the dermatophytes, there is no evidence of natural resistance to any of these drugs by *C. albicans*.

Drying agents such as gentian violet, Castellani's paint, and aluminum chloride (20%) have limited application because of their irritant effect, discoloration of the skin, and low efficiency in eradicating *C. albicans*. Taking those limitations into consideration, I prefer Castellani's paint because of its superior drying capacity. The same drawbacks apply to the quinolines—such as iodochlorhydroxyquin—except that the irritant effect is minimal.

Treatment Based on Clinicoanatomic Infection

Intertriginous Areas. The naturally occluded areas such as perineum, interdigital spaces of the toes and third interdigital space of the hands, the axillae, and the inframammary regions are more susceptible to development of candidiasis. The basic prerequisite for yeast overgrowth, namely humidity and maceration, should be controlled by drying out these surfaces with adequate ventilation or the use of a non-starch-containing, absorbent powder. The application of one of the polyene or imidazole group of medications in a cream formulation twice a day for 2 to 3 weeks is usually adequate. My choice is miconazole cream twice a day for 3 weeks. Talcum powder can be used prophylactically after a bath to prevent recurrences, especially during hot and humid weather. Hygiene is important, especially in cases of perineal infections. If relapses are frequent, a course of oral treatment with polyenes (nystatin) or an imidazole (ketoconazole) might be advisable to reduce overgrowth of *C. albicans* in the gut. Since oral nystatin is safer than ketoconazole, I prefer the former to treat these cases.

Chronic Paronychia. Chronic paronychia as a manifestation of candidiasis is normally treated with topical medications, in contrast to tinea unguium where topical therapy is ineffective. It is a therapeutic challenge because of the inability of the patient to avoid exposure to humidity and trauma and because of the relative inaccessibility of the nail fold to receive an adequate concentration of the antifungal medication. The use of thymol, 4 to 5%, in chloroform or alcohol, or the immersion of the affected finger in alcohol for several minutes are helpful measures to reduce the moisture content of the affected area. Liquid preparations of polyene or imidazole will enhance penetration of the antifungal agent by capillary diffusion into the nail fold. This medication, preceded by the drying agent, should be applied three times a day for 2 months. Compliance, therefore, is poor and relapses, frequent. The use of the oral imidazole, ketoconazole, should be limited to severe cases with multiple nail involvement because of possible adverse effects.

Chronic Mucocutaneous Candidiasis. CMS presents another therapeutic challenge since immunologic unresponsiveness on the part of the host is invariably present. Topical therapy is usually ineffective, and this syndrome is probably the best indication for the use of ketoconazole orally. Oral nystatin is not effective because it has only a local effect in reducing colonization of the gut, but it does not have a systemic effect to prevent fungemia in these patients.

Oral Treatment of Dermatomycoses

Oral therapy for the dermatomycoses is confined to the use of griseofulvin and ketoconazole. Griseofulvin is effective only for dermatophytes, whereas the broad antifungal spectrum of ketoconazole serves to treat all dermatomycoses. Because of its adverse effects, however, ketoconazole should not be used to treat tinea versicolor or dermatophytoses that are responsive to griseofulvin. Its use, therefore, should be confined to CMC and severe cases of dermatophytoses that are resistant to griseofulvin. It should be stressed that ketoconazole has not been approved for use in tinea versicolor or der-

TABLE 3 Oral Therapy for Dermatomycoses

	Dose/Day	*Duration (months)*	*Response*
Griseofulvin*			
Dermatomycoses			
Tinea capitis	500 mg	2	Good
Tinea barbae	250 mg	2	Good
Tinea corporis	250 mg	1	Good
Tinea pedis (moccasin type)	500 mg	3	Variable
Tinea unguium			
Fingernails	250 mg	8	Good
Toenails	500 mg	12	Poor
Ketoconazole†			
Mucocutaneous candidiasis	200 mg (single dose)	Periodic to indefinite	Palliative: good Cure: poor
Dermatophytoses‡			
Tinea unguium			
Fingernails	200 mg	8	Good
Toenails	200 mg	12	Poor
Tinea pedis (moccasin type)	200 mg	3	Good

* 250 mg tablet, ultramicrosize.
† 200 mg tablet.
‡ Griseofulvin-resistant.

matophytoses. Table 3 provides guidelines for oral therapy for dermatomycoses with griseofulvin and ketoconazole.

Dermatophytoses that require oral therapy include tinea unguium, chronic noninflammatory tinea pedis (moccasin type) with or without palmar involvement, tinea capitis and barbae, and extensive tinea corporis. In general any extensive, chronic, noninflammatory tinea could be amenable to oral therapy. Although 80 percent of cases with tinea unguium of the fingernails respond to oral therapy (6 to 9 months), the success rate of this drug for infections of the toenails rarely warrants its use. Less than 20 percent of cases of tinea unguium of toenail will clear with continuous treatment for more than a year. The moc-

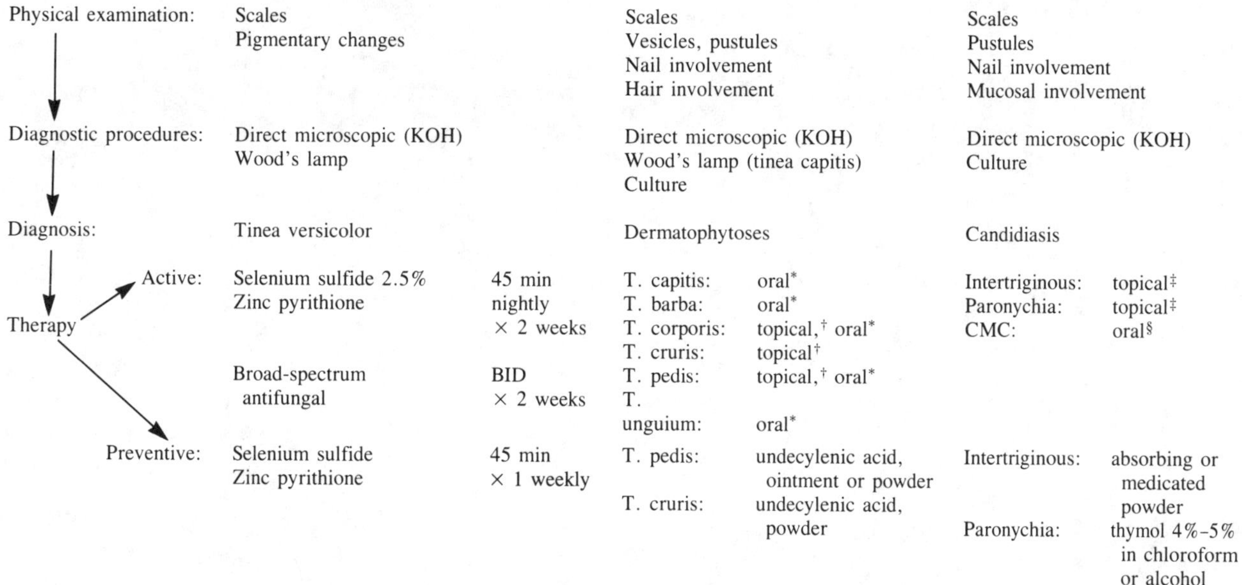

Physical examination:
Scales
Pigmentary changes
Scales
Vesicles, pustules
Nail involvement
Hair involvement
Scales
Pustules
Nail involvement
Mucosal involvement
Diagnostic procedures:
Direct microscopic (KOH)
Wood's lamp
Direct microscopic (KOH)
Wood's lamp (tinea capitis)
Culture
Direct microscopic (KOH)
Culture
Diagnosis:
Tinea versicolor
Dermatophytoses
Candidiasis
Therapy
Active:
Selenium sulfide 2.5%
Zinc pyrithione
45 min
nightly
× 2 weeks
Broad-spectrum
antifungal
BID
× 2 weeks
T. capitis: oral*
T. barba: oral*
T. corporis: topical,† oral*
T. cruris: topical†
T. pedis: topical,† oral*
T. unguium: oral*
Intertriginous: topical‡
Paronychia: topical‡
CMC: oral§
Preventive:
Selenium sulfide
Zinc pyrithione
45 min
× 1 weekly
T. pedis: undecylenic acid, ointment or powder
T. cruris: undecylenic acid, powder
Intertriginous: absorbing or medicated powder
Paronychia: thymol 4%-5% in chloroform or alcohol

* Oral therapy: griseofulvin (see Table 3 for dose and duration).
† Topical therapy: clotrimazole, miconazole, econazole, ciclopirox, haloprogin, tolnaftate.
‡ Clotrimazole, micanazole, econazole, ciclopirox, nystatin, haloprogin.
§ Ketoconazole (see Table 3 for dose and duration).

Figure 1 Evaluation and management of patients infected with dermatomycoses.

casin type of tinea pedis and the two foot–one hand tinea are also recalcitrant to therapy and usually require 3 months of continuous treatment.

Griseofulvin

The absorption of this drug from the gut depends on the size of the particle. The ultramicrosize griseofulvin will be absorbed more predictably and can be taken with or between meals. The drug is delivered to the skin by deposition in keratin-producing epidermal cells of skin, hair, and nails, and via sweat secretions.

Griseofulvin should not be given to patients with acute,intermittent or variegate porphyria or hepatocellular failure. Compensatory increases in the dose of oral anticoagulants, such as Coumadin, should be instituted since griseofulvin decreases their anticoagulant effect. Barbiturates compete with the absorption of griseofulvin and should not be used concomitantly. Common side effects are headaches and gastrointestinal distress, which are dose dependent. Hypersensitivity and photosensitivity reactions are rare. Except for tinea unguium, all infections with dermatophytes will clear with 1 to 3 months of therapy in doses of 250 to 500 mg daily of ultramicrosize griseofulvin (see Table 3). Therapy should continue until there is evidence of clinical and microbiologic cure. Since prolonged, high doses of griseofulvin produce frequent headaches, I instruct the patient to take 500 mg daily for 1 week and continue with 250 mg daily. Clinical and mycologic evaluations are performed on a monthly basis until cure is obtained.

Ketoconazole

This oral, water-soluble, lipophilic imidazole interferes with ergosterol synthesis and disrupts the cell membrane of fungi. It should be taken after a meal since its absorption is enhanced by an acid stomach. Its broad antifungal spectrum and its oral administration anticipated that this drug was going to be the choice for most mycoses. Because of related adverse effects, however, enthusiasm to treat the dermatophytoses, has been tempered. Furthermore, except for the occasional case of griseofulvin-resistant dermatophytoses, ketoconazole does not seem to offer therapeutic benefit over griseofulvin. The best indication for ketoconazole is CMS as well as several systemic mycoses. The drug is supplied as 200 mg tablets, and the usual dose is 1 tablet daily. Although adverse reactions are uncommon, its effect on the liver and endocrine glands precludes its use in most of the dermatomycoses. Abnormal hepatic function tests, hepatitis, and several cases of hepatic necrosis have been reported. Gynecomastia as a result of inhibition of sterol synthesis has also been reported and is dose dependent. A single, daily dose, rather than divided doses, is recommended to prevent prolonged inhibition of adrenal and testicular function in humans.

NOSOCOMIAL INFECTIONS

CATHETER-ASSOCIATED URINARY TRACT INFECTION

JOHN W. WARREN, M.D.

Much of the clinical and research attention directed at catheter-associated bacteriuria has been directed toward the catheter as a means of entry for organisms into the urinary tract. The catheter may, however, play other roles in the development and maintenance of bacteriuria. The catheter and the intravesical balloon may, through mechanical and/or chemical factors, cause erosion and inflammation of the urethral and bladder mucosa. Additionally, the presence of the catheter may cause bacterial adherence properties of uroepithelial cells to change. Once bacteriuria has developed, the catheter acts as a foreign body at the site of infection, thus diminishing the clearance of the infecting organisms. The lumen of the catheter, via the accumulation of adherent organisms and of encrustations formed of other urinary constituents, may become a microenvironment for these organisms, thus allowing them a continuous access to the urinary tract itself. Furthermore, these encrustations may cause a partial or complete obstruction of urine flow, converting an asymptomatic bacteriuria into a symptomatic one and, perhaps, into bacteremia. Finally, the catheter may obstruct periurethral structures with complications of prostatic and epididymal infections.

Although there are many indications for placement of a tube into the urinary bladder to drain urine, the four main indications are (*1*) hemodynamic monitoring of acutely ill patients; (*2*) pelvic or abdominal surgery; (*3*) bladder outlet obstruction; and (*4*) urinary incontinence. The first two, output measurement and pelvic or abdominal surgery, almost always involve short-term use. The third, bladder outlet obstruction, usually requires transient use if the obstruction can be corrected. The fourth, the management of incontinence, may also be a temporary indication, e.g., for the patient undergoing anesthesia. These temporary indications appear to be commonest for patients in acute care hospitals where the mean and median duration of catheterization is 2 to 4 days. About 10 percent of patients are catheterized during their hospital stay and 10 to 20 percent of catheterized patients become bacteriuric. Although only 1 to 2 percent of these bacteriuric catheterized patients develop bacteremia, the large number of catheterized patients means that the instrumented urinary tract is the most frequent source of gram-negative rod bacteremia in hospitalized patients.

Because the risk of bacteriuria is 5 to 10 percent per day once a urethral catheter is in place, the majority of patients with a catheter in place for 30 days or more are bacteriuric, usually with several organisms. Although difficult to document through published accounts, the main indications for long-term urinary catheterization (30 days or more) are (*1*) bladder outlet obstruction that cannot be corrected by surgery and (*2*) incontinence of urine. The latter is probably the commoner indication. These patients, in whom catheters may be in place for months and years, generally reside in chronic care facilities such as nursing homes.

Evidence is developing that a subtle but important distinction should be made between management techniques for short-term and long-term catheters. The goal of medical management of the patient with a short-term catheter is to postpone the development of bacteriuria. The long-term catheterized patient is almost always bacteriuric, and the goal of medical care might be best termed the prevention of complications of bacteriuria.

DIAGNOSIS OF INFECTION

Many studies of catheter-associated urinary tract infections have required a minimum of 100,000 colony forming units (CFU) per milliliter of urine aspirated from the distal catheter to establish a diagnosis. However, some investigators have arbitrarily selected lower concentrations. Recent studies have suggested that the majority of organisms initially present in catheter urine in concentrations of even 100 CFU per milliliter or less will, over succeeding days, reach concentrations of at least 100,000 CFU per milliliter. This suggests, at least for patients catheterized for only several days, that organisms present even in small numbers in catheter urine represent actual residence in the urine and not contamination. This understanding may or may not have impact upon therapeutic decisions, but is of epidemiologic assistance in dating the incidence of bacteriuric episodes.

But does the presence of an organism in urine aspirated from the distal catheter mean that the organism is present in the bladder as well? Recent studies have found that the majority of bacterial species isolated from catheter urine were also isolated from bladder urine, obtained either by suprapubic aspiration or by removal of the old catheter and insertion of a new one. However, in some patients, a bacterial species was found in catheter urine but not in bladder urine, and in other patients, catheter urine contained the same species of bacteria, but at higher concentrations, than bladder urine. These findings suggest that the most accurate practical means of assessing the presence of bacteria in bladder urine of a catheterized patient is to culture urine draining from a newly replaced catheter. Otherwise, an assessment of isolates obtained from urine aspirated through an indwelling catheter, particularly one in place for a long period, should be viewed only as an approximation of the microbiologic status of bladder urine.

SHORT-TERM CATHETERIZATION

Prevention

Because of the frequency of catheter use and of associated bacteriuria, many efforts have been directed towards prevention or, more accurately, posponement of bacteriuria. By far the most important modification of the venerable catheter has been the closed system, one in which the catheter and collecting tube empty into a receptacle in such a way that urine is always contained within a lumen and protected from the possibly contaminated environment. Although no well-designed controlled trial comparing open with closed catheter systems has been reported, the closed system appears to be associated with a much lower incidence of bacteriuria and has become the standard of care.

Nevertheless, bacteriuria remains the most frequent complication of the use of even closed-system urethral catheters. The risk of bacteriuria is directly associated with female gender, age, duration of catheterization, and presence of periurethral colonization with gram-negative bacteria or enterococci. There are three possible routes of entry for bacteria into the catheter lumen and/or bladder. One route is that by which the catheter acts as a foreign body traversing the urethra from its external orifice to the interior of the bladder. Organisms in the periurethral area may move along the mucous sheath between the catheter's exterior surface and the urethral mucosa and enter the bladder directly. If a closed catheter system is used and maintained well, this route may be the commonest. Other means of bacterial entry involve breaking the integrity of the closed catheter system, either at the disconnectable junction between the catheter and the collection tube or by contamination of the collection bag.

Understanding these origins of catheter-associated bacteriuria has led to several modifications of the closed catheter system in an attempt to prevent or postpone bacteriuria. Only two types of modification appear to be useful. The first is simply a strict adherence to maintaining a closed catheter system, for instance, by the use of a catheter-collection tube junction, which is difficult or impossible to disconnect. The other practice resulting in a lower incidence of bacteriuria has been the use of systemic antibiotics. However, antimicrobial use is associated only with postponement, and the eventual bacteriuria is commonly caused by organisms resistant to the antibiotic used.

Most of the modifications that have been attempted, but that have not reliably reduced the incidence of bacteriuria, include localized use of antiseptics or antimicrobial agents. These ineffective uses of antibacterial substances have included applications to the periurethral area, lubrication for the catheter, impregnation or coating of the catheter, irrigation continuously or periodically of the catheter, and instillation into the collection bag.

Undoubtedly the most effective means of preventing catheter-associated bacteriuria is by preventing the use of the catheter itself. Careful assessment of the patient's needs may reveal that the catheter may not be necessary at all or, if deemed so, for only a short duration. Furthermore, alternatives to indwelling urethral catheters that are dictated by the indications for catheterization are available. For patients with bladder outlet obstruction, intermittent catheterization is a possible alternative. For patients in whom urinary retention is not a problem, condom catheters in males and incontinence clothing in females and males may be used. Suprapubic catheters have been used in gynecologic, urologic, and other types of pelvic or abdominal surgery. None of these alternatives have been well studied in prospective, randomized, controlled trials.

Treatment

Once a urethral catheter is in place, the techniques noted above are only means by which catheter-associated bacteriuria can be postponed. Consequently, given the 5 to 10 percent daily incidence of bacteriuria, some patients catheterized for even short periods will become bacteriuric. I have rarely been compelled to treat patients as long as they remain catheterized and asymptomatic. However, because a recent study has reported excess mortality related to catheter-associated bacteriuria which could not be explained by other confounding factors this posture may have to be modified as further data are developed. Until that time, I suggest that patients with catheter-associated bacteriuria, while asymptomatic and still catheterized, not be treated with antibiotics. However, if the patient becomes symptomatic with fever and/or signs of bacteremia, I would treat as outlined in the chapter on bacteremia, even while the patient has a catheter still in place. Similarly, for the occasional patient with lower abdominal pain or other symptoms suggestive of symptomatic lower urinary tract infection, I recommend treatment with an oral antibiotic active in vitro against the bacteriuric organisms and in doses as outlined in the chapter on urinary tract infections.

I would not, however, treat the asymptomatic catheterized bacteriuric patient. If one would not treat such an infection even if identified, then why identify it? In other words, why culture the urine of patients with indwelling catheters if no action is to be taken on the basis of the results? Although this is a reasonable course for many patients, I believe a urine culture should be performed in several instances. The first is the case of the patient who is to undergo urologic surgery. Because such surgery is associated with a risk of bacteremia with the urinary tract as the source, I believe that most bacteriuric patients should be treated for the bacteriuria before and during the procedure. Second, I recommend once or twice a week surveillance urine cultures of catheterized patients in intensive care units. This will allow the early identification and possible control of an antibiotic-resistant organism that could be transmitted to other patients. Third, I recommend the culture of catheter urine of all patients immediately prior to removal of the catheter. If this culture has organisms in any concentration, I recommend a follow-up urine culture of the now noncatheterized patient within the next week. Although some patients will clear their bacteriuria once the catheter is removed, others will not. I recommend treatment of the latter group if follow-up cultures reveal bacteriuria.

LONG-TERM CATHETERIZATION

The indications for long-term catheterization (30 days or more) are usually either chronic urinary incontinence or urinary retention that is not correctable by surgery. Patients with these problems commonly reside in nursing homes or other chronic care facilities, and relatively little attention has been directed towards this type of associated bacteriuria. Because most long-term catheters in use are closed drainage systems like those used in acute care hospitals, the assumption has been made that many aspects of epidemiology, transmission, and pathogenesis of catheter-associated urinary tract infections are similar to those in the patient with the better-studied short-term catheter. However, two differences are quite clear. The first is that the types of organisms causing bacteriuria in long-term catheterized patients include unfamiliar uropathogens such as *Providencia stuartii, Providencia rettgeri, Morganella morganii*, as well as the better known *Escherichia coli, Proteus mirabilis, Pseudomonas aeruginosa*, and enterococcus. The second is that complications in addition to fever, acute pyelonephritis, and bacteremia occur. These include local periurinary infections such as urethritis, periurethral abscess, epididymitis, prostatitis, prostatic abscess, perivesical abscess, and perinephric abscess as well as complications of a more chronic nature such as urinary tract stones, vesicoureteral reflux, chronic tubulointerstitial nephritis, and renal failure. Much of this information is derived from studies of patients with spinal injuries. Whether one can extrapolate to the less well-studied but larger population of aged long-term catheterized patients is unclear.

Because preventive techniques only postpone but do not actually prevent bacteriuria, virtually all patients catheterized for long periods of time are bacteriuric. Indeed, most such patients have a polymicrobial bacteriuria with a variety of aerobic gram-negative rods and gram-positive cocci. Consequently, in addition to establishing and maintaining appropriate catheter hygiene in the care of these patients, the medical community should devote attention towards preventing the complications of the omnipresent and usually polymicrobial bacteriuria.

However, guidelines for the management of catheterized patients with bacteriuria have not been well developed. Antibiotics active in vitro against the organism(s) present can be expected to eradicate three-fourths of these organisms. However, reinfection commonly occurs, often with organisms resistant to the antibiotics used.

Methenamine preparations have been widely used in chronically catheterized patients, but are ineffective. This conclusion is based not only upon clinical studies but also upon the understanding that methenamine must be hydrolyzed to formaldehyde in order to be effective. At least 60 minutes of exposure to an acidic urine is necessary for the accumulation of a formaldehyde concentration high enough to inhibit bacterial growth. Urine constantly draining through an unobstructed catheter does not accumulate in the bladder for a sufficiently long period to allow an adequate concentration of formaldehyde to form. Nevertheless, several studies have indicated that although bacteriuria per se was not affected, catheterized patients receiving methenamine tended to have lower incidences of symptomatic urinary tract infections, perhaps associated with lower incidences of catheter obstructions. This intriguing finding may not be due to antimicrobial activity of methanamine, but, rather, to a biochemical alteration of salt solubility in the urine.

Another practice that may prevent catheter obstruction and the subsequent development of symptomatic urinary tract infection is periodic irrigation of the catheter. However, because such irrigation jeopardizes the closed nature of the present catheter systems, this procedure should not be practiced until appropriate trials are performed.

Perhaps even more for patients with indications for long-term urine drainage assistance, alternatives to urethral catheters should be sought. The incontinent patient can be managed with condom catheters or diapers. The probable advantage in the lower incidence of bacteriuria and its complication must be balanced against greater nursing effort and potential for skin breakdown. For the patient with urinary retention, suprapubic or intermittent methods of catheterization are available. These alternatives to long-term catheterization require appropriate controlled trials to evaluate acute and chronic complications, mortality, patient comfort, nursing acceptance, and medical cost.

INTRAVENOUS CATHETER-ASSOCIATED INFECTION

DAVID R. SNYDMAN, M.D

Infections associated with intravenous catheters occur in approximately 1 percent of hospitalized patients. Catheter-related infections may result in cellulitis, wound infection at the intravenous site, suppurative thrombophlebitis, and bacteremia. Every vascular catheter carries a risk of bacteremia. The risk of infection is influenced by many factors, including the patient's susceptibility (burned and immunocompromised patients carrying the highest risk), site of placement of the catheter (use of the cutdown or lower limb carrying the highest risk), the use of the catheter for total parenteral nutrition or central venous pressure determination, and, most important, the duration of catheterization. The risk of local infection at the catheter entrance site increases from 1 percent at 24 hours after placement to about 5 percent if the catheter is left in place for 4 days. Risk of bacteremia from a catheter infection increases from 0.1 percent at 24 hours after placement to 2 percent at 4 days. Risk of infection appears to be lowest in patients who have steel needles, but this lower risk may be attributable to a shorter duration of catheterization rather than any inherent safety of the steel needle.

The insertion of the catheter in a blood vessel results in a fibrin sheath, which envelops the catheter in the first 24 to 48 hours. Since normal skin defense mechanisms are bypassed, organisms from the skin may migrate down the fibrin sheath and gain access to the vein itself. Thrombogenicity may play a role in the development of infection. The source of bacteria in catheter-related infections is most commonly the patient's own skin flora. Occasionally, the flora from the hands of personnel inserting the catheter or from contaminated disinfectants may contaminate the wound.

As one might expect, *S. aureus* and *S. epidermidis* are the commonest pathogens implicated in intravenous catheter-associated infections. Aerobic gram-negative rods and *Candida* are also being recognized more frequently.

DIAGNOSIS

In catheter-related infections, the affected area will usually have erythema and tenderness. The vein itself may be swollen or thrombosed. However, all inflammation about the vein may not necessarily be caused by infection. Chemical irritation from the intravenous solution, the tape, or local antibiotic ointments may result in local inflammation. The diagnosis of intravenous catheter-associated infection requires cultural confirmation, preferably using the semiquantitative methods described below.

Although most laboratories still culture a vascular catheter qualitatively by incubating the catheter tip in liquid medium, semiquantitative culture of the surface of that part of the catheter that traverses the skin-wound interface is the most sensitive and specific method to distinguish true infection from colonization. The skin around the catheter entrance site should be cleaned with an alcohol wipe and allowed to dry before catheter removal. For short catheters, the entire segment can be removed. For longer catheters, a 5- to 7-cm section of the intracutaneous segment should be cultured as well as the tip. Using sterile technique, the laboratory should transfer the segment to a standard blood-agar plate, where the segment should be rolled back and forth four times. Multiple studies from several institutions have shown that growth of more than 15 colonies on a culture plate suggests infection rather than simple colonization. Most catheter-related bacteremias will be associated with several hundred or more colonies cultured from the catheter.

If pus can be expressed from the wound, it should be gram-stained and cultured separately. If an intravenous-site infection is suspected, but pus is not evident, the vein may be compressed at a site proximal to the insertion site in order to express purulence that may be present around a thrombus; pressure should be applied by milking the vein toward the insertion site. If a palpable "cord" is present, but pus is not evident, it may be useful to insert a large-gauge syringe and aspirate the area. If the aspiration is "dry" we have occasionally found it useful to inject nonbacteriostatic saline and then reaspirate the material for culture.

THERAPY

The first goal for therapy of intravenous catheter-related infections is the removal of the catheter itself (Fig. 1). If mild local phlebitis is all that is present, removal of the catheter and administration of oral antibiotics may be all that is necessary for therapy. If the patient does not have sepsis with rigors, high fever, and/or hypotension, but has severe local phlebitis with low-grade fever, I usually choose a cephalosporin, such as cefazolin, that has good activity against *Staphylococcus aureus* and *Staphylococcus epidermidis*. An appropriate dose would be 1 g intravenously every 8 hours in patients with normal renal function. In the cephalosporin-allergic patient or in a hospital where methicillin resistance is a nosocomial problem, vancomycin, 500 mg intravenously every 6 hours, would be an appropriate alternative. If purulent material is present, Gram stain of the material should guide the therapy.

Generally, removal of the catheter and administration of intravenous antibiotics over 3 to 5 days should suffice in the majority of cases. If the patient has persistent symptoms of fever or persistent bacteremia while on therapy, suppurative phlebitis should be considered (see special considerations below).

In patients with hypotension, where the catheter may be the source of sepsis, I would cover more broadly with a combination of either cefazolin or vancomycin, in the dosages noted earlier, along with gentamicin, 2 mg per kilogram loading dose, then 1.5 mg per kilogram intravenously every 8 hours.

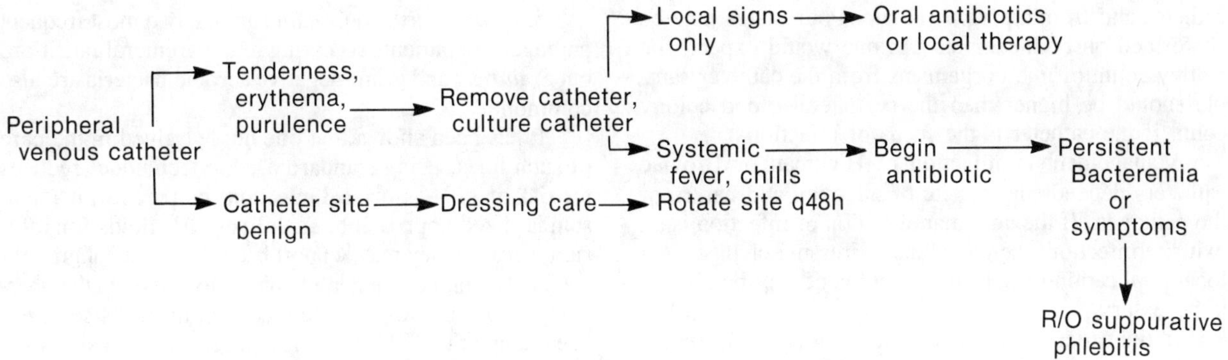

Figure 1 Management of peripheral venous catheter.

PREVENTION

The single most important preventive measure is routine replacement at a different site of all intravenous catheters at 48 to 72 hours. Other guidelines to prevent catheter-associated infection include handwashing by personnel prior to insertion, preparation of the intravenous site with an antiseptic—1 to 2 percent tincture of iodine (chlorhexidine, iodophors, or 70 percent alcohol are acceptable alternatives)–prior to insertion, and use of the upper extremity for catheter insertion. A sterile dressing, not tape, should be used to cover the insertion site, and the catheter should be secured at the entrance site. The insertion date should be recorded in an easily accessible place.

Antibiotic ointment applied to the insertion site will decrease the local infection risk, but may be unnecessary for peripheral catheters that are changed routinely every 48 to 72 hours. Use of the newer nonocclusive dressings has not been shown to reduce the rate of phlebitis or local infection; furthermore, several studies have shown increased bacterial colonization rates at catheter insertion sites. Central catheters and cutdowns differ from peripheral catheters in that they should be inserted under sterile conditions (gloves and drapes) using aseptic technique. Antibiotic ointment applied locally to the insertion site is required for these types of catheters and clearly reduces the infection risk. Manipulations of the system, such as flushing, should be avoided.

SUPPURATIVE PHLEBITIS

This condition represents a more extreme form of catheter-related infection in which the vein becomes an abscess seeding the bloodstream with microorganisms. Burned patients are the group in which this entity is most frequently encountered, but this condition may occur as a complication of any intravenous catheter insertion or of intravenous drug abuse. Suppurative phlebitis may be insidious in onset with little or no inflammation about the infected vein. Local signs may be slight. Persistent bacteremia in the face of adequate antibiotic therapy or septic pulmonary emboli may be the only clue that the vein is involved.

S. aureus is still the commonest pathogen causing suppurative phlebitis due to an intravenous catheter. Aerobic gram-negative organisms or *Candida* appear to be commoner among thermally injured patients. Diagnosis rests on a strong clinical suspicion. Aspiration of pus from the affected vein is diagnostic. Treatment usually requires ligation and excision of the affected vein along with antibiotic therapy. In the patient for whom surgery cannot be performed, we have been able to treat suppurative phlebitis with heparin and appropriate antibiotics.

BROVIAC AND HICKMAN CATHETERS

These catheters are silasic catheters designed for long-term use. They are surgically inserted, tunnelled, and anchored with a Dacron cuff. Their use has eased the management of bone marrow recipients and facilitated the use of home chemotherapy, home intravenous antibiotics, and home parenteral nutrition in a variety of patients. The risk of infection with a Broviac or Hickman catheter is substantial, with a rate of approximately one infection per 100 patient-catheter days of use. The patient may develop infection at the exit site, within the subcutaneous tunnel, or in the deep veins with suppurative phlebitis. Bacteremia may be the only manifestation of infection.

The most frequent pathogens are *S. epidermidis* and *S. aureus*; however infection with gram-negative rods, *Candida*, and corynebacteria have been reported.

In the absence of local signs such as erythema or pus at the exit site, recognition of Hickman-line infections may be difficult in the typically febrile, granulocytopenic patient. In the case of *S. aureus* or *S. epidermidis* bacteremia, the catheter should always be the presumed focus; the diagnostic problem of bacteremia with gram-negative bacteria becomes more difficult. One method to assess the likelihood that the catheter is the source of infection is the use quantitative pour-plate cultures in which a simultaneous sample of blood for culture is drawn through the catheter and from a peripheral site. Pour plates may be performed on both samples. As one would expect, the colony count of microorganisms from the catheter sample should be higher than the peripheral blood colony count if the catheter is the focus of infection.

Management of infection of Hickman or Broviac catheters depends on the site of infection and nature of the pathogen. If the only manifestation of infection is an exit site infection, then local daily dressing changes and local application of polysporin ointment may be all that is necessary.

In the patient who is bacteremic with *S. epidermidis* or *S. aureus*, an attempt may be made to treat with systemic antimicrobial agents while leaving the catheter in place. Many patients infected with these organisms have been successfully treated while leaving the line in place. It is important to determine whether the patient is cured of infection by ensuring that blood cultures remain sterile while the patient is receiving therapy. If bacteremia persists, then the line must be removed.

In patients in whom gram-negative bacteria or *Candida* have been documented to be the cause of infection and for whom the line has been implicated as the site, it has generally been necessary to remove the line in order to cure the infection. Patients with Hickman catheters who develop suppurative phlebitis of the great veins are particularly difficult management problems. They require catheter removal, appropriate antibiotics, and anticoagulation.

TOTAL PARENTERAL NUTRITION

Intravenous catheters used for total parenteral nutrition (TPN) carry the highest risk for infection, in part related to the bacterial and fungal growth-promoting properties of the TPN solution. The risk of bacteremia or fungemia approaches 3 to 5 percent, and the risk of local infection may be fourfold higher.

These lines must be treated with strict asepsis. Violation of the line for purposes other than TPN has been associated with a threefold increase in infection risk. A strong association with skin colonizaton and the development of subsequent catheter-associated infection has been well documented by several investigators.

S. epidermidis and *Candida* are the two most frequent pathogens in patients receiving total parenteral nutrition, but *S. aureus* and gram-negative aerobic bacteria are also common.

It has been shown that one nurse trained in the care of such lines, using standard aseptic technique, reduces the risk of TPN-associated infection compared with a nonstandardized approach to such lines. All fluids for infusion, because they may support bacterial or fungal growth, need to be admixed under a laminar flow hood in the pharmacy. No additives may be placed in the TPN solution. We change the TPN dressings and inspect the site three times per week. At the time of dressing change, we apply iodophor-containing ointment to the site.

A vexing management problem in the patient receiving TPN is the development of fever. We and others have instituted skin site surveillance cultures at the time of each dressing change. Virtually all such patients in whom catheter-related infection develops have microbial colonizaton at the skin-vascular interface prior to infection. If persistent colonization occurs, then the TPN catheter should be strongly considered as the source of infection and the catheter should be removed and replaced in another site.

Management of infections of the TPN catheter should be similar to the management of other catheter-related infections, except that one needs to recognize that *Candida* is a more frequent pathogen. Candidemia is always worrisome in such debilitated patients. Although some authors have had success in the management of TPN-associated candidemia with catheter removal alone, there has been well-documented examples of endophthalmitis or osteomyelitis following ''transient'' catheter-related fungemia. Therefore, I advocate low-dose amphotericin therapy, aiming for 200 to 500 mg total dose given over a 10 to 20 day period. If deep tissue infection is not documented, it is reasonable to stop amphotericin therapy at this low dosage. Endophthalmitis has been documented to occur up to 5 weeks after candidemia; therefore, it is incumbent upon the physician to assure adequate follow-up to rule out deep tissue invasion. If deep tissue invasion is documented, then the patient should be managed with a longer course of amphotericin (see chapter *Antifungal Chemotherapy*).

POSTOPERATIVE WOUND INFECTION

RICHARD A. GARIBALDI, M.D.
JOSEPH J. KLIMEK, M.D.

Despite recent advances in our understanding of the pathogenesis, risk factors, and strategies for the prevention of postoperative wound infections, these infections remain a significant cause of morbidity and mortality for hospitalized patients. Although there is no national surveillance of postoperative infections, it is estimated that there are more than one million cases each year in the United States. In addition to morbidity and mortality, surgical wound infections are responsible for prolonged hospital stays and significant increases in health care costs. The direct and indirect costs attributable to these infections reach as high as ten billion dollars annually. The occurrence of a wound infection more than doubles the cost of hospitalization for a surgical procedure.

EPIDEMIOLOGY

Several factors are associated with an increased risk of postoperative wound infection. The most important of these risk factors is the degree of endogenous or exogenous wound contamination that occurs during the surgical procedure. This observation has prompted clinicians to group surgeries by their expected degrees of contamination in order to calculate risks and compare wound infection rates. A clean wound is a nontraumatic wound in which neither the respiratory, alimentary, nor genitourinary tracts are entered and in which no break in technique is evident. These wounds are usually elective, closed primarily, and require no drains. Clean-contaminated wounds involve surgeries in which the gastrointestinal or respiratory tracts are entered, but in which there is no significant intraoperative spillage. Contaminated surgeries include procedures in which acute inflammation is encountered or in which gross spillage from a hollow viscus occurs. Open, fresh, traumatic wounds and operations with major breaks in aseptic technique are included in this category. Dirty wounds involve surgeries in which grossly purulent material is present or a perforated viscus is found.

This classification scheme enables clinicians to estimate the relative probability that a specific type of surgical wound will become infected during the postoperative period. Clean wounds have a 1 to 5 percent risk of infection; clean-contaminated, 8 to 11 percent; contaminated, 15 to 17 percent; and dirty, more than 27 percent. Even though this system is helpful in grouping relatively similar surgical procedures, marked variation in infection rates occurs within each group for specific operations. Thus, within the clean wound classification, the rate of infection following a simple cholecystectomy (3% to 5%) is more than twice that for an inguinal hernia repair (1% to 2%).

Rates of wound infection are also influenced by a variety of other surgery-related and host-related risk factors. Surgical technique is a factor that is difficult to define, but is critical to the pathogenesis of infection. Meticulous attention to operative detail, gentle handling of tissue, maintenance of local blood supply, insistence on complete hemostasis, careful use of cautery, avoidance of hematoma formation, obliteration of dead space, removal of devitalized tissue, use of fine, nonabsorbable suture material, precise suturing, proper use of drains, and careful wound closure play a major role in the prevention or development of wound infection. The duration of the surgical procedure is an independent risk factor that identifies higher risk surgeries, even though longer surgeries are not necessarily associated with poorer technique, greater complexity, or higher levels of intraoperative contamination.

Host factors also play a major role in identifying patients at high risk for wound infections. In general, patients with more debilitating underlying diseases are at increased risk for infection. Thus, patients with poor nutritional status, patients with diabetes mellitus or major organ system failure, those receiving immunocompromising drugs, those who require prolonged preoperative stays to prepare for surgery, and patients with active infections at distant sites are at increased risk. The exact mechanism by which these host factors increase susceptibility to wound infection is not totally clear, but presumably involves a combination of impaired phagocytic function, compromised blood supply, diminished tissue integrity, and poor wound healing.

DEFINITION OF WOUND INFECTION

Surgical wound infections are classified as either superficial incisional infections or deep wound infections; minor stitch abscesses are generally not included as postoperative wound infections.

Infection of the incisional site and underlying tissues usually begins as an inflammatory process with infiltration by red cells, leukocytes, and macrophages. It is characterized by clinical findings of erythema, edema, and local tenderness. At this stage, the diagnosis of wound infection may be difficult because these signs and symptoms may also reflect natural host responses to the trauma of surgery. However, with a wound infection, suppuration soon becomes evident, with liquefaction of tissue and accumulation of local purulence. Wound infection is defined by the presence of purulent drainage, whether or not pathogenic bacteria are recovered by culture. Incisional sites that are inflamed and have serous drainage from which bacteria are recovered are classified as possibly infected wounds.

Deep wound infections are often more insidious and difficult to diagnose than incisional infections. Loculated pus deep in a surgical site is often suggested by systemic symptoms that develop 5 days or more after the surgical procedure and that are characterized by generalized malaise, unexplained fever, or leukocytosis with a left shift. Signs of local tenderness, mass formation, wound cellulitis, purulent drainage, or dehiscence may focus attention on the prior surgical site as a source of infection. Sometimes the identification of a deep wound infection requires the use of computerized tomography, ultrasound, or nuclear medicine scanning techniques.

MICROBIOLOGY OF WOUND INFECTION

Knowledge of the pathogenesis and epidemiology of wound infections provides insight into the reasons why certain bacteria cause infections following specific classes of surgery. During clean surgery, exogenous bacteria from the patient, surgical team member, or environment contaminate the open wound intraoperatively. The exact route of contamination (direct contact or airborne spread) is not clearly delineated. Infections following these surgeries are usually caused by normal skin flora with such organisms as *Staphylococcus epidermidis, Staphylococcus aureus* or streptococci. Clean procedures that involve the implantation of prosthetic materials and surgeries involving extensive dissection are at increased risk for infections with these organism.

For clean-contaminated, contaminated, and dirty surgeries, a wide variety of pathogenic bacteria have been implicated as causes of postoperative infection. Specific etiologic organisms reflect the endogenous flora of the internal structure that has been transected, perforated, or traumatized. Oftentimes these infections involve mixed aerobic or aerobic/anaerobic flora. Thus, infections following colon surgery typically involve fecal bacteria such as *Escherichia coli*, other Enterobacteriaceae, *Bacteroides fragilis*, or other anaerobic bacteria. Deep postoperative infections that occur in patients who have been hospitalized for a prolonged period or who have received prior antibiotics are more likely to involve antibiotic-resistant bacteria such as enterococci, *Pseudomonas auerginosa, Enterobacter* species, or nonmirabilis *Proteus*. Deep pelvic infections following surgeries in which the vagina has been entered usually involve mixed anaerobic/aerobic organisms including *B. fragilis* and Enterobacteriaceae; however, in addition, other vaginal flora including *Chlamydia trachomatis* or *Mycoplasma hominis* may occasionally be implicated as causes of postoperative infection.

Data from the National Nosocomial Infection Study (NNIS) published by the Centers for Disease Control in the mid- and early 1970s showed that the commonest bacterial isolates from surgical wound infections were *S. aureus* and *E. coli* (Table 1). More recent surveillance data from NNIS and individual hospitals reflect the emergence of relatively resistant bacteria in wound infection cultures. For instance, at Hartford Hospital from 1982 to 1984, *E. coli* was recovered less frequently and *S. epidermidis* and enterococci were isolated more frequently than in the earlier CDC surveys.

Rarely, contaminated products or devices may be sources of pathogenic microorganisms that can contaminate and infect the surgical wound. Cases of prosthetic value endocarditis with *Mycobacterium chelonei* and *Mycobacterium fortuitum* have been traced to porcine valves that were contaminated prior to surgical insertion. Contaminated elastoplast bandages used over dressings to wrap incision sites can be sources of wound infection caused by fungi of the genus *Rhizopus*. These fungi are ubiquitous in nature and do not invade healthy, intact tissue. However, given close contact with a fresh incisional site, they are able to induce a local infection. Other classes of microorganisms such as viruses, parasites, rickettsiae, spirochetes, or actinomyces rarely have been implicated as causes of postoperative wound infection.

TABLE 1 Time Trend of Pathogens Recovered from Postoperative Wound Infections, 1970–1984

Organism	*NNIS* 1970*	*NNIS 1975*	*NNIS 1979*	*HH† 1982–1984*
S. aureus	21	17	15	18
E. coli	20	15	13	9
P. aeruginosa	10	4	6	10
S. epidermidis	7	6	5	17
Streptococci	6	2	3	1
Proteus species	6	8	6	7
Enterococci	6	9	10	14
Enterobacter species	5	4	4	6
Klebsiella species	5	6	5	--
Serratia	1	1	2	3
Candida	1	1	1	--
Bacteroides	--	6	3	4
Acinetobacter	--	--	--	4
Other	11	11	13	17
No organism cultured	11	9	15	--

Note: Data represent the percent of infections in which the organism was recovered.
* NNIS: National Nosocomial Infection Study.
† HH: Hartford Hospital.

MANAGEMENT OF THE INFECTED SURGICAL WOUND

The cornerstone in the management of a superficial or deep postoperative wound infection is the initiation of effective drainage, debridement of the devitalized tissue, and removal of foreign material. Oftentimes, drainage occurs spontaneously; but, sometimes it must be accomplished by a second surgical procedure to open the wound, explore the wound cavity, irrigate the wound contents, and drain the involved area. Drainage should be continued until the entire cavity is closed, thus preventing the development of another closed-space infection. After incision and drainage, the wound should not be closed by primary intention. Instead, it should be packed loosely with a fine mesh gauze and left open until all signs of inflammation are absent, purulent drainage ceases, and good granulation tissue is evident. Secondary closure is the accepted practice for the surgical treatment of infected wounds.

Although antibiotics are important in treating bacterial infections at other sites, their role for postoperative wound infections has often been overstated. For these infections, antimicrobial agents should be regarded as an adjunct to surgery. Their primary importance is to prevent further tissue damage, treat bacteremia, and prevent bacterial seeding at distant metastatic sites. The avascular nature of the deep wound infection or abscess, low pH, anaerobic environment, and presence of necrotic debris make antibiotics relatively ineffective. Loculated pus must be drained by either open surgery or percutaneous aspiration and tube insertion.

The antibiotic(s) selected empirically to treat an established wound infection should be active against the most likely infecting pathogens. Etiologic bacteria may be suggested by gram-stained smears of purulent wound drainage. Specimens should be cultured to establish a specific etiologic agent, which can be tested for antimicrobic sensitivities. Whenever possible, specimens for staining and culture should consist of fresh pus. Culture material should never be obtained from dressings that have covered the wound for indeterminant periods. Specimens collected by aspirating loculated pus or tissue biopsies are more accurate for identifying pathogenic bacteria than surface smears. Surface cultures often are contaminated with nonpathogenic skin flora that may complicate their interpretation. Anaerobic bacteria can only be recovered from aspirated or biopsied specimens. In order to isolate anaerobes, pus should be aspirated into an airless syringe and plated as soon as possible on appropriate media for anaerobic culture. Carelessness in obtaining the wound specimen is a more frequent problem than laboratory error when culture results are ambiguous. Blood cultures may also be useful in identifying a specific etiologic pathogen.

In emergent situations, the Gram stain may provide the clinician with useful information on which to base the choice of empiric antimicrobics while awaiting definitive culture results. Gram-stained specimens may suggest staphylococcal or streptococcal infection (gram-positive cocci), clostridia (gram-positive rods), enteric aerobic gram-negative bacteria (plump, gram-negative rods), or *Bacteroides* species (long, thin, gram-negative bacilli). When empiric antibiotics are needed to treat a patient with wound sepsis, the choice is often broad-spectrum (e.g., gentamicin and oxacillin or gentamycin and clindamycin). If there is resistance to gentamicin at the institution, tobramycin or amikacin may be substituted. Once a specific etiologic pathogen has been identified, the antibiotics can be selected according to susceptibility test results for maximal in vitro antibacterial activity.

Superficial wound infections caused by gram-positive cocci are often treated with oral antibiotics such as dicloxacillin or cephalexin. Deep infections caused by gram-positive cocci usually respond to intravenous semisynthetic penicillins or cephalosporin antibiotics. More than 90 percent of *S. aureus* are resistant to penicillin, but are susceptible to penicillin derivatives such as oxacillin or nafcillin, cephalosporins, and clindamycin. First-generation cephalosporins appear to be more active against *S. aureus* than later-generation cephalosporins. Occasionally, methicillin-resistant *S. aureus* or *S. epidermidis* may be identified as a cause of wound infection; vancomycin is considered the drug of choice for these isolates. Each clinician should know the prevalence of methicillin-resistant isolates for his or her institution. In most hospitals, less than 1 percent of *S. aureus* are methicillin-resistant; whereas in others, the percentage of resistant isolates may be as great as 30 percent. Infections with *S. epidermidis* may sometimes be treated with penicillin, although semisynthetic penicillins are usually considered the drugs of choice. In most hospitals, 30 to 40 percent of clinically significant *S. epidermidis* isolates are methicillin-resistant and must be treated with vancomycin. Wound infections with group A beta-hemolytic streptococci can be extremely devastating and rapidly progressive; intravenous aqueous penicillin is the drug of choice for these infections. Enterococci are often found in mixed intraabdominal infection. These infections can be treated with ampicillin. For clinically severe enterococcal infections, a combination of ampicillin and an aminoglycoside such as gentamicin are recommended. Penicillin-allergic patients can be treated with vancomycin and an aminoglycoside.

The presence of gram-positive rods on Gram stain suggests infection with a clostridial species. These infections usually respond to penicillin. They are commonest following traumatic injuries or biliary surgery. If these infections are not recognized promptly, the clinical picture of gas gangrene may develop with associated systemic toxicity and high case-fatality ratio. Penicillin therapy must be considered an adjunct to wide surgical excision, removal of dead tissue, and exposure to an aerobic environment. When available, hyperbaric oxygen is useful to improve tissue oxygenation and to help the surgeon distinguish viable from nonviable muscle. The use of clostridial antitoxin has not been shown to enhance recovery.

Deep wound infections with aerobic gram-negative bacilli are treated with either a cephalosporin or aminoglycoside antibiotics. The choice of a specific aminoglycoside (gentamicin, tobramycin, or amikacin) should be guided by the usual pattern of antibiotic susceptibilities for gram-negative isolates at that particular hospital. First-generation cephalosporins such as cefazolin are active against most strains of *E. coli, Klebsiella,* and *Proteus mirabilis*. The newer-generation cephalosporins, such as cefotaxime, ceftizoxime, and ceftriaxone, extend the spectrum of these antibiotics to most of the other Enterobacteriaceae. Cefoperazone is very active against most isolates of *P. aeruginosa*. However, the cephalosporins as a group have little or no activity against enterococci and, with the exception of cefoxitin, are less active than other agents against *B. fragilis*. We use these agents only when the bacteria isolated from the wound are shown to be susceptible, or when the patient is at high risk for aminoglycoside nephrotoxicity.

Deep infections of the abdomen or pelvis frequently are mixed and contain anaerobic as well as aerobic pathogens. *B. fragilis* is particularly troublesome because of its relative resistance to aminoglycosides, semisynthetic penicillins, and most cephalosporins. However, several agents are available that are very active against *B. fragilis*. These agents can be used in combination with aminoglycosides for deep abdominal or pelvic infections. Agents used in combination with the aminoglycosides for mixed infections include clindamycin, metronidazole, chloramphenicol, and the broad-spectrum penicillins such as piperacillin, mezlocillin, or ticarcillin. Some investigators have suggested the use of newer-generation cephalosporins such as cefoxitin or cefotaxime alone for the treatment of intra-abdominal infection. Oftentimes, single-agent therapy with these antimicrobics is effective. However, patients treated with monotherapy must be observed carefully for the emergence of resistant pathogens such as enterococci, *P. aeruginosa*, or resistant *B. fragilis*. Patients who have been previously treated with cephalosporins or who have been hospitalized for prolonged periods prior to infection should be treated with combination therapy that includes an appropriate aminoglycoside and an antianaerobic antibiotic active against *B. fragilis*. Our preference is a combination of gentamicin and ticarcillin.

The duration of antimicrobial therapy depends on the

rapidity of resolution of the clinical signs and symptoms of infection. Superficial infections may respond to drainage and antibiotics almost immediately. If intravenous antibiotics are used originally, these patients can be quickly switched to oral agents. Treatment usually is continued for 7 to 10 days. The course of deep surgical wound infections is more variable. The source of the original sepsis must be identified and treated surgically. Drainage should be continued until evidence or purulence is resolved. The wound should be maintained open until granulation occurs; then it should be allowed to heal secondarily. Intravenous antibiotics should be prescribed while signs and symptoms of active infection are present. Antibiotics are usually continued for 7 to 10 days following clinical resolution. These wounds must be closely monitored for signs and symptoms suggestive of loculated pus that might necessitate an additional drainage procedure.

PREVENTION

Many wound infections are potentially preventable. Techniques for prevention are based on an awareness of the sources of bacteria that contaminate the operative wound and risk factors that increase the patient's susceptibility to infection. It has been shown by prospective, controlled trials that prophylactic, systemic antibiotics are effective in preventing infections in clean-contaminated and contaminated surgeries. For bowel surgeries, mechanical cleansing of the gastrointestinal tract with laxatives and/or enemas coupled with gut sterilization by oral antibiotics further decrease the likelihood of endogenous intraoperative contamination. Systemic prophylaxis is also prescribed for clean surgeries in which prosthetic devices are inserted because of the disastrous clinical consequences of infections in these patients.

Prophylactic antibiotics should be limited to the immediate perioperative period. They should be administered intravenously one-half to one hour prior to the surgical incision, readministered during prolonged surgeries according to the half-life of the particular agent, and discontinued within 24 hours. Peak blood and tissue levels should be reached and maintained for the duration of the surgery. A first-generated cephalosporin such as cefazolin (1 g every 8 hours for three doses) is an excellent, cost-effective choice for prophylaxis in most surgical procedures. Newer cephalosporins with longer half-lives may be shown to be equally effective and cost saving if they are administered as a single, preoperative dose.

Several infection control techniques have been suggested as logical strategies to lessen the likelihood of intraoperative wound contamination and thereby decrease the incidence of postoperative infection. Avoidance of razor shaves, use of antiseptic showers and skin preps, surgical scrubs, gloves, laminar-air-flow operating rooms, antibiotic wound irrigations, antibiotic impregnated beads, disposable gown and drape materials, foot wipes, and ultraviolet lights have been advocated as possible adjunctive measures to prevent infections. However, few of these techniques have been subjected to rigorous clinical trials and therefore few scientific data are available on which to judge their efficacy. Of these practices, only the avoidance of razor shaves prior to surgery has been shown to have a significant impact on subsuent infection rates.

Host-related risk factors are more difficult to modify. The presence of chronic, debilitating underlying diseases may predispose patients to an increased risk of surgical infection. The care of underlying diseases should be optimal at the time of surgery. Diabetes should be controlled; active infections should be treated. If possible, nutritional depletion should be corrected with oral protein calorie supplementation. Proper preparation of the patient prior to surgery may have a significant impact on subsequent complications.

Careful attention must be given to modifiable host risk factors, strategies to reduce levels of intraoperative wound contamination, surgery-related risk factors, and operative technique if we are to further reduce the morbidity, costs, and mortality of postoperative wound infections.

SYSTEMIC PROPHYLACTIC ANTIBIOTICS IN SURGERY

JAN V. HIRSCHMANN, M.D.

GENERAL PRINCIPLES

Prophylactic antibiotics can reduce the frequency and the enormous costs of postoperative wound infections in many surgical procedures, but maximal benefit occurs only when certain principles govern their use. For an operation to warrant antimicrobial prophylaxis, the adverse consequences of infection must exceed the costs of the antibiotics used. These costs include not only the price of the drug and its administration, but also those arising from toxic and allergic reactions to the agents, the development of antibiotic-resistant infections, and the effect of widespread antimicrobial use on hospital flora and subsequent nosocomial infections.

To justify the routine administration of prophylactic antibiotics, the surgical procedure must have frequent or extraordinarily severe postoperative infections. Because the risk of wound infections varies considerably according to the type of procedure, operations have been classified into four groups: clean, clean-contaminated, contaminated, and dirty.

Clean procedures constitute about 75 percent of all operations and have an expected wound infection rate of less than 5 percent, in most centers less than 2 percent. By definition, these wounds are nontraumatic, with no break in sterile technique, and no entry into the respiratory, alimentary, or genitourinary tracts. Postoperative wound infections are not only infrequent, but also usually minor, requiring local measures for treatment and no prolonged hospitalization or antimicrobial therapy. The costs of antimicrobial prophylaxis in clean procedures exceed the costs of infectious complications, with one major exception—the insertion of prosthetic devices, such as artificial joints or cardiac valves. The wound infection rate in these operations is higher because, in the presence of these foreign bodies, infection occurs with lower numbers of organisms than usual and with bacteria like *Staphyloccocus epidermidis* that are ordinarily not pathogens. Furthermore, the consequences of infected prostheses are severe: hospitalization is lengthy, antimicrobial therapy is prolonged, and removal of the prosthesis is usually necessary.

Clean-contaminated procedures, constituting 15 percent of all operations, have an expected wound infection rate of 10 percent but in certain procedures it approaches 40 percent. These operations involve entry into the alimentary or respiratory tract, the vagina, or uninfected urinary or biliary tracts. For those procedures where transection occurs across a mucosal surface that normally harbors a teeming population of bacteria, such as the upper airway or the large bowel, the wound infection rate is very high, and prophylaxis is clearly justified.

Contaminated cases, about 5 percent of operative procedures, have a wound infection rate of about 20 percent. Such cases involve fresh trauma, a major break in sterile technique, gross spillage from the gastrointestinal tract, or acute, nonpurulent inflammation.

Dirty operations have a wound infection rate of 30 to 40 percent and involve traumatic wounds with retained, devitalized tissue, foreign bodies, fecal contamination, or delayed treatment. Also included are operations for acute bacterial infections, perforated viscera, or transection of clean tissue to drain pus. Because inflammation, infection, or severe bacterial contamination are already present at the time of surgery in contaminated or dirty operations, antimicrobial agents function as treatment rather than prophylaxis, and different principles of antibiotic administration apply. Thus, prophylaxis deals with clean and clean-contaminated cases only.

The major discoveries from both experimental and clinical investigations relate to the timing and duration of drug administration. To be effective, prophylactic antibiotics must be present in adequate concentration in the wound tissue concurrent with or only shortly after contamination occurs. Antimicrobial agents begun after this brief "decisive period" fail to prevent wound infections. The practical conclusion is that the prophylactic antibiotic must be given shortly before or during the operation, not afterwards. Postoperative doses alone are ineffective. A second principle is that postoperative doses following preoperative or intraoperative antibiotics are unnecessary. Effective tissue levels of the agent must persist for the duration of contamination, but this contamination ceases at the time of wound closure. Accordingly, for most procedures a single dose of an agent given just before surgery provides adequate coverage. Only for prolonged operations is a second (intraoperative) dose appropriate.

A third major principle is that the antibiotic chosen for prophylaxis should be active against the major pathogens likely to be encountered in a specific operation. The agent need not be effective against all possible contaminating organisms, but must be able to reduce the number below the level required to cause infection.

Cephalosporins have been especially popular prophylactic agents because of their wide spectrum of activity, infrequent adverse effects, and extensive promotion by drug companies. Most trials have investigated cephalosporins rather than other agents for these reasons. Their efficacy and safety have been impressive. For most surgical procedures, a first-generation cephalosporin is the drug of choice. Because cefazolin has some special advantages, it has emerged as the preferred agent. Unlike cephalothin, it can be given intramuscularly and has the additional benefit of high serum levels and a long half-life. Because cefazolin and other first-generation cephalosporins are inactive against *Bacteroides fragilis*, cefoxitin, a second-generation cephalosporin effective against this organism, should be used when *B. fragilis* is a frequent cause of postoperative infections. These procedures include colorectal surgery and appendectomies. Otherwise, second-generation cephalosporins have no advantage and are much more expensive than cefazolin. Third-generation cephalosporins such as moxalactam and cefotaxime are unjustified as prophylactic agents. They are much more expensive, and their activity against unusual gram-negative bacilli confers no advantage since these organisms are extremely uncommon causes of wound infections in clean and clean-contaminated surgery.

PROPHYLAXIS IN SPECIFIC SURGICAL PROCEDURES

Abdominal Surgery

Gastroduodenal

Ordinarily, the stomach and duodenum have a relatively sparse flora of aerobic organisms because the low pH from gastric acidity and the vigorous intestinal motility discourage bacterial growth. With impairment of either of these protective mechanisms, aerobic bacteria, including gram-negative bacilli, flourish, and the wound infection rate, ordinarily negligible in gastroduodenal surgery, rises substantially. The indications for prophylactic antibiotics, therefore, are obstruction; hemorrhage, where blood buffers the acid; gastric ulcer and malignancy, where both acidity and motility decrease; and chronic use of H-2 blockers, such as cimetidine, which markedly reduce acid secretion.

Biliary Tract

The wound infection rate following biliary tract surgery is low unless the bile is infected. Situations where bile cultures are likely to be positive include common duct obstruction, previous biliary tract surgery, patient age greater than 70 years, and acute cholecystitis. Patients in these circumstances should receive antimicrobial prophylaxis against the likely organisms, usually *Escherichia coli, Klebsiella* species, and various streptococci.

Appendectomy

Agents effective against *B. fragilis* alone or also against coliforms, especially *E. coli*, reduce the frequency of wound infections following appendectomy. For patients with a normal or inflamed appendix, a single preoperative or intraoperative dose of cefoxitin suffices; patients with appendiceal perforation or abscess require postoperative antibiotics to eradicate the established infection.

Colorectal

Postoperative wound sepsis is very common following colorectal surgery, even with preceding mechanical bowel preparation using liquid diet, cathartics, and enemas. The commonest infecting organisms are *E. coli* and *B. fragilis*. Oral or parenteral agents active against these bacteria markedly reduce infectious complications. Some regimens have employed nonabsorbable oral agents to reduce the concentration of intraluminal bacteria below that necessary to cause infection when minor spillage of bowel contents occurs; other programs have used parenteral agents to provide effective tissue levels to prevent infection when such contamination develops. The distinction between these two approaches is partly fallacious: oral agents are absorbed in sufficient quantity to yield measurable tissue levels, and parenteral agents, even if given immediately before surgery, reduce the concentration of intraluminal intestinal bacteria.

Oral programs have included an agent effective against coliforms—usually an aminoglycoside such as neomycin or kanamycin—and one active against *B. fragilis* such as erythromycin or metronidazole. Oral doxycycline alone is effective against both types of organisms. Alternatively, a parenteral regimen using cefoxitin, doxycycline, or a combination of an aminoglycoside and clindamycin or metronidazole has also been effective. Whether a combination of oral and parenteral agents together is superior to either alone remains unsettled. A reasonable approach for elective colorectal surgery is a combination of oral erythromycin and neomycin supplemented with a single preoperative dose of cefoxitin. For emergency surgery, bowel obstruction, or other circumstances where the oral route is not feasible, cefoxitin should be used alone in a single dose.

Cardiothoracic Surgery

Valvular

The serious consequences of prosthetic valve endocarditis justify the use of a prophylactic agent effective against the usual causes of this infection: *Staphylococcus aureus, S. epidermidis*, and, less commonly, coliforms. The most important element in preventing endocarditis and other postoperative infections is to have effective serum levels sustained throughout the operation. Cefazolin given every 4 hours during the procedure is an excellent choice, but cefonicid, with its very long serum half-life, may have a special advantage in protracted cases where a single, preoperative dose would provide satisfactory serum and tissue levels.

Coronary Artery Bypass

Unless there is a concomitant valvular surgery, endocarditis is a rare complication. Sternal wound infections, with the serious potential of sternal osteomyelitis, however, seem to be frequent, and several studies have shown a significant reduction with use of prophylactic antibiotics. *S. aureus* is the commonest pathogen, but, especially with contaminated or inadequate topical antiseptic preparation of the chest, other organisms can be responsible.

Pacemaker Implantation

Skin flora, usually *S. aureus* or *S. epidermidis*, causes pacemaker pocket infections. Prophylactic antibiotics can reduce their incidence significantly.

Noncardiac Thoracic Surgery

Several trials of prophylaxis in noncardiac thoracic surgery have reached conflicting conclusions about its benefit. It is not clear what factors predispose to postoperative infectious complications. A reasonable approach may be to give a first-generation cephelosporin for major lung resection, but its efficacy remains unsettled.

Peripheral Vascular Surgery

Vascular grafts of the abdominal aorta or of the lower extremities through a groin incision have fewer complicating infections with prophylactic antibiotics than without. *S. aureus* is the major pathogen. Surgery of the brachiocephalic vessels requires no prophylaxis, since the incidence of the postoperative infections is very low.

Obstetrical and Gynecologic Surgery

Vaginal Hysterectomy

Prophylactic antibiotics reduce the incidence of febrile morbidity defined as temperature greater than 38 °C on two separate occasions at least 6 hours apart—excluding the first 24 hours following surgery. Studies have employed this criterion because the determination of the presence of a wound infection is so difficult following vaginal hysterectomy. Although there are numerous possible causes of this postoperative fever, infectious complications—urinary tract infections, pelvic cellulitis, vaginal cuff infections, and infected hematoma or abscess—apparently account for most cases. Several antimicrobial agents have been effective in reducing febrile morbidity, but a first-generation cephalosporin enjoys the widest use. The bacteriology of the pelvic infections is predominantly aerobic and anaerobic gram-positive organisms, nonfragilis *Bacteroides* species, and coliforms.

Abdominal Hysterectomy

The preponderance of studies illustrates the value of prophylactic antibiotics in abdominal hysterectomy, although the incidence of febrile morbidity is usually less than in vaginal hysterectomies. The infecting flora appears to be the same.

Cesarean Section

With ruptured membranes at the commencement of labor, the risk of postoperative infection, predominantly endometritis, increases. In these circumstances prophylactic antibiotics significantly reduce infectious complications. To avoid administering antibiotics to the baby, the agent may be given after cord clamping without any diminution in efficacy.

Head and Neck Surgery

Because the saliva contains an abundant flora of aerobic and anaerobic organisms, infections following neck incision through the oral or pharyngeal mucosa are common and usually polymicrobial. The usual bacteria found include streptococci, staphylococci, *Klebsiella* species, anaerobic gram-positive cocci, and nonfragilis *Bacteroides* species. A cephalosporin significantly reduces these infectious complications.

Orthopedic Surgery

Joint Replacement

Skin flora, such as *S. aureus* and *S. epidermidis*, diphtheroids, and *Propionibacterium acnes*, causes the preponderance of infections complicating total joint replacement. Although studies have examined only total hip replacement where prophylactic antistaphylococcal agents significantly reduce deep infections, implantation of any artificial joint seems to warrant antimicrobial prophylaxis.

Hip (Proximal Femoral) Fractures

Proximal femoral fractures repaired by nails, plates, or other orthopedic hardware have a low incidence of postoperative wound infection (5% to 8%), but the frequency of these serious infections is significantly reduced by prophylactic antistaphylococcal agents.

Genitourinary Surgery

Prostatectomy

In patients with sterile preoperative urine, the incidence of postoperative bacteriuria following prostatecto-

TABLE 1 Systemic Prophylactic Antibiotics in Surgery

Procedure	*Recommended Antibiotic*	*Preoperative Adult Dosage**
Gastroduodenal surgery (high-risk patients only)	Cefazolin	1 g IM or IV
Biliary tract surgery (high-risk patients only)	Cefazolin	1 g IM or IV
Appendectomy	Cefoxitin	1 g IV
Colorectal surgery	Oral: erythromycin and neomycin	1 g each at 1 PM, 2 PM, and 11 PM the day before surgery
	Parenteral: cefoxitin	1 g IV
Open heart surgery	Cefazolin *or*	1 g IV q4h throughout procedure
	Cefonicid (for prolonged procedure)	1 g IV before surgery
Pacemaker implantation	Cefazolin	1 g IM or IV
Pulmonary resection	Cefazolin	1 g IM or IV
Peripheral vascular surgery (abdominal aortic graft, lower extremity graft through groin incision)	Cefazolin	1 g IM or IV
Vaginal or abdominal hysterectomy	Cefazolin	1 g IM or IV
Cesarean section (high-risk patients only)	Cefazolin	1 g IV after cord clamping
Head and neck surgery (incision through oral or pharyngeal mucosa)	Cefazolin	1 g IM or IV
Joint replacement or internal fixation of proximal femoral fracture	Cefazolin	1 g IM or IV

* Single dose except where noted otherwise.

my is about 25 percent. Although prophylactic antibiotics can reduce this to less than 5 percent, they do not diminish the frequency of postoperative fever and gram-negative bacillary sepsis. Since postoperative bacteriuria is often asymptomatic and self-limited, prophylactic antibiotics do not seem to be indicated.

Neurosurgery

Several studies failed to demonstrate any benefit for prophylactic antibiotics in the insertion of ventricular shunts for hydrocephalus. Other neurosurgical procedures have had too little investigation to determine whether antimicrobial prophylaxis is warranted in them.

INDEX

F

G

H

N

O

X

Y

Z